KU-509-568

Veterinary Immunology

Veterinary Immunology

NINTH EDITION

IAN R. TIZARD

BVMS, PhD, DACVM (Hons), DSc (Hons)

Richard M. Schubot Professor of Exotic Bird Health
and Professor of Immunology
Department of Veterinary Pathobiology
College of Veterinary Medicine and Biomedical
Sciences
Texas A&M University
College Station, Texas

3251 Riverport Lane
St. Louis, Missouri 63043

VETERINARY IMMUNOLOGY, NINTH EDITION ISBN: 978-1-4557-0362-3
Copyright © 2013, 2009, 2004, 2000, 1996, 1992, 1987, 1982, 1977 by Saunders, an imprint of Elsevier Inc.

All rights reserved. No part of this publication may be reproduced or transmitted in any form or by any means, electronic or mechanical, including photocopying, recording, or any information storage and retrieval system, without permission in writing from the publisher. Details on how to seek permission, further information about the Publisher's permissions policies and our arrangements with organizations such as the Copyright Clearance Center and the Copyright Licensing Agency, can be found at our website: www.elsevier.com/permissions.

This book and the individual contributions contained in it are protected under copyright by the Publisher (other than as may be noted herein).

Notices

Knowledge and best practice in this field are constantly changing. As new research and experience broaden our understanding, changes in research methods, professional practices, or medical treatment may become necessary.

Practitioners and researchers must always rely on their own experience and knowledge in evaluating and using any information, methods, compounds, or experiments described herein. In using such information or methods they should be mindful of their own safety and the safety of others, including parties for whom they have a professional responsibility.

With respect to any drug or pharmaceutical products identified, readers are advised to check the most current information provided (i) on procedures featured or (ii) by the manufacturer of each product to be administered, to verify the recommended dose or formula, the method and duration of administration, and contraindications. It is the responsibility of practitioners, relying on their own experience and knowledge of their patients, to make diagnoses, to determine dosages and the best treatment for each individual patient, and to take all appropriate safety precautions.

To the fullest extent of the law, neither the Publisher nor the authors, contributors, or editors, assume any liability for any injury and/or damage to persons or property as a matter of products liability, negligence or otherwise, or from any use or operation of any methods, products, instructions, or ideas contained in the material herein.

Library of Congress Cataloging-in-Publication Data

Tizard, Ian R.
Veterinary immunology / Ian Tizard.—9th ed.
p. ; cm.
Includes bibliographical references and index.
ISBN 978-1-4557-0362-3 (pbk.: alk. paper)
I. Title.
[DNLM: 1. Animal Diseases—immunology. 2. Animal Population Groups—immunology. 3. Immune System Diseases—veterinary. SF 757.2]
636.0896079—dc23

2011039847

Vice President: Linda Duncan
Content Strategy Director: Penny Rudolph
Content Manager: Shelly Stringer
Content Development Specialist: Brandi Graham
Publishing Services Manager: Pat Joiner-Myers
Designer: Amy Buxton

Working together to grow
libraries in developing countries

www.elsevier.com | www.bookaid.org | www.sabre.org

ELSEVIER   BOOK AID International   Sabre Foundation

Printed in China

Last digit is the print number: 9 8 7 6 5 4 3 2

To Devon and Trevor

Preface

A pair of recurring themes discussed in the preface of almost all previous editions is the centrality of immunology in veterinary medicine and the vast amount of new data being generated. Some things don't change, so I will not belabor the point that immunology is important and we are indeed drowning in a sea of data. This combination can be frustrating for both teachers and students. The time allocated to immunology in the veterinary curriculum has, in many cases, been reduced to suboptimal levels at a time when a knowledge of immunology remains central to the practice of veterinary medicine. Although it is essential therefore to rigorously control the amount of information contained in a textbook such as this, there are limits, beyond which it is inappropriate to go. Immunology is broad and complex, and the educated veterinarian needs more than a superficial knowledge of the subject.

One result of the vast increase in data, and a major change in this edition, is the recognition that the immune system is not simply the sum of a series of discrete signaling pathways. Immunology is not a linear subject. On the contrary, it is a complex set of responses that result from the interactions of a network of thousands of different molecules. Multiple ligands simultaneously stimulate many receptors that in turn activate several signaling pathways. These pathways then interact, showing cross-talk, feedback-enhancing loops, and multiple complex and diverse regulatory processes.

The readers' task, therefore, is not to learn the innumerable details but rather to attempt to fix in their mind the major reactions and routes and the overall pattern of reactions (not the pathways but the major highways). Students are recommended not to focus on the details (and trust me, I've left out most of them) but to first seek at an overall picture. Students should feel free to alter chapter order and jump between subjects. As a complex interactive network, there is really no beginning or end to immunology.

A second very major change in this edition is my belated recognition that we live in a world dominated by microbes. We are not microbiologically sterile creatures but rather form complex "superorganisms" with our own dense, complex, microbial populations. The immune system governs our relationships with this microbial world and determines our survival in the presence of huge numbers of microbes. The body's microflora influences many important disease states, including both allergic and autoimmune diseases. It affects the development of the immune system, and the immune system also modulates the composition of the microbial flora. With this has come the realization that the gut flora controls the development of the immune system, the development of autoimmune diseases, and even metabolic consequences such as obesity. Try not to lose sight of this microbial background.

Significant Changes in This Edition

The overall arrangement of the text has changed little, although three new chapters have been added. The inflammation chapter has been split in two, with one chapter focusing on the detection of invaders and a second chapter on the mediators of inflammation. This reflects the enormous amount of new information on pattern-recognition receptors and the ways in which they warn the body of microbial invasion. The importance of illness and the systemic response to inflammation have also been recognized by splitting this material off as a new chapter. Finally, the growing recognition of the significance of natural killer cells in many areas of immunology now warrants a separate chapter unlinked to tumor immunology.

The flood of new information has come from many directions. The greatest amount has probably come in the area of inflammation and the recognition of invaders by pattern-recognition receptors. Other growth areas include resistance to infection, such as, vaccine use, especially with respect to duration of immunity; the effects of old age on immunity; and both antiviral and parasitic immunity. New information is being generated on immunological diseases in areas such as atopic dermatitis and the complex reactions associated with allergic disease, inflammatory bowel disease, and the pathogenesis of autoimmune diseases, especially rheumatoid arthritis and systemic lupus erythematosus. The importance of adipose tissue in immunity and inflammation is now discussed, an essential topic considering both the epidemic of obesity in domestic pets and the extraordinary growth rates expected of domestic livestock. Even something that has been well recognized for many years, such as neutrophil phagocytosis, has been shown to have unexpected complexity with the description of antigen-trapping neutrophil nets. Likewise, the description of lymph node conduits has important new information about the capture and processing of antigens within these organs.

New topics discussed in addition to the above include pathways involving type I and related hypersensitivities, the explosive growth in our understanding of new cytokines, pattern-recognition receptors, autophagy, the roles of vitamins A and D in immunity, tumor-associated inflammation, lymph node structure and dynamic functions, Th17 and other T-cell subsets, natural killer cells, immunity to fungi, bacterial and viral suppression of the immune system, and the extensive linkages between adaptive and innate immunity. Devil facial tumor disease is now described, as are bovine neonatal pancytopenia and foal immunodeficiency syndrome.

Diagnostic tests described now include sections on the analysis of data from enzyme-linked immunosorbent assay tests. Molecular techniques such as the polymerase chain reaction can no longer be ignored despite the fact that they do not involve the use of immunology. Almost all the figures have been redrawn, and more than 30 new ones have been added.

Finally, readers are strongly encouraged to visit the Evolve website for this text. Although this website is constantly evolving and improving, you will be able to find a collection of more than 450 multiple-choice questions (with the answers!) keyed to each chapter; a set of flash cards also linked to chapters; all the text figures available for downloading; a small collection of animations kindly provided by Dr. Abdul Abbas; and all the chapter references keyed to PubMed. You will also find a monthly update of new information gleaned from the current veterinary immunology literature. This too is arranged according to the book chapters and will ensure that you remain current in this rapidly expanding and exciting field.

Ian Tizard

Acknowledgments

As always, a book such as this could not be written without the support of colleagues and family. Among my colleagues who took the time to review chapters are Drs. Ann Kier, Jeffrey Musser, Susan Payne, Mike Crisitello, Shuping Zhang, Loren Skow, and Robert Kennis.

Writing a book takes away, of course, from the time allocated to other tasks. I am especially grateful to my assistant, Debra Turner, who keeps my research program functioning when I am irreversibly immersed in writing.

I would also like to acknowledge the professionalism and assistance provided by the staff at Elsevier, especially my content strategists, Heidi Pohlman and Shelly Stringer; my content development strategists, Kate Dobson and Brandi Graham; and my production managers Cassie Carey and Pat Joiner-Myers.

Finally, of course, I must thank my wife Claire for her continuing encouragement and support, without which none of this would be possible.

Ian Tizard

Contents

1

The Defense of the Body

Key Points

- The immune system protects animals against microbial invasion and is therefore essential for life.
- Multiple mechanisms are needed to ensure freedom from invasion. These include physical barriers that exclude invaders, innate immunity that provides rapid initial protection, and adaptive immunity that provides prolonged effective immunity.
- These major defensive mechanisms are linked together to form complex interacting networks. As a result, changes in one area may result in diverse effects in many other areas of immunity.
- One form of adaptive immunity is mainly directed against bacterial invaders and is mediated by antibodies. Antibodies are proteins that circulate in body fluids, especially in the bloodstream. They bind to bacteria and mark them for destruction.
- Another form of adaptive immunity is mainly directed against viruses. It is called cell-mediated immunity. This employs cells that destroy abnormal cells such as those infected by viruses.
- The adaptive immune system can remember prior exposure to foreign invaders and mount a faster and more effective response on subsequent exposure to that invader. This ensures an animal's health and survival in the face of continuing microbial challenge.

The animal body contains all the components necessary to sustain life. It is warm, moist, and rich in nutrients. As a result, animal tissues are extremely attractive to microorganisms that seek to invade the body and exploit these resources for themselves. The magnitude of this microbial attack can be readily seen when an animal dies. Within a few hours, especially when warm, a body decomposes rapidly as bacteria invade its tissues. On the other hand, the tissues of living, healthy animals are highly resistant to microbial invasion since their survival depends on their preventing the damage caused by microbial invaders. The defense of the body is encompassed by the discipline of immunology and is the subject of this book.

Because effective resistance to infection is critical, the body dare not rely on a single defense mechanism alone. To be effective and reliable, multiple defense systems must be available. Some may be effective against many different invaders. Others may destroy specific organisms. Some act at the body surface to exclude invaders. Others act deep within the body to destroy organisms that have breached the outer defenses. Some defend against bacterial invaders, some against viruses that live inside cells, and some against large invaders such as protozoa, fungi or parasitic worms and insects. The protection of the body depends upon a complex system of overlapping and interlinked defense mechanisms that collectively destroy or control almost all invaders. A failure in these defenses either because the immune system is destroyed (as occurs in acquired immune deficiency syndrome [AIDS]) or because the invading organisms can overcome or evade the defenses will result in disease and possibly death. An effective

1

immune system is not simply a useful system to have around; it is essential to life.

The immune system can be thought of as an interactive network in which the presence of foreign invaders causes diverse changes that generate an expanding set of responses through multiple pathways that eventually result in activation of the defenses, elimination of the invaders, and subsequent increased resistance to infection. Most of the complexity of the immune system stems from the fact that none of its pathways is truly independent. Pathways interact and intersect. Apparently unrelated cells talk to each other. Invasion results not in a single response but in multiple responses involving many different cell types, many different molecules, and many different organs. Cells respond to multiple stimuli simultaneously, and the cellular response is generated by signals derived from multiple interacting signaling pathways. Collectively, however, it is these signals and responses that keep us alive in a microbial world.

A Brief History of Veterinary Immunology

An awareness of the importance of the defense of the body against microbial invasion could not develop until the medical community accepted the concept of infectious disease. When infections such as smallpox or plague spread through early human societies, many people died, but some individuals recovered. It was rarely noticed that these recovered individuals remained healthy during subsequent outbreaks—a sign that they had developed immunity. Nevertheless, by the 12th century, the Chinese had observed that persons who recovered from smallpox were resistant to further attacks of this disease. Being practical people, they therefore deliberately infected infants with smallpox by inserting scabs from infected individuals into small cuts in their skin. Those infants who survived the resulting disease were protected from smallpox in later life. The risks inherent in this procedure were acceptable in an era of high infant mortality. On gaining experience with the technique it was found that using scabs from the mildest smallpox cases minimized the hazards. As a result, mortality due to smallpox inoculation (or variolation) dropped to about 1% compared with a mortality of about 20% in clinical smallpox cases. Knowledge of variolation spread westward to Europe by the early 18th century and was soon widely employed.

Outbreaks of rinderpest (then called cattle plague) had been a common occurrence throughout Western Europe since the ninth century and inevitably killed huge numbers of cattle. Since none of the traditional remedies appeared to work and the skin lesions in affected animals vaguely resembled those seen in smallpox, it was suggested in 1754 that inoculation might help. This process involved soaking a piece of string in the nasal discharge from an animal with rinderpest and then inserting the string into an incision in the dewlap of the animal to be protected. The resulting disease was usually milder than natural infection, and the inoculated animal became resistant

□ Box 1-1 | **Eradication of Rinderpest**

Rinderpest, a lethal virus disease of cattle, has been eradicated. The global rinderpest eradication program began in 1993 and was based on effective vaccination. Originally widespread across Eurasia and Africa, the last outbreak of this lethal disease of cattle and related animals occurred in Kenya in 2002. The program was declared completed in June 2011 after many years careful surveillance. Rinderpest is caused by a virus related to human measles and canine distemper. The virus affects many body systems, especially the gastrointestinal tract, and kills ruminants in 6 to 12 days. Animals that recover are immune for life. In the early 20th century, rinderpest wiped out vast numbers of African wildlife and cattle and led to the death of many people who depended on cattle for survival. Indeed, rinderpest has been claimed to be "the greatest natural calamity ever to befall the African continent." Once an economical and effective vaccine was developed, it became possible to prevent the spread of this disease. Widespread, well-designed vaccination campaigns gradually reduced the range of this disease until it was eventually eradicated. The success of the rinderpest vaccination campaign represents yet another triumph of the science of immunology.

to the disease. The process proved very popular, and skilled inoculators traveled throughout Europe inoculating cattle and branding them to show that they were protected against rinderpest (Box 1-1).

In 1798, Edward Jenner, an English physician, demonstrated that material from cowpox lesions could be substituted for smallpox in variolation. Since cowpox does not cause severe disease in humans, its use reduced the risks incurred by variolation to insignificant levels. The effectiveness of this procedure, called vaccination (*vacca* is Latin for "cow") was such that it was eventually used in the 1970s to eradicate smallpox from the world.

Once the general principles of inoculation were accepted (even though nobody had the faintest idea how it worked), attempts were made to use similar procedures to prevent other animal diseases. Some of these techniques were effective. Thus, material derived from sheep pox was used to protect sheep in a process called ovination and was widely employed in Europe. Likewise, inoculation for bovine pleuropneumonia consisted of inserting a small piece of tissue from an infected lung into a cut in the tail. The tail fell off within a few weeks, but the animal became immune! Although the process was effective, infected material from the tail also spread the disease and delayed its eradication. On the other hand, administration of cowpox scabs to the nose of puppies to prevent canine distemper, although widely employed, was a complete failure.

The general implications of Jenner's observations on cowpox and the importance of reducing the ability of an immunizing organism to cause disease were not realized until 1879. In that year, Louis Pasteur in France investigated fowl cholera, a

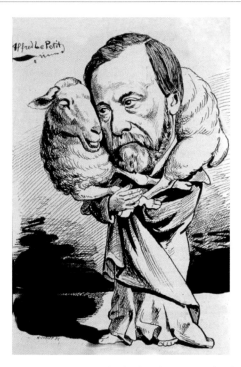

FIGURE 1-1 Louis Pasteur made the key discoveries that led to the development of vaccines against infectious agents. This drawing shows him as the good shepherd "Le bon Pasteur," reflecting his discovery of a vaccine against anthrax, 1882.

(Copyright Institut Pasteur. With permission.)

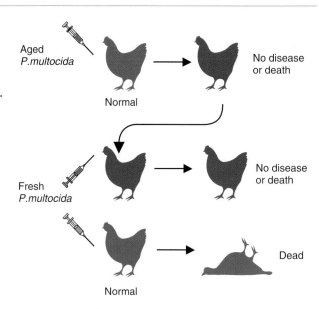

FIGURE 1-2 Pasteur's fowl cholera experiment. Birds inoculated with an aged culture of *Pasteurella multocida* did not die. However, when subsequently inoculated with a fresh culture of virulent *P. multocida*, the birds were found to be protected. It was this experiment that launched the science of immunology.

disease caused by the bacterium now called *Pasteurella multocida* (Figure 1-1). Pasteur had a culture of this organism that was accidentally allowed to age on a laboratory bench while his assistant was on vacation. When the assistant returned and tried to infect chickens with this aged culture, the birds remained healthy (Figure 1-2). Saving money, Pasteur retained these chickens and subsequently used them for a second experiment in which they were challenged again, this time with a fresh culture of *P. multocida* known to be capable of killing chickens. To Pasteur's surprise the birds were resistant to the infection and did not die. In a remarkable intellectual jump, Pasteur immediately recognized that this phenomenon was similar in principle to Jenner's use of cowpox for vaccination. In vaccination, exposure of an animal to a strain of an organism that will not cause disease (an avirulent strain) can provoke an immune response. This immune response will protect the animal against a subsequent infection by a disease-producing (or virulent) strain of the same, or closely related, organism. Having established the general principle of vaccination, Pasteur first applied it to anthrax. He made anthrax bacteria *(Bacillus anthracis)* avirulent by growing them at an unusually high temperature. These attenuated organisms were then used as a vaccine to protect sheep against challenge with virulent anthrax bacteria. Pasteur subsequently developed a successful rabies vaccine by drying spinal cords taken from rabies-infected rabbits and using the dried cords as his vaccine material. The drying process effectively rendered the rabies virus avirulent (and probably killed much of it).

Although Louis Pasteur used only living organisms in his vaccines, it was not long before Daniel Salmon and Theobald Smith, working in the United States, demonstrated that dead organisms could make effective vaccines. They showed that a heat-killed culture of a bacterium called *Salmonella choleraesuis* (then called *Bacillus suipestifer* and believed to be the cause of hog cholera) could protect pigeons against the disease caused by that organism. A little later, Von Behring and Kitasato in Germany showed that filtrates taken from cultures of the tetanus bacillus *(Clostridium tetani)* could protect animals against tetanus even though they contained no bacteria. Thus bacterial products, in this case tetanus toxin, were also protective.

By 1900 many vaccines had been developed, and the development of immunity to infectious diseases of animals was a well-recognized phenomenon. Since then, immunologists have determined the molecular and cellular basis of this antimicrobial immunity. With this understanding has come the ability to use immune mechanisms to enhance resistance to infectious diseases. The role of the immune system in many different disease processes has been clarified. While much has been learned, much remains to be investigated. It is the current state of immunology as it relates to those species of interest to veterinarians that is the subject of this book.

Microbial Invasion

The world is full of microorganisms. These include bacteria, viruses, fungi, protozoa, and helminths (worms). As they struggle to survive, many microorganisms find the animal body to be a rich source of nutrients and a place to shelter. Enormous numbers of them colonize body surfaces, especially within the intestine or on the skin. These organisms, called commensals, do not seek to invade the body and do not normally cause disease. Other, more aggressive organisms try to invade animal tissues. This is normally prevented, or at least controlled by our immune defenses. If these organisms succeed in invading the body and overcoming the immune defenses, they may cause disease. The invaders will survive provided they can avoid the host's immune system for sufficient time to replicate and transmit their progeny to a new host. While it is essential for an animal to control invading organisms, infectious agents are under even more potent selective pressure. They must find a host or die. Organisms that cannot evade or overcome the immune defenses will not survive and will be eliminated.

An organism that can cause disease is said to be a pathogen. Remember, however, that only a small proportion of the world's microorganisms are associated with animals, and very few of these can overcome the immune defenses and become pathogens. Pathogenic microorganisms also vary greatly in their ability to invade the body and cause disease. This ability is termed virulence. Thus a highly virulent organism has a greater ability to cause disease than an organism with low virulence. If a bacterium can cause disease almost every time it invades a healthy individual, even in low numbers, it is considered a primary pathogen. Examples of primary pathogens include canine distemper virus; human immunodeficiency virus (HIV), which causes AIDS; and *Brucella abortus*, the cause of contagious abortion in cattle. Other pathogens may be of such low virulence that they only cause disease if administered in very high doses or if the immune defenses of the body are impaired first. These are opportunistic pathogens. Examples of opportunistic pathogens include bacteria such as *Mannheimia hemolytica* and fungi such as *Pneumocystis jiroveci*. These organisms rarely cause disease in healthy animals.

The Body's Defenses

The defenses of the body, collectively called the immune system, consist of complex, interacting networks of biochemical and cellular reactions. For descriptive purposes, it is convenient to divide this network into discrete pathways. Nevertheless, the reader should be aware that these biochemical and cellular pathways are extensively interlinked. No immune response is restricted to a single biochemical mechanism or pathway. The entry of a pathogen or vaccine into the animal body can alter the expression of a very large number of molecules. Understanding immunity requires an understanding of dynamic immunological networks. These networks possess redundancies and multiple simultaneous mechanisms working together to ensure microbial destruction. This of course maximizes their efficiency and minimizes the chances of any individual microbe successfully evading those defenses.

Physical Barriers

Because the successful exclusion of microbial invaders is essential for survival, it is not surprising that animals use many different defense strategies. The body employs multiple, overlapping layers of defense (Figure 1-3). As a result, an organism that has succeeded in breaking through the first defenses is then confronted with the need to overcome a second, higher barrier, and so forth. The first and most obvious of these defenses are the physical barriers to invasion. Thus intact skin provides an effective barrier to microbial invasion. If skin is damaged, microbes may invade; however, wound healing ensures that this is repaired very rapidly. On other body surfaces, such as in the respiratory and gastrointestinal tracts, simple physical defenses include the "self-cleaning" processes: coughing, sneezing, and mucus flow in the respiratory tract; vomiting and diarrhea in the gastrointestinal tract; and urine flow in the urinary system. The presence of a huge population of commensal bacteria on the skin and in the intestine also excludes many potential invaders. Well-adapted commensal organisms adapted to living on body surfaces can easily outcompete poorly adapted pathogenic organisms.

Innate Immunity

Physical barriers, although essential in excluding invaders, cannot be totally effective in themselves. Given time and persistence, an invading microorganism will eventually overcome mere physical obstacles. Nevertheless most microbial attempts at invasion are blocked before they can result in disease. This is the task of the innate immune system. All animals and plants, even the simplest, need to exclude microbial invaders. As a result, many different innate defense mechanisms have evolved over time. The mammalian innate immune system is therefore a collection of distinct subsystems that work through diverse mechanisms. All respond rapidly with cells or chemicals to block microbial invasion and minimize tissue damage (Figure 1-4). Innate immunity is activated immediately when

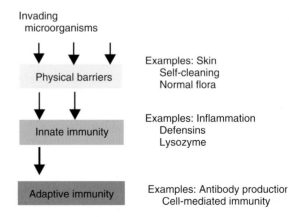

FIGURE 1-3 The three major barriers that protect an animal's body against microbial invasion. Each barrier provides a more effective defense than the previous one.

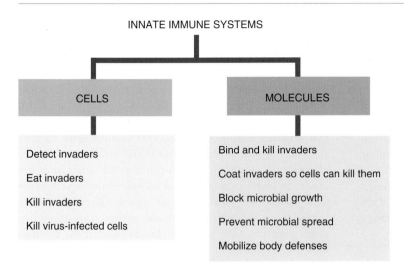

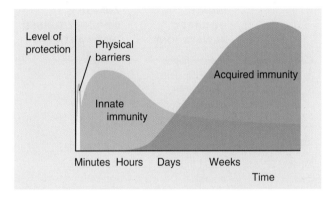

FIGURE 1-4 The innate immune system consists of a collection of multiple subsystems. They can be divided into the cells that largely eat and kill invaders and the molecules that bind and kill the invaders.

a pathogen penetrates the epithelial barriers, it ideally lasts for just a few hours, and is directed toward the rapid elimination of the pathogen. Innate immune mechanisms in general rely on the fact that microbes such as bacteria and viruses differ structurally and chemically from normal animal tissues. Animals make molecules that can kill invaders directly or promote their destruction by defensive cells. Some of these molecules circulate all the time, whereas the production of others is induced by the presence of bacteria, viruses, or damaged tissues.

Other subsystems employ sentinel cells that can detect the molecules commonly associated with invading microorganisms. Sentinel cells recruit other cells, called leukocytes, that can destroy most invading organisms. Other innate subsystems include the complement system, a set of complex enzyme pathways that are lethal to invaders. Some of the cells involved in inflammation may also help repair damaged tissues once the invading microbes have been destroyed.

The innate immune system is a network of "hard-wired" subsystems that lack any form of memory, and as a result, each infection episode is treated identically. The intensity and duration of innate responses such as inflammation therefore remain unchanged no matter how often a specific invader is encountered. These responses also come at a price: the pain of inflammation and the development of sickness largely result from the activation of innate immune pathways. On the other hand, the multiple subsystems of the innate immune system are "on call" and ready to respond immediately when an invader is detected.

Adaptive Immunity

Inflammation and the other subsystems of the innate immune system are critical to the defense of the body. Animals that cannot mount effective innate responses will die from overwhelming infections. Nevertheless, these innate mechanisms cannot offer the ultimate solution to the defense of the body. What is really needed is a defense system that can recognize and destroy invaders and then learn from the process, so that

FIGURE 1-5 The time course of innate and adaptive immunity. Physical barriers provide immediate protection. Innate mechanisms provide rapid protection that keeps microbial invaders at bay until adaptive immunity can develop. It may take several days or even weeks for adaptive immunity to become effective.

if they invade again, they will be destroyed even more effectively. In this system, the more often an individual encounters an invader, the more effective will be its defenses against that organism. This type of response is the function of the adaptive immune system, so called since it adapts itself to the requirements of the animal. (This is also called the acquired immune system.) The adaptive immune system takes several days or weeks to become effective (Figure 1-5). Although it develops slowly, when an animal eventually develops adaptive immunity to an invader, the chances of successful invasion by that organism decline precipitously, and the animal is said to be immune. The adaptive immune system is a complex and sophisticated system that provides the ultimate defense of the body. Its essential nature is readily seen when it is destroyed. The loss of adaptive immunity leads inevitably to uncontrolled infections and death.

A key difference between the innate and adaptive immune systems lies in their use of cell surface receptors to recognize foreign invaders (Table 1-1). The cells of the innate system use a limited number of preformed receptors that bind to molecules commonly expressed on many different microbes. In contrast, the cells of the adaptive immune system generate enormous numbers of completely new, structurally unique receptors. These receptors can bind to an enormous array of foreign molecules. Because the binding repertoire of these receptors is generated randomly, they are not predestined to recognize any specific foreign molecule but collectively recognize some of the molecules on almost any invading microorganism.

The adaptive immune system not only recognizes foreign invaders but also destroys them and retains the memory of the encounter. If the animal encounters the same organism a second time, the adaptive immune system responds more rapidly and more effectively. Such a sophisticated system must of necessity be complex.

One reason for this complexity is the great diversity of potential invaders, including bacteria, viruses, fungi, protozoa, and helminths (worms). These invaders may be classified into two broad categories. One category consists of the organisms that originate outside the body. This includes most bacteria and fungi as well as many protozoa and invading helminths. The second category consists of organisms that originate or live inside the body's own cells. These include viruses and intracellular bacteria or protozoa. These require different defensive strategies, so the adaptive immune system consists of two major branches. One branch is directed against the extracellular (or exogenous) invaders. Soluble proteins called antibodies promote the destruction of these invaders. This type of immune response is sometimes called a *humoral immune response* since antibodies are found in body fluids (or "humors"). The second major branch of the adaptive immune system is directed against the intracellular (or endogenous) invaders. Specialized cells are required to destroy these infected or abnormal cells since antibodies do not work inside cells. This type of response is therefore called a *cell-mediated immune response.*

◻ Table 1-1 | Comparison of Innate and Adaptive Immunity

	INNATE IMMUNITY ALWAYS "ON"	ADAPTIVE IMMUNITY TURNED ON BY ANTIGENS
Cells engaged	Macrophages, dendritic cells neutrophils, natural killer cells	T and B cells
Evolutionary history	Ancient	Recent
Onset	Rapid (minutes to hours)	Slow (days to weeks)
Specificity	Common microbial structures	Unique antigens
Potency	May be overwhelmed	Rarely overwhelmed
Memory	None	Significant memory
Effectiveness	Does not improve	Improves with exposure

Antibody-Mediated Immune Responses

Soon after Louis Pasteur discovered that it was possible to produce immunity to infectious agents by vaccination, it was recognized that the substances that provided this immunity could be found in blood serum (Figure 1-6). For example, if serum is taken from an immune horse that has been previously vaccinated against tetanus (or has recovered from tetanus) and then injected into a normal horse, the recipient animal will become temporarily resistant to tetanus (Figure 1-7).

The protective molecules found in the serum of immune animals are proteins called antibodies. Antibodies against

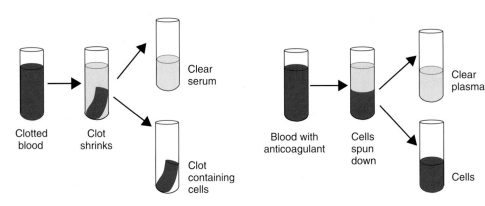

FIGURE 1-6 The difference between serum and plasma. Plasma is obtained when blood is not allowed to clot, and the cells are sedimented by centrifugation. In contrast, when blood is allowed to clot, the clot gradually contracts, releasing clear serum. Plasma therefore contains blood-clotting proteins that are absent from serum.

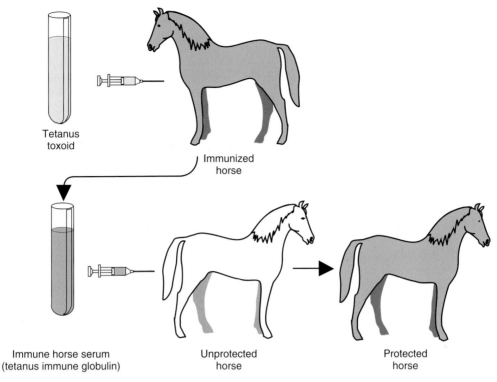

FIGURE 1-7 Immunity to tetanus can be transferred to a normal horse by means of serum derived from an immunized horse. This clearly demonstrates that antibodies in serum are sufficient to confer immunity to tetanus in horses.

tetanus toxin are not found in normal horses but are produced following exposure to tetanus toxin as a result of infection or vaccination. Tetanus toxin is an example of a foreign substance that stimulates an adaptive immune response. The general term for such a substance is *antigen*. If an antigen is injected into an animal, antibodies will be produced that can bind to that antigen and ensure its destruction. Antibodies are highly specific and can bind only to the antigen that stimulates their production. For example, the antibodies produced in response to tetanus toxin bind only tetanus toxin. When the antibodies bind, they "neutralize" the toxin so that it is no longer toxic. In this way antibodies protect animals against the lethal effects of tetanus infection.

The time course of the antibody response to tetanus toxin can be examined by taking blood samples from a horse at intervals after injection of a low dose of the toxin. The blood is allowed to clot, and the clear serum is removed. The amount of antibody in the serum may be estimated by measuring its ability to neutralize a standard amount of toxin. After a single injection of toxin into an unexposed horse, no antibody is detectable for several days (Figure 1-8). This lag period lasts for about 1 week. When antibodies eventually appear, their levels climb to reach a peak by 10 to 20 days before declining and disappearing within a few weeks. The amount of antibody formed, and therefore the amount of protection conferred, during this first or primary response is relatively small.

If sometime later a second dose of toxin is injected into the same horse, the lag period before the antibody response can be detected lasts for no more than 2 or 3 days. The amount of

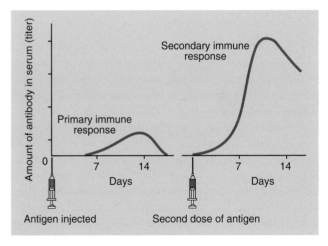

FIGURE 1-8 The characteristic time course of the adaptive immune response to an antigen as measured by serum antibody levels. Note the differences between a primary and a secondary immune response. These differences account for the success of the adaptive immune responses.

antibody in serum then rises rapidly to a high level before declining slowly. Antibodies may be detected for many months or years after this injection. A third dose of the antigen given to the same animal results in an immune response characterized by an even shorter lag period and a still higher and more prolonged antibody response. As will be described later in this book, the antibodies produced after repeated injections are better able to bind and neutralize the toxin than those produced early in the immune response. The enhancement of the immune responses to infectious agents by repeated injections of antigen forms the basis of vaccination.

The response of an animal to a second dose of antigen is very different from the first in that it occurs much more quickly, antibodies reach much higher levels, and the response persists much longer. This secondary response is specific in that it can be provoked only by a second dose of an antigen. A secondary response may be provoked many months or years after the first injection of antigen, although its size tends to decline as time passes. A secondary response can also be induced even though the response of the animal to the first injection of antigen was so weak as to be undetectable. These features of the secondary response indicate that the antibody-forming system possesses the ability to "remember" previous exposure to an antigen. For this reason, the secondary immune response is sometimes called an anamnestic response (*anam-nesko* is Greek for "memory"). It should be noted, however, that repeated injections of antigen do not lead indefinitely to greater immune responses. The levels of antibodies in serum are regulated, so that they eventually stop rising after multiple doses of antigen or exposure to many different antigens.

Cell-Mediated Immune Responses

If a piece of living tissue such as a kidney or a piece of skin is surgically removed from one animal and grafted onto another of the same species, it usually survives for a few days before being rejected by the recipient. This process of graft rejection is significant because it demonstrates the existence of a mechanism whereby foreign cells, differing only slightly from an animal's own normal cells, are rapidly recognized and destroyed. Even cells with minor structural abnormalities may be recognized as foreign by the immune system and destroyed though they are otherwise apparently healthy. These abnormal cells include aged cells, virus-infected cells, and some cancer cells. The immune response to foreign cells as shown by graft rejection demonstrates that the immune system can identify and destroy abnormal cells.

If a piece of skin is transplanted from one dog to a second, unrelated, dog, it will survive for about 10 days. The grafted skin will initially appear to be healthy, and blood vessels will develop between the graft and its host. By 1 week, however, these new blood vessels will begin to degenerate, the blood supply to the graft will be cut off, and the graft will eventually die and be shed (Figure 1-9). If the experiment is repeated and a second graft is taken from the original donor and placed on the same recipient, the second graft will survive for no more than a day or two before being rejected. Thus the rejection of a first graft is relatively weak and slow and analogous to the primary antibody response, whereas a second graft stimulates very rapid and powerful rejection similar in many ways to the

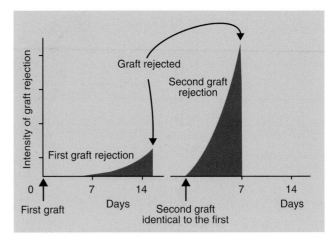

FIGURE 1-9 The characteristic time course of the rejection of a foreign skin graft. The intensity of the rejection process is much more severe when a secondary response is mounted. Notice how similar this diagram is to Figure 1-8.

secondary antibody response. Graft rejection, like antibody formation, is a specific adaptive immune response in that a rapid secondary reaction occurs only if the second graft is from the same donor as the first. Like antibody formation, the graft rejection process also involves immunological memory since a second graft may be rapidly rejected many months or years after loss of the first.

However, graft rejection is not entirely identical to antibody-mediated immunity because it cannot be transferred from a sensitized to a normal animal by means of serum. The ability to mount a secondary reaction to a graft can only be transferred between animals by living cells. The cells that do this are called lymphocytes and are found in the spleen, lymph nodes, or blood. The process of graft rejection is mediated primarily by lymphocytes and not by serum antibodies. It is a good example of a cell-mediated immune response.

Mechanisms of Adaptive Immunity

In some ways the adaptive immune system may be compared to a totalitarian state in which foreigners are expelled, citizens who behave themselves are tolerated, but those who "deviate" are eliminated. While this analogy must not be carried too far, clearly such regimes possess a number of characteristic features. These include border defenses and a police force that keeps the population under surveillance and promptly eliminates dissidents. In the case of the adaptive immune system, the antibody-mediated responses would be responsible for keeping the foreigners out, whereas the cell-mediated responses would be responsible for stopping internal dissent. Organizations of this type also tend to develop a pass system, so that foreigners or dissidents not possessing certain identifying features are rapidly detected and dealt with.

Similarly, when a foreign antigen enters the body, it first must be trapped and processed so that it can be recognized as being foreign. If so recognized, this information must be conveyed either to the antibody-forming system or to the cell-mediated immune system. These systems must then respond by the production of specific antibodies or cells that are capable of eliminating the antigen. The adaptive immune system must also remember this event so that the next time an animal is exposed to the same antigen, its response will be faster and more efficient. The immune system also learns how to make antibodies or cells that can bind more strongly to the invader. In our totalitarian state analogy, the police force would be trained to recognize selected foreigners or dissidents and respond more promptly when they are encountered.

It must be emphasized, however, that just as human societies and responses are very complex and involve the interactions of thousands of individuals, so too is the immune system. While, for reasons of simplicity we consider discrete processes and pathways, the system should be thought of as a very complex interactive network. Thousands of different molecules interact in many ways and are subject to multiple influences. Thus its behavior can rarely be completely explained by examining just a few of its components. The pathways involved interact with each other, sometimes in a very complex manner. Likewise the immune response is not simply a function of the individual animal. The invading microbe, its virulence, its ability to evade defenses, and its interactions with other microbes all lead to variations in a host's immune response.

For introductory purposes, we can consider that the adaptive immune system consists of several major components (Figure 1-10). Thus it is triggered by cells that can trap and process antigen and then present it for recognition to the cells of the immune system. These cells can recognize and respond to the processed antigen since they possess specific antigen receptors. Some of these cells, once activated by antigen, will produce specific antibodies, whereas others will participate in the cell-mediated immune responses against the antigen. Other cells retain the memory of the event and react rapidly to that specific antigen if it is encountered at a later time. Finally, there are cells that regulate this response and ensure that it functions at an appropriate level.

All of these cell populations can be recognized within the body. Antigen is trapped, processed, and presented by several cell types, including dendritic cells and macrophages. Lymphocytes called B and T cells have specific receptors for foreign antigen and are thus able to bind the processed antigen and respond appropriately. Lymphocytes also function as memory cells and therefore initiate a secondary immune response. The lymphocytes that mediate the cell-mediated responses are T cells. The lymphocytes that mediate the antibody-mediated responses are B cells. The immune response is mainly regulated by populations of T cells. Those that promote immune responses are called helper T cells. Those that inhibit immune responses are called regulatory T cells.

In subsequent chapters we will first review the mechanisms involved in innate immunity. Following that, we will review

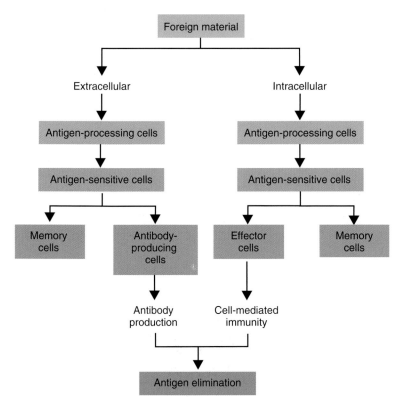

FIGURE 1-10 A simple flow diagram showing the essential features of the adaptive immune responses.

LIVERPOOL JOHN MOORES UNIVERSITY
LEARNING SERVICES

adaptive immunity in detail and examine each of its basic components in turn. We will then examine the role of the immune system in protecting animals against microbial invasion. We will also see what happens when the immune system functions abnormally, either excessively or inadequately.

Where to Go for Additional Information

Many veterinary journals carry articles of interest to immunologists. Some of the most important include the following: *American Journal of Veterinary Research, Animal Genetics, Australian Veterinary Journal, Canadian Journal of Veterinary Research, Developmental and Comparative Immunology, Fish and Shellfish Immunology, Journal of the American Veterinary Medical Association, Journal of Comparative Pathology, Journal of Small Animal Practice, Journal of Veterinary Internal Medicine, Research in Veterinary Science, Vaccine, Veterinary Dermatology, Veterinary Immunology and Immunopathology, The Veterinary Journal, Veterinary Pathology, The Veterinary Record,* and *Veterinary Research.*

For information on new developments in basic immunology (with occasional papers on subjects of veterinary interest), the reader should review journals such as *Cell Host and Microbe, Clinical and Experimental Immunology, European Journal of Immunology, Infection and Immunity, Immunity, Immunogenetics, Immunology, Journal of Immunology, Journal of Leukocyte Biology, Molecular Immunology, Nature, Nature Immunology, Nature Reviews Immunology, New England Journal of Medicine, Proceedings of the National Academy of Sciences, Science, Trends in Immunology,* and *Vaccine.*

As in many scientific fields, the World Wide Web can be a very useful source of information about veterinary immunology, although care should be taken to verify the information provided. Some important sites include PubMed (http://www.ncbi.nlm.nih.gov/sites/entrez), which provides rapid access to scientific journals, and the Comparative Immunoglobulin workshop (http://www.medicine.uiowa.edu/cigw/), which provides current information on immunoglobulin structures. Readers may also wish to look at the websites of the American Association of Veterinary Immunologists (http://www.theaavi.org/) or national Immunology organizations such as the American Association of Immunologists (www.aai.org/) and the British Society for Immunology (http://www.immunology.org)/.

Innate Immunity: The Recognition of Invaders

Key Points

- Two types of signal trigger the body's innate defenses. One signal generated by the presence of invading microorganisms is detected by sensing their characteristic surface molecules, or nucleic acids. These are called pathogen-associated molecular patterns (PAMPs).
- Cells also detect molecules released from damaged tissues and broken cells. These are called damage-associated molecular patterns (DAMPs) or alarmins.
- Both PAMPs and DAMPs bind to pattern-recognition receptors (PRRs) on cell surfaces or located within cells.
- PRRs are found on many different cell types. The most important of these "sentinel" cells are macrophages, dendritic cells, and mast cells.
- A major group of PRRs is called toll-like receptors (TLRs).
- Signals generated when PAMPs bind TLRs activate sentinel cells and stimulate them to secrete many different molecules. Some of these molecules are proteins called cytokines that "turn on" the inflammatory process.
- These molecules trigger local increases in blood flow, attract defensive cells such as neutrophils, and increase blood vessel permeability, allowing antimicrobial molecules and cells to flood affected tissues.

Infectious agents such as bacteria and viruses multiply rapidly. A single bacterium with a doubling time of 50 minutes can produce about 500 million offspring within 24 hours. If these microorganisms invade the body, they must be recognized and destroyed before they can overwhelm the defenses. Time is of the essence, and delay can be fatal. The body must therefore employ fast-reacting mechanisms as its first line of defense against invaders. These mechanisms need to be on constant standby and respond promptly at the first signs of microbial invasion. These mechanisms constitute the innate immune system. Because all multicellular organisms are subject to microbial attack, innate immunity has developed in both animals and plants, in vertebrates and in invertebrates. Innate immune mechanisms have arisen in different ways and at different times in response to different threats. As a result, the innate immune system consists of many diverse subsystems.

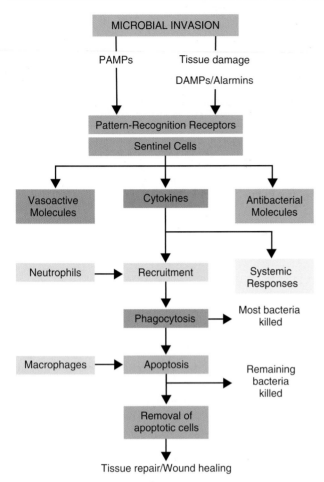

FIGURE 2-1 An overview of the essential features of acute inflammation, an innate mechanism for focusing cells and other defensive mechanisms. It is triggered by microbial invasion and tissue damage.

The most important of these innate subsystems is the process we call inflammation.

Inflammation concentrates defensive cells and antimicrobial molecules at sites of microbial invasion and tissue damage. These defensive cells are the white blood cells (leukocytes) that circulate constantly in the bloodstream. Inflammation triggers the migration of leukocytes, from the bloodstream to sites of invasion where they attack and destroy invaders. Likewise, many protective proteins, such as antibodies and complement components, are normally found only in blood and can only enter tissues during inflammation. Inflammation is therefore a mechanism by which defensive cells and proteins are focused on sites of microbial invasion. Together, they destroy the invaders and then repair any subsequent tissue damage (Figure 2-1).

How Invaders Are Recognized

The innate immune system is activated when the body senses that it is under attack. This involves recognizing alarm signals generated by two pathways. Alarm signals are generated either by invading microorganisms (exogenous signals) or by dead and dying cells (endogenous signals). Exogenous signals consist of molecules produced by microbial invaders. Collectively, these are called pathogen-associated molecular patterns (PAMPs). Endogenous signals consist of molecules released from damaged, dead, or dying cells. These are collectively called damage-associated molecular patterns (DAMPs). Together, the DAMPs and PAMPs are recognized by pattern-recognition receptors (PRRs) on sentinel cells located throughout the body. Once recognized, they activate the innate immune system.

Pathogen-Associated Molecular Patterns

Microbes not only grow very fast but also are highly diverse and can mutate and change many of their surface molecules very rapidly. For this reason, the innate immune system does not attempt to recognize all possible microbial molecules. Rather, the body uses receptors that can bind and respond to abundant, essential molecules that are common to many different microorganisms but are absent from normal animal tissues. Because they play essential roles, they tend not to change rapidly. They are essential for microbial survival, and as a result, are commonly shared by entire classes of pathogens. They are, in effect, widely distributed molecular patterns. For example, the walls of Gram-positive bacteria are largely composed of peptidoglycans (chains of alternating *N*-acetylglucosamine and *N*-acetylmuramic acid cross-linked by short peptide side chains) (Figure 2-2). Gram-positive bacterial cell walls also contain lipoteichoic acids. The cell walls of Gram-negative bacteria consist of peptidoglycans covered by a layer of lipopolysaccharide (LPS). Acid-fast bacteria are covered in glycolipids. Yeasts have a mannan- or β-glucan–rich cell wall. Viruses, in contrast, grow within infected host cells, so the main targets of antiviral PRRs are unique viral nucleic acids.

Many different PRRs are used to ensure as complete coverage as possible of PAMPs. Most are cell-associated receptors found on cell membranes, within the cytosol, and within cytoplasmic vesicles. Soluble receptors also circulate in the bloodstream (Figure 2-3). Examples of PRRs include the toll-like receptors (TLRs), the retinoic acid-inducible gene (RIG)-1-like receptors (RLRs), nucleotide-binding oligomerization domain (NOD)-like receptors (NLRs), and the C-type lectin receptors (CLRs). CLRs are soluble proteins primarily involved in the capture and uptake of invading bacteria. The others, in contrast, are receptors that activate intracellular signaling cascades.

Toll-like Receptors

The most important family of PRRs consists of the TLRs (Box 2-1). Some TLRs are located on cell surfaces, where they are responsible for recognizing extracellular invaders such as bacteria and fungi. Other TLRs are located within the cells, where they are responsible for detecting intracellular invaders such as

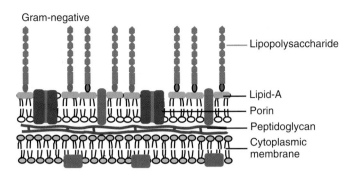

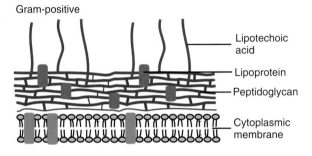

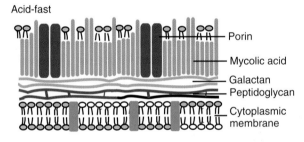

FIGURE 2-2 The major structural features of the cell walls of Gram-negative, Gram-positive, and acid-fast bacteria. It is these conserved structural molecules that serve as pathogen-associated molecular patterns and are recognized by pattern-recognition receptors such as the toll-like receptors.

viruses. TLRs are a critical first line of defense against bacterial, viral, and fungal invaders and play a vital role in microbial sensing.

TLRs are expressed by many different cell types. Most importantly, they are expressed on sentinel cells located on or near the surface of the body. Sentinel cells include macrophages, mast cells, and dendritic cells, as well the epithelial cells that line the respiratory and intestinal tracts.

TLRs are transmembrane glycoprotein receptors. Mammals possess 10 or 12 different functional TLRs (TLR1 to TLR10 in humans and cattle and TLR1 to TLR9 and TLR11 to TLR13 in mice) (Table 2-1). The cell surface TLRs (TLR1, 2, 4, 5, and 11) mainly recognize bacterial and fungal proteins, lipoproteins, and lipopolysaccharides. The intracellular TLRs (TLR3, 7, 8, 9, and 10), in contrast, recognize viral and bacterial nucleic acids. For example, TLR4 on the cell surface recognizes lipopolysaccharides on Gram-negative bacteria. TLR2 recognizes peptidoglycans, lipoproteins, and a glycolipid called lipoarabinomannan from *Mycobacterium tuberculosis,* whereas TLR5 recognizes flagellin, the major protein of bacterial flagella. TLR9 is an intracellular sensor of bacterial DNA and is triggered by intracellular bacteria. Other intracellular receptors, such as TLR3 and TLR7, recognize viral double-stranded

□ **Box 2-1 Toll-like Receptors**

This strange name alludes to the original discovery of a protein called "Toll" in fruit flies *(Drosophila)*. This protein was necessary for proper embryological development. In its absence, the flies developed abnormally, and the German researchers who first saw these abnormal flies exclaimed "Toll!" (amazing, or weird!). This protein was subsequently found to be necessary for antifungal immunity in *Drosophila* species. When the first pattern-recognition receptor in mammals was identified, it was found to be similar in sequence and structure to the *Drosophila* toll protein, hence "toll-like receptors."

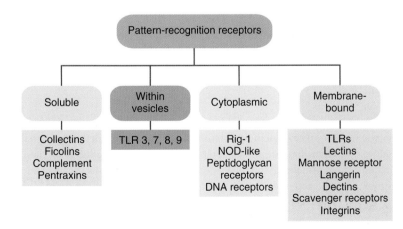

FIGURE 2-3 There are many different pattern-recognition receptors found in the body. Most are found on or within cells. Others are soluble molecules that circulate in the bloodstream.

□ Table 2-1 | Pathogen-Associated Molecular Patterns Recognized by the Mammalian Toll-like Receptors

TLR	LOCATION	LIGAND	SOURCE OF LIGAND
TLR1	Cell surface	Triacylated lipoprotein	Bacteria
TLR2	Cell surface	Lipoproteins	Bacteria, viruses, parasites
TLR3	Intracellular	dsRNA	Viruses
TLR4	Cell surface	LPS	Bacteria, viruses
TLR5	Cell surface	Flagellin	Bacteria
TLR6	Cell surface	Diacylated lipoprotein	Bacteria, viruses
TLR7	Intracellular	ssRNA	Viruses, bacteria
TLR8	Intracellular	ssRNA	Viruses, bacteria
TLR9	Intracellular	CpG DNA, dsDNA	Viruses, bacteria, protozoa
TLR10	Intracellular	Unknown	Unknown
TLR 11	Cell surface	*Toxoplasma* profilin-like molecule	Protozoa
TLR12 and TLR13	Found in mice, not humans		Unknown

CpG, cytosine-guanosine; *LPS*, lipopolysaccharide; *TLR*, toll-like receptor.

(ds) ribonucleic acid (RNA), whereas TLR7 and TLR8 recognize viral single-stranded (ss) RNA. Most TLRs are usually homodimers formed by identical paired peptide chains. They may also form heterodimers using dissimilar chains. For example, one TLR2 chain can associate with a TLR6 chain, and this heterodimer can then recognize bacterial diacylated lipopeptides. A TLR2 chain also associates with a TLR1 chain to recognize mycobacterial triacylated lipopeptides. Given the number of possible TLR chain combinations, it is believed that the presently known TLRs can collectively recognize almost all PAMPs. TLR11 is different from the other TLRs. It is found only on dendritic cells, macrophages, and epithelial cells in the mouse urinary tract, where it recognizes bacteria and PAMPs from protozoan parasites (Box 2-2).

When a PAMP binds to its corresponding TLR, signals are passed to the cell. Multiprotein signaling complexes are formed, signal transduction cascades are initiated, and as a result, pro-inflammatory molecules are produced by the cell. Each step in the process involves multiple biochemical reactions involving many different proteins, and the precise signaling pathway employed differs between TLRs. For example, the cell surface TLRs use different pathways than the intracellular TLRs. All TLRs except TLR3 use an adaptor protein called MyD88 to activate three major transcription factors, nuclear factor kappa-B (NF-κB), MAP kinase (MAPK), and IRF3 (Figure 2-4). NF-κB and MAPK activate the genes for three major proteins, interleukin-1 (IL-1), interleukin-6 (IL-6), and tumor necrosis factor-alpha (TNF-α) IRF3 activates the gene for

□ Box 2-2 | **TLRs and Diarrhea in German Shepherd Dogs**

The critical role of TLRs is to trigger the initial steps in resistance to microbial invaders. If they are ineffective, an animal may show increased susceptibility to infections. For example, inflammatory bowel disease is especially common in German Shepherd dogs. Genetic analysis of a large number of these dogs suffering from inflammatory bowel disease showed that several single-nucleotide polymorphisms (SNPs) in the *TLR4* and *TLR5* genes were significantly associated with the occurrence of this disease. It is likely that in German Shepherd dogs, changes in their TLR4 and TLR5 have reduced their ability to defend against bacterial invasion in the intestine. This results in a predisposition to enteric infections, as shown by diarrhea and vomiting.

Data from Kathrani A, House A, Catchpole B, et al: Polymorphisms in the TLR4 and TLR5 gene are significantly associated with inflammatory bowel disease in German shepherd dogs, *PloS One* 5:e15740, 2010.

another protein, interferon-β. (For additional details on signal transduction, see Chapter 8.) The proteins produced by these sentinel cells are all classed as cytokines, proteins that regulate the activities of cells involved in the defense of the body. The cytokines are produced as inactive precursors and then

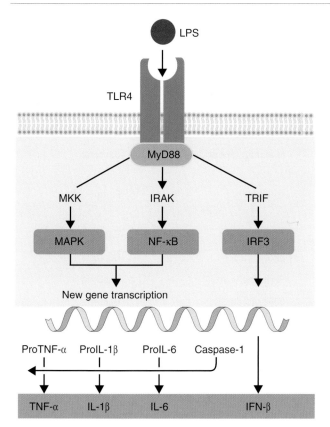

FIGURE 2-4 Binding of a pathogen-associated molecular pattern such as lipopolysaccharide to a toll-like receptor generates a signaling cascade involving three major signaling molecules and activating several transcription factors. These include MAPK, NF-κB, and IRF3. These transcription factors activate the genes for the three major cytokines, IL-1, IL-6, and TNF-α, as well as the activating enzyme caspase-1. The TRIF complex turns on another transcription factor, IRF3, that activates the gene for the antiviral cytokine, IFN-β.

activated by an enzyme called caspase-1. The production of caspase-1 is triggered by a protein complex called an inflammasome (Box 2-3).

Caspases are proteolytic enzymes (the cysteinyl aspartate–specific proteinases) that play key roles in the initiation of inflammation. Many, such as caspase-1, -4, -5, and -12, are activated by signals generated by TLRs. Caspase-1 is most important because it acts on the inactive precursors to generate active cytokines. These cytokines trigger the next phase of the inflammatory response. Different TLRs trigger the production of different cytokine mixtures, and different PAMPs trigger distinctly different responses even within one cell type. For example, TLRs that recognize bacterial molecules tend to trigger the production of cytokines optimized to combat bacteria; those that recognize viral molecules produce antiviral cytokines, and so forth. TLRs not only trigger innate responses such as inflammation but also begin the process of "turning on" the adaptive immune system. For example, stimulation of TLR4 makes macrophages and their close relatives, the

□ Box 2-3 | **Inflammasomes**

When the cytosolic NOD-like receptors are triggered by pathogen binding, they initiate a series of reactions by which several cellular proteins bind together to form large multiprotein complexes called inflammasomes. The inflammasome then recruits an enzyme, caspase-1, and activates it. Caspase-1 in turn acts on pro-IL-1, pro-IL-6, and TNF-α to generate the active forms of these cytokines. Several different inflammasomes have been characterized, each generated by a different set of pathogens, containing slightly different subcomponents and thus presumably generating different cytokines and proinflammatory molecules. In humans, inherited defects in some inflammasome components are linked to certain diseases characterized by uncontrolled inflammation.

dendritic cells, produce cytokines that are potent stimulators of immune cells (Chapter 10).

TLRs are also expressed on the bone marrow stem cells that are the source of leukocytes. Bacterial lipopolysaccharides binding to TLR4 on stem cells stimulates the bone marrow to increase leukocyte production. An increase in leukocyte numbers in the blood (the white cell count), is therefore a consistent feature of infectious diseases. The intracellular TLRs detect the presence of viral nucleic acids. When triggered, they synthesize antiviral cytokines, collectively called type I interferons (IFNs). The interferons are proteins that activate genes encoding antiviral proteins and pathways and so "interfere" with viral growth.

RIG-1-like Receptors

Retinoic acid inducible gene (RIG)-like receptors (RLRs) are another family of PRRs expressed within the cytosol. They recognize viral dsRNA. Because viral dsRNA differs structurally from mammalian RNA, RLRs can discriminate between viral and normal mammalian RNA. Once triggered, the RLRs activate caspases and trigger signaling pathways, leading to the production of type I IFNs.

NOD-like Receptors

Nucleotide-binding oligomerization domain (NOD)-like receptors (NLRs) are a family of PRRs that can also detect pathogens within the cytosol (Table 2-2). Although TLRs and NLRs differ in their location and function, they share similar structures for microbial sensing and cooperate to trigger host responses to invaders. NOD1 recognizes bacterial peptidoglycans, whereas NOD2 recognizes muramyl dipeptide and serves as a general sensor of intracellular bacteria. Binding to either NLR activates the NF-κB pathway and triggers the production of proinflammatory cytokines. NOD2 also triggers

☐ Table 2-2 | Other Mammalian Pattern-Recognition Receptors

RECEPTOR	LOCATION	LIGAND	SOURCE OF LIGAND
RLRs			
RIG-1	Intracellular	Short dsRNA	RNA viruses
NLRs			
NOD1	Cytoplasm	Peptidoglycans	Bacteria
NOD2	Cytoplasm	Muramyl dipeptide	Bacteria
CLRs			
Dectins	Cell surface	Glucans	Fungi
Others			
Mannose-fucose receptor	Cell surface	Glycoproteins	Bacteria
CD14	Cell surface	LPS	Bacteria
Peptidoglycan recognition proteins	Cell surface	Peptidoglycans	Bacteria
CD1	Cell surface	Glycolipids	Bacteria
CD36	Cell surface	Lipoproteins	Bacteria
CD48	Cell surface	Fimbria	Bacteria

the production of the antimicrobial proteins known as defensins (Chapter 3).

C-type Lectin Receptors

Lectins are proteins that bind carbohydrates. The C-type lectins require Ca^{2+} for this binding, hence their name. At least 1000 C-type lectins have been identified in animals. They are found on many different cell types and serve multiple functions. Some are cell surface PRRs that can recognize the carbohydrates on bacteria, fungi, and some viruses. The major cell surface lectins involved in pathogen recognition are dectin-1, dectin-2, and DEC205. These dectins recognize β-glucans on fungal cell walls and play an important role in antifungal defense. They promote the intracellular destruction of fungi. Dectin-1 is expressed by bovine macrophages, monocytes, and dendritic cells. Bovine dectin-2 is expressed in large amounts on Langerhans cells in the skin (Chapter 10). DEC205 is expressed on bovine dendritic cells. Another C-type lectin, the macrophage mannose receptor, is expressed on macrophages and recognizes numerous diverse pathogens, such as the yeasts *Candida albicans* and *Pneumocystis jiroveci*, the protozoa *Leishmania*, and viruses such as bovine viral diarrhea virus.

The sentinel cells—macrophages, mast cells, and dendritic cells—have many other receptors that can recognize microbial molecules and trigger innate defenses. These include mannan receptors that bind carbohydrates, CD36 that binds lipoproteins, and CD1 that binds glycolipids (Box 2-4).

☐ Box 2-4 | **The CD System**

When advances in immunology made it possible to produce highly specific antibodies against individual cell surface proteins (Chapter 9), it was soon shown that mammalian cells possessed hundreds of different surface proteins. Initially, each protein was given a specific name and often an acronym as well. It soon became clear, however, that such a system was unworkable. In an attempt to classify these proteins, a system has been established that assigns each protein to a numbered cluster of differentiation (CD). In many cases, a defined CD denotes a protein of specific function. For example, the protein CD14 binds bacterial lipopolysaccharide. As of October 2010, numbers up to CD360 have been assigned. Unfortunately, CD numbers provide no clue to a molecule's function. In practice, therefore, immunologists tend to use a mixed system employing both a CD number and an abbreviation that denotes the function of a molecule. For example, CD32 is also called FcγR1. A list of selected CD molecules can be found in Appendix 1.

Microbial Pathogen-Associated Molecular Patterns

As described earlier, PAMPs are conserved molecular structures (or patterns) that occur in a diverse range of potential microbial invaders. They include lipopolysaccharides, peptidoglycans, and nucleic acids.

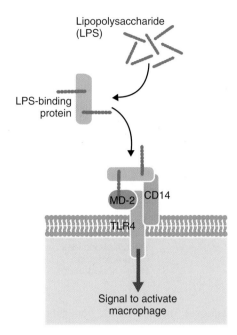

FIGURE 2-5 Bacterial lipopolysaccharide cannot bind directly to TLR4. It must first bind to lipopolysaccharide-binding protein and then to two other proteins, MD-2 and CD14, before it can bind and activate cells such as macrophages.

Bacterial Lipopolysaccharides

Lipopolysaccharides are ubiquitous structural components of the cell walls of many bacteria, especially Gram-negative ones. TLR4 does not bind LPS directly but only after they have been linked to three other proteins. These proteins are called MD-2 (myeloid differentiation factor-2), LPS-binding protein (LBP), and CD14. The CD14 interacts with TLR4 in such a way that it decreases the specificity of these reactions and enables both rough and smooth strains of bacteria to be recognized (Figure 2-5). Binding of LPS to the CD14/TLR4/MD-2 complex activates macrophages and triggers cytokine production. The LPS subsequently dissociates from CD14 and binds to lipoproteins, where its toxic activities are lost. CD14 also binds many other microbial molecules, including lipoarabinomannans from mycobacteria, mannuronic acid polymers from *Pseudomonas*, and peptidoglycans from *Staphylococcus aureus*.

Bacterial Peptidoglycans

Peptidoglycans are polymers of alternating *N*-acetyl glucosamine and *N*-acetyl muraminic acid that are major constituents of the cell walls of both Gram-positive and Gram-negative bacteria. Several PRRs can recognize these peptidoglycans, including some TLRs, NODs, and CD14. Peptidoglycan recognition proteins (PGRPs) are PRRs that induce the production of proinflammatory and antimicrobial peptides. Although first identified in arthropods, they have since been found in humans, mice, cattle, and pigs. In pigs, they are expressed constitutively in the skin, bone marrow,

intestine, liver, kidney, and spleen. One member of this family, bovine PGRP-S, can kill microorganisms in which the peptidoglycan is either buried (Gram-negative bacteria) or absent (*Cryptococcus*), raising questions about its precise ligand. PGRP-S also binds bacterial lipopolysaccharides and lipoteichoic acids. It is found in the large granules of neutrophils, and these neutrophils release PGRP-S when exposed to bacteria. Thus, PGRP-S probably plays a significant role in the resistance of cattle to bacterial infections.

Bacterial DNA

Bacterial deoxyribonucleic acid (DNA) can stimulate innate immunity because it is structurally different from eukaryotic DNA. Thus, it differs from the animal's DNA in that much of it consists of the dinucleotide, unmethylated cytosine-guanosine (CpG). (The cytosine in eukaryotic DNA is normally methylated, but this is not the case in bacteria.) These unmethylated CpG dinucleotides can bind and trigger TLR9. Bacterial DNA also contains deoxyguanosine (dG) nucleotides. These dG nucleotides form structures other than the usual double helix. They also bind to TLR9 and trigger production of cytokines such as TNF-α, IL-6, and IL-12.

Viral Nucleic Acids

Viruses are very simple organisms, usually consisting of a nucleic acid core surrounded by a layer of proteins, the capsid, and possibly a lipid envelope. Viruses have few characteristic structures. However, viral nucleic acids are structurally different from those found in animals so that intracellular PRRs can recognize them. Thus, TLR9 detects dsDNA and CpG DNA; TLR8 and TLR7 detect ssRNA; and TLR3 detects dsRNA. TLR9 therefore binds DNA from viruses and intracellular bacteria, whereas TLR7 and TLR8 bind ssRNA from viruses such as vesicular stomatitis virus. TLR3, in contrast, mainly binds dsRNA from viruses such as reoviruses, but it can also recognize some ssRNA and some dsDNA viruses as well. TLR7 and TLR9 predominantly activate MyD88-mediated signaling pathways and trigger production of inflammatory cytokines and type I IFNs. TLR3, in contrast, does not use MyD88 but rather another signaling molecule, the Tir-domain-containing adaptor protein inducing IFN-β (TRIF). The TRIF pathway activates the transcription factor IRF3, which in turn, activates the genes for inflammatory cytokines and IFN-β (see Figure 2-3). Intracellular RLRs detect and respond to viral dsRNA.

Damage-Associated Molecular Patterns

Inflammation can be triggered not only by microbial infection but also by physical trauma and tissue damage. The PRRs such as the TLRs recognize not only PAMPs from invading

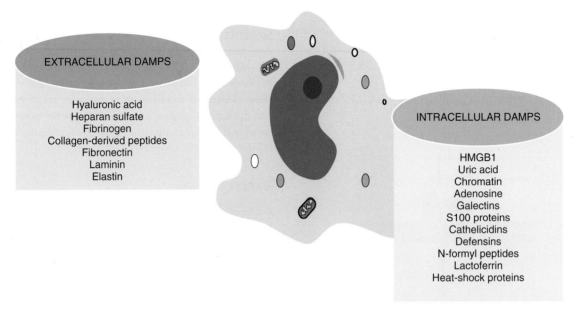

FIGURE 2-6 Damage-associated molecular patterns that trigger innate immune responses. They are derived from both intracellular and extracellular sources.

microorganisms but also molecules that escape from dead, dying, and damaged tissues. These molecules, collectively called DAMPs or alarmins, may be released when cells die (intracellular) or generated when connective tissue is damaged (extracellular) (Figure 2-6). Others may be produced by stimulated sentinel cells. Some of these DAMPs have potent antimicrobial properties. Others may recruit and activate cells of the innate immune system and promote adaptive immune responses.

Some intracellular DAMPs are released by the mitochondria of dying cells. Mitochondria are cytoplasmic organelles that generate energy for cells. They have evolved from intracellular bacteria and retain many of their original bacterial features. For example, they have their own DNA that resembles that in bacteria, being rich in unmethylated CpG. When cells die, therefore, damaged mitochondria may be recognized as the bacteria they once were. Their DNA and proteins trigger PRRs such as TLR9 and formyl peptide receptors on neutrophils. In animals suffering severe trauma, mitochondrial DNA is released from damaged tissues into the bloodstream. The resulting proinflammatory cascade is an initiating factor for septic shock (Chapter 6).

One of the most important intracellular DAMPs is called high mobility group box protein-1 (HMGB1) (Figure 2-7). HMGB1 normally binds DNA molecules and ensures that they fold correctly. However, HMGB1 is also a potent trigger of inflammation. Thus, it is secreted by macrophages that have been activated by lipopolysaccharides or cytokines such as IFN-γ. HMGB1 also escapes from broken cells. HMGB1 binds to both TLR2 and TLR4 and so sustains and prolongs inflammation. It induces the secretion of inflammatory cytokines from macrophages, monocytes, neutrophils, and endothelial

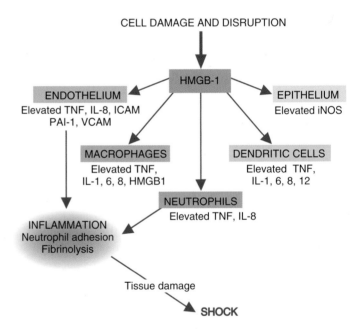

FIGURE 2-7 The properties of HMGB1. Released from "broken" cells, it triggers many of the cells associated with inflammation and triggers systemic responses to tissue damage, perhaps even causing septic shock.

cells. Administration of HMGB1 to animals causes fever, weight loss, anorexia, acute lung injury, arthritis, and even death. HMGB1 plays a role in tissue repair because it stimulates the growth of new blood vessels. It also has potent antimicrobial activity. Detection of elevated levels of HMGB1 in blood suggests the presence of acute inflammation somewhere in the body. Many other molecules released from broken cells can act as intracellular DAMPs. These include adenosine and adenosine triphosphate, uric acid, S100 proteins (a family of calcium-binding proteins involved in cell growth and tissue injury), and heat-shock proteins.

An important extracellular DAMP is heparan sulfate. This molecule is normally found in cell membranes and the extracellular matrix but is shed into tissue fluids following injury. Heparan sulfate binds and triggers TLR4. Other examples of extracellular DAMPs include hyaluronic acid, fibronectin, and peptides from collagen and elastin (see Figure 2-6).

Soluble Pattern-Recognition Receptors

Although the TLRs, NLRs, and RLRs are expressed on cell surfaces, many soluble PRRs can also bind PAMPs. Since many bacterial PAMPs are glycoproteins and polysaccharides, lectins can act as PRRs and play important roles in innate immunity. Mammalian lectins are diverse and are classified into many different families. Three extracellular lectin families, P-, S-, and C-type lectins, are involved in innate immunity.

P-type lectins are also called pentraxins. Pentraxins are formed by five protein subunits arranged in a ring. Two are important acute-phase proteins: C-reactive protein (CRP) and serum amyloid P (SAP) (Chapter 6). They are called acute-phase proteins because their blood levels climb greatly during infections or after trauma. Pentraxins have multiple biological functions, including activation of complement and stimulation of leukocytes. They bind to microbial carbohydrates such as LPS in a calcium-dependent manner and activate the classical complement pathway by interacting with C1q (Chapter 7). They also interact with neutrophils, monocyte-macrophages, and NK cells and augment their activities.

The galectins are extracellular S-type lectins. Their name derives from their specificity for galactosides. They play a role in inflammation by binding leukocytes to the extracellular matrix.

C-type lectins (collectins), as described previously, are a very large family of proteins with many different roles. All require calcium to bind to carbohydrates. Each end of a collectin molecule has a distinct function; the C-terminal domain binds to carbohydrates, whereas the N-terminal domain interacts with cells or complement components, thereby exerting their biological effect. The most important of the soluble C-type lectins is mannose-binding lectin (MBL). MBL is found in high levels in serum. MBL has multiple carbohydrate-binding sites that bind oligosaccharides, such as *N*-acetylglucosamine, mannose, glucose, galactose, and *N*-acetylgalactosamine. This binding is relatively weak, but multiple binding sites give it a high functional activity. As a result, MBL binds very strongly to bacteria such as *Salmonella enterica* and *Listeria monocytogenes*. It binds to *Escherichia coli* with moderate affinity. MBL

binds strongly to yeasts such as *C. albicans* and *Cryptococcus neoformans*. It can bind viruses such as influenza A as well as parasites such as *Leishmania*. MBL plays an important role in activating the complement system (Chapter 7). There are two forms of MBL in the pig: MBL-A and MBL-C. These can bind to *Actinobacillus suis* and *Haemophilus parasuis*. Some European pig breeds may express very low levels of MBL-C and hence suffer from increased disease susceptibility. Bacteria coated by MBL are readily ingested by phagocytic cells through their cell surface receptors. The collectins are especially important in the defense of young animals whose adaptive immune system is not capable of mounting an efficient response.

Multiple C-type lectins, such as the surfactant proteins SP-A and SP-D, are also produced in the lungs. Six different soluble collectins (conglutinin, MBL, pulmonary surfactant proteins [SP-A, SP-D], and collectins-46 [CL-46 and CL-43]) have been identified in mammals. However, conglutinin, CL-46, and CL-43 have been identified only in Bovidae.

Other soluble collectins include the ficolins, a family of lectins (H-, L-, and M-ficolins) produced by the liver and some lung cells. These, too, can bind bacterial carbohydrates and are able to activate the complement system (Chapter 7). There are also many cell-associated lectins. DC-SIGN, for example, is a lectin expressed on macrophages and dendritic cells (Chapter 10). Not only does it recognize bacterial carbohydrates, but it also recognizes carbohydrates expressed on T cells. It is used by dendritic cells to interact with T cells. Cell-associated lectins also include dectin-1 and dectin-2, which act as PRRs for fungal glucans; the macrophage mannose-fucose receptor (CD220), a transmembrane lectin that can bind bacterial carbohydrates and mediates nonopsonic phagocytosis; and langerin, a C-type lectin found on Langerhans cells in the skin.

Sentinel Cells

The cells whose primary function it is to recognize and respond to invading microbes are called sentinel cells. The major sentinel cell types, namely macrophages, dendritic cells, and mast cells, are scattered throughout the body but are found in highest numbers just below body surfaces at sites where invading microorganisms are most likely to be encountered. All these cells are equipped with multiple, diverse PRRs, so they can detect and then respond rapidly to both PAMPs and DAMPs. Other cell types scattered throughout the body, such as epithelial cells, endothelial cells, and fibroblasts, can serve as sentinel cells when opportunity arises.

Macrophages

The most important sentinel cells are macrophages. Macrophages scattered throughout the body can capture, kill, and destroy microbial invaders. Macrophages have multiple other functions and so consist of multiple different subpopulations. Macrophages are described in detail in Chapter 5.

Dendritic Cells

The second major population of sentinel cells consists of dendritic cells, so called because many possess long, thin cytoplasmic processes called dendrites. Dendritic cells are a heterogeneous population of cells, many of which are closely related to, or derived from, macrophages. They are discussed in detail in Chapter 10.

Mast Cells

A third population of sentinel cells are the mast cells. Long known to play a key role in allergies, it has now been recognized that they also trigger inflammation in conventional situations. They are described in detail in Chapter 28.

For sources of additional information, please visit http://evolve.elsevier.com/tizard/immunology/

3

Innate Immunity: Proinflammatory and Antimicrobial Mediators

Key Points

- Three major proinflammatory cytokines produced by sentinel cells are tumor necrosis factor-α, interleukin-1, and interleukin-6.
- Stimulation of toll-like receptors (TLRs) and other pattern-recognition receptors (PRRs) activates the sentinel cells and trigger secretion of these cytokines.
- Sentinel cells and damaged cells produce many other molecules that trigger and maintain inflammation.
- Some inflammatory molecules are secreted by nerves.
- Collectively, these molecules trigger local increases in blood flow, attract defensive cells such as neutrophils, promote increased vascular permeability leading to tissue swelling, and kill invading microorganisms.

Acute inflammation develops within minutes after tissues are damaged. The damaged tissue generates three types of signal. First, broken cells release molecules (or damage-associated molecular patterns [DAMPs]) that trigger the release of cytokines, chemokines, and enzymes from sentinel cells. Second, invading microbes provide molecules (pathogen-associated molecular patterns [PAMPs]) that trigger additional sentinel cell responses. Third, pain due to tissue damage causes sensory nerves to release bioactive peptides. This complex mixture of molecules collectively attracts defensive white blood cells (leukocytes) and at the same time act on blood vessels, resulting in increased local blood flow.

Products of Sentinel Cells

Macrophages, dendritic cells, and mast cells are activated when PAMPs or DAMPs bind to their pattern-recognition receptors (PRRs). As a result, they synthesize and secrete a mixture of molecules that trigger inflammation, inhibit microbial growth, and initiate the first steps in adaptive immunity. Mediator molecules are released by the signaling cells and diffuse to nearby receiving cells, where they bind to receptors and trigger their responses. The cells of the immune system can synthesize and secrete hundreds of different proteins that control the immune responses in this way. These proteins are called cytokines. Cytokines affect many different cell types, and cells rarely secrete a single cytokine at a time. This complexity results in a cytokine network,—a web of different signals transmitted among the cells of the immune system mediated by complex mixtures of cytokines.

Cytokines

When exposed to infectious agents or their PAMPs, sentinel cell signaling pathways activate the genes that result in the synthesis and secretion of three major cytokines. These are, tumor necrosis factor-α (TNF-α), interleukin-1 (IL-1), and IL-6. TNF-α is produced very early in inflammation, and this is followed by waves of IL-1 and then by IL-6. Activated sentinel cells also secrete a large number of small chemotactic proteins called chemokines. These chemokines attract defensive cells to sites of microbial invasion. At the same time, stimulated sentinel cells synthesize enzymes such as nitric oxide synthase 2 (NOS2) that in turn generates oxidants such as nitric oxide (NO). They also make the enzyme cyclooxygenase-2 (COX-2) that generates inflammatory lipids such as the prostaglandins and leukotrienes. When produced in sufficient quantities to reach the brain and liver, these molecules cause a fever and sickness behavior and promote an acute-phase response (Chapter 6). If the sentinel cells detect the presence of damaged or foreign DNA or RNA, such as that from viruses,

they will also secrete the antiviral type I interferons, IFN-α and IFN-β (Chapter 26).

Tumor Necrosis Factor-α TNF-α is a protein of 17 Da produced by sentinel cells in response to TLR stimulation. TNF-α can also be produced by stimulated endothelial cells, T cells, B cells, and fibroblasts. It is produced in both soluble or membrane-bound forms. The membrane-bound form is cleaved from the cell surface by a protease called TNF-α convertase. The soluble TNF-α released in this way triggers the release of chemokines and cytokines from nearby cells and promotes the adherence, migration, attraction, and activation of leukocytes (Figure 3-1). Later, TNF-α facilitates the transition from innate to adaptive immunity by enhancing antigen presentation and T cell activation. TNF-α production is stimulated not only through the toll-like receptors (TLRs) but also by molecules secreted by nerves such as the neurotransmitter neurokinin-1.

TNF-α is an essential mediator of inflammation because in combination with IL-1 it triggers changes in the vascular endothelial cells that line small blood vessels. A local increase in TNF-α causes the classic signs of inflammation, including heat, swelling, pain, and redness. Circulating TNF-α can depress cardiac output, induce microvascular thrombosis, and cause capillary leakage. TNF-α acts on neutrophils (key defensive cells in inflammation; see Chapter 4) to enhance their ability to kill microbes. It attracts neutrophils to sites of tissue

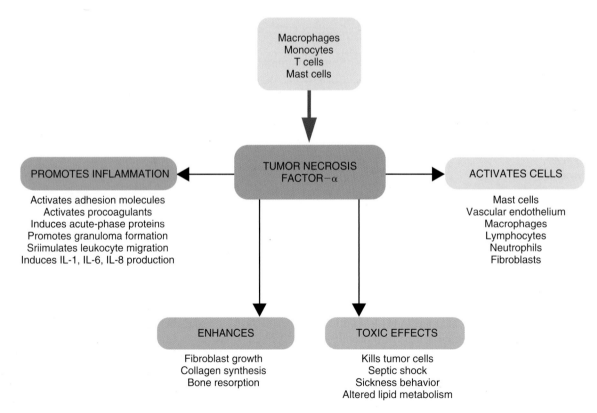

FIGURE 3-1 The origins and some of the biological activities of tumor necrosis factor-α.

damage and increases their adherence to vascular endothelium. It stimulates macrophage phagocytosis and oxidant production. It amplifies and prolongs inflammation by promoting macrophage synthesis of other mediators such as NOX2 and COX-2, and it also activates mast cells. TNF-α induces macrophages to increase its own synthesis together with that of IL-1. As its name implies, TNF-α can kill some tumor cells and virus-infected cells. In high doses, TNF-α may cause septic shock (Chapter 6). There are two TNF receptors: TNFR1 is found on most cells, where it can bind both soluble and cell-associated TNF; and TNFR2 is restricted to the cells of the immune system and responds only to cell-associated TNF.

Based on sequence, functional, and structural similarities, cytokines may be grouped into families. For example, the TNF family consists of multiple proteins, several of which share the ability to kill cells. Other important members include TNF-β (or lymphotoxin) (Chapter 18); CD40L (Chapter 14); FasL (CD95L) (Chapter 18); and TRAIL (Chapter 19).

Interleukin-1 When stimulated through CD14 and TLR4, sentinel cells such as macrophages also produce IL-1α and IL-1β. IL-1β is produced as a large precursor protein that is cleaved by caspase-1 to form the active 17.5-kDa molecule. Ten- to 50-fold more IL-1β is produced than IL-1α, and whereas IL-1β is secreted, IL-1α remains attached to the cell. Therefore, IL-1α only acts on cells in direct contact with the macrophage (Figure 3-2). Transcription of IL-1β messenger RNA (mRNA) occurs within 15 minutes of ligand binding. It reaches a peak 3 to 4 hours later and levels off for several hours before declining. Like TNF-α, IL-1β acts on nearby cells to initiate and amplify inflammation. Thus it acts on vascular endothelial cells to make them adhesive for neutrophils. IL-1 also acts on other macrophages to stimulate their synthesis of NOS2 and COX-2.

During severe infections, IL-1β circulates in the bloodstream where, in association with TNF-α, it is responsible for sickness behavior. Thus it acts on the brain to cause fever, lethargy, malaise, and lack of appetite. It acts on muscle cells to mobilize amino acids, causing pain and fatigue. It acts on liver cells to induce the production of new proteins, called acute-phase proteins, that assist in the defense of the body (Chapter 6).

The most important IL-1 receptors are CD121a and CD121b. CD121a is a signaling receptor, whereas CD121b is not. CD121b thus inhibits IL-1 functions. Soluble CD121b can bind IL-1 and acts as an IL-1 antagonist. IL-1 activity is also regulated by

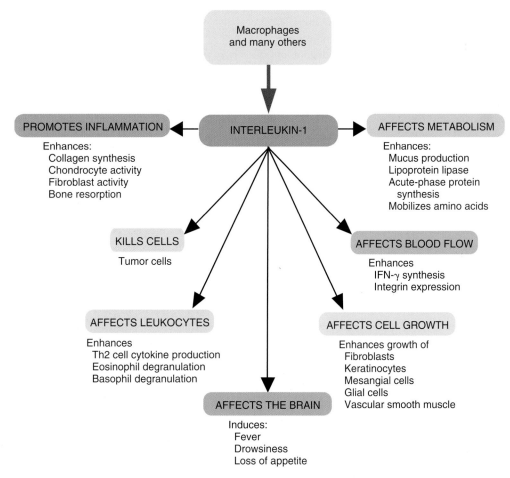

FIGURE 3-2 The origins and some of the biological activities of interleukin-1.

IL-1 receptor antagonist (IL-1RA), an inactive molecule that binds and blocks CD121a. IL-1RA is therefore an important regulator of IL-1 activity and inflammation. It reduces mortality in septic shock and graft-versus-host disease and has antiinflammatory effects (Chapter 6).

IL-1 is a member of a family of cytokines that regulate innate immune responses. Other family members include IL-1RA, IL-18, IL-33, IL-36, IL-37, and possibly IL-38 (Chapter 8 and Appendix 3). All these cytokines signal through a group of closely related receptors. IL-1 and IL-18 are produced as precursor proteins that require activation by inflammatory caspases. Other members of the IL-1 family that play a role in innate immunity include IL-36, which has a proinflammatory effect, and IL-37, which has an antiinflammatory effect.

Interleukin-6 IL-6 is a 22- to 28-kDa glycoprotein produced by macrophages, T cells, and mast cells. Its production is triggered by bacterial endotoxins, IL-1, and TNF-α. IL-6 affects both inflammation and adaptive immunity. It promotes some aspects of inflammation, especially in response to tissue damage and severe infections since it is a major mediator of the acute-phase reaction and of septic shock (Chapter 6). It is an important mediator in antibacterial resistance. It has been suggested that IL-6 regulates the transition from a neutrophil-dominated process early in inflammation to a macrophage-dominated process later. It is also produced by muscles during exercise. IL-6 also has an antiinflammatory role in that it inhibits some activities of TNF-α and IL-1 and promotes the production of IL-1RA as well as a suppressive cytokine called IL-10 (Chapter 20). The IL-6 receptor is a heterodimer consisting of two proteins, gp130 and IL-6R, found on T cells, neutrophils, macrophages, hepatocytes, and neurons.

Chemokines

Chemokines are a family of at least 50 small (8- to 10-kDa) chemotactic cytokines. They coordinate the migration of cells and hence dictate the course of many inflammatory and immune responses (Table 3-1). Chemokines are produced by sentinel cells, including macrophages and mast cells. They are classified into four families on the basis of their amino acid sequences (Figure 3-3). For example, the CC, or α, chemokines have two contiguous cysteine (C) residues, whereas the CXC, or β, chemokines have two cysteine residues separated by another amino acid (X). (Chemokine nomenclature is based on this classification, each molecule or receptor receiving a numerical designation. Ligands have the suffix "L" [e.g., CXCL8], whereas receptors have the suffix "R" [e.g., CXCR1].)

CXCL8 (or IL-8) is produced by macrophages or mast cells. CXCL8 attracts and activates neutrophils, releasing their granule contents and stimulating their respiratory burst (Chapter 4). Another important CXC chemokine is CXCL2 (macrophage inflammatory protein-2, MIP-2), which is secreted by macrophages and also attracts neutrophils.

☐ **Table 3-1 | Nomenclature of Some Selected Chemokines and Their Receptors**

CURRENT NAME	OLD NAME	RECEPTOR
α Family		
CCL2	MCP-1	CCR2
CCL3	MIP-1α	CCR1, CCR5
CCL4	MIP-1β	CCR5
CCL5	RANTES	CCR1, CCR3, CCR5
CCL7	MCP-3	CCR3
CCL8	MCP-2	CCR3
CCL11	Eotaxin	CCR3
CCL13	MCP-4	CCR3
CCL20	MIP-3α	CCR6
CCL22	MDC	CCR4
CCL26	Eotaxin 3	CCR3
CCL28	MEC	CCR3
β Family		
CXCL1	GRO1	CXCR2
CXCL7	MDGF	CXCR2
CXCL8	IL-8	CXCR1, CXCR2
CXCL12	SDF	CXCR4
CXCL13	BCA-1	CXCR5
γ Family		
XCL1	Lymphotactin	XCR1
δ Family		
CX3CL1	Fractalkine	CX3CR1

CC chemokines act predominantly on macrophages and dendritic cells. Thus CCL3 and CCL4 (MIP-1α and -1β) are produced by macrophages and mast cells. CCL4 attracts CD4+ T cells, whereas CCL3 attracts B cells, eosinophils, and cytotoxic T cells. CCL2 (monocyte chemotactic protein-1, MCP-1) is produced by macrophages, T cells, fibroblasts, keratinocytes, and endothelial cells. It attracts and activates monocytes, stimulating their respiratory burst and lysosomal enzyme release. CCL5 (RANTES) is produced by T cells and macrophages. It attracts monocytes, eosinophils, and some T cells. It activates eosinophils and stimulates histamine release from basophils. Regakine-1 is a CC chemokine found in bovine serum that acts with CXCL8 and C5a to attract neutrophils and enhance inflammation.

Two chemokines fall outside the CC and CXC families. A C (only one cysteine residue) or γ chemokine, called XCL1 (or lymphotactin), is chemotactic for lymphocytes. Its receptor is

XCR1. A CXXXC (two cysteines separated by three amino acids) or δ chemokine, called CX3CL1 or fractalkine, triggers adhesion by T cells and monocytes. Its receptor is CX3CR1.

Most chemokines are produced by sentinel cells in infected or damaged tissues and attract other cells to sites of inflammation or microbial invasion. It is likely that the chemokine mixture produced by damaged or infected tissues regulates the precise composition of the inflammatory cell populations. In this way, the body can adjust the inflammatory response to provide the most effective way of destroying different microbial invaders. Many chemokines, such as CXCL4, CCL20, and CCL5, are structurally similar to the antimicrobial proteins called defensins and, like them, have significant antibacterial activity. Chemokines play a major role in infections and inflammation in domestic animal species. They regulate immune cell trafficking. They have been detected in many inflammatory diseases, including pneumonia (bovine

pasteurellosis), bacterial mastitis, arthritis, and endotoxemia. Impaired neutrophil migration is associated with specific CXCR2 genotypes and may lead to increased susceptibility to mastitis in cattle.

Inflammatory Mediators

In its classic form, acute inflammation is said to have five major symptoms (or cardinal signs): heat, redness, swelling, pain, and loss of function. These symptoms result from changes in small blood vessels brought about by "vasoactive" molecules (Figure 3-4). Immediately after injury, the blood flow through small capillaries at the injection site decreases. This gives leukocytes an opportunity to bind to the blood vessel walls. Shortly thereafter, the small blood vessels in the damaged area dilate, and blood flow to the injured tissue increases greatly. While the blood vessels are dilated, they also leak, so that fluid moves from the blood into the tissues, where it causes edema and swelling.

At the same time as these changes in blood flow are occurring, cellular responses are also taking place. Changes in the endothelial cells lining blood vessel walls permit neutrophils and monocytes to adhere. If the blood vessels are damaged, blood platelets may also bind to the injured sites and release vasoactive and clotting molecules. Inflamed tissues swell as a result of leakage of fluid from blood vessels. This leakage occurs in two stages. First, there is an immediate increase in leakage caused by vasoactive molecules produced by sentinel cells, damaged tissues, and nerves (Table 3-2). The second phase of increased leakage occurs several hours after the onset of inflammation, at a time when the leukocytes are beginning to emigrate. Endothelial and perivascular cells contract so that they pull apart and allow fluid to escape through the intercellular spaces. After the invading agent is eliminated, the inflammatory process is terminated, and blood flow returns to normal.

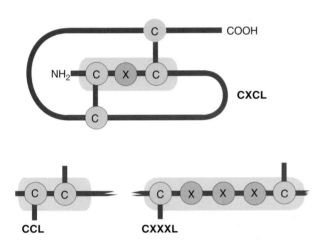

FIGURE 3-3 The classification of chemokines is based on the location and spacing of their cysteine (C) residues and their separation by other (X) amino acids.

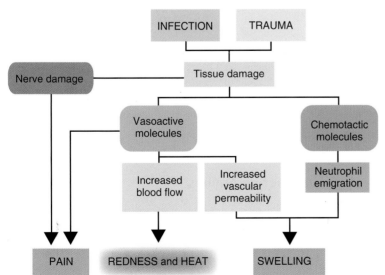

FIGURE 3-4 The major signs of acute inflammation and how they are generated.

□ Table 3-2 | Some Vasoactive Molecules Produced During Acute Inflammation

MEDIATOR	MAJOR SOURCE	FUNCTION
Histamine	Mast cells and basophils, platelets	Increased vascular permeability, pain
Serotonin	Platelets, mast cells, basophils	Increased vascular permeability
Kinins	Plasma kininogens and tissues	Vasodilation Increased vascular permeability, pain
Prostaglandins	Arachidonic acid	Vasodilation, increased vascular permeability
Thromboxanes	Arachidonic acid	Increased platelet aggregation
Leukotriene B$_4$	Arachidonic acid	Neutrophil chemotaxis Increased vascular permeability
Leukotrienes C, D, E	Arachidonic acid	Smooth muscle contraction Increased vascular permeability
Platelet-activating factor	Phagocytic cells	Platelet secretion Neutrophil secretion Increased vascular permeability
Fibrinogen breakdown products	Clotted blood	Smooth muscle Neutrophil chemotaxis Increased vascular permeability
C3a and C5a	Serum complement	Mast cell degranulation Smooth muscle contraction Neutrophil chemotaxis (C5a)

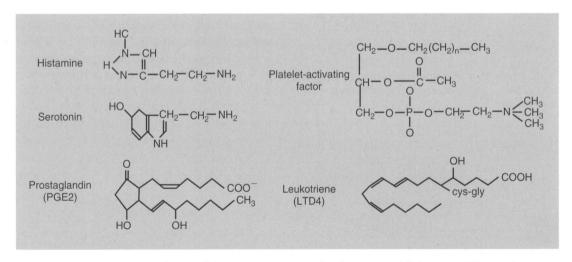

FIGURE 3-5 Structure of some of the major vasoactive molecules generated during acute inflammation.

Vasoactive molecules come from multiple sources. Some are derived from inactive precursors in plasma. Others are derived from sentinel cells such as macrophages and mast cells; from leukocytes such as neutrophils, basophils, and platelets; or from damaged tissue cells. Stimulated sensory nerves may also produce neurotransmitters that cause vasodilation and increased permeability.

Vasoactive Amines

One of the most important of the vasoactive molecules released by mast cells is histamine (Figure 3-5). The two major types of histamine receptor, H1 and H2, are expressed on nerve cells, smooth muscle cells, endothelial cells, neutrophils, eosinophils, monocytes, dendritic cells, and T and B cells. When histamine binds to H1 receptors, it stimulates endothelial cells to produce nitric oxide, a potent vasodilator. At the same time, histamine causes blood vessel leakage, leading to fluid escape into tissues and local edema. Histamine also upregulates TLR expression on sentinel cells.

Serotonin (5-hydroxytryptamine, 5-HT), a derivative of the amino acid tryptophan, is another amine released and is found in the mast cells of some rodents and the large domestic herbivores. Serotonin normally causes a vasoconstriction that results in a rise in blood pressure (except in cattle, in which it is a vasodilator). It has little effect on vascular permeability, except in rodents, in which it induces acute inflammation.

Vasoactive Peptides

Vasoactive peptides are generated by proteolysis of inactive precursors. For example, mast cell proteases act on the complement components C3 and C5 to generate two small (15-kDa) peptides called C3a and C5a (Chapter 7). These molecules, collectively called anaphylatoxins, promote histamine release from mast cells. C5a is also a potent attractant for neutrophils and monocytes. Mast cell granules contain proteases called kallikreins. These act on proteins called kininogens to generate small vasoactive peptides called kinins. The most important of the kinins is bradykinin. Kinins not only increase vascular permeability, they also stimulate neutrophils and trigger pain receptors, and they may have defensin-like antimicrobial activity. Neuropeptides such as substance P and neurokinin produced by sensory nerves also cause pain and trigger vasodilation and increased permeability. A peptide called calcitonin gene–related peptide (CGRP) is the most abundant of these neurotransmitters. It is a potent vasodilator and inducer of pain. These neuropeptides may promote additional mediator release from mast cells and platelets.

Vasoactive Lipids

When tissues are damaged or sentinel cells stimulated, their phospholipases act on cell wall phospholipids to produce arachidonic acid. The enzyme 5-lipoxygenase then converts this arachidonic acid to biologically active lipids called leukotrienes (Figure 3-6). Another enzyme, called cyclooxygenase, converts arachidonic acid to a second family of vasoactive lipids called prostaglandins. The collective term for all these complex lipids is eicosanoids.

Four leukotrienes play a central role in inflammation by promoting leukocyte recruitment, survival, and activation. The most important of these, leukotriene B_4 (LTB_4), is a neutrophil attractant and activator produced by neutrophils, macrophages, and mast cells. LTB_4 also stimulates eosinophil chemotaxis and random motility. Leukotrienes C_4, D_4, and E_4, in contrast, increase vascular permeability and collectively cause slow smooth muscle contraction. All three contain the amino acid cysteine conjugated to the lipid backbone, so they are called cysteinyl leukotrienes. They are produced by mast cells,

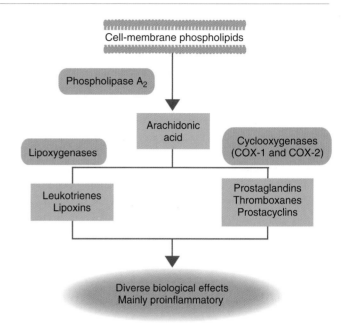

FIGURE 3-6 Production of leukotrienes and prostaglandins by the actions of lipoxygenase and cyclooxygenase on arachidonic acid. Both prostaglandins and leukotrienes may have proinflammatory or antiinflammatory activity depending on their chemical structure.

eosinophils, and basophils. The cytokine interleukin-13 upregulates production of LTD_4 and its receptor, whereas LTD_4 upregulates IL-13 production. This feedback loop is a major contributor to severe inflammation.

There are four groups of proinflammatory prostaglandins: PGE_2, PGF_2, the thromboxanes (TxA_2, PGA_2), and the prostacyclins (PGI_2). Although prostaglandins can be generated by most nucleated cells, the prostacyclins are produced by vascular endothelial cells and the thromboxanes by platelets. The biological activities of the prostaglandins vary widely, and since many different prostaglandins are released in inflamed tissues, their net effect on inflammation may be complex.

As neutrophils enter inflamed tissues, they use the enzyme 15-lipoxygenase to produce lipoxins from arachidonic acid. These oxidized eicosanoids inhibit neutrophil migration. Thus, as inflammation proceeds, there is a gradual switch in production from proinflammatory leukotrienes to antiinflammatory lipoxins. The rise in PGE_2 in tissues also inhibits 5-lipoxygenase activity and eventually suppresses inflammation.

Activated neutrophils also produce a phospholipid called platelet-activating factor (PAF). PAF is produced by mast cells, platelets, neutrophils, and eosinophils. It makes endothelial cells even stickier and thus enhances neutrophil adhesion and emigration. PAF aggregates platelets and makes them release their vasoactive molecules and synthesize thromboxanes. It acts on neutrophils in a similar fashion. Thus it promotes neutrophil aggregation, degranulation, chemotaxis, and release of oxidants.

The Coagulation System

When blood vessels dilate and fluid leaks from the bloodstream into the tissues, the blood coagulation system is activated. Platelet aggregation accelerates this process. Activation of the coagulation system generates large quantities of thrombin, the main clotting enzyme. Thrombin acts on fibrinogen in tissue fluid and plasma to produce insoluble fibrin. Fibrin is therefore deposited in inflamed tissues, where it forms a barrier to the spread of infection. Activation of the coagulation cascade also initiates the fibrinolytic system. This leads to activation of plasminogen activator, which in turn generates plasmin, a potent fibrinolytic enzyme. In destroying fibrin, plasmin releases peptide fragments that attract neutrophils.

Antimicrobial Molecules

The products of sentinel cells do two things: They increase vascular permeability and blood flow and at the same time attract white blood cells (leukocytes) to sites of microbial invasion and/or tissue damage. These leukocytes initially consist primarily of neutrophils, but these are followed by a wave of macrophages. Their function is to kill microbial invaders as fast and as completely as possible. To this end, many of these cells produce a multitude of antimicrobial molecules.

Peptides

Antimicrobial peptides are widely distributed throughout the plant and animal kingdoms, and more than 800 have been identified to date. Different species tend to employ their own specific set of peptides that have evolved in response to their microbiological environment (Box 3-1). Although structurally diverse, these peptides usually contain multiple arginine and lysine residues, making them cationic, and can form amphipathic structures; that is, they have both hydrophobic and hydrophilic regions. The hydrophobic regions can insert themselves into the lipid-rich membranes of bacteria, whereas the other regions can form channel-like pores or simply cover the membrane. This results in membrane disruption and microbial death. The cationic antimicrobial peptides can kill most species of bacteria as well as some fungi, protozoa, enveloped viruses, and tumor cells. The fact that they kill microorganisms rather than host cells is thought to be due to their interactions with microbial phospholipids, lipopolysaccharides, or teichoic acids.

Antimicrobial peptide production is concentrated in sites where microbes are most likely to be encountered. These include organelles within neutrophils and macrophages (Chapter 4) and sites within secondary lymphoid organs (Chapter 12). Epithelial cells of the skin and respiratory, alimentary, and genitourinary tracts also synthesize many antimicrobial peptides.

The defensins are typical antimicrobial peptides containing 28 to 42 amino acids arranged in a β-sheet that contains three

□ **Box 3-1 | The Big Picture**

The complete bovine genome has been sequenced, and unexpectedly, it was found that cattle possess unusually large numbers of genes associated with innate immunity (see Box 6-1). For example, they have 10 cathelicidin genes, compared with only 1 in humans and mice. They have about 106 defensin genes, compared with 30 to 50 in humans and mice. They have many more interferon genes than other species, including a hitherto undescribed family, IFN-X (Chapter 26). It has been suggested that this duplication and divergence of genes involved in innate immunity may be a consequence of the load of microorganisms in the rumen and the resulting increased need to prevent microbial invasion. Alternatively, these new genes may be necessary since living within dense herds may promote infectious disease transmission between individuals and thus requires a more effective immune system. Additionally, cattle show substantial differences from other mammals in the genes related to lactation. Many of these lactation-associated genes, such as those for serum amyloid A, β$_2$-microglobulin, and the cathelicidins, are also related to innate immunity. Finally, the cattle genome contains 10 lysozyme genes, largely expressed in the abomasum and gastrointestinal tract. It is speculated that they may play a role in killing bacteria entering the intestine from the rumen.

Elsik CG, Tellam RL, Worley KC, et al: The genome sequence of taurine cattle: a window to ruminant biology and evolution, *Science* 324:522–527, 2009.

or four disulfide bonds. More than 50 different mammalian defensins have been identified. The vertebrate defensins are classified as α-, β-, or θ-defensins based on their origin and on the number and position of these disulfide bonds. The α-defensins account for about 15% of the total protein in neutrophil granules. In cattle, at least 13 different α-defensins are produced by neutrophils alone. They are also found in the granules of Paneth cells in the small intestine (see Figure 22-3). The β-defensins are expressed in the epithelial cells that line the airways, skin, salivary gland, and urinary system. Theta defensin is a circular peptide that is found only in primate neutrophils. Defensins may be produced at a constant rate (constitutively) by some cells or in response to microbial infection. Some defensins attract monocytes, immature dendritic cells, and T cells. All defensins identified so far can kill or inactivate some bacteria, fungi, or enveloped viruses. Some defensins may also neutralize microbial toxins such as the toxins of *Bacillus anthracis, Corynebacterium diphtheriae,* and staphylokinase from *Staphylococcus aureus.* Although present in normal tissues, defensin concentrations increase in response to infections. For example, calves infected with *Cryptosporidium parvum* or *Mycobacterium paratuberculosis* show a significant increase in cryptdin production. *Mannheimia haemolytica* infection in bovine lungs induces increased defensin expression in airway epithelium. The equine defensin DEFA1 is an enteric defensin exclusively produced in Paneth cells. It has potent activity against the major horse pathogens, especially *Rhodococcus equi* and *Streptococcus equi*.

The second major class of antibacterial peptides in neutrophil granules is the cathelicidins. These are peptides ranging from 12 to 80 amino acids in size with a broad range of antibacterial activity. They are stored within cells in an inactive form attached to a precursor peptide and released following cleavage of the precursor molecule. They are named using acronyms or amino acid symbols followed by the number of amino acids they contain. Humans and mice have only one cathelicidin gene, whereas the pig, cow, and horse have multiple cathelicidin genes. Porcine cathelicidin PR-39 has been shown to promote wound repair, angiogenesis, and neutrophil chemotaxis. The bovine cathelicidin BMAP-28 induces apoptosis in some cells and may serve to get rid of unwanted cells. Canine cathelicidin K9CATH has broad-spectrum activity against both Gram-positive and Gram-negative bacteria. Many cathelicidins have been given specific names such as protegrins, novispirin, and ovispirin.

Other families of antibacterial peptides include the serprocidins and the granulysins. Serprocidins are antimicrobial serine proteases found in the primary granules of neutrophils. Granulysins are peptides produced by cytotoxic T cells and natural killer (NK) cells (Chapters 18 and 19). In addition to their antibacterial functions, granulysins attract and activate macrophages. Two other important antibacterial proteins are bactericidal permeability–increasing protein (BPI) and calprotectin. BPI is a major constituent of the primary granules of human and rabbit neutrophils. It kills Gram-negative bacteria by binding to lipopolysaccharides and damaging their inner membrane. Calprotectin is found in neutrophils, monocytes, macrophages, and epidermal cells. It forms about 60% of neutrophil cytosolic protein and is released in large amounts into blood and tissue fluid in inflammation.

The production of some antimicrobial proteins by epithelial cells is regulated by cytokines of the innate and adaptive immune systems. In particular, the cytokines produced by Th17 cells, IL-17 and IL-22, are crucial regulators of antimicrobial peptide production in the intestine and lungs (Chapter 22). Likewise, IL-1 stimulates epithelial cells to produce antimicrobial proteins. Antimicrobial peptides can also regulate cytokine production. For example, lactoferrin stimulates macrophage production of IL-18, whereas some cathelicidins stimulate production of IL-6, IL-8, and IL-10. Some defensins can block IL-1 production by endotoxin-treated macrophages.

Lysozyme

The enzyme lysozyme cleaves the bond between *N*-acetyl muraminic acid and *N*-acetyl glucosamine and destroys cell wall peptidoglycans in Gram-positive bacteria. Lysozyme is found in all body fluids except cerebrospinal fluid and urine. It is present in large amounts in inflammatory tissue fluid. It is absent from bovine neutrophils and tears. It is found in high concentrations in tears of other mammals and in egg white. Although many of the bacteria killed by lysozyme are nonpathogenic, it might reasonably be pointed out that this susceptibility could account for their lack of pathogenicity. Lysozyme is found in high concentrations in neutrophil granules and accumulates in areas of acute inflammation, including sites of bacterial invasion. Lysozyme is also a potent opsonin, binding to bacterial surfaces and facilitating phagocytosis in the absence of specific antibodies and under conditions in which its enzyme activity is ineffective (Chapter 4).

Complement

The complement system is an innate defense subsystem that consists of a complex mixture of enzymes, regulatory proteins, and receptors that plays a major role in innate antimicrobial immunity. This system, described in detail in Chapter 7, can be activated simply by exposing microbial cell walls to serum proteins since the complement components also recognize PAMPs. It can also be activated when antibodies bind to microbial cell walls. Once activated, complement components, especially C3, the third component, bind irreversibly to bacteria and initiate bacterial killing or phagocytosis.

For sources of additional information, please visit http:// evolve.elsevier.com/tizard/immunology/

4

Innate Immunity: Neutrophils and Phagocytosis

Key Points

- The first cells attracted to sites of inflammation are neutrophils.
- Cytokines activate vascular endothelial cells so that neutrophils in the bloodstream will stop, attach, and then migrate toward sites of microbial invasion and tissue damage.
- Neutrophils bind, phagocytose, and kill invading microorganisms.
- Microorganisms must usually be opsonized before they can be efficiently ingested and killed. The most effective opsonins are antibodies and complement.
- Ingested microorganisms are killed by potent oxidants through a process called the respiratory burst, by antibacterial proteins called defensins and by lytic enzymes.
- Neutrophils are short-lived cells that cannot undertake prolonged or multiple phagocytosis.

Although physical barriers such as the skin exclude many organisms, such barriers are not impenetrable, and microbial invaders often gain access to body tissues. Once recognized by sentinel cells, signals are generated that attract leukocytes. These leukocytes kill and eat the invaders. This process is called phagocytosis (Greek for "eating by cells").

The prime purpose of inflammation is to ensure that invading phagocytic cells intercept and destroy invading microbes as rapidly and efficiently as possible.

The defensive cells of the body circulate in the bloodstream, where they are collectively called leukocytes (white cells). These leukocytes are derived from pluripotent stem cells located in the bone marrow (Figure 4-1). All types of leukocytes, including neutrophils, monocytes, lymphocytes, and dendritic cells, originate from bone marrow (myeloid) stem cells, and all help defend the body. Two types of leukocytes specialize in killing and eating invading microorganisms. These cells, called neutrophils and macrophages, originate from a common stem cell but look very different and have different, but complementary, roles. Thus neutrophils respond and eat invading organisms very rapidly but are incapable of sustained phagocytic effort. Macrophages, in contrast, move more slowly but are highly effective phagocytes and are capable of repeated phagocytosis. In this chapter, we review the properties of neutrophils and their role in inflammation and innate immunity. We will examine macrophages in the next chapter.

Leukocyte Classification

Examination of a stained blood smear reveals many different types of leukocyte. Those that have a cytoplasm filled with granules are called granulocytes (Figure 4-2). Granulocytes also have a characteristic lobulated, irregular nucleus, so that they are described as "polymorphonuclear" (as opposed to the single rounded nucleus of "mononuclear" cells such as macrophages). Granulocytes are classified based on the staining properties of their granules. Cells whose granules take up basic dyes such as hematoxylin are called basophils; those whose granules take up acidic dyes such as eosin are called eosinophils; and those that take up neither basic nor acidic dyes are called neutrophils. All

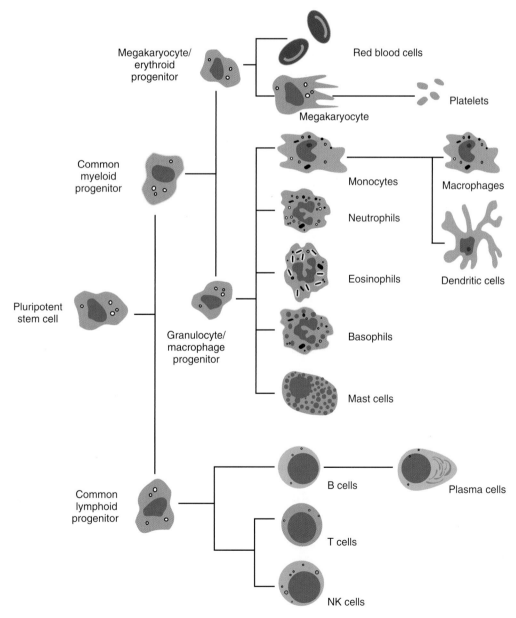

FIGURE 4-1 The origin of cells from the bone marrow. Note that lymphoid cells originate from different stem cells than the cells of the myeloid system. Note too that cells such as eosinophils and basophils are probably closely related despite significant morphological differences.

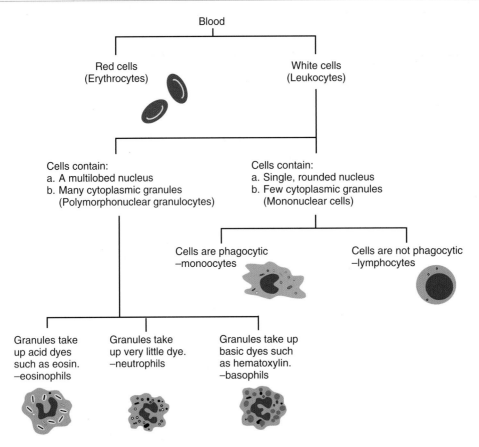

FIGURE 4-2 Differentiation and nomenclature of the cells found in blood. Leukocytes are first differentiated on the basis of their nuclear shape. Polymorphonuclear cells are then differentiated on the basis of their granule staining. Lymphocytes and macrophages are differentiated on the basis of nuclear shape and extent of cytoplasm. Note that tone cannot identify the different subpopulations of lymphocytes on the basis of their morphology.

three populations play important roles in the defense of the body.

Neutrophils

The predominant blood leukocyte is the polymorphonuclear neutrophil granulocyte, otherwise called the neutrophil (Figure 4-3). About two thirds of the hematopoietic activity of the bone marrow is devoted to neutrophil production. Neutrophils are formed by bone marrow stem cells at a rate of about 8 million per minute in normal humans; they migrate to the bloodstream and about 12 hours later move into the tissues. They live for only a few days and must therefore be constantly replaced. Neutrophils constitute about 60% to 75% of the blood leukocytes in most carnivores, about 50% in the horse and 20% to 30% in cattle, sheep, and laboratory rodents. Normally, however, circulating neutrophils account for only 1% to 2% of the total population. The vast majority are sequestered in capillaries within the liver, spleen, lungs, and bone marrow. During bacterial infections, the numbers of circulating neutrophils may increase 10-fold as the stored cells are released from the bone marrow and other organs.

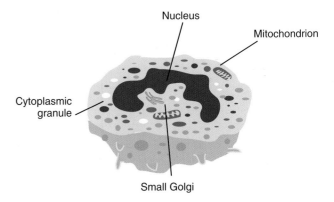

FIGURE 4-3 The major structural features of a neutrophil. Note the characteristic nucleus and the plentiful cytoplasmic granules.

The production of neutrophils is regulated by a cytokine called granulocyte colony-stimulating factor (G-CSF) and their loss by their rate of apoptosis. Normal neutrophils migrate to tissues, where they eventually become apoptotic and are then phagocytosed by macrophages. The production of G-CSF is regulated by their rate of apoptosis. Thus dying neutrophils are removed by macrophages. These macrophages produce

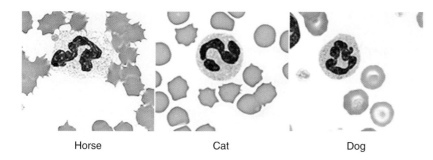

Horse   Cat   Dog

FIGURE 4-4 Neutrophils in peripheral blood smears. These cells are about 10 μm in diameter. Giemsa stain.

(Courtesy Dr. M.C. Johnson.)

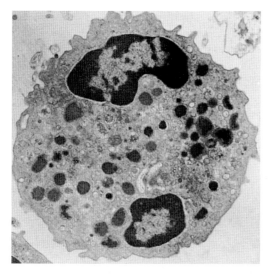

FIGURE 4-5 Transmission electron micrograph of a rabbit neutrophil. Note the two lobes of the nucleus and the granule-filled cytoplasm.

(Courtesy Dr. S. Linthicum.)

interleukin-23 (IL-23) so that, as neutrophils die, IL-23 production increases. IL-23 promotes IL-17 production by lymphocytes (Th17 cells; Chapter 20). IL-17 stimulates G-CSF production and stem cell activity. As a result, the rate of neutrophil production matches the rate of their removal by apoptosis. Toll-like receptors (TLRs) are also expressed on myeloid stem cells. During microbial infections, pathogen-associated molecular patterns (PAMPs) such as lipopolysaccharides bind to these TLRs and trigger the stem cells to produce more neutrophils. TLRs thus provide a mechanism whereby neutrophil availability increases rapidly in response to infection.

Structure

Neutrophils suspended in blood are round cells about 10 to 20 μm in diameter. They have a finely granular cytosol at the center of which is an irregular sausage-like or segmented nucleus (Figure 4-4). The chromatin within the nucleus is condensed and compacted so that neutrophils do not divide. Electron microscopy shows three major types of enzyme-rich granules in the cytosol (Figure 4-5). Primary (azurophil) granules contain enzymes such as myeloperoxidase, lysozyme, elastase, β-glucuronidase, and cathepsin B. Secondary (specific) granules lack myeloperoxidase but contain lysozyme and collagenase and the iron-binding protein lactoferrin. Tertiary granules contain gelatinase. These granules are synthesized at different stages in the cell's development. Thus primary granules are synthesized at the promyelocyte stage, secondary granules at the myeloid stage, and tertiary granules late in the development process. Granules formed early in development are rarely exocytosed, whereas tertiary granules are readily exocytosed. Because neutrophil granules contain a complex mixture of bactericidal molecules, the cells may regulate their release at inflammatory sites to ensure that they are appropriate. Neutrophil granule proteins enhance monocyte adherence to vascular endothelium, trigger macrophages to secrete cytokines, and activate dendritic cells, thus promoting antigen presentation. Neutrophil secretory vesicles and granule membranes also serve as storage sites for receptors and other membrane-integrated proteins. Mature neutrophils have a small Golgi apparatus, some mitochondria, a few ribosomes, and a little rough endoplasmic reticulum.

Emigration from the Bloodstream

Circulating neutrophils are normally confined to the bloodstream so that in normal tissues, neutrophils are simply carried along by the flow. In inflamed tissues, however, molecules released by dead and dying cells cause these fast moving cells to slow down, stop, bind to blood vessel walls, and emigrate into the tissues. This emigration is triggered by molecules that affect both the endothelial cells that line blood vessel walls and the neutrophils themselves.

Changes in Endothelial Cells

In aggregate, the endothelial cells that line all blood vessels collectively have a huge surface area (estimated at 4000 square meters in humans) and thus serve as a broad sensor of microbial invasion. When bacterial products such as LPS or damage-associated molecular patterns (DAMPs) from damaged tissues such as thrombin or histamine reach the capillary endothelium, they stimulate the cells to express a glycoprotein called P-selectin (CD62P) on their surface. P-selectin is normally stored in cytoplasmic granules but can move to the cell surface within minutes after cell stimulation. Once expressed, the P-selectin can bind a protein called L-selectin (CD62L) on the surface of passing neutrophils. At first, this binding is transient because the neutrophils readily shed their L-selectin. Nevertheless, the neutrophils gradually slow, roll along the endothelial cell surface as they lose speed, and eventually come to a complete stop (Figure 4-6). This mainly happens in venules where the vessel wall is thin and the diameter sufficiently small to permit the neutrophils to make firm contact with the endothelium.

Changes in Neutrophils

As neutrophils roll along the endothelial surface, the second stage of adhesion occurs. Platelet-activating factor (PAF), secreted by the endothelial cells, triggers the rolling neutrophils to express an adhesive protein called CD11a/CD18 or leukocyte function–associated antigen-1 (LFA-1). LFA-1 is an integrin that binds to an intercellular adhesion molecule-1 (ICAM-1 or CD54) on the endothelial cells (Figure 4-7). This strong

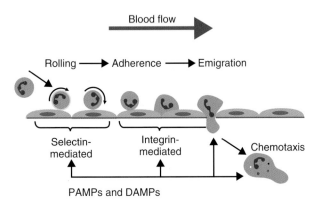

FIGURE 4-6 The stages of neutrophil adhesion and emigration from blood vessels. Changes in vascular endothelial cells are triggered by tissue damage and microbial invasion. Selectins on endothelial cells tether neutrophils and stimulate them to roll. When they come to a halt, integrins bind them firmly to vascular endothelial cells and signal them to emigrate into tissues.

binding brings the neutrophil to a complete stop and attaches it firmly to the vessel wall despite the shearing force of the blood flow. Adherent neutrophils also secrete small amounts of elastase. The elastase removes CD43 (leukosialin), an anti-adhesive protein, from the neutrophil surface, permitting the cells to bind even more strongly.

After several hours, endothelial cells activated by IL-1, IL-23, or tumor necrosis factor-α (TNF-α) express the strongly adhesive E-selectin (CD62E). IL-1 and IL-23 also induce endothelial cells to produce the chemokine CXCL8, and this attracts still more neutrophils. TNF-α stimulates endothelial cells to secrete IL-1. It also promotes vasodilation, procoagulant activity, and thrombosis and increases the expression of adhesion proteins and chemotactic molecules.

Neutrophils themselves increase vascular permeability and open up gaps between endothelial cells as a result of endothelial cell contraction and disruption of intercellular junctions. They secrete the chemokines CXCL1, 2, 3, and 8 in response to the binding of LFA-1 to endothelial ICAM-1. Neutrophil phospholipase A2 releases arachidonic acid, which is converted to leukotriene A_4. This is subsequently processed by endothelial cells to produce permeability-inducing thromboxane A_2 and leukotriene C_4. Neutrophil-derived oxidants also increase vascular permeability.

Integrins

Many cell surface proteins make cells stick together, but the most important of these are the integrins. There are several families of integrins. Each consists of paired protein chains (heterodimers) using a unique α chain linked to a common β chain. For example, three β_2-integrins are found on neutrophils. Their α chain, called CD11a, b, or c, is linked to a common β_2 chain (CD18). Therefore, these three integrins are called CD11a/CD18, CD11b/CD18, and CD11c/CD18. As described previously, LFA-1 on activated neutrophils binds to ICAM-1 on capillary endothelial cells. CD11b/CD18 also binds leukocytes to endothelial cells and is a receptor for some components of the complement system (complement receptor 3, CR3) (Chapter 7).

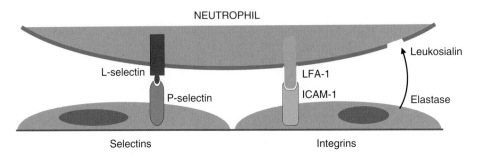

FIGURE 4-7 A simplified view of the proteins and their ligands engaged in neutrophil-vascular endothelial cell binding. Selectins are carbohydrate-binding proteins that bind other glycoproteins. This selectin-mediated binding is weak and temporary. Subsequently, integrins on leukocytes, especially CD11a/18, bind strongly to their ligand ICAM-1 on vascular endothelial cells. Elastase secreted by endothelial cells removes leukosialin, thus permitting the neutrophil to bind strongly to the endothelial cell.

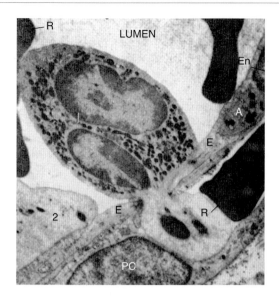

FIGURE 4-8 Inflamed venule of a rat. Cell 1 is a neutrophil pushing its way through a capillary wall to reach the surrounding tissues. *R,* red blood cells; *E,* endothelium; *PC,* periendothelial cell; cells 2 and 3 are also neutrophils.

(From Marchesi VT, Florey HW: Electron micrographic observations on the emigration of leucocytes. *Q J Exp Physiol* 45:343, 1960.)

Emigration

After binding to blood vessel walls and coming to a complete stop, neutrophils emigrate into the surrounding tissues under the influence of chemoattractants (Figure 4-8). Most migrating neutrophils squeeze between the endothelial cells, but about 20% actually pass through endothelial cells. They produce proteases to get through the basement membrane. They then crawl toward any invading microbes becoming activated in the process. Since neutrophils are the most mobile of all the blood leukocytes, they are the first cells to arrive at damaged tissues.

Phagocytosis

Once they reach sites of microbial invasion, neutrophils eat and destroy invading bacteria through phagocytosis. Although a continuous process, phagocytosis can be divided into discrete stages: activation, chemotaxis, adherence, ingestion, and destruction (Figure 4-9).

Activation

Neutrophils attack and destroy invading organisms after they have become "activated." Thus, when neutrophils bind to endothelial cells and receive the dual signal of integrin binding together with stimulation by TNF-α, CXCL8, or C5a, they secrete elastase, defensins, and oxidants. The elastase promotes their adhesiveness. The oxidants activate tissue proteases, which in turn cleave more TNF-α from macrophages. The TNF-α, in turn, attracts more neutrophils.

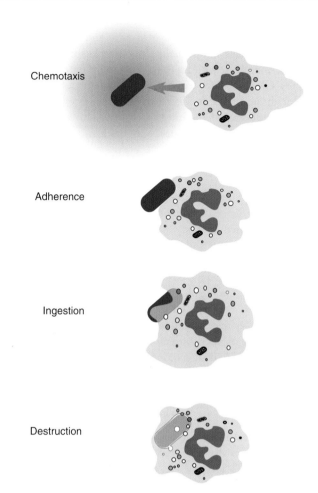

FIGURE 4-9 The different stages in the process of phagocytosis. While in fact a continuous process, this division into stages provides a useful method of analyzing the process.

Chemotaxis

Neutrophils do not wander randomly but crawl directly toward invading organisms and damaged tissues attracted by chemotactic molecules. These chemoattractants diffuse from sites of microbial invasion and form a concentration gradient. Neutrophils crawl toward the area of highest concentration—the source of the material. The moving cells generate projections (lamellipodia) at their leading edge. Chemoattractant receptors are distributed over the neutrophil surface, but the formation of lamellipodia is driven by the higher concentration of attractants at the cell's leading edge.

Microbial invasion and tissue damage generate many different chemoattractants. These include a peptide called C5a, generated by activation of complement (Chapter 7); a peptide called fibrinopeptide B, derived from fibrinogen; and hydrogen peroxide. A damage-triggered gradient of H_2O_2 is established within 5 minutes of wounding, just preceding the movement of the first neutrophils toward a wound. Other chemoattractants include chemokines (Chapter 3) and lipids such as leukotriene B_4. Invading bacteria release peptides with formylated methionine groups that are very attractive to the neutrophils of some mammals. Thus, migrating neutrophils receive a multitude of signals drawing them toward sites of invasion and tissue damage.

Not all animals have equally responsive neutrophils. For example, some cattle with a specific genotype of the chemokine receptor CXCR2 show reduced neutrophil migration compared with normal cattle. Cows with this genotype also show reduced expression of the integrin chains CD18 and CD11b and as a result decreased resistance to mastitis.

Adherence and Opsonization

Once a neutrophil encounters a bacterium, it must "catch" it. This does not happen spontaneously because both cells and bacteria suspended in body fluids usually have a negative charge (zeta potential) and repel each other. The electrostatic charge on the bacteria must be neutralized by coating them with positively charged molecules. Molecules that coat bacteria in this way and promote phagocytosis are called opsonins. This word is derived from the Greek word for "sauce," implying perhaps that they make the bacterium "tastier" for the neutrophil. Examples of such opsonins include mannose-binding lectin, some complement components, and most importantly, antibodies (Chapter 16).

Antibodies, the major proteins of the adaptive immune system, are by far the most effective opsonins. They coat bacteria, bind them to receptors on phagocytic cells, and trigger their ingestion. Antibody receptor–mediated phagocytosis (or type I phagocytosis) is triggered by the binding of antibody-coated bacteria to receptors on the neutrophil (Figure 4-10). CD32 is an example of such an antibody receptor. The ligand of CD32 is a site on the Fc region of antibody molecules (Chapter 16). CD32 is therefore an example of an Fc receptor

(FcR). (Since there are several different Fc receptors, CD32 is classified as FcγRII.) However, as pointed out previously, antibodies are not produced until several days after the onset of an infection, and the body must therefore rely on innate opsonins for immediate protection. CD35 (or complement receptor-1, CR1) binds the complement component C3b. CR1 is found not only on neutrophils but also on other granulocytes, monocytes, red cells, and B cells. Linking of C3b-coated particles to neutrophil CD35 results in attachment but may not necessarily trigger ingestion.

The surface of phagocytic cells is also covered with many pattern-recognition receptors (PRRs) that can recognize their ligands on the surface of infectious agents. Thus neutrophils have mannose receptors or integrins that can bind directly to bacteria.

Another important mechanism that promotes contact between bacteria and neutrophils is trapping. Normally bacteria are free to float away when they encounter a neutrophil suspended in blood plasma. If, however, a bacterium is lodged in tissues or trapped between a neutrophil and another cell surface and thus prevented from floating away; it can be readily ingested. This process is called surface phagocytosis.

Although it has generally been assumed that neutrophils must ingest bacteria before killing them, they can also trap and kill extracellular bacteria. Thus neutrophils can undergo a form of cell death termed NETosis as an alternative to apoptosis or necrosis. After activation by CXCL8 or lipopolysaccharides, neutrophils may release their nuclear contents, extruding large strands of decondensed nuclear DNA and associated proteins into the extracellular fluid. These form a network of extracellular fibers called neutrophil extracellular traps (NETs) (Figure 4-11). The extracellular DNA net is coated with antimicrobial

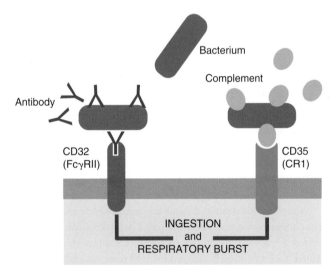

FIGURE 4-10 The opsonization of a bacterium by antibodies and complement. Binding of these ligands to their receptors triggers ingestion and the respiratory burst. The antibody receptor is called CD32, and the complement receptor is called CD35. Type 1 phagocytosis is mediated by antibodies through CD32. Type 2 phagocytosis is mediated by complement through CD35.

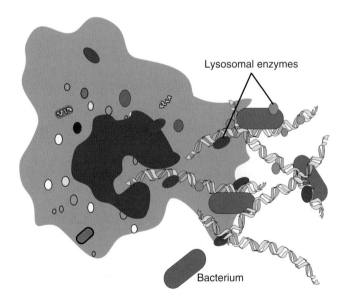

FIGURE 4-11 The structure of neutrophil extracellular traps (NETS). NETS are composed of a network of DNA strands to which are attached neutrophil lysosomal enzymes such as myeloperoxidase, cathepsins, and elastases.

proteins, including histones and granule components such as elastase, myeloperoxidase, lactoferrin, and gelatinase since the granules disintegrate at the same time the nuclei dissolve. As a result, the DNA Net not only physically captures bacteria but can also kill them and destroy their virulence factors. NETs are abundant in sites of acute inflammation and are also found in mastitic milk. They trap and kill many different bacteria, fungi such as *Candida albicans* and protozoa such as *Leishmania amazonensis* and *Eimeria bovis* (Figure 4-12). NETs may be very important in containing microbial invaders, acting as physical barriers, capturing large numbers of bacteria, and so preventing their spread.

Ingestion

As neutrophils crawl toward a chemotactic source, a lamellipod advances first, followed by the main portion of the cell. The cytosol of the lamellipodia contain a filamentous network of actin and myosin whose state determines the fluidity of the cytoplasm. When a neutrophil meets a bacterium, the lamellipod flows over and around the organism, and binding occurs between opsonins on the organism and receptors on the neutrophil surface (Figure 4-13). When antibody-coated microbes bind to neutrophil CD32, they trigger polymerization of actin.

As a result, actin-rich lamellipodia extend from the cell to engulf the particle (type I phagocytosis).

In complement-mediated phagocytosis, particles sink into the neutrophil without lamellipodia formation, suggesting that the ingestion process is fundamentally different from that mediated by antibodies (type II phagocytosis). Binding of these receptors enables a cup-like structure to cover the organism. The bacterium is eventually drawn into the cell, and as it is engulfed, it becomes enclosed in a vacuole called a phagosome. The ease of ingestion depends on the properties of the bacterial surface. Neutrophils readily flow over lipid surfaces so that hydrophobic bacteria, such as *Mycobacterium tuberculosis*, are readily ingested. In contrast, *Streptococcus pneumoniae*, a cause of pneumonia in humans, has a hydrophilic capsule. It is poorly phagocytosed unless made hydrophobic by opsonization. The progressive covering of a bacterium by the linkage of cell receptors with ligands on the bacterial surface has been likened to a zipper. A third type of ingestion occurs with bacteria such as *Legionella pneumophila* and *Borrelia burgdorferi*. In these cases, a single lamellipod may wrap itself several times around the organism. This is called coiling phagocytosis.

Destruction

Neutrophils destroy ingested bacteria through two distinct processes. One involves the generation of potent oxidants—the respiratory burst. The other involves release of lytic enzymes and antimicrobial peptides from intracellular granules (Box 4-1).

The Respiratory Burst Within seconds of binding a bacterium, neutrophils increase their oxygen consumption nearly

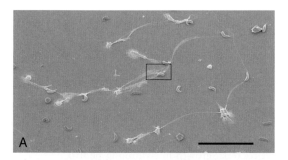
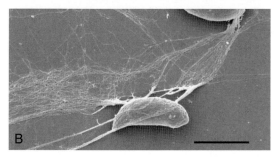

FIGURE 4-12 NETs formed by bovine neutrophils co-cultured with sporozoites of the protozoan parasite, *Eimeria bovis*. **A,** Several sporozoites can be seen sticking to a network of fibers originating from dead and disrupted neutrophils (scale bar, 50 μm). **B,** At higher magnification, it can be seen that the NETs consist of a meshwork of filaments, many of which are attached to a sporozoite (scale bar, 5 μm).

(From Behrendt JH, Ruiz A, Zahner H, et al: Neutrophil extracellular trap formation as innate immune reactions against the apicomplexan parasite *Eimeria bovis*, Vet Immunol Immunopathol 133:1–8, 2010.)

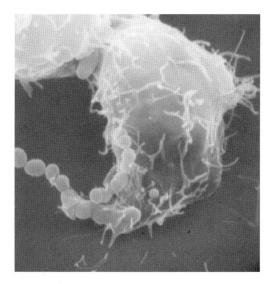

FIGURE 4-13 A scanning electron micrograph of a bovine milk neutrophil ingesting *Streptococcus agalactiae*. Note how a film of neutrophil cytoplasm appears to flow over the surface of the bacterium. Original magnification ×5000.

◻ Box 4-1 | **Autophagy**

Phagocytosis, as described in this chapter, involves the ingestion, killing, and digestion of extracellular particles such as invading bacteria. Cells can also destroy microorganisms or unwanted cellular proteins or organelles present within the cytosol by the process of autophagy (Figure 4-16). Autophagy is a form of cellular self-digestion. The particle to be digested, such as an intracellular microbe or a damaged organelle, is first enclosed within a double membrane to form a cytosolic vesicle called an autophagosome. This then fuses with the lysosomes, whose enzymes then digest the contents of the autophagosome. The macromolecules are then released back into the cytosol, where they are available for reuse. Autophagy can be triggered by starvation to provide more amino acids for protein synthesis, but it can also be used to selectively remove organelles such as mitochondria, misfolded and aggregated proteins, and intracellular infectious agents. Thus TLR7 or FcγR signaling from phagosomes can initiate their targeting by the autophagy system, possibly by acting through the NOX system. Disorders of autophagy are associated with cancer, neurodegeneration, microbial infections, and ageing.

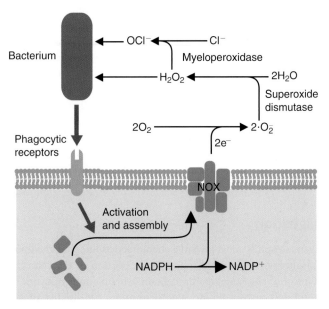

FIGURE 4-14 The major features of the respiratory burst pathway in neutrophils. The process is triggered by binding of opsonized bacteria to phagocytic receptors such as CD32. It results in the assembly of the multicomponent enzyme NADPH oxidase (NOX) in the membrane of the phagosome. Once assembled, NOX catalyses the generation of singlet oxygen. In association with other enzymes such as superoxide dismutase and myeloperoxidase, bactericidal products such as hydrogen peroxide (H_2O_2) and hypochloride ions (OCl^-) are then generated.

100-fold. This results from activation of a cell surface enzyme complex called NADPH oxidase (NOX). The subcomponents of the NOX complex are separated in resting cells, but when a neutrophil encounters TNF-α or is exposed to other inflammatory stimuli, the NOX complex is assembled and activated (Figure 4-14). Activated NOX converts NADPH (the reduced form of NADP, nicotinamide adenine dinucleotide phosphate) to NADP$^+$ with the release of electrons. A molecule of oxygen accepts a donated electron, generating a superoxide anion (the dot in $^•O_2^-$ denotes the presence of an unpaired electron):

$$NADPH + 2O_2 \xrightarrow{\text{NOX}} NADP^+ + H^+ + 2^•O_2^-$$

The two superoxide anions interact spontaneously (dismutate) to generate one molecule of H_2O_2 under the influence of the enzyme superoxide dismutase:

$$2^•O_2^- + 2H^+ \xrightarrow{\text{superoxide dismutase}} H_2O_2 + O_2$$

The hydrogen peroxide is converted to bactericidal compounds through the action of myeloperoxidase. Myeloperoxidase catalyzes the reaction between hydrogen peroxide and intracellular halide ions (Cl^-, Br^-, I^-, or SCN^-) to produce hypohalides:

$$H_2O_2 + Cl^- \xrightarrow{\text{myeloperoxidase}} H_2O + OCl^-$$

Plasma Cl^- is used in most inflammatory sites except in milk and saliva, where SCN^- is also employed. Hypochlorous acid (HOCl) is the major product of neutrophil oxidative metabolism. Because of its reactivity, HOCl is rapidly

consumed in multiple reactions. As long as H_2O_2 is supplied (neutrophils can generate H_2O_2 for up to 3 hours after triggering), myeloperoxidase will generate HOCl. HOCl kills bacteria by unfolding and aggregating their proteins and oxidizing their lipids, and it enhances the bactericidal activities of the lysosomal enzymes. (Remember that HOCl is the active ingredient of household bleach and is commonly used to prevent bacterial growth in swimming pools.)

There are minor quantitative differences in neutrophil activity between the domestic species, especially in the intensity of the respiratory burst. For example, sheep neutrophils appear to produce less superoxide than human or bovine neutrophils. Neutrophils also have safety mechanisms to detoxify oxidants and minimize collateral damage. Thus they contain large amounts of glutathione, which reduces the oxidants. Redox-active metals such as iron can be bound to lactoferrin to minimize OH formation, and antioxidants such as ascorbate and vitamin E interrupt these reactions.

Lytic Enzymes Once a bacterium is ingested by a neutrophil, the cell's granules (or lysosomes) migrate through the cytoplasm, fuse with the maturing phagosome, and release their enzymes. (The complete vacuole is then called a phagolysosome.) The rise in ionic strength within phagosomes releases elastase and cathepsin G from their sulfated proteoglycan matrix (Figure 4-15). Other lysosomal enzymes include

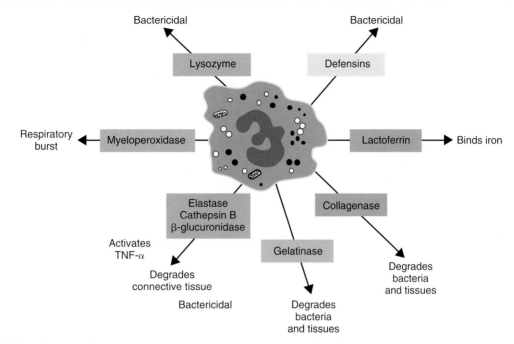

FIGURE 4-15 Some of the enzymes and other antibacterial molecules found in the cytoplasmic granules of neutrophils.

lysozyme, proteases, acid hydrolases, and myeloperoxidase. The enzymes that accumulate in phagosomes can digest bacterial walls and kill most microorganisms, but, as might be expected, variations in susceptibility are observed. Gram-positive bacteria susceptible to lysozyme are rapidly destroyed. Gram-negative bacteria such as *Escherichia coli* survive somewhat longer since their outer wall is resistant to digestion. Lactoferrin, by binding iron, may deprive bacteria of this essential nutrient and limit bacterial growth (Chapter 25). Some organisms such as *Brucella abortus* and *Listeria monocytogenes* can interfere with phagosomal maturation in such a way that they do not come into contact with the lysosomal enzymes and can therefore grow inside phagocytic cells. Neutrophil enzymes released into tissues cleave membrane-bound TNF-α from macrophages. The TNF-α attracts and activates yet more neutrophils.

Cytokines Under the influence of bacterial products such as lipopolysaccharides, neutrophils secrete cytokines such as IL-1α, IL-1β, IL-1RA, TNF-α, IL-6, CXCL8 (IL-8), IL-10, and transforming growth factor-β (TGF-β). Although individual neutrophils produce only small quantities of these cytokines, they invade inflammatory sites in large numbers, so their total contribution may be significant.

Surface Receptors

Cells must interact with many molecules in their environment. To this end, they express many different cell surface receptors. As mentioned in Box 2-4, cell surface glycoproteins are classified by the cluster of differentiation (CD) system. Neutrophils

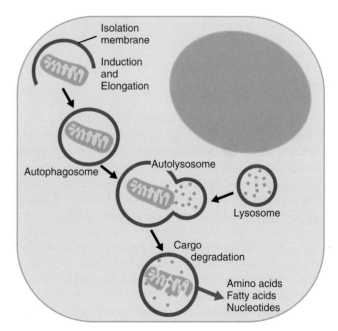

FIGURE 4-16 The process of autophagy. The self-ingestion of parts of a cell. The autophagosome forms within the cytoplasm and encloses the organelle or microbe to be destroyed. Lysosomes fuse with the autophagosome to form an autolysosome. The contents are degraded and recycled. This is a way to get rid of old, damaged organelles as well as intracellular bacteria.

carry many different CD molecules on their surface (Figure 4-17). The most relevant of these proteins are the receptors for opsonins and those that attach neutrophils to blood vessel walls. Other neutrophil surface molecules include receptors for inflammatory mediators such as leukotrienes, complement

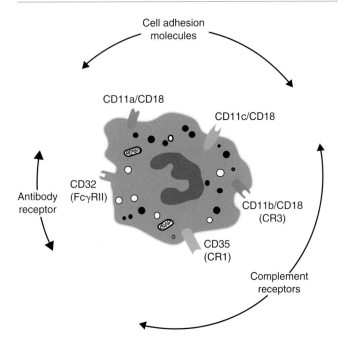

Cell adhesion
molecules

CD11a/CD18

CD11c/CD18

Antibody
receptor

CD32
(FcγRII)

CD11b/CD18
(CR3)

CD35
(CR1)

Complement
receptors

FIGURE 4-17 Some of the major surface receptors on neutrophils and their functions.

components such as C5a, chemokines, and cytokines (see Box 4-2).

Fate

Neutrophils are short-lived terminally differentiated cells with a high rate of spontaneous apoptosis. They have a limited reserve of energy that cannot be replenished. Most neutrophils survive only a few days. They are therefore most active immediately after release from the bone marrow but are rapidly exhausted and can undertake only a limited number of phagocytic events. Apoptosis occurs in the presence of inflammatory stimuli, especially oxidants. This may also involve the formation of NETs of exocytosed DNA. Apoptotic neutrophils are removed by the cells of the mononuclear phagocytic system. When dendritic cells ingest apoptotic neutrophils infected with bacteria, they secrete TGF-β, IL-6, and IL-23. As described previously, this IL-23 stimulates the differentiation

◻ **Box 4-2** | **Intercellular Transfer of Cell Membranes**

Under some circumstances, cells may exchange fragments of surface membrane together with their receptors and thus change their phenotype. The newly acquired membrane proteins can alter the function of the recipient cells. Leukocytes appear to be especially adept in this regard, and inflammation appears to provide them with many opportunities to acquire membrane proteins from necrotic and apoptotic cells. Examples include the transfer of MHC class II proteins from dendritic cells to B cells, T cells, macrophages, and neutrophils. This may permit the recipient cells to act as antigen presenters. Neutrophils appear to be especially prone to acquire new surface proteins. These acquired proteins alter the neutrophil phenotype and may promote some neutrophil functions. The process occurs through membrane exchange and only takes a few minutes. These changes in cell surface receptors obviously have the potential to modify neutrophil functions. For example, this may explain why some neutrophils may express functional T cell receptors!

Data from Puellmann K., Kaminski WE, Vogel M, et al: A variable immunoreceptor in a population of human neutrophils, *Proc Natl Acad Sci U S A* 103:14441–14446, 2006.

of Th17 cells that promote the production of more neutrophils. Conversely, ingestion of uninfected apoptotic neutrophils triggers the secretion of IL-10 and TGF-β, promoting the production of regulatory T cells and suppressing immune responses (Chapter 20).

Thus neutrophils may be considered a first line of defense, converging rapidly on invading organisms and destroying them promptly but being incapable of sustained effort. The second line of defense is the mononuclear phagocyte system. DAMPs released by neutrophil degranulation or death, promote the recruitment and activation of both macrophages and dendritic cells, augmenting both the innate and adaptive immune responses (see Figure 2-6).

For sources of additional information, please visit http:// evolve.elsevier.com/tizard/immunology/

5

Innate Immunity: Macrophages and Recovery from Inflammation

Key Points

- Macrophages migrate to sites of inflammation after neutrophils. They eat and kill any surviving microbial invaders.
- Macrophages also eat dead and dying neutrophils and thus prevent damage caused by escaping neutrophil enzymes.
- Macrophages generate the powerful oxidizing agent, nitric oxide.
- Macrophages effectively remove foreign particles from the bloodstream and the respiratory tract.
- Macrophages begin the healing process in damaged tissues.
- Macrophages are essential antigen-presenting cells for the adaptive immune system.

Although neutrophils act as a first line of defense, mobilizing rapidly, converging on, and eating and killing invading microorganisms with enthusiasm, they cannot, by themselves, ensure that all invaders are killed. The body therefore employs a "backup" system employing phagocytic cells collectively known as macrophages. As phagocytic cells, macrophages differ from neutrophils in their speed of response, which is slower; in their antimicrobial abilities, which are greater; and in their ability to initiate adaptive immunity. They also act as sentinel cells and initiate tissue repair. Unlike neutrophils, which are specialized for a single task—the killing of invading organisms—macrophages have diverse functions. For this reason, many different macrophage subpopulations are recognized. It should also be pointed out that the use of two phagocytic cell systems permits cooperation between neutrophils and macrophages to enhance many aspects of innate immunity. The neutrophils tend to be of greater importance in killing extracellular pathogens, whereas the macrophages dominate in the fight against intracellular pathogens.

Macrophages

Macrophages not only detect and kill invading microorganisms, but when stimulated, they also secrete a mixture of cytokines that promote both innate and adaptive immune responses; they control inflammation; and they contribute directly to the repair of damaged tissues by removing dead, dying, and damaged cells and assist the healing process. Their name is derived from the fact that they are "large-eating" cells (Greek *macro, phage*).

Macrophage function and structure are highly variable, and this variation has given rise to a confusing nomenclature. Immature macrophages circulate in the bloodstream, where they are called monocytes. When monocytes emigrate into tissues, they become macrophages. Macrophages are found in connective tissue, where they are called histiocytes; those found lining the sinusoids of the liver are called Kupffer cells; those in the brain are microglia. The macrophages in the alveoli of the lungs are called alveolar macrophages, whereas those in the capillaries of the lung are called pulmonary intravascular macrophages. Large numbers are found in the sinusoids of the spleen, bone marrow, and lymph nodes. Irrespective of their name or location, they are all macrophages and all are part of the mononuclear phagocyte system (Figure 5-1).

Structure

In suspension, monocytes are round cells about 15 nm in diameter. They possess abundant cytoplasm, at the center of which is a single large nucleus that may be round, bean shaped,

or indented (Figure 5-2). Their central cytoplasm contains mitochondria, large numbers of lysosomes, some rough endoplasmic reticulum, and a Golgi apparatus, indicating that they can synthesize and secrete proteins (Figures 5-3 and 5-4). In living cells, the peripheral cytoplasm is in continuous movement, forming and reforming veil-like ruffles. Many macrophages show variations in this basic structure. For example, blood monocytes have round nuclei, which elongate as the cells mature. Alveolar macrophages contain very little rough endoplasmic reticulum, but their cytoplasm is full of granules. The microglia of the central nervous system have rod-shaped nuclei and very long cytoplasmic processes (dendrites) that are lost when the cell encounters tissue damage.

Life History

Mononuclear phagocytes develop from common myeloid stem cells in the bone marrow (Figure 5-5). During monocyte development, the myeloid stem cells give rise in sequence to monoblasts, promonocytes, and eventually to monocytes, all under the influence of cytokines called colony-stimulating factors. Monocytes enter the bloodstream and circulate for about 3 days before entering tissues and developing into macrophages. They form about 5% of the total leukocyte population in blood. It is unclear whether there are subpopulations of monocytes and whether these give rise to the specialized macrophage populations. The stage at which they leave the bloodstream may determine their function. Tissue macrophages either originate directly from monocytes or arise by division within tissues. They are relatively long-lived cells, replacing themselves at a rate of about 1% per day unless activated by inflammation or tissue damage. Macrophages may live for a long time after ingesting inert particles, such as the carbon in tattoo ink, although they may fuse together to form multinucleated giant

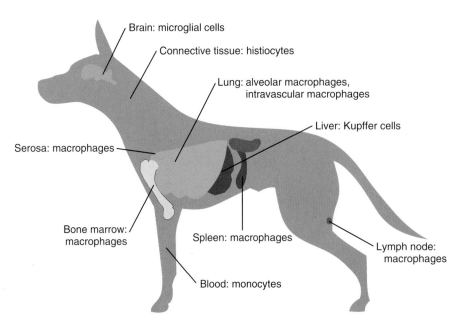

FIGURE 5-1 The location of the major populations of cells of the mononuclear phagocyte system.

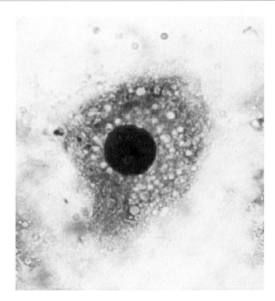

FIGURE 5-2 A typical bovine macrophage. Original magnification ×500.

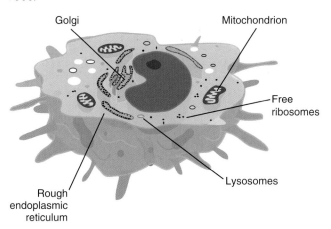

Golgi

Mitochondrion

Free ribosomes

Lysosomes

Rough endoplasmic reticulum

FIGURE 5-3 The major structural features of a macrophage.

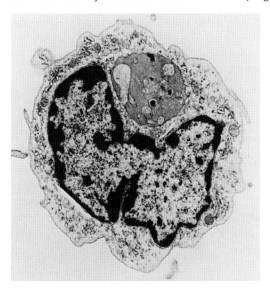

FIGURE 5-4 Transmission electron micrograph of a normal rabbit macrophage. The nature of the large inclusion is unknown.

(Courtesy Dr. S. Linthicum.)

cells in their attempts to eliminate the foreign material. Myeloid stem cells may also, when appropriately stimulated, give rise to dendritic cells. Indeed, these cells are so closely related that many investigators consider that dendritic cells are simply specialized macrophages optimized for antigen processing and presentation (Chapter 10).

Functions

Sentinel Cells

As described in Chapter 2, macrophages express many different pattern-recognition receptors (PRRs) and readily detect and respond to invading bacteria and viruses. In addition to effective phagocytosis, they respond by producing complex cytokine mixtures. The most important of these are interleukin-1 (IL-1), IL-6, IL-12, IL-18, and tumor necrosis factor-α (TNF-α) (Figure 5-6).

Inflammation

Macrophages recognize tissue damage, promote the recruitment of neutrophils, and regulate the processes by which neutrophils recruit monocytes. As sentinel cells, macrophages promote neutrophil emigration from blood vessels. The release of high-mobility group band protein-1 (HMGB1) and other damage-associated molecular patterns (DAMPs) from damaged tissues stimulates resident macrophages to produce TNF-α and IL-6 as well as neutrophil chemotactic chemokines, CXCL8, CCL3, and CCL4 and reactive oxygen species.

Exosomes are small cytoplasmic vesicles, about 50 to 100 nm in diameter, that can transmit signals between cells. They are released by stimulated macrophages, dendritic cells, and B cells. These exosomes carry with them a mixture of immunostimulatory and proinflammatory molecules. They can spread through the extracellular fluid, where they interact with nearby cells. Thus exosomes from macrophages containing bacteria can express bacterial cell wall components such as glycopeptidolipids and other pathogen-associated molecular patterns (PAMPs) on their surfaces. As a result, the exosomes can bind to PRRs on nearby neutrophils and macrophages, leading to MyD88-dependent release of TNF-α, CCL5, and iNOS and promoting more inflammation.

Phagocytosis

When microbial invasion occurs and inflammation develops, blood monocytes respond by binding to vascular endothelial cells in a manner similar to neutrophils. Thus adherence and rolling are triggered by selectin binding, and the cells are brought to a gradual halt by integrins binding to ligands on vascular endothelial cells. The monocytes bind to endothelial cell intracellular adhesion molecule 1 (ICAM-1), using β_2-integrins and then emigrate into the tissues. Within the tissues these cells are called macrophages. Several hours

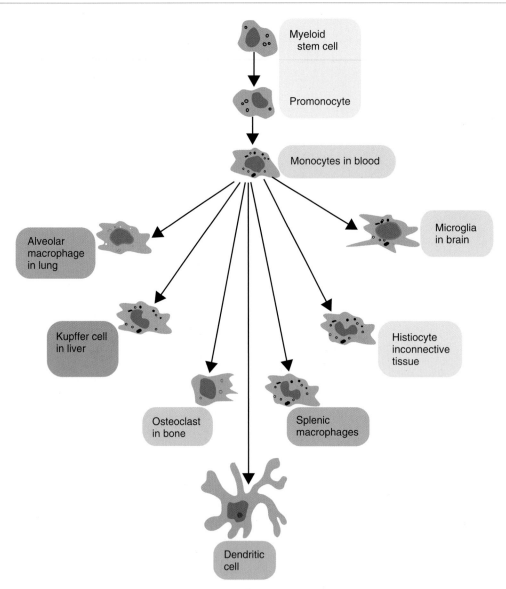

FIGURE 5-5 The origin and development of macrophages. Monocytes in blood can differentiate into many different types of macrophage. They can also differentiate into dendritic cells.

after neutrophils have entered an inflammatory site, the macrophages arrive. These macrophages are attracted not only by bacterial products and complement components such as C5a but also by DAMPs from damaged cells and tissues. Once neutrophils have emigrated into tissues, they also attract macrophages. Thus neutrophil granules contain macrophage chemoattractants such as azurocidin, defensins, and cathelicidins. Activated neutrophils and endothelial cells produce monocyte chemoattractant protein-1 (CCL2) under the influence of IL-6. Neutrophils are the martyrs of the immune system: they reach and attack foreign material first, and in dying they attract macrophages to the site of invasion. Phagocytosis by macrophages is similar to the process in neutrophils. Macrophages destroy bacteria by both oxidative and nonoxidative mechanisms. In contrast to neutrophils, however, macrophages can undertake sustained, repeated phagocytic activity. In addition,

macrophages release collagenases and elastases that destroy nearby connective tissue. They release plasminogen activator that generates plasmin, another potent protease. Thus macrophages can "soften up" the local connective tissue matrix and permit more effective penetration of the damaged tissue. Macrophages phagocytose both apoptotic neutrophils and their exosomes. The contents of neutrophil granules are not always destroyed but may be carried to macrophage endosomes where they can continue to inhibit the growth of bacteria. Thus neutrophils can enhance the effectiveness of macrophages in host defense.

Generation of Nitric Oxide In some mammals, especially rodents, cattle, sheep, and horses (but not in humans, pigs, goats, or rabbits), microbial PAMPs trigger macrophages to synthesize inducible nitric oxide synthase (iNOS or NOS2).

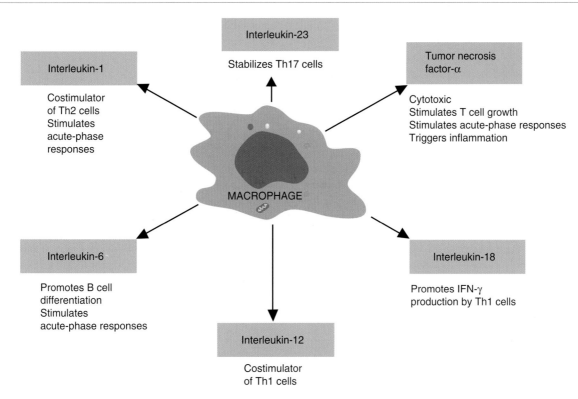

FIGURE 5-6 Some of the most important cytokines produced by macrophages and their functions.

This enzyme acts on L-arginine using NADPH and oxygen to produce large amounts of nitric oxide (nitrogen monoxide, NO) and citrulline (Figure 5-7). Nitric oxide alone is not highly toxic, but it can react with superoxide anion to produce potent oxidants such as peroxynitrite and nitrogen dioxide radical.

$$\underset{\substack{\text{Nitric}\\\text{oxide}}}{NO} + O_2^- \rightarrow \underset{\substack{\text{Peroxynitrite}\\\text{anion}}}{OONO^-} \rightarrow HOONO \rightarrow OH + \underset{\substack{\text{Nitrogen}\\\text{dioxide}\\\text{radical}}}{NO_2^-}$$

Not all macrophages generate nitric oxide. Those that do are called M1 cells, and their primary function is host defense. The sustained production of NO permits M1 macrophages to kill bacteria, fungi, protozoa, and some helminths. Nitric oxide also binds to metal-containing enzymes such as ribonucleotide reductase and impedes DNA synthesis. It also blocks mitochondrial heme-containing respiratory enzymes.

A second population of macrophages, called M2 cells, does not produce NO but instead converts arginine to ornithine using the enzyme arginase. These two macrophage populations play different roles in defending the body. M1 cells defend against microbial invaders and produce proinflammatory cytokines. M2 cells have opposite effects: they reduce inflammation and produce cytokines that suppress immune responses. M2 cells thus promote blood vessel formation, tissue remodeling, and tissue repair. M1 cells are produced early in the inflammatory process when inflammation is required. M2 cells, on the other hand, tend to appear late in the process when healing is required.

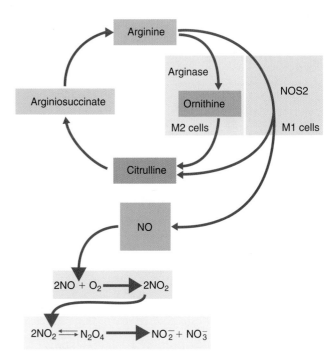

FIGURE 5-7 The two pathways of arginine metabolism in macrophages. The production of nitric oxide through the use of nitric oxide synthase 2 is a major antimicrobial pathway and the key feature of M1 macrophages. The use of arginase to produce ornithine, however, reduces the antimicrobial activities of M2 cells.

Activation

Although macrophages are potent phagocytes, their activities may be greatly enhanced by several activating pathways. Molecules that trigger macrophage activation include PAMPs such as lipopolysaccharides, CpG DNA, microbial carbohydrates, and heat-shock proteins as well as many DAMPs. Different levels of activation are recognized, depending on the triggering agent, and some bacteria, such as *Mycobacterium tuberculosis*, are better able to activate macrophages than others. Thus when monocytes first move into inflamed tissues, they produce increased amounts of lysosomal enzymes, increase phagocytic activity, increase the expression of antibody and complement receptors, and secrete more proteases (Figure 5-8). The cytokines produced by these macrophages, especially TNF-α and IL-12, activate a population of lymphocytes called natural killer (NK) cells (Chapter 19). The NK cells in turn secrete interferon-γ (IFN-γ), which activates macrophages still further. IFN-γ upregulates many different genes, especially the gene for NOS2. The *NOS2* gene can be upregulated 400-fold by a combination of IFN-γ and mycobacteria. As a result of this

increased NO production, activated M1 macrophages become very potent killers of bacteria.

Receptors

Macrophages express many different receptors on their surface (Figure 5-9). All are glycoproteins. Some are PRRs, such as the toll-like receptors (TLRs) and the mannose-binding receptor (CD206). CD206 can bind mannose or fucose on bacterial surfaces and permit macrophages to ingest nonopsonized bacteria.

Macrophages have many receptors for opsonins. For example, CD64 is a high-affinity antibody receptor expressed on macrophages and to a lesser extent on neutrophils. Like other antibody receptors, CD64 binds the Fc region of antibody molecules and thus is called an Fc receptor (FcγRI). Its expression is enhanced by IFN-γ-induced activation. Human macrophages also carry two low-affinity antibody receptors, CD32 (FcγRII) and CD16 (FcγRIII). Cattle and sheep macrophages have a unique Fc receptor called Fcγ 2R, which can bind particles coated with a specific type of antibody called immunoglobulin

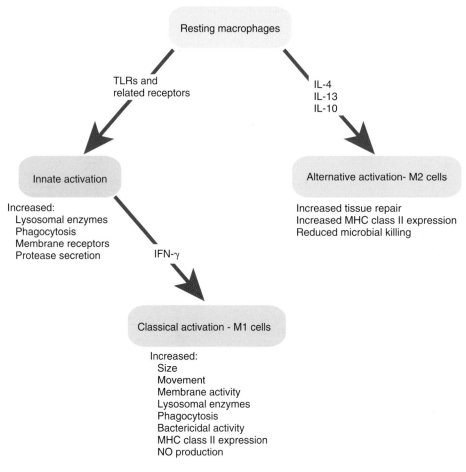

FIGURE 5-8 The progressive activation of macrophages can involve three pathways. Thus macrophages can become classically activated M1 cells by exposure to microbial products and subsequent exposure to Th1 cytokines such as IFN-γ. Alternatively, they may undergo "alternative activation" on exposure to Th2 cytokines and become M2 cells.

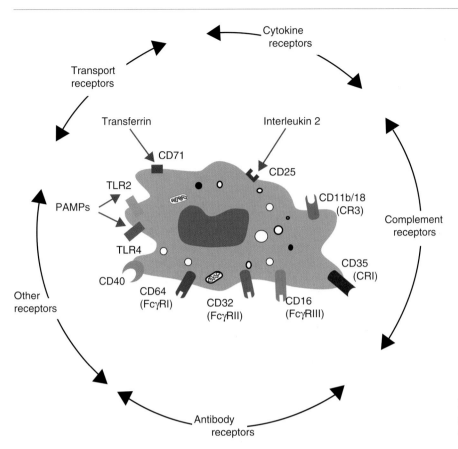

FIGURE 5-9 Some of the major surface receptors expressed by macrophages and their functions.

G2 (IgG2) (Chapter 16). Macrophages also have receptors for complement components. These include CD35 (CR1) and CD11b/CD18, both of which are C3b receptors.

Cell surface integrins bind macrophages to other cells, to connective tissue molecules such as collagen and fibronectin, and to some complement components. CD40 is used by macrophages to communicate with lymphocytes. Its ligand (CD40L or CD154) is found on T cells. Thus T cells can activate macrophages via CD40.

Fate of Foreign Material

Macrophages are located throughout the body and can detect and capture bacteria or fungi invading by many different routes. For example, bacteria injected intravenously are rapidly removed from the blood. Their precise fate depends on the species involved. In dogs, rodents, and humans, 80% to 90% are trapped and removed in the liver. The bacteria are removed by the macrophages (Kupffer cells) that line the sinusoids of the liver. The process occurs in two stages. Bacteria are first phagocytosed by blood neutrophils. These neutrophils are then ingested and destroyed by the Kupffer cells. These processes thus resemble acute inflammation in which neutrophils are primarily responsible for destruction of invaders, whereas the macrophages are responsible for preventing damage caused by apoptotic neutrophils (Table 5-1). In ruminants, pigs, horses,

□ Table 5-1 | Sites of Clearance of Particles from the Blood in Domestic Mammals

SPECIES	LOCALIZATION (%)	
	LUNG	LIVER/SPLEEN
Calf	93	6
Sheep	94	6
Dog	6.5	80
Cat	86	14
Rabbit	0.6	83
Guinea pig	1.5	82
Rat	0.5	97
Mouse	1.0	94

Selected data from Winkler GC: Pulmonary intravascular macrophages in domestic animal species: review of structural and functional properties, *Am J Anat* 181:223, 1988; and Chitko-McKown CG, Blecha F: Pulmonary intravascular macrophages, a review of immune properties and functions, *Ann Rech Vet* 23:201–214, 1992.

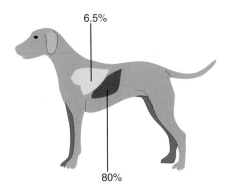
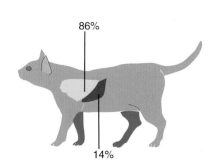

FIGURE 5-10 The different routes by which bacteria are cleared from the bloodstream in the dog and cat expressed as percentages of an administered dose. Dogs mainly use Kupffer cells in the liver. Cats mainly employ pulmonary intravascular macrophages.

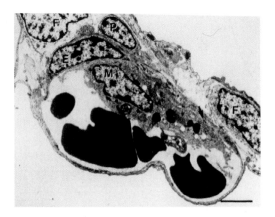

FIGURE 5-11 An intravascular macrophage *(M)* from the lung of a 7-day-old pig. The cell has numerous pseudopods, electron-dense siderosomes, phagosomes, and lipid droplets. It is closely attached to the thick portion of the air-blood tissue barrier that contains fibroblasts *(F)* and a pericyte *(P)* between basal laminae of the capillary endothelium *(E)* and the alveolar epithelium. At sites of close adherence, intercellular junctions with subplasmalemmal densities are seen *(arrow)*. Bar = 2 μm. Original magnification ×8000.

(From Winkler GC, Cheville NF: Postnatal colonization of porcine lung capillaries by intravascular macrophages: an ultrastructural morphometric analysis, *Microvasc Res* 33:224–232, 1987.)

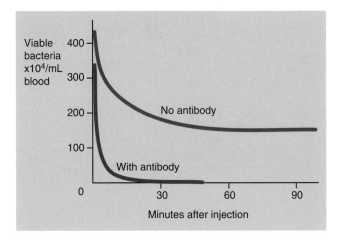

FIGURE 5-12 The clearance of bacteria from the blood (in this case *Escherichia coli* from piglets). In the absence of antibodies, bacteria are slowly and incompletely removed.

and cats, particles are mainly removed from the bloodstream by macrophages that line the endothelium of lung capillaries (pulmonary intravascular macrophages) (Figures 5-10 and 5-11).

In species in which hepatic clearance is important, large viruses or bacteria may be cleared completely by a single passage through the liver (Figure 5-12). The spleen also filters blood. It is a more effective filter than the liver, but since it is much smaller, it traps much less material. There are also differences in the type of particle removed by the liver and spleen. Splenic macrophages have antibody receptors (CD64) so that particles opsonized with antibody are preferentially removed in the spleen. In contrast, phagocytic cells in the liver express CD35, a receptor for C3, the third component of complement, so that particles opsonized by C3 are preferentially removed in the liver. The clearance of particles from the blood is regulated by soluble opsonins such as fibronectin, or mannose-binding lectin. Experimentally, if an animal is injected intravenously with a very large dose of particles such as colloidal carbon, these opsonins are temporarily depleted, and other particles (such as bacteria) will not be removed from the bloodstream. In this situation, the mononuclear-phagocytic system is said to be "blockaded."

Removal of organisms from the bloodstream is greatly enhanced if they are opsonized by specific antibodies. If antibodies are absent or the bacteria possess an antiphagocytic polysaccharide capsule, the rate of clearance is decreased. Some molecules, such as bacterial endotoxins, estrogens, and simple lipids, stimulate macrophage activity and therefore increase the rate of bacterial clearance. Corticosteroids and other drugs that depress macrophage activity depress the clearance rate.

Soluble Proteins Given Intravenously

Unless carefully treated, protein molecules in solution tend to aggregate spontaneously. If such a protein solution is injected intravenously, neutrophils, monocytes, and macrophages

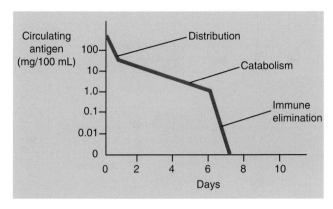

FIGURE 5-13 The clearance of a soluble antigen from the bloodstream. Note the three phases of this clearance.

rapidly remove these protein aggregates. Unaggregated protein molecules remain in solution and are distributed evenly through the animal's blood. Small proteins (<60 kDa) also spread throughout the extravascular tissue fluids. Once distributed, these proteins are catabolized, resulting in a slow but progressive decline in its concentration. Within a few days, however, the animal will mount an immune response against the foreign protein. Antibodies combine with the antigen; phagocytic cells remove these antigen-antibody complexes from the blood; and the protein is rapidly eliminated (Figure 5-13).

This triphasic clearance pattern of redistribution, catabolism, and immune elimination may change according to circumstances. For example, if the animal has not been previously exposed to a protein antigen, it takes between 5 and 10 days before immune elimination occurs. If, on the other hand, the animal has been primed by prior exposure to the protein, a secondary immune response will occur in 2 to 3 days, and the catabolic phase will be short. If antibodies are present at the time of antigen administration, immune elimination is immediate, and no catabolic phase is seen. If the injected material is not antigenic, or if an immune response does not occur, catabolism will continue until all the material is eliminated.

Fate of Material Administered by Other Routes

When foreign material is injected into a tissue, some local damage and inflammation are bound to occur, and DAMPs are released. As a result, neutrophils and macrophages migrate toward the injection site and phagocytose the injected material. Some, however, will be captured by dendritic cells. The material captured by macrophages and the dendritic cells will be processed and used to initiate an adaptive immune response. Antibodies and complement (Chapter 7) interact with the antigenic material, generating chemotactic factors that attract still more phagocytic cells and hastening its final elimination. In the skin, a web of antigen-trapping dendritic cells called Langerhans cells may trap foreign molecules and present them directly to lymphocytes. For this reason, intradermal injection

of antigen may be most effective in stimulating an immune response.

Soluble material injected into a tissue is redistributed by the flow of tissue fluid through the lymphatic system. It eventually reaches the bloodstream, so its final fate is similar to intravenously injected material. Any aggregated material present is phagocytosed by neutrophils or tissue macrophages or by the macrophages and dendritic cells of lymph nodes through which the tissue fluid flows.

Digestive Tract Digestive enzymes normally break macromolecules passing through the intestine into small fragments. However, some molecules may remain intact and pass through the intestinal epithelium (Chapter 22). Bacterial polysaccharides and molecules that associate with lipids are especially effective in this respect since they are absorbed in chylomicrons. Particles that enter the blood from the intestine are removed by macrophages in the liver, whereas those particles entering the intestinal lymphatics are trapped in the mesenteric lymph nodes.

Respiratory Tract The fate of inhaled particles such as dust or aerosol droplets depends on their size. Large particles (>5 μm in diameter) stick to the mucous layer that covers the respiratory epithelium from the trachea to the terminal bronchioles (see Figure 22-6). These particles are then removed by the flow of mucus toward the pharynx or by coughing. Very small particles that reach the lung alveoli are ingested by alveolar macrophages, which carry them back to the bronchoalveolar junction; from there, they are also removed by the flow of mucus. Nevertheless, some material may be absorbed from the alveoli. Small particles absorbed in this way are cleared to the draining lymph nodes, whereas soluble molecules enter the bloodstream and are distributed throughout the body. When large amounts of dust are inhaled, as occurs in workers exposed to industrial dusts or in cigarette smokers, the alveolar macrophage system may be "blockaded" and the lungs made more susceptible to microbial invasion.

Recovery from Inflammation

Once invading organisms have been destroyed, the tissue response must switch from a killing process to a repair process. Thus as inflammation progresses, macrophages change their properties (Figure 5-14). The first macrophages are activated in the classical manner by TNF-α to kill invading bacteria. However, these M1 macrophages eventually convert to M2 cells and develop antiinflammatory properties. Thus the same cell can act in a proinflammatory manner at the beginning of an infection but switch to antiinflammatory activities once the infection is overcome.

Inflammation is also resolved by an active process mediated by several polyunsaturated fatty acid–derived lipids related to the leukotrienes. Two of these, resolvin E1 and protectin D1, activate inflammation resolution programs.

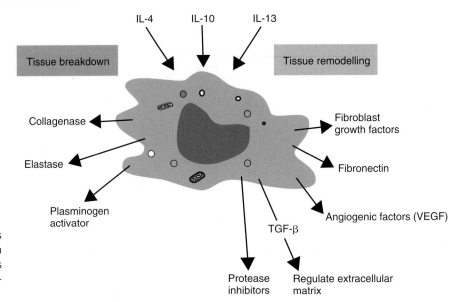

FIGURE 5-14 The role of M2 macrophages in tissue breakdown and tissue repair in wound healing. In effect, damaged tissues must be removed before repair and remodeling can begin.

Produced by endothelial cells, they promote phagocyte removal by regulating phagocyte infiltration and promoting macrophage ingestion of apoptotic neutrophils. Changes in chemokine composition such as increased CCR5 expression lead to removal of the chemoattractants CCL3 and CCL5. These chemokines are also destroyed by tissue metalloproteases. Apoptotic neutrophils exercise negative feedback by releasing lactoferrin that suppresses neutrophil recruitment. Dying neutrophils attract scavengers. Thus phagocytosis of apoptotic neutrophils by macrophages triggers the release of vascular endothelial growth factor (VEGF) that is crucial for revascularization and wound repair. Once generated, M2 cells secrete SLP1, a serine protease inhibitor. This molecule inhibits the release of elastase and oxidants by TNF-α-stimulated neutrophils and inhibits the activity of the elastase. SLP1 also protects the antiinflammatory cytokine transforming growth factor-β (TGF-β) from breakdown, and TGF-β inhibits the release of TNF-α.

Even in normal healthy animals, many cells die every day and must be promptly removed. This is the function of macrophages. For example, dying neutrophils release the nucleotides adenosine triphosphate and uridine triphosphate. These attract macrophages that move rapidly toward the apoptotic cells. Macrophages "palpate" any neutrophils that they encounter. If the neutrophil is healthy, the cells separate. If, however, the neutrophil is dead or dying, the macrophage remains in contact and eats the neutrophil. This interaction operates through the adhesion protein CD31 (Figure 5-15). Thus CD31 on a neutrophil binds to CD31 on a macrophage. If the neutrophil is healthy, it sends a signal to the macrophage, causing it to disengage. On the other hand, if the neutrophil fails to signal, it will be eaten. It is interesting to note that this failure in CD31 signaling occurs long before a neutrophil begins to leak its enzyme contents and cause damage. Likewise the macrophages that consume these neutrophils do not release cytokines or vasoactive lipids. Ingestion of apoptotic neutrophils

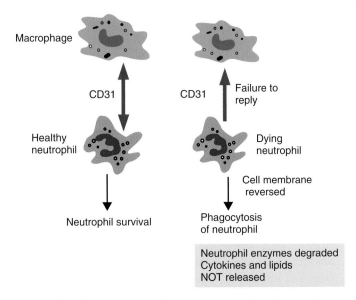

FIGURE 5-15 The removal of apoptotic neutrophils. The reaction is initiated by interactions between CD31 on neutrophils and macrophages. If the neutrophil fails to reply when interrogated by a macrophage, it will be ingested and destroyed.

does, however, cause the macrophages to secrete more TGF-β, which in turn promotes tissue repair. Phagocytosis is thus an efficient way of removing apoptotic neutrophils without causing additional tissue damage or inflammation.

By secreting IL-1β, macrophages attract and activate fibroblasts. These fibroblasts enter the damaged area and secrete collagen. Once sufficient collagen fibers have been deposited, their synthesis stops. This collagen is then remodeled over several weeks or months as the tissue returns to normal. The reduced oxygen tension in dead tissues stimulates macrophages to secrete cytokines such as VEGF that promote the growth of new blood vessels. Once the oxygen tension is restored to normal, new blood vessel formation ceases.

Chronic infections, chemical insults, parasites

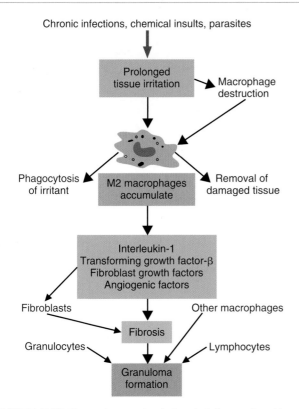

FIGURE 5-16 The pathogenesis of chronic inflammation. Macrophages undergoing prolonged stimulation may switch from an M1 to an M2 phenotype. M2 cells secrete cytokine mixtures that not only promote wound healing, but also promote the "walling-off" of persistent irritants by fibroblasts and extracellular matrix. Other cell types are attracted to the persistent antigen. Their precise composition will vary with the antigens involved.

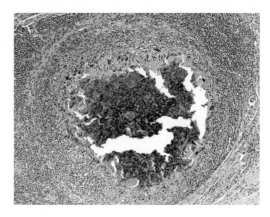

FIGURE 5-17 A granulomatous inflammatory reaction around a degenerating tapeworm cyst in a bovine heart. The mass of cells around the central organism is a mixture of macrophages and fibroblasts serving to wall it off from the rest of the body. Original magnification ×250.

(Courtesy Dr. John Edwards.)

The final result of this healing process depends on the effectiveness of the inflammatory response. If the cause is rapidly and completely removed, healing will follow uneventfully. If tissue health is not restored, either because the invaders are not eliminated or because tissue repair is inadequate, inflammation may persist and become a damaging, chronic condition. Examples of persistent invaders include bacteria such as *M. tuberculosis*, fungi such as *Cryptococcus* species, parasites such as liver fluke, or inorganic material such as asbestos crystals. Macrophages, fibroblasts, and lymphocytes may accumulate in large numbers around the persistent material for months or years. Because they resemble epithelium in histological sections, these accumulated macrophages are called epithelioid cells. Epithelioid cells may fuse and form multinucleated giant cells as they attempt to enclose particles too large to be ingested by a single macrophage.

In all these cases, the persistence of foreign material results in the continual arrival of new M2 macrophages that continue to attract fibroblasts and stimulate the deposition of collagen. The chronic inflammatory lesion that develops around this foreign material is called a granuloma (Figure 5-16). Granulomas consist of granulation tissue—an accumulation of macrophages, lymphocytes, fibroblasts, loose connective tissue, and new blood vessels. The term *granulation tissue* is derived from the granular appearance of this tissue when cut. The "granules" are in fact new blood vessels. If the irritant is antigenic (e.g., some persistent bacteria, fungi, and parasites), the granuloma may contain many lymphocytes as well as macrophages, fibroblasts, and probably some neutrophils, eosinophils, and basophils (Figure 5-17). The chronically activated M2 cells within these granulomas secrete IL-1, which stimulates collagen deposition by fibroblasts and eventually "walls off" the lesion from the rest of the body. If the persistent foreign material is not antigenic (e.g., silica, talc, or mineral oil), few neutrophils or lymphocytes will be attracted to the lesion. Epithelioid and giant cells, however, continue their attempts to destroy the offending material. If the material is toxic for macrophages (as is asbestos), leaking enzymes may lead to chronic tissue damage, local fibrosis, and scarring.

Chronic granulomas, whether due to immunological or foreign body reactions, are clinically important since they may enlarge and destroy normal tissues. In liver fluke infestations, for example, death may result from the gradual replacement of normal liver cells by fibrous tissue formed as a result of the persistence of the parasites.

For sources of additional information, please visit http:// evolve.elsevier.com/tizard/immunology/

6

Systemic Responses to Inflammation

Chapter Outline

Key Points

- Inflammation is not only a local tissue reaction but also a systemic reaction involving the whole body.
- Cytokines secreted by sentinel cells cause a fever and are responsible for the diverse behavioral changes that we call sickness.
- Excessive production of these cytokines (a cytokine storm) can lead to the development of a lethal shock syndrome.
- Excessive, chronic release of inflammatory cytokines may result in tissue deposition of insoluble misfolded proteins called amyloid.

In one sense, inflammation is a very local response, focused on sites of tissue damage or microbial invasion, but it also has significant systemic effects on other, distant parts of the body. If the local inflammation is minor, such systemic effects may not even be noticed. If, however, inflammation is extensively affecting multiple organ systems, or if the microbial invader succeeds in spreading throughout the body, these systemic effects become clinically significant. Collectively we call them sickness. It need hardly be pointed out that in veterinary medicine, it is these signs of sickness that commonly draw the attention of an owner to an animal's illness.

Systemic Innate Responses

Hematopoietic stem cells (HSCs) proliferate in response to systemic infections as the body needs to replenish its effector cells. This response is mediated by multiple cytokines including the interferons and tumor necrosis factor-α (TNF-α). The type I interferons have a direct effect on HSCs and stimulate them to proliferate in response to viral infections. TNF-α has a similar effect and is necessary for HSC maintenance. Since HSCs express TLRs, especially toll-like receptor 2 (TLR2) and TLR4, it is possible that bacterial pathogen-associated molecular patterns (PAMPs) may directly promote HSC proliferation.

Sickness Behavior

When an animal is invaded by pathogens, a generalized response may occur—a response that we call sickness. The subjective feelings of sickness—malaise, lassitude, fatigue, loss of appetite, and muscle and joint pains—along with a fever, are signs of a systemic innate immune response. They reflect a change in the body's priorities as it fights off the invaders. Microbial PAMPs acting through the pattern-recognition receptors (PRRs) of phagocytic cells stimulate the production of interleukin-1β (IL-1β), IL-6, and TNF-α. All three of these cytokines signal to the brain (Figure 6-1). They use two routes. One route is through the neurons that serve damaged tissue. IL-1 receptors are expressed on these sensory neurons, especially the vagus nerve. Sensory stimulation by IL-1β through the vagus nerve can trigger afferent signaling to the brain. (IL-1 will not trigger a fever if the vagus nerve is cut.) Lipopolysaccharide (LPS) and TLR4 can also trigger these vagal signals. They therefore trigger fever, nausea, and other sickness responses in the brain. The second route involves cytokines that either diffuse into the brain from the bloodstream or are produced within the brain. Microglial cells express TLR4, whereas neurons express TNF receptors. These cytokines can act on neurons or microglial cells to modify behavior and, for example, alter pain perception. As a result, anti-TNF antibodies can greatly reduce the pain associated with rheumatoid arthritis (Chapter 36).

The most obvious of the brain's responses to infection is the development of a fever. IL-1, IL-6, and TNF-α all trigger changes in body temperature. These cytokines induce the expression of cyclooxygenase-2 (COX-2) in the hypothalamus that results in prostaglandin production, which causes the body's thermostatic set-point to rise. In response, animals conserve heat by vasoconstriction and increase heat production by shivering, thus raising their body temperature until it reaches the new set-point. This fever enhances some components of the immune responses. For example, it enhances transendothelial neutrophil migration and chemotaxis and increases neutrophil accumulation within tissues. It also accelerates caspase-dependent neutrophil apoptosis. Raised body temperatures cause dendritic cells to mature; enhance the circulation of lymphocytes; and promote the secretion of IL-2. Fever range temperatures enhance the survival of T cells by inhibiting their apoptosis. In addition to causing a fever, inflammatory cytokines, especially IL-1, promote the release of sleep-inducing molecules in the brain. Increased lethargy is commonly associated with a fever and may, by reducing the energy demands of an animal, increase the efficiency of defense and repair mechanisms. IL-1 also suppresses the hunger centers of the brain and induces the loss of appetite associated with

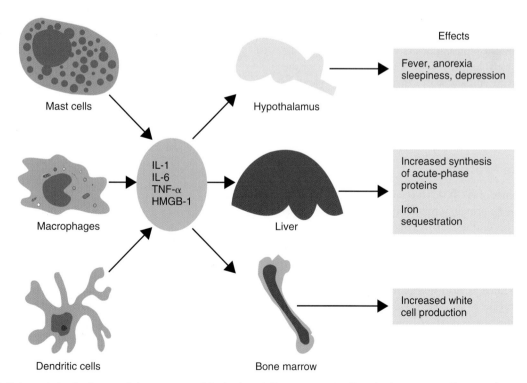

FIGURE 6-1 Sickness behavior is part of the response of the body to inflammatory stimuli. Multiple systemic effects are due to the four major cytokines secreted by sentinel cells, mast cells, macrophages, and dendritic cells. The major sickness-inducing cytokines are IL-1, IL-6, TNF-α, and HMGB1.

infections. The benefits of this are unclear, but it may permit the animal to be more selective about its food. If the anorexia persists, it can have an adverse effect on animal growth and production.

High-mobility group band protein-1 (HMGB1) (Chapter 3) is a potent sickness-inducing cytokine. Although IL-1, IL-6, and TNF-α have long been known to cause septic shock and sickness behavior, it is now clear that these three molecules induce HMGB1 release from macrophages several hours after initiation of sickness. It enters secretory lysosomes and is then released slowly from the cells. HMGB1 has been implicated in food aversion and weight loss by its actions on the hypothalamic-pituitary axis. It mediates endotoxin lethality, arthritis, and macrophage activation. The inflammation induced by necrotic cells is caused in part by the release of HMGB1 from disrupted nuclei and damaged mitochondria.

Metabolic Changes

In addition to their effects on the nervous and immune systems, IL-1, IL-6, and TNF-α act on skeletal muscle to increase protein catabolism and release amino acids. Although this eventually results in muscle wastage, the newly available amino acids are available for increased antibody and cytokine synthesis. Other systemic responses include the development of a neutrophilia (elevated blood neutrophils) as a result of enhanced stem cell activity, weight loss due to muscle wasting and loss of adipose tissue, and the production of many new proteins (acute-phase proteins) that help fight infection.

Animals exposed to chronic, low doses of TNF-α lose weight and become anemic and protein depleted. This occurs because TNF-α inhibits the synthesis of enzymes necessary for the uptake of lipids by preadipocytes and causes mature adipocytes to lose stored lipids. TNF-α is thus responsible for the weight loss seen in animals with cancer or chronic parasitic and bacterial diseases. Weight loss is a common response to infection (and sometimes to vaccination) and is therefore of considerable significance to livestock producers.

Acute-Phase Proteins

Under the influence of IL-1β, TNF-α, and especially IL-6, liver hepatocytes increase protein synthesis and secretion. New proteins may also be synthesized in lymph nodes, tonsils, and spleen as well as in blood leukocytes. This increase begins about 90 minutes after injury or systemic inflammation and subsides within 48 hours (Figure 6-2). It may also occur following prolonged stress such as road transportation or confinement. Because this increase is associated with acute infections and inflammation, the newly produced proteins are called acute-phase proteins. About 30 acute-phase proteins have been recognized, and many are important components of the innate immune system. They include soluble PRRs, complement components, clotting molecules, protease inhibitors, and iron-binding proteins. Different mammals produce different sets of acute-phase proteins (Figure 6-3).

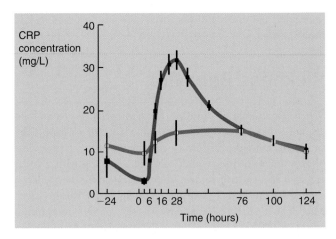

FIGURE 6-2 The rise in C-reactive protein levels in six dogs following anesthesia and surgery *(red line)* and in six dogs undergoing anesthesia alone *(blue line).*

(From Burton SA, Honor DJ, Mackenzie AL, et al: C-reactive protein concentration in dogs with inflammatory leukograms, *Am J Vet Res* 55:615, 1994.)

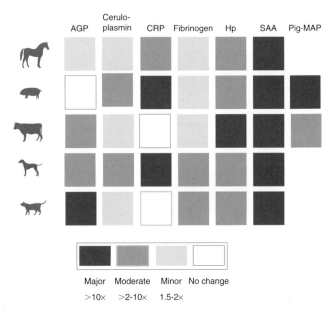

FIGURE 6-3 Species differences in the major acute-phase proteins produced by the domestic mammals.

Soluble Pattern-Recognition Receptors

C-reactive protein (CRP) is the major acute-phase protein produced in primates, rabbits, hamsters, and dogs and is important in pigs. CRP is a pentraxin (P-type lectin) and has a pentameric structure with two faces (five 20-kDa units). One face binds phosphocholine, a common side chain found in all cell membranes and many bacteria and protozoa. The other face binds to the antibody receptors FcγRI and FcγRIIa on the surface of neutrophils. CRP thus promotes the phagocytosis and removal of damaged, dying, or dead cells in addition to microorganisms. CRP can bind to bacterial polysaccharides and glycolipids and to damaged cells, where it activates the classical complement pathway. (Its name derives from its ability to bind and precipitate the C-polysaccharide of *Streptococcus pneumoniae*.) CRP also has an antiinflammatory role since it inhibits neutrophil superoxide production and degranulation and blocks platelet aggregation. CRP may therefore promote healing by reducing damage and enhancing the repair of damaged tissue. The functions of CRP may differ between species. For example, in lactating cows, the level of CRP in serum rises two- to five-fold for unknown reasons.

Serum amyloid P (SAP) is the major acute-phase protein in rodents. It is a pentraxin related to CRP. Like CRP, it is a soluble PRR, where one face of the molecule can bind nuclear constituents such as DNA, chromatin, and histones as well as cell membrane phospholipids. The other face can bind and activate C1q and thus activate the complement system through the classical pathway. Other soluble PRRs that are also acute-phase proteins include LPS-binding protein in cattle, CD14 in humans and mice, and C-type lectins such as mannose-binding lectin and conglutinin in other species.

Iron-Binding Molecules

One of the most important factors that determines the success or failure of bacterial invasion is the availability of iron. Many pathogenic bacteria, such as *Staphylococcus aureus*, *Escherichia coli*, *Bacillus anthracis*, *Pasteurella multocida*, and *Mycobacterium tuberculosis*, require large amounts of iron for growth since iron forms the key catalytic site in many of their enzymes. Animals, however, also require iron to survive. As a result, microbe and host compete for the same metal.

Iron concentrations within animal tissues are normally very low. Mammalian blood has just 10^{-26} M free iron since almost all available iron is bound to proteins. These iron-binding proteins include transferrin, lactoferrin, hepcidin, siderocalin, haptoglobin, and ferritin. Because many pathogenic bacteria such as *Salmonella* species and mycobacteria require iron for growth, withholding iron through the use of potent iron-binding proteins is an effective innate defense mechanism (Box 6-1).

When bacteria invade the body, intestinal iron absorption ceases. Liver cells secrete transferrin and haptoglobin, and there is increased incorporation of iron into the liver. Haptoglobin is a major acute-phase protein in ruminants, horses, and cats. It can rise from virtually undetectable levels in normal calves to as high as 1 mg/mL in calves with acute respiratory disease. Haptoglobin binds iron molecules and makes them unavailable to invading bacteria, thus inhibiting bacterial proliferation and invasion. Haptoglobin also binds free hemoglobin, thus preventing its oxidation of lipids and proteins.

A similar situation occurs in the mammary gland when, in response to bacterial invasion, milk neutrophils release their stores of lactoferrin. The lactoferrin binds free iron and makes it unavailable to the bacteria. Despite the reduced availability of iron, some bacteria, such as *M. tuberculosis*, *B. anthracis*, and *E. coli*, can still invade the body because they produce their own potent iron-binding proteins (siderophores) that can

> □ Box 6-1 | **Genes That Control Innate Immunity**
>
> Innate resistance to many intracellular organisms such as the mycobacteria, *Brucella* species, *Leishmania* species, and *Salmonella typhimurium* is controlled in part by a gene called *Slc11a1*. (This is an abbreviation for solute carrier family 11, member a1. It was previously called *Nramp1*). After phagocytosis, *Slc11a1* is acquired by the phagosomal membrane. It then acts to pump divalent metals, especially Fe^{2+}, out of the phagosome and inhibits the growth of intracellular parasites by depriving them of iron. Thus resistance-associated alleles of this gene inhibit the intracellular replication of many intracellular pathogens. For example, macrophages from cattle with the resistant allele have a higher level of this transporter protein and, by reducing iron availability, can effectively reduce the growth of intracellular *Brucella abortus*. The difference between the resistant and susceptible alleles appears to be associated with polymorphisms in the *Slc11a1* gene.

remove the iron from transferrin or lactoferrin. In effect, the body and the bacteria engage in a competition for iron molecules. Mycobacteria use their siderophore carboxymycobactin to strip iron from mammalian ferritin. The result of this competition may determine the outcome of the infection. When serum iron levels are elevated, as occurs after red cell destruction, animals may become more susceptible to bacterial infections.

Mammals may also capture iron by stealing bacterial siderophores. Thus during bacterial infections, the mammalian liver, spleen, and macrophages synthesize a protein called lipocalin 2. Lipocalin 2 (also called siderocalin) binds the bacterial siderophore enterochelin with very high affinity. Lipocalin 2 is essential for limiting the growth of enterochelin-producing bacteria such as *E. coli* but does not affect the growth of bacteria that employ other methods to acquire iron.

Less than 10% of our daily needs are met by dietary iron. The rest is derived from aged or damaged erythrocytes by macrophages. Macrophages phagocytose these erythrocytes and catabolize the hemoglobin using hemoxygenase. They release the iron obtained from hemoglobin into the circulation via a cell surface iron-carrier protein called ferroportin. This iron efflux is suppressed by hepcidin (Figure 6-4). Hepcidin is produced by hepatocytes under the influence of IL-1 and IL-6. Hepcidin binds to ferroportin, triggering its internalization, ubiquitination, and subsequent degradation. Hepcidin also suppresses intestinal iron absorption by downregulating ferroportin expression on enterocytes. In healthy individuals, hepcidin production is also regulated by systemic iron availability or by erythropoietic signals and hypoxia. In inflammation, however, IL-6 and IL-1 stimulate the hepcidin promoter through its JAK/STAT receptor. As a result, hepcidin increases, ferroportin decreases and a hypoferremia develops, iron availability for red blood cell production drops, and chronically

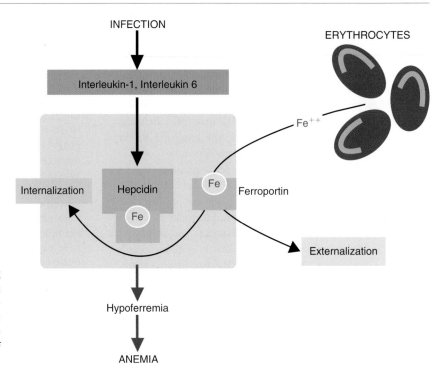

FIGURE 6-4 The role of hepcidin in regulating iron availability. This protein prevents iron efflux from cells by binding to ferroportin and triggering its degradation. The net effect is to retain iron within cells, making it unavailable for hemoglobin synthesis and leading to the development of anemia.

infected animals become anemic—the anemia of infection. Ferroportin inhibits iNOS synthesis and therefore reduces nitric oxide production by macrophages.

Other iron-binding acute-phase proteins include transferrin (important in birds) and hemopexin. Activation of macrophages by interferon-γ (IFN-γ) leads to downregulation of macrophage iron acquisition through transferrin receptors and depriving intracellular bacteria of needed iron.

Protease Inhibitors

Some serum protease inhibitors such as α_1-antitrypsin, α_1-antichymotrypsin, and α_2-macroglobulin are acute-phase proteins in many mammals. All of these may inhibit neutrophil proteases in sites of acute inflammation. For example, major acute-phase protein (MAP) is a major protease inhibitor in pigs and a moderate one in cattle.

Other Acute-Phase Proteins

α_1-Acid glycoprotein is a minor acute-phase protein in cattle. Neutrophils exposed to activating agents such as phorbol myristate acetate rapidly release their stores of α_1-acid glycoprotein. This protein inhibits the respiratory burst and may reduce the damage caused by excessive inflammation.

Serum amyloid A (SAA), a serum protein of 15 kDa, is the major acute-phase protein in cattle, cats, and horses and is also important in humans and dogs. Thus equine SAA concentrations rise several hundred–fold during noninfectious arthritis, whereas canine SAA concentrations increase up to 20-fold in bacterial disease. LPS induces a 1000-fold increase in SAA in

mice. The functions of SAA are unclear, but it binds to TLR2 and may also be an endogenous TLR4 agonist. This leads to NF-κB activation and the production of multiple inflammatory cytokines. SAA also carries cholesterol to the liver before secretion in bile. It recruits lymphocytes to inflammatory sites and induces enzymes that degrade the extracellular matrix. SAA is a chemoattractant for neutrophils, monocytes, and T cells. It increases significantly in mastitic milk. Other acute-phase proteins include ceruloplasmin, haptoglobin, and fibrinogen in sheep and CRP, SAA, haptoglobin, sialic acid, and ceruloplasmin in pigs.

Some protein levels fall during acute inflammation. These are called "negative" acute-phase proteins. Two of the most important are albumin and transferrin. The albumin serves as a source of amino acids that can be used on demand, such as during infections and inflammation.

Acute-Phase Proteins as "Biomarkers" of Disease

It is possible to identify animals with severe infections or inflammation by measuring acute-phase proteins in their blood. This may be of benefit, for example, in antemortem meat inspections by identifying those animals that are suffering from inapparent inflammation or infection and hence are not fit to eat. In cattle, haptoglobin is a major acute-phase protein and increases especially in chronic infections such as mastitis, enteritis, pneumonia, traumatic pericarditis, and endometritis. A mammary-associated isoform of SAA (M-SAA3) is elevated in mastitis. The acute-phase response in sheep is similar to that in cattle.

Pigs with tail lesions due to biting had elevated levels of CRP, SAA, and haptoglobin compared with control pigs. These tail lesions were associated with increased carcass condemnation.

In cats, blood SAA levels increase 10- to 50-fold in inflammatory conditions such as feline infectious peritonitis (FIP). They are also elevated in diabetes mellitus, infectious diseases, injury, and cancer. α_1-Acid glycoprotein also increases in FIP, although this is usually less than 10-fold. It also increases in calicivirus, chlamydiosis, feline leukemia, and feline immunodeficiency virus infections. Haptoglobin usually increases 2- to 10-fold and is especially high in FIP.

In dogs, CRP is the major acute-phase protein, increasing 100-fold in infectious diseases such as babesiosis, leishmaniasis, parvovirus infection, and colibacillosis. Levels of acute-phase protein increase moderately in canine inflammatory bowel disease. CRP, haptoglobin, and SAA are significantly elevated in the cerebrospinal fluid and serum of dogs with canine steroid-responsive arteritis-meningitis (Chapter 35). In pregnant dogs, haptoglobin, ceruloplasmin, and fibrinogen levels increase midway through gestation.

Systemic Inflammatory Response Syndrome

After massive tissue damage, excessive amounts of cytokines, HMGB1, mitochondrial components, and oxidants may escape into the bloodstream and trigger a lethal form of shock known as systemic inflammatory response syndrome (SIRS). Released DAMPs may activate large numbers of sentinel cells and as a result generate very large quantities of inflammatory mediators. The most important of these are TNF-α, IFN-γ, CXCL8, and IL-6. These cytokines in turn trigger the activation of additional T cells and the release of additional cytokines, leading to even more cell destruction (Box 6-2). This "cytokine storm" may result in severe illness and even death. The most important of these cytokine storms results from tissue trauma or burns that damage large numbers of cells. However, many virus infections, such as influenza and dengue, can also trigger cell destruction, leading to excessive cytokine release and death.

Bacterial Septic Shock

Septic shock is the name given to the SIRS caused by severe bacterial infections. It accounts for about 9% of human deaths in the United States and is a correspondingly important cause of animal deaths. Animals or humans with mild infections develop the characteristic signs of sickness such as fevers, rigors, myalgia, depression, headache, and nausea as a result of cytokine release. Severe infections, however, may cause excessive triggering of TLRs leading to a massive and uncontrolled release of HMGB1. Other cytokines involved are TNF-α and IL-1β, with IFN-γ, IL-6, and CXCL8 (IL-8) in a supporting role.

□ **Box 6-2 | Macrophage Migration Inhibitory Factor**

Macrophage migration inhibitory factor (MIF) was one of the earliest cytokines identified because it suppresses the random movement of macrophages. It is unique in that it is secreted both by the anterior pituitary gland in the brain and by T cells. Its production by T cells is triggered by proinflammatory cytokines and LPS. The secreted MIF binds to its receptor, CD74, on antigen-presenting cells such as dendritic cells, endothelial cells, and macrophages. It stimulates Th1 cells to produce large amounts of proinflammatory cytokines, such as TNF-α, IFN-γ, IL-1β, IL-6, and IL-8, as well as NO, prostaglandins, and leukotrienes. MIF is produced by the pituitary in stressed animals. These cytokines contribute to the development of SIRS while counteracting any protective effects induced by glucocorticoids. Neutralization of MIF protects against LPS-induced shock.

These cytokines in turn stimulate expression of nitric oxide synthase 2 (NOS2), leading to an increase in serum nitric oxide, and of COX-2, leading to prostaglandin and leukotriene synthesis. This vastly excessive cytokine production leads to severe acidosis, fever, lactate release in tissues, an uncontrollable drop in blood pressure, elevation of plasma catecholamines, and eventually renal, hepatic, and lung injury and death. Tissue damage, severe systemic inflammation, and the release of damaged cell fragments all act to raise blood levels of tissue factor, a key initiator of coagulation. Vascular endothelial cell apoptosis may trigger their detachment from the basement membrane. The cytokines activate vascular endothelial cells so that procoagulant activity is enhanced, leading to blood clotting. The nitric oxide causes vasodilation and a drop in blood pressure. The prostaglandins and leukotrienes cause increases in vascular permeability. This combination results in enhanced coagulation. Simultaneous downregulation of anticoagulant systems occurs as a result of reduced antithrombin synthesis (it is a "negative" acute-phase protein), whereas fibrinolysis is reduced owing to increased synthesis of inhibitors of plasminogen activator. All these changes promote intravascular coagulation and capillary thrombosis (Figure 6-5). The widespread damage to vascular endothelium eventually causes organ failure.

Multiple-organ dysfunction syndrome is the end stage of severe septic shock. It is characterized by hypotension, insufficient tissue perfusion, uncontrollable bleeding, and organ failure caused by hypoxia, tissue acidosis, tissue necrosis, and severe local metabolic disturbances. The severe bleeding is due to disseminated intravascular coagulation.

The sensitivity of mammals to septic shock varies greatly. Species with pulmonary intravascular macrophages (cat, horse, sheep, and pig) tend to be more susceptible than dogs and

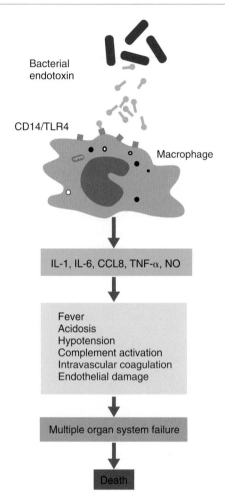

FIGURE 6-5 The pathogenesis of the systemic inflammatory response syndrome. In effect, the syndrome results from overexpression of multiple cytokines. These cytokines are toxic in high doses.

rodents, which lack pulmonary intravascular macrophages and are relatively insusceptible to lung injury. It is of interest to note that in foals with sepsis, *TLR4* gene expression is greatly increased, and a poorer prognosis is associated with increased expression of IL-10.

Bacterial Toxic Shock

Some strains of *S. aureus* produce enterotoxins that bind and stimulate T cell antigen receptors (Figure 6-6). These toxins may thus stimulate up to 20% of an animal's T cells, causing them to secrete enormous quantities of IL-2 and IFN-γ. These in turn stimulate production of TNF-α and IL-1β. This leads to the development of a fever, hypotension, collapse, skin lesions, and damage to the liver, kidney, and intestines with multiple-organ dysfunctions called toxic shock syndrome. A similar syndrome has also been observed in some streptococcal infections. In these cases, streptococcal M-protein binds to fibrinogen. The M-protein–fibrinogen complexes bind to endothelial cell integrins and trigger a respiratory burst. This causes an increase in vascular permeability

and hypercoagulability, leading to toxic shock characterized by hypotension and disseminated intravascular coagulation.

Graft-versus-Host Disease

Another syndrome characterized by excessive production of cytokines, especially TNF-α, is graft-versus-host disease. In this disease, described in more detail in Chapter 32, donor lymphocytes attack the tissues of the graft recipient. TNF-α from these cells causes mucosal destruction, leading to ulceration, diarrhea, and liver destruction.

Protein Misfolding Diseases

Amyloidosis is the name given to the deposition of insoluble proteins in tissues. These deposits appear as amorphous, eosinophilic, hyaline proteins in cells and tissues (Figure 6-7). Amyloid is produced as a result of errors in the folding of newly formed protein chains. These misfolded chains eventually aggregate to form insoluble fibrils. Electron microscopy shows that amyloid proteins consist of protein fibrils, formed by peptide chains cross-linked to form β-pleated sheets (Figure 6-8). This molecular conformation makes amyloid proteins extremely insoluble and almost totally resistant to proteases. Consequently, once deposited in cells or tissues, amyloid deposits are almost impossible to remove. Amyloid infiltration eventually leads to gradual cell loss, tissue destruction, and death. Amyloidosis may be systemic when it involves multiple organs, or it may be localized, involving only a single organ.

Many different proteins can misfold and form amyloid. For example, amyloidosis may develop when infection or inflammation causes a sharp rise in the concentration of the acute-phase protein, SAA. A 76-amino acid proteolytic fragment of SAA can accumulate, misfold, aggregate, and be deposited in multiple organs. This material, one of the most common forms in domestic animals, is called reactive amyloid. Reactive amyloidosis is associated with chronic inflammation in diseases such as mastitis, osteomyelitis, abscesses, traumatic pericarditis, metritis, gangrenous pneumonia, and tuberculosis (Figure 6-9). Reactive amyloidosis is a major cause of death in animals repeatedly immunized for commercial antiserum production. Familial amyloidosis of Shar-Pei dogs consists of reactive amyloid deposited following chronic immune-mediated arthritis.

Multiple myelomas are plasma cell tumors that secrete antibodies, especially antibody light chains (Chapter 15). Huge quantities of antibody light chains and their fragments are produced, and their misfolding results in the deposition of immunogenic amyloid. Although immunogenic amyloid is the most common form of amyloid in humans, it is very rare in domestic animals.

Several forms of localized amyloidosis are recognized in domestic animals; for example, old dogs may suffer from vascular amyloidosis, in which amyloid is deposited in the media

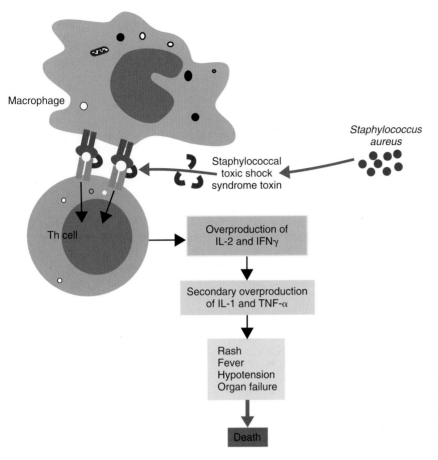

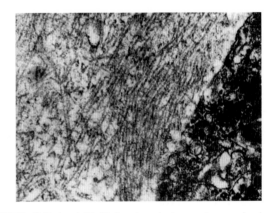

FIGURE 6-6 The pathogenesis of staphylococcal toxic shock syndrome. The toxic shock syndrome toxin is a potent superantigen that acts as a powerful stimulant of IL-1 and TNF-α production.

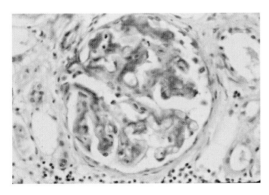

FIGURE 6-7 Secondary amyloid deposited in a glomerulus. The red dye (Congo red) specifically binds to amyloid fibrils. Original magnification ×400.

FIGURE 6-8 Amyloid fibrils. An electron micrograph showing bundles of paired amyloid fibrils deposited parallel to a cell membrane.

(Courtesy Dr. E.C. Franklin. From Franklin EC, and Zucker-Franklin D. Current concepts of amyloid: *Adv Immunol* 15:249-304, 1972.)

of leptomeningeal and cortical arteries. An inherited form of amyloid has been described in Abyssinian cats. Tumor-like amyloid nodules and subcutaneous amyloid have been reported in horses, but in general, amyloid deposits are found in the liver, spleen, and kidneys, particularly within glomeruli. In humans, amyloid fibrils are deposited in the neurons of patients with Alzheimer's disease.

Misfolded proteins may be transmissible (Box 6-3). They form the prion proteins that cause spongiform encephalopathies such as bovine spongiform encephalopathy (BSE) and scrapie. Prions are protease-resistant forms of cellular proteins. In the case of BSE, the prion is a misfolded and aggregated form of a cellular protein PrP^c that is important for normal macrophage functions. These prion proteins normally play a role in resistance to intracellular bacteria such as *Brucella* species.

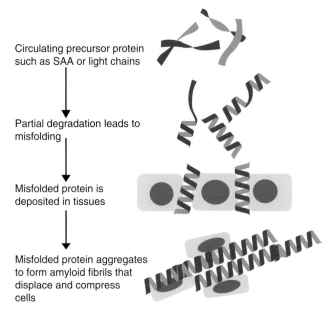

Circulating precursor protein such as SAA or light chains

Partial degradation leads to misfolding

Misfolded protein is deposited in tissues

Misfolded protein aggregates to form amyloid fibrils that displace and compress cells

FIGURE 6-9 The pathogenesis of reactive amyloid fibril deposition. Misfolded proteins aggregate to form insoluble fibrils.

□ **Box 6-3** | **Transmissible Amyloidosis?**

AA amyloidosis is unusually common in captive cheetahs and poses a significant threat to the species' survival. On investigation, however, it was found that cheetahs suffering from amyloidosis excreted AA amyloid fibrils in their feces. These fecal amyloid fibers could be purified and injected into mice, where they were much more effective than tissue amyloid in inducing amyloidosis. Thus cheetahs appear to transmit AA amyloid in their feces. This material may cause disease in mice that happen to ingest cheetah feces. It is also possible that amyloidosis may develop in cheetahs that happen to eat these mice! It may also be that other cheetahs may acquire the amyloidosis by fecal contamination of cuts or abrasions. Given that cheetahs are genetically homogeneous and tend to suffer from many chronic inflammatory diseases, they may be more susceptible to amyloidosis than other species. The transferred amyloid might simply enhance an ongoing disease. Thus AA amyloidosis in cheetahs may be a prion disease.

Data from Zhang B, Une Y, Fu X, Yan J et al: Fecal transmission of AA amyloidosis in the cheetah contributes to high incidence of disease, *Proc Natl Acad Sci U S A* 105:7263–7268, 2008.

It is of interest to note that even reactive amyloidosis is somewhat "transmissible" since inoculation of AA proteins into an animal will hasten the development of amyloidosis. Amyloid proteins likely act by providing a substrate on which other misfolded proteins can be deposited. There is evidence that foie gras prepared from duck or goose liver can transmit AA amyloidosis when fed to mice. Similarly, silk fibers formed from a protein composed of β-sheets, may promote amyloidosis when injected into mice!

For sources of additional information, please visit http://evolve.elsevier.com/tizard/immunology/

7

Innate Immunity: The Complement System

□ Chapter Outline

Key Points

- The complement system plays multiple roles in both innate and adaptive immunity.
- Complement proteins are found in normal serum.
- The complement system may be activated through three different pathways: two innate pathways, the alternative pathway and the lectin pathway, and one adaptive pathway, the classical pathway.
- The innate pathways are activated by recognizing microbial pathogen-associated molecular patterns (PAMPs). The classical pathway is activated by antibodies bound to foreign antigens.
- Complement components, especially C3b, bind covalently to invading microbes and opsonize them.
- Complement components may form a terminal complement complex and punch holes in microbes.
- The complement system triggers inflammation through the release of the potent chemoattractant C5a.
- Deficiencies of some complement components lead to increased susceptibility to infections.

The complement system is a major innate defense system. Although its main role is to protect against infections, complement can also regulate inflammatory processes, remove damaged or altered cells, send "danger" signals to the body, and regulate adaptive immune responses. It is involved in the clearance of immune complexes, angiogenesis, mobilization of stem cells, tissue regeneration, and lipid metabolism. As with other innate mechanisms, inappropriate activation of the complement system can contribute to various immune and inflammatory diseases.

Protection from infection requires that the innate immune system respond to invasion as rapidly as possible. An important component of this early response is the complement system. The complement system is a complex interacting network that consists of many interacting pattern-recognition proteins, proteases, serum proteins, receptors, and regulators (Figure 7-1). Complement proteins are activated through pathways that

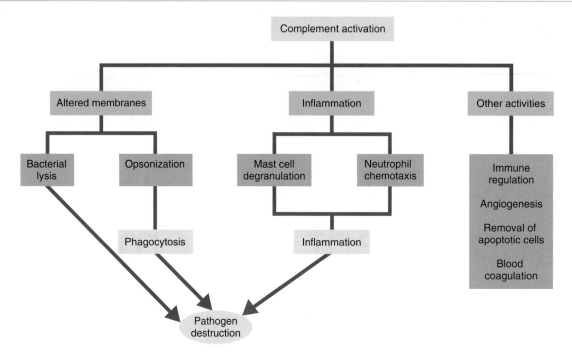

FIGURE 7-1 The functions of the complement system. Complement may either alter microbial membranes or trigger inflammation. Either way, it hastens the elimination of microbial invaders and is thus a key component of the innate immune system. It has multiple other functions as well.

cause some molecules to bind covalently (and hence irreversibly) to the surface of invading microbes. Once bound, these proteins can destroy the invaders. The complement system is inactive in healthy, uninfected animals. It is activated by either pathogen-associated molecular patterns (PAMPs) on the surface of infectious agents or by antigen-bound antibodies. Because the complement system is so potent, it must be carefully regulated and controlled. This in turn makes for significant complexity.

The complement system consists of sets of inactive proteins that are activated in a stepwise manner. Three major steps are involved. First, the complement system must be activated. Second, a key protein called C3b must be generated. Third, a terminal complement complex is assembled through an amplification pathway. Once activated, the complement system generates multiple effector molecules. The progression of complement activation and the delivery of these effector molecules are carefully regulated. The first step, the triggering of complement activation, can occur by three different mechanisms, referred to as the alternative, the lectin, and the classical pathways (Figure 7-2). The alternative and lectin pathways are activated directly by microbial carbohydrates—typical examples of the pattern-recognition pathways that trigger innate immunity. The classical pathway, in contrast, is an evolutionary recent pathway activated when antibodies bind to the surface of an organism and thus works only in association with adaptive immune responses. Although complement has been conventionally regarded as a series of linear pathways, like other areas of immunology, it should properly be regarded as a network with several key hubs.

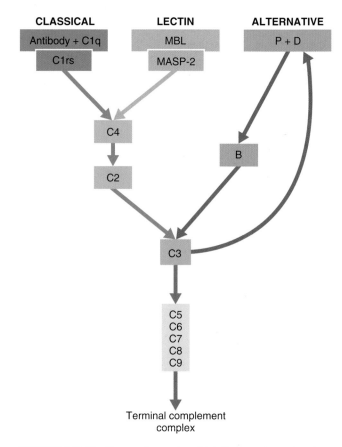

FIGURE 7-2 The three pathways by which the complement system can be activated.

Complement Proteins

The 30 or more proteins that form the complement system are either labeled numerically with the prefix C (e.g., C1, C2, C3) or designated by letters of the alphabet (B, D, P, and so forth). Some are found free in serum, whereas others are cell-surface receptors. Complement components account for about 5% to 10% of the proteins in blood serum. The size of complement components varies from 24 kDa for factor D to 460 kDa for C1q. Their serum concentrations in humans vary between 20 μg/mL of C2 and 1300 μg/mL of C3 (Table 7-1). Complement components are synthesized at multiple sites throughout the body. Most C3, C6, C8, and B components are made in the liver, whereas C2, C3, C4, C5, B, D, P, and I are made by macrophages. Neutrophil granules may store large quantities

▢ Table 7-1 | Complement Components

NAME	MW (kDa)	SERUM CONCENTRATION (mg/mL)
Classical Pathway		
C1q	460	80
C1r	83	50
C1s	83	50
C4	200	600
C2	102	20
C3	185	1300
Alternate Pathway		
D	24	1
B	90	210
Terminal Components		
C5	195	70
C6	120	65
C7	120	55
C8	160	55
C9	70	60
Control Proteins		
C1-INH	105	200
C4BP	550	250
H	150	480
I	88	35
Ana INH	310	35
P	4×56	20
S	83	500

of C6 and C7. As a result, these components are readily available for defense at sites where macrophages and neutrophils accumulate.

Activation Pathways

The Alternative Pathway

The alternative pathway of complement activation is an evolutionary ancient pathway. It is triggered when microbial cell walls interact with complement components in the bloodstream. It is a key component of innate immunity.

The most important complement protein is called C3. C3 is a disulfide-linked heterodimer with α and β chains. It is synthesized by liver cells and macrophages and is the complement component of highest concentration in serum. C3 possesses a highly reactive thioester side chain, that, when activated, binds to the surface of microbes and marks them for destruction by immune cells. The activation of the C3 thioester must be carefully regulated to ensure that it does not bind to normal tissues. To prevent such accidents, the thioester group in unactivated C3 is hidden inside the folded molecule.

In healthy normal animals, C3 breaks down slowly but spontaneously into two fragments called C3a and C3b (Figure 7-3). This opens up the C3b molecule to expose the thioester group. The thioester then generates a carbonyl group that binds the C3b irreversibly to carbohydrates and proteins on nearby cell surfaces (Figure 7-4). The breakdown of C3 also exposes binding sites for a protein called factor H. When factor H binds to these sites, a protease called factor I degrades the C3b, blocking further activity and generating two fragments, iC3b and C3c. iC3b binds receptors found on circulating leukocytes (Figure 7-5). It stimulates these cells to engulf pathogens and activate inflammatory cells. The final breakdown product of C3, C3dg, targets pathogens to surface receptors on B cells and so promotes antibody production (Chapter 15).

The rapid destruction of cell-bound C3b depends on binding by factor H, which depends in turn on the nature of the target surface. When factor H interacts with normal cells, glycoproteins rich in sialic acid and other neutral or anionic polysaccharides enhance its binding to C3b, factor I is activated, and the C3b is destroyed. In a healthy individual, therefore, factors H and I destroy C3b as fast as it is generated.

In contrast, bacterial cell walls lack sialic acid. When C3b is deposited on these surfaces, factor H cannot bind, factor I is inactivated, and the bound C3b therefore persists. In this case, the opening of C3b on an activating surface exposes a binding site for another complement protein called factor B. As a result, a complex called C3bB is formed. The bound factor B is then cleaved by a protease called factor D, releasing a soluble fragment called Ba and leaving C3bBb attached to the bacteria. This bound C3bBb is a protease whose preferred substrate is C3. (It is therefore called the alternative C3 convertase.) Factor D can only act on factor B after it has bound to C3b but not before. This constraint is called substrate

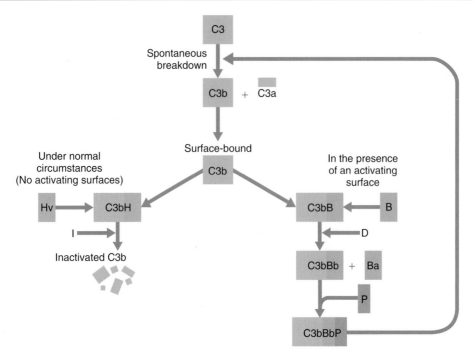

FIGURE 7-3 The alternative complement pathway. Surface-bound C3b may either be destroyed, as normally happens, or activated by the presence of an activating surface.

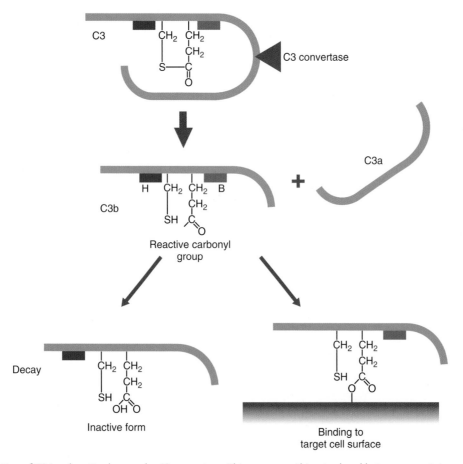

FIGURE 7-4 Activation of C3 involves its cleavage by C3 convertase. This exposes a thioester bond between a cysteine and a glutamine. This bond breaks to form a reactive carbonyl group that enables the molecule to bind covalently (and hence irreversibly) to target cell surfaces. Removal of C3a also reveals the binding sites for factor H and factor B.

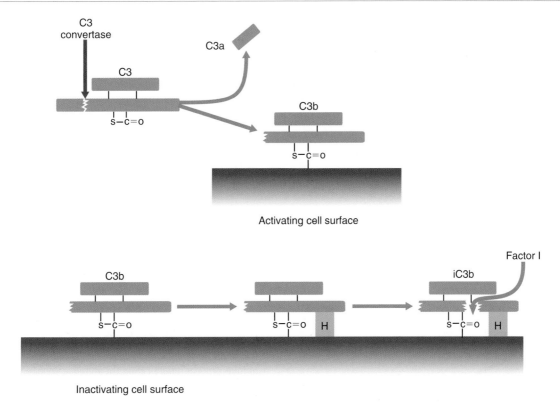

FIGURE 7-5 Activated C3 binds to cell surfaces. This C3b is normally inactivated by the actions of factors H and I. However, factor H must first be activated by binding to the surface. In the absence of factor H, factor I will not work. In this case, C3b persists and activates the terminal complement pathway.

modulation, and it occurs at several points in the complement pathways. It ensures that the activities of enzymes such as factor D are confined to the correct molecules.

The alternative C3 convertase, C3bBb, can act on C3 to generate more C3b. C3bBb is, however, very unstable, with a half-life of only 5 minutes. If another protein, called factor P (or properdin), binds to the complex, it forms C3bBbP with a half-life of 30 minutes. Since C3b thus serves to generate more C3bBbP, the net effect of all this is that a positive loop is generated where increasing amounts of C3b are produced and irreversibly bound to the surface of the invading organism. Properdin also recognizes several PAMPs and damage-associated molecular patterns (DAMPs) on foreign and apoptotic cells. Despite its name, the alternative complement pathway accounts for 80% to 90% of all complement activated even if initially triggered by the classical or lectin pathway.

The Lectin Pathway

The second method of activating the complement system involves the use of soluble pattern-recognition molecules that recognize microbial carbohydrates. These lectins bind to microbes and then activate proteases that activate complement. Like the alternative pathway, this is an innate pathway triggered simply by the presence of bacterial PAMPs (Figure 7-6).

These activating lectins include mannose-binding lectin (MBL) and the ficolins. MBL can attach to bacteria, fungi, parasitic protozoa, and viruses by binding to mannose or N-acetylglucosamine on microbial cell walls. It does not bind to mammalian glycoproteins. Once bound, MBL activates a serum protease called MASP-2. (MASP stands for MBL-associated serine protease.) Activated MASP-2, in turn, acts on the complement component C4, splitting it into C4a and C4b. This exposes a thioester group on the C4b that generates a reactive carbonyl group that covalently attaches the C4b to the microbial surface (Figure 7-7). Another complement component, C2, then binds to C4b to form a complex, C4b2. The bound C2 is then cleaved by MASP-2 to generate C4b2b (Box 7-1).

Cell-bound C4b2b is a protease that splits C3 to generate C3a and C3b and exposes the thioester group on the C3b. The activation of C3b by C4b2b is a major step because each C4b2b complex can generate as many as 200 C3b molecules. Since these reactions are usually confined to the microenvironment close to microbial surfaces, newly formed C3b will bind to nearby microbes. The bound C3b then binds C5 and cleaves it to C5a and C5b. The complement pathway then can proceed to completion and the killing of the organism by terminal complement complexes.

The MBL–MASP-2 pathway is ancient, having existed for at least 300 million years. Although in many ways it duplicates

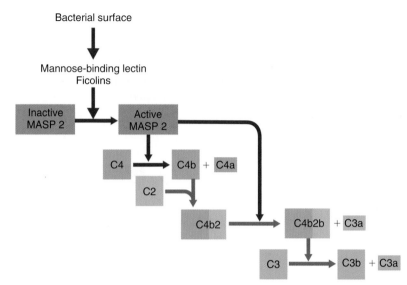

FIGURE 7-6 Complement activation by the lectin pathway.

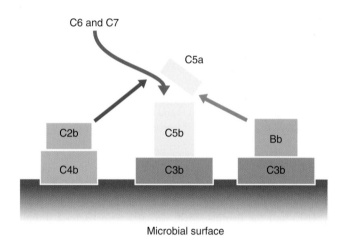

FIGURE 7-7 The two C3 convertases, C4b2b and C3bBb, act on C5 when it is linked to C3b and cleave off a small peptide called C5a. In so doing they reveal a site that binds C6 and C7.

□ Box 7-1 | **The Defense Collagens**

C1q and mannose-binding lectin (MBL) are members of a unique protein family called the defense collagens with similar structures and functions. Other members of this family include surfactant protein A, adiponectin, conglutinin, and ficolin. These are soluble lectins characterized as containing a conserved collagen-like region as well as a carbohydrate recognition domain. Like C1q, they commonly polymerize. These proteins serve as soluble pattern-recognition receptors. They can bind to foreign pathogens and subsequently interact with phagocytic cells or complement. Thus MBL recognizes mannose-containing carbohydrates. On binding to their ligands, they trigger an immediate protective response such as activation of complement systems or promotion of phagocytosis.

the alternative pathway, it is an example of the way the body uses redundant mechanisms to ensure protection.

The Classical Pathway

The classical complement pathway (Figure 7-8) is usually triggered by clusters of antibody molecules on the surface of a foreign organism. It is thus associated with adaptive immune responses. Unlike the immediate alternate and lectin pathways, the classical pathway cannot be triggered until antibodies are made, which may occur as late as 7 to 10 days after infection. Nevertheless, once activated, it is a very effective complement-activating pathway.

When antibody molecules bind an antigen they expose active sites on their Fc regions. If several antibody molecules are clustered on the surface of an organism, the multiple exposed active sites can collectively trigger classical complement pathway activation.

The first component of the classical complement pathway is a protein complex called C1. C1 consists of three proteins (C1q, C1r, C1s) bound together by calcium. C1q looks like a six-stranded whip when viewed by electron microscopy (Figure 7-9). Two molecules of C1r and two of C1s form a structure located between the C1q strands. C1q is activated when at least two of its strands bind to complement-activating sites on clustered antibody molecules. Binding to antibodies causes a conformational change in C1q that is transmitted to C1r. As a result, C1r exposes an active proteolytic site that acts on C1s to convert that molecule to an active enzyme.

Single, antigen-bound molecules of immunoglobulin M (IgM) or paired, antigen-bound molecules of IgG are needed to activate C1. The polymeric IgM structure readily provides two closely spaced complement-activating sites. In contrast, at least two IgG molecules must be closely clustered to have the same effect. Thus IgG is much less efficient than IgM in activating the classical pathway. C1 may also be activated directly

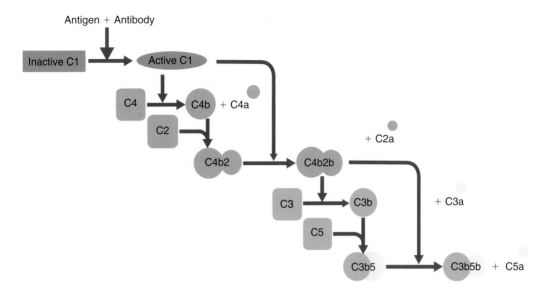

FIGURE 7-8 The basic features of the classical complement pathway.

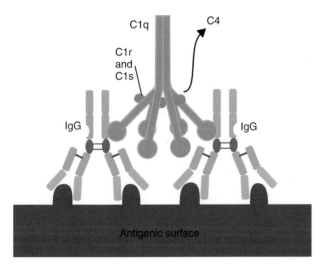

FIGURE 7-9 The structure of C1 and its role in interacting with antibodies to initiate the classical complement pathway.

by some viruses, or by bacteria such as *Escherichia coli* and *Klebsiella pneumoniae*. It can also be activated by cell surface–bound pentraxins such as C-reactive protein (CRP).

Activated C1s cleaves C4 into C4a and C4b. C2 then binds to C4b to form C4b2. Activated C1s then splits the bound C2, generating a small peptide fragment C2a and active C4b2b. C1s cannot act on soluble C2; the C2 must first be bound to C4b before it can be cleaved (another example of substrate modulation). Active C4b2b is a potent protease that cleaves C3 and is therefore called classical C3 convertase. C3b generated in this way binds and activates C5. Subsequent reactions lead to formation of the terminal complement complex and microbial killing.

In addition to binding immune complexes, C1q can also bind to apoptotic and necrotic cells, extracellular matrix proteins, pentraxins such as CRP, amyloid and prion proteins, and

DNA. However, all these substances with the exception of immune complexes can also bind the complement inhibitors C1-BP and factor H so that full complement activation does not occur. If these inhibitory processes are blocked, uncontrolled complement activation may lead to unwanted inflammation.

The Amplification Pathway

All surface-bound C3 convertases, regardless of their origin, can induce the next step in complement activation, the amplification pathway (Figure 7-10). Once C5 binds to C3b, substrate modulation occurs, and the C5 can be cleaved by C3bBb (Figure 7-11). The convertases cleave C5 (195 kDa) into a small fragment called C5a (15 kDa), leaving a large fragment C5b attached to the C3b. This cleavage also exposes a site on C5b that can bind two new proteins, C6 and C7, to form a multimolecular complex called C5b67 (Figure 7-12). The C5b67 complex can then insert into the microbial cell membrane. Once inserted in the surface of an organism, the complex binds a molecule of C8. Twelve to 18 C9 molecules then aggregate with the C5b678 complex to form a tubular structure called the terminal complement complex (TCC), also called the membrane attack complex (MAC). The TCC inserts into microbial cell membranes and punches a hole in the invader. If sufficient TCCs are formed on an organism, it will be killed by osmotic lysis. These TCCs can be seen by electron microscopy as ring-shaped structures on the microbial surface with a central electron-dense area surrounded by a lighter ring of poly C9 (see Figure 7-12). (In practice, there are very few examples of this lethal effect since many pathogens have a cell wall resistant to lysis or can interfere with TCC assembly. Nonlethal consequences such as opsonization are probably more significant.)

Much more important than TCC-mediated lysis are the potent proinflammatory effects of the small released peptides

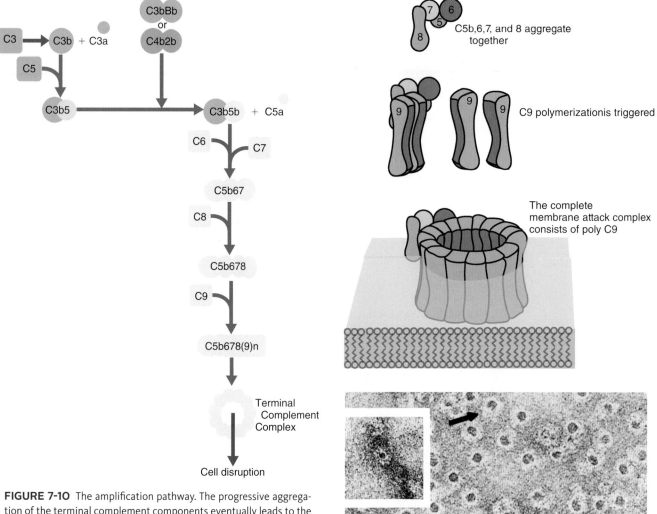

FIGURE 7-10 The amplification pathway. The progressive aggregation of the terminal complement components eventually leads to the polymerization of C9 and the assembly of a terminal complement complex.

FIGURE 7-12 Formation of poly C9 by the terminal complement pathway and an electron micrograph of poly-C9 complement lesions on an erythrocyte membrane. The *insert* shows a mouse complement lesion. The *arrow* points to a possible C5b678 complex. Compare these lesions to the T cell polyperforins in Figure 18-9.

(From Podack ER, Dennert G: Assembly of two types of tubules with putative cytolytic function by cloned natural killer cells, *Nature* 302(5907):442-445, 1983.)

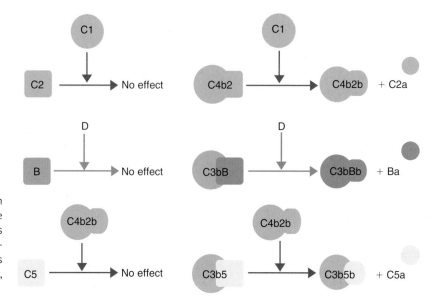

FIGURE 7-11 Substrate modulation is one way in which the complement system is regulated. The target for a protease cannot be cleaved unless it is first bound to another protein. Examples of substrate modulation include the cleavage of factors C2, B, and C5 only after they have bound to C4, C3, and C3, respectively.

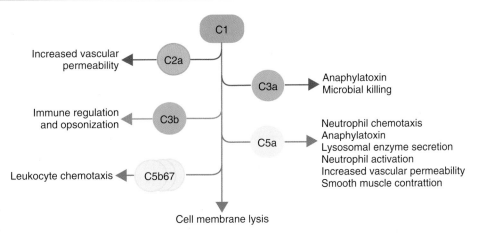

FIGURE 7-13 Some of the biological consequences of complement activation.

C3a and C5a. These peptides degranulate mast cells and stimulate platelets to release the vasoactive molecules histamine and serotonin. Both trigger inflammation through their cell surface receptors (C3aR and C5aR). They are powerful chemoattractants for neutrophils and macrophages. They increase vascular permeability, causing lysosomal enzyme release from neutrophils and thromboxane release from macrophages (Figure 7-13). C3a and its inactivated derivative C3a-des Arg can kill bacteria. Thus C3a is an efficient killer of *E. coli*, *Pseudomonas aeruginosa*, *Enterococcus faecalis*, and *Streptococcus pyogenes*. C3a acts like other antimicrobial peptides by disrupting bacterial membranes. (C3a and C5a are also called anaphylatoxins since, when injected in sufficient amounts, they can kill an animal in a manner similar to anaphylaxis [Chapter 28].)

Regulation of Complement Activation

The consequences of complement activation are so significant and potentially dangerous that each of the activation pathways must be carefully controlled by soluble and cell-bound regulatory proteins (Figure 7-14).

The most important regulator of the classical pathway is C1-inactivator (C1-INH), a glycoprotein that inhibits several proteases in the classical and lectin pathways. C1-INH blocks the activities of active C1r and C1s. Other regulatory proteins control the activities of the C3 and C5 convertases. Some compete with the MASPs for the binding sites on MBL and ficolins. CD55, or decay accelerating factor, is a glycoprotein expressed on the surface of red blood cells, neutrophils, lymphocytes, monocytes, platelets, and endothelial cells. CD55 binds to the convertases and accelerates their decay. Its function is to protect normal cells from complement attack. Other proteins that accelerate degradation of the convertases include factor H and C4-binding protein (C4BP) found in plasma and CD35 (CR1) and CD46 found on cell membranes. Control of the amplification pathway is mediated by three

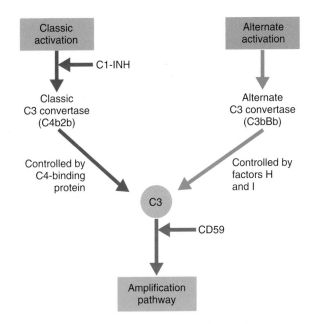

FIGURE 7-14 Basic control mechanisms of the complement system.

glycoproteins: vitronectin, clusterin, and, most important, CD59 (protectin). They all inhibit assembly of the TCC by blocking C5b678 insertion and C9 polymerization.

Complement Receptors

Five receptors for C3 or its fragments are expressed on cells. These are called CR1 (CD35), CR2 (CD21), CR3 (CD11a/CD18), CR4 (CD11c/CD18), and CRIg.

CR1 is found on primate red cells, neutrophils, eosinophils, monocytes, macrophages, B cells, and some T cells. It binds C3b and C4b as well as the C3b breakdown product, iC3b. Red cell CR1 accounts for 90% of all CR1 in the blood. In primates, CR1 removes immune complexes (antigen-antibody-complement complexes) from the circulation. (Immune complexes bind to CR1 on red cells, and the coated red cells are then removed in the liver and spleen [Chapter 30].) Deficiencies of complement components or their receptors may allow circulating immune complexes to accumulate in organs such as kidney and cause damage. For example, some patients with the autoimmune disease systemic lupus erythematosus have a CR1 deficiency and are thus unable to remove these immune complexes effectively. C3-deficient dogs develop immune complex–mediated kidney lesions for the same reason (Chapter 30).

CR2 (CD21) is found on most B cells. It binds a breakdown fragment of C3 called C3d. CR2 forms a complex with CD19. This complex regulates B cell responses (see Figure 15-10). B cells require stimulation by C3d acting through CR2 to respond optimally to antigens.

CR3 (CD11a/CD18) is an integrin that binds iC3b. It is found on macrophages, neutrophils, and natural killer cells. A genetic deficiency of CR3 (leukocyte adherence deficiency, LAD) has been described in humans, cattle, and dogs in which affected individuals experience severe recurrent infections (Chapter 37).

CR4 (CD11c/CD18) is another integrin found on neutrophils, T cells, natural killer cells, a few platelets, and macrophages. It binds breakdown fragments of C3.

CRIg is expressed on tissue macrophages including Kupffer cells in the liver. It has an affinity for C3b and iC3b and is a receptor for the C3-dependent opsonization of blood-borne pathogens.

Other Consequences of Complement Activation

Although microbial destruction mediated by terminal complement complexes is the most obvious beneficial activity of the complement system, its protective effects go far beyond this, and complement contributes to the body's defenses in many ways.

Opsonization

Microbes of course normally lack complement regulators so that uncontrolled complement activation occurs on their surface. This leads to proinflammatory signaling, opsonization, phagocytosis, and in some organisms, especially Gram-negative bacteria and some parasites, TCC assembly and cell lysis. C3b and C4b bound covalently to a microbial surface effectively tag it as foreign and so serve as very potent and effective opsonins. Phagocytic cells express CR1 and tissue macrophages also express CRIg. C3b-coated organisms will bind strongly to these cells and undergo type II phagocytosis (Chapter 4). If for some reason these organisms cannot be ingested, neutrophils may secrete their lysosomal enzymes and oxidants into the surrounding tissue fluid. These molecules then cause inflammation and tissue damage—a reaction classified as type III hypersensitivity (Chapter 30). Given the long evolutionary

history of the complement system, it is not surprising that many bacteria have evolved mechanisms to neutralize the effects of complement (Chapter 25)

Removal of Apoptotic Cells

Complement also contributes to postinflammatory healing by promoting the removal of apoptotic cells and immune complexes. Apoptotic cells lose their complement inhibitors CD46 and CD59. As a result, they can be opsonized by C3b and C4b and removed by phagocytosis. Apoptotic cells bind CRP that can then bind C1q, leading to classical pathway activation. Properdin (factor P) also binds to apoptotic T cells, resulting in C3b-mediated opsonization and destruction.

Inflammation

The anaphylatoxins, C3a and C5a, enhance TLR-induced production of the three proinflammatory cytokines, TNF-α, IL-1β, and IL-6. After binding to their receptors, they interact with toll-like receptor 2 (TLR2), TLR4, and TLR9. Conversely, TLR stimulation enhances cellular expression of C3aR and C5aR.

Blood Coagulation

The complement system enhances blood coagulation and inhibits fibrinolysis. Thus C5a induces the expression of tissue factor and plasminogen activator inhibitor I. Likewise, components of the clotting system amplify the complement system. Activated clotting factor XII can activate the classical pathway through C1 cleavage. Thrombin directly acts on C5 to generate C5a.

Chemotaxis

The complement system is a major contributor to acute inflammation. For example, activation of the complement system by any of its pathways generates several potent chemotactic peptides, including C5a and C5b67 (Table 7-2). C5b67 is chemotactic for neutrophils and eosinophils, whereas C5a attracts not only neutrophils and eosinophils but also macrophages and

◻ **Table 7-2** ◱ **Complement-Derived Chemotactic Factors**

FACTOR	TARGET
C3a	Eosinophils
C5a	Neutrophils, eosinophils, macrophages
C567	Neutrophils, eosinophils
Bb	Neutrophils
C3e	Promotes leukocytosis

basophils. When C5a attracts neutrophils, it stimulates their respiratory burst and upregulates CR1 and integrin expression.

Immune Regulation

Complement regulates humoral immunity. Thus C3d enhances adaptive responses when bound to antigen. When an antigen molecule binds to a B cell antigen receptor, any attached C3d will bind to CD21/CD19 on the B cell surface. (Remember that several hundred C3 molecules may attach to an antigen as a result of C3 convertase activity.) Binding to CD21/CD19 enhances B cell antigen receptor signaling and is an important stimulatory pathway for mature B cells (Chapter 15). Conversely, depletion of C3 is associated with reduced B cell responses. Coating of antigens with C3d also permits them to bind to CR2 on dendritic cells and so influences antigen presentation. In the absence of C3, immune complexes will not localize on follicular dendritic cells in germinal centers (Chapter 10).

Complement Genes

The genes coding for the complement proteins are scattered throughout the genome. However, two major gene clusters have been identified. Thus the genes for C4, C2, and factor B are located within the major histocompatibility complex class III region. Likewise, the genes for C4BP, CD55, CD35, CD21, CD46, and factor H are linked within the RCA (regulation of complement activation) cluster.

Complement components, like other proteins, may occur in different allelic forms. The precise number varies between components and species. For example, bovine factor H has three alleles, equine C3 has six, and canine C3 has two. Canine C6 has seven alleles, and porcine C6 has 14. Eleven alleles of canine C7 have been identified, whereas canine C4 has at least five. There is an association among C4-4 allele expression, low serum C4 levels, and the development of autoimmune polyarthritis in dogs. Feline and equine C4 each have at least four alleles.

Complement Deficiencies

Canine C3 Deficiency

Because the complement system is an essential defensive mechanism, complement deficiencies increase susceptibility to infections. The most severe of these diseases occurs in individuals deficient in C3. For example, a colony of Brittany Spaniels with an autosomal recessive C3 deficiency has been described (Figure 7-15). Dogs that are homozygous for this trait have no detectable C3, whereas heterozygous animals have C3 levels that are approximately half normal. Heterozygous animals are clinically normal. The homozygous-deficient animals have

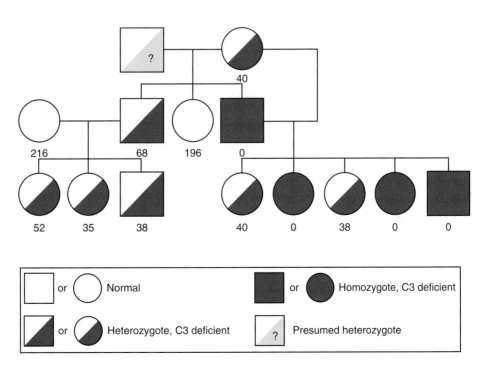

FIGURE 7-15 Inheritance of a C3 deficiency in a colony of Brittany Spaniels. The number below each circle or square represents the animal's C3 level as a percentage of a standard reference serum. The mean level in healthy spaniels was 126. (*Squares* denote males, *circles* denote females.)

(From Winkelstein JA, Cork LC, Griffin DE, et al: Genetically determined deficiency of the third component of complement in the dog, *Science* 212:1169–1170, 1981.)

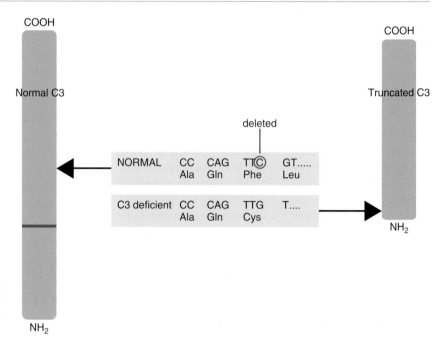

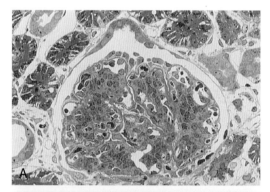

FIGURE 7-16 The mutation that results in canine C3 deficiency. Deletion of a cytosine results in a frame shift and premature termination of transcription of the C3 gene.

lower IgG levels than normal, and their ability to make antibodies against defined antigens is reduced. These dogs tend to make more IgM and less IgG. They experience recurrent sepsis, pneumonia, pyometra, and wound infections. The organisms involved include *Clostridium* species, *Pseudomonas* species, *E. coli*, and *Klebsiella* species. Some affected dogs develop amyloidosis, and many develop immune complex–mediated kidney disease (Chapter 30). The mutation responsible for this deficiency (deletion of a single cytosine) shortens the C3 chain as a result of a frameshift and the generation of a premature stop codon (Figure 7-16).

Porcine Factor H Deficiency

Factor H is a critical component of the alternative complement pathway. It normally inactivates C3b as soon as it is generated and so prevents excessive alternative pathway activation. If an animal fails to make factor H, C3b will be generated in an uncontrolled fashion. Factor H deficiency has been identified as an autosomal recessive trait in Yorkshire pigs. Affected piglets are healthy at birth and develop normally for a few weeks. However, eventually they fail to thrive, stop growing, become anemic, and die of renal failure.

On autopsy, multiple petechial hemorrhages are seen on the surface of the kidneys, accompanied by atrophy of the renal papillae. On light microscopy, alterations are seen in the renal glomeruli, that is, mesangial cell proliferation and capillary basement membrane thickening (Figure 7-17). On electron microscopy, extensive intramembranous electron-dense deposits are found within the glomerular basement membranes (Figure 7-18). This is typical of type II membranoproliferative glomerulonephritis (Chapter 30). Indirect immunofluorescence tests demonstrate massive deposits of C3 but no

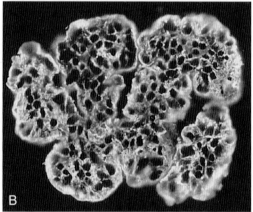

FIGURE 7-17 A, A thin section of the glomerulus of a piglet with factor H deficiency. Note the thickened basement membrane and increased numbers of mesangial cells, hence the name membranoproliferative glomerulonephritis. **B,** An immunofluorescence photomicrograph of another glomerulus from a factor H–deficient piglet. This is stained with fluorescent anti-C3. The bright fluorescence indicates the presence of C3 deposited in this glomerulus. Compare this figure with Figure 28-10.

(**A,** Courtesy of Johan H. Jansen; **B,** from Jansen JH, Hogasen K, Mollnes TE: Extensive complement activation in hereditary porcine membranoproliferative glomerulonephritis type II (porcine dense deposit disease, *Am J Pathol* 143:1356–1365, 1993.)

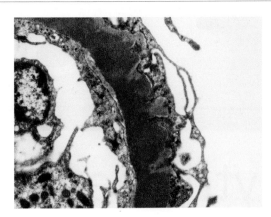

FIGURE 7-18 Electron micrograph showing dense intramembranous deposits in the glomerulus of a piglet with factor H deficiency.

(From Jansen JH: Porcine membranoproliferative glomerulonephritis with intramembranous dense deposits (porcine dense deposit disease, *APMIS* 101:281–289, 1993.)

immunoglobulins in the basement membranes. C3 can be found in the glomeruli before birth, but the morphological changes (mesangial proliferation and intramembranous dense deposits) are never seen before 5 days of age. These pigs have no plasma C3.

Nephritic piglets are almost totally deficient in factor H (2% of normal levels), whereas heterozygotes have half the normal levels. If factor H is replaced by plasma transfusions, the progress of the disease can be slowed and piglets survive longer. Since heterozygotes are readily detected by measurement of plasma C3, this disease can be eradicated from affected herds.

Other Complement Deficiencies

Mannose-binding lectin deficiency has been described in children, in whom it results in increased susceptibility to infection. It has not yet been described in domestic animals. In contrast to the severe effects of a C3 deficiency, congenital deficiencies of other complement components in laboratory animals or humans are not necessarily lethal. Thus individuals with C6 or C7 deficiencies have been described who are quite healthy. Apparently healthy C6-deficient pigs have been described. The lack of discernible effect of these deficiencies suggests that the terminal portion of the complement pathway leading to TCC formation may not be biologically essential.

For sources of additional information, please visit http://evolve.elsevier.com/tizard/immunology/

8

Cell Signaling: Cytokines and Their Receptors

□ Chapter Outline

Key Points

- The immune responses result from multiple interactions among many different cell populations.
- One way that these cells interact is by secreting specialized signaling molecules such as cytokines and hormones.
- These signaling molecules bind to specific receptors on target cells.
- When signaling molecules bind to their receptors, transcription factors are generated. These transcription factors then activate the transcription of selected genes.
- As a result of changes in gene transcription, new proteins are produced and secreted, and affected cells alter their behavior, perhaps by dividing or even dying on command.

The immune systems form complex networks involving many different cell types, each sending and receiving multiple messages from many different sources. Intercellular signals are transmitted in two general ways. One method is called volume transmission. In volume transmission, a mediator molecule is released by the signaling cell and diffuses through the extracellular fluid to the receiving cell, where it binds to cell surface receptors. The second method, called network transmission, occurs when two cells come into direct contact using complementary receptors. Signals are then transmitted directly between these two receptors.

Irrespective of how the signals are transmitted, by signaling through appropriate receptors, target cells can be directed to behave in a specific manner. They may be told to divide or stop dividing; they may be stimulated to secrete their own signaling molecules or express new receptors; they may be told to commit suicide. Each cell may be exposed to many different signaling molecules at any one time. The target cell must

integrate these signals and respond appropriately. In this chapter, we review the signaling molecules secreted by cells, the receptors that receive these signals, and the way in which the received signals are interpreted by the receiving cell.

The cells of the immune system can synthesize and secrete hundreds of different proteins that control the immune responses by communicating among cells. These proteins are called cytokines (Box 8-1). Cytokines differ from conventional hormones in several important respects. For example, unlike conventional hormones, which tend to affect a single target cell type, cytokines can affect many different cell types. Second, immune system cells rarely secrete a single cytokine at a time. For instance, macrophages secrete at least four interleukins (IL-1, IL-6, IL-12, IL-18) as well as tumor necrosis factor-α (TNF-α). Third, cytokines are "redundant" in their biological activities in that many different cytokines have similar effects. For example, IL-1, TNF-α, TNF-β, IL-6, high mobility group box protein-1 (HMGB1), and the chemokine CCL3 all act on

□ Box 8-1 | **Properties of Cytokines**

- Short-lived proteins
- Highly diverse structures and receptors
- Can act locally and/or systemically
- Pleiotropic: affect many different cells
- Redundant: exhibit biologically overlapping functions
- Carefully regulated
- Toxic in high doses

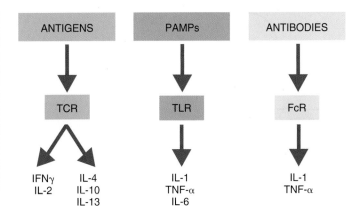

FIGURE 8-1 Three of the most important pathways that trigger cytokine release are the combination of antigens with their receptors on T and B cells, the combination of PAMPs with toll-like receptors on sentinel cells; and the combination of antibodies with Fc receptors on phagocytic cells.

the brain to cause a fever. Finally, cytokine-mediated signals are transient, and the messages delivered may vary over time as the cytokine environment changes.

Cytokine Nomenclature

The nomenclature and classification of the cytokines is not based on any systematic relationship among these proteins. Many were originally named after their cell of origin or the bioassay used to identify them.

The interleukins, for example, are cytokines that mediate signaling between lymphocytes and other leukocytes. They are numbered sequentially in the order of their discovery. Because their definition is so broad, the interleukins are a heterogeneous mixture of proteins with little in common except their name. As of 2011, 37 different numbered interleukins have been described. As might be expected, we know a lot about some of these molecules and very little about others. Likewise, some are clearly critical to a successful immune response, whereas others appear to be much less essential.

The interferons are cytokines produced in response to virus infection or immune stimulation. Their name is derived from the fact that they interfere with viral RNA and protein synthesis and so have antiviral activity (Chapter 26). There are three types of interferon. Type I interferons are a diverse family, the most important of which are interferon-α (IFN-α) and IFN-β. There is a single type II interferon, called IFN-γ. Three type III interferons (IFN–λ) have been identified. Type I interferons are primarily antiviral with a secondary immunoregulatory role. For type II and type III interferons such as IFN-γ and IFN–λ, the reverse is the case. Many type I interferons also play an important role in the maintenance of pregnancy.

TNFs are cytokines secreted by macrophages and T cells. As their name suggests, they can kill tumor cells, although this is not their primary function. Thus TNF-α is the key mediator of acute inflammation. The TNFs belong to a large family of related cytokines, the TNF superfamily, which is involved in immune regulation and inflammation. Other important members of the TNF superfamily include CD178 (also called CD95L or Fas ligand) (Chapter 18), and CD154 (CD40 ligand) (Chapter 14).

Many cytokines are growth factors (or colony-stimulating factors) and regulate blood cell production by regulating stem cell activities. They thereby ensure that the body is supplied with sufficient cells to defend itself.

Chemokines are a family of at least 50 small cytokines that play an important role in leukocyte chemotaxis, circulation, migration, and activation, especially in inflammation. A typical example of a chemokine is CXCL8 (also known as IL-8). Chemokines are described in detail in Chapter 3.

Cytokine Functions

Cytokines are produced in response to many different stimuli. Examples of these stimuli include antigens acting through the T cell or B cell antigen receptors; antigen-antibody complexes acting through antibody receptors (FcR); pathogen-associated molecular patterns (PAMPs) such as lipopolysaccharides acting through toll-like receptors (TLRs); and other cytokines acting through cytokine receptors (Figure 8-1).

Cytokines act on many different cellular targets. They may, for example, bind to receptors on the cell that produced them and thus have an autocrine effect. Alternatively, they may bind only to receptors on nearby cells; this is called a paracrine effect. Some cytokines may spread throughout the body, affecting target cells in distant locations, and thus have an endocrine effect (Figure 8-2).

When cytokines bind to receptors on target cells, they affect cell behavior. They may induce the target cell to divide or differentiate, or they may stimulate the production of new proteins. Alternatively they may inhibit these effects—preventing division, differentiation, or new protein synthesis. Most cytokines act on many different target cell types, perhaps inducing different responses in each one, a feature that is called pleiotropy. Conversely, many different cytokines may act on a single target, a feature known as redundancy. For example, IL-3,

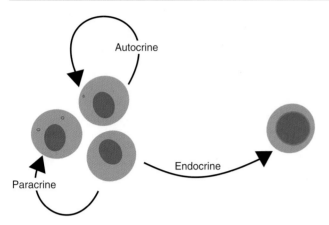

FIGURE 8-2 The distinction among autocrine, paracrine, and endocrine effects. Cytokines differ from hormones in that most of their effects are autocrine or paracrine, whereas hormones usually act on distant cells in an endocrine fashion.

□ Table 8-1 | Molecular Classification of Selected Cytokines

STRUCTURAL FAMILIES	STRUCTURE	EXAMPLES
Group 1	Four α helix bundle	IL-2, -3, -4, -5, -6, -7, -9, -11, -13, -15, -21, -23, -30; GM-CSF, erythropoietin, G-CSF, prolactin, leptin
	IFN subfamily	IFN-α/β, IFN-γ, IFN–λ
	IL-10 subfamily	IL-10, -19, -20, -22, -24, -26
Group 2	β Sheets	TNFs; TGF-β; IL-1α, -1β, -18
Group 3	α Helices and β sheets	Chemokines
Group 4	Mixed motifs	IL-12
Ungrouped	Unique structures	IL-17A-F, -14, -16

IL-4, IL-5, and IL-6 all affect B cell function. Some cytokines work best when paired with other cytokines in a process called synergy. For example, the combination of IL-4 and IL-5 stimulates B cells to make immunoglobulin E (IgE) and hence triggers an allergic response. Synergy can also occur in sequence when, for example, one cytokine induces the target cell to express the receptor for another cytokine. Finally, some cytokines have opposing effects and may antagonize the effects of others. The best example of this is the mutual antagonism of IL-4 and IFN-γ.

Cytokine Structure

Cytokines are complex proteins with many diverse structures. They are classified based on these structures (Table 8-1). Thus the largest family, the group I cytokines (or hematopoietins), consist of four α helices bundled together. This family includes many different interleukins as well as growth hormone and leptin. Within the group I cytokines are two major subfamilies, the interferon subfamily and the IL-10 subfamily. Group II cytokines consist of long-chain β-sheet structures. They include the TNFs, the IL-1 family, and transforming growth factor-β (TGF-β). Group III cytokines are small proteins with both α helices and β sheets. These include the chemokines and related molecules. Group IV cytokines use mixtures of domains with mixtures of structural motifs and include the IL-12 family. Many cytokines, such as the IL-17 family, IL-14, and IL-16, are structurally unique proteins and do not belong to any of these major structural families.

Patterns may also be seen in the biological activities of these cytokines. Thus group I cytokines tend to be involved in immune regulation or stem cell regulation. Group II cytokines are mainly involved in the growth and regulation of cells, cell death, and inflammation. Group III cytokines are involved in inflammation. The activities of the group IV cytokines depend on their subcomponents. For example, IL-12 is formed by a combination of a group I structure with a stem cell receptor, but it acts like a group I cytokine.

Cytokine Receptors

Cytokines act through cell surface receptors. These receptors consist of at least two functional units, one for ligand binding and one for signal transduction (Figure 8-3). These units may or may not be on the same protein chain. Cytokine receptors can also be classified into classes based on their structure.

One class of receptor includes the channel-linked receptors, which act as transmitter-gated ion channels. Thus the receptor itself is a channel, and binding of its ligand opens that channel, allowing ions to pass through it. Channel-linked receptors are found in inflammatory and immune cells, but their roles are unclear. They do not serve as cytokine receptors.

A second class of receptor consists of proteins that also act as tyrosine kinases (Figure 8-4). These are typically growth factor and cytokine receptors. In these cases, binding of the ligand to two adjacent receptors forms an active dimer. The ligand-binding site, the membrane-spanning region, and the tyrosine kinase are usually separate domains of a single protein. Thus when the ligand binds to the extracellular domain, the receptor chains dimerize so that the two tyrosine kinases are brought together and activate each other. These kinases phosphorylate tyrosine residues on other proteins or even the receptor itself (autophosphorylation). Since many of these other proteins are also tyrosine kinases, phosphorylation also converts them to an active state. In this way a cascade of expanding phosphorylations develops within the cell (Figure 8-5).

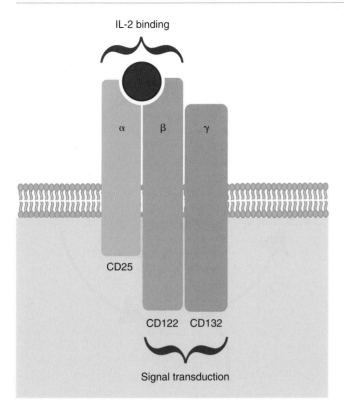

FIGURE 8-3 The structure of a cytokine receptor—in this case, the IL-2 receptor complex. The complete trimer serves as a high-affinity receptor, whereas the β–γ dimer serves as a low-affinity receptor. Note that different receptor components each serve different functions.

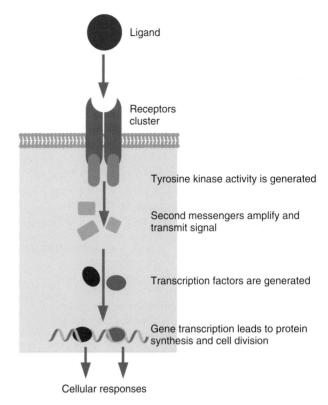

FIGURE 8-4 A generic view of signal transduction involving the activation of tyrosine kinases. Although receptor signaling varies in its details and intricacy, the overall process of signal transduction has some consistent features as shown here.

Phosphorylation triggers changes in cellular activities (Box 8-2). Many cytokines and other immunological signals operate through this type of receptor (especially through tyrosine kinases of the src family).

A related class of receptor consists of proteins that are not themselves tyrosine kinases but can activate tyrosine kinases associated with the receptors. This type of receptor is also widely employed in the cells of the immune system. Examples of tyrosine kinase–linked receptors include the T cell antigen receptor (TCR) and the B cell antigen receptor (BCR). Some of these tyrosine kinases may transfer their phosphate groups to transcription factors within the nucleus and activate them. Others act indirectly through the production of second messenger molecules.

A large class of receptors are coupled to membrane-bound guanosine triphosphate (GTP)–binding proteins, called G-proteins. G-proteins act as chemical switches and so control many different cellular processes. When the receptor is inactive, they bind guanosine diphosphate (GDP). When bound to their ligand they exchange the GDP for GTP (Figure 8-6). The activated G-protein then activates other substrates, resulting in a biological response. The GTP is rapidly hydrolyzed to GDP so that the G-protein is then turned off. The targets of G-proteins include ion channels, enzymes such as adenylate cyclase, phospholipase C, and some protein kinases.

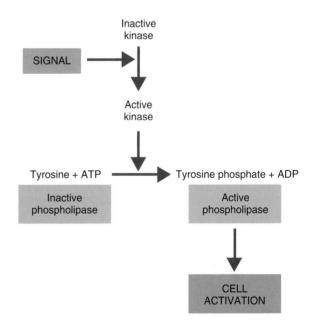

FIGURE 8-5 The key to signal transduction and cellular activation is the phosphorylation of the amino acid tyrosine by the actions of a tyrosine kinase. For example, phosphorylation of tyrosine by a protein kinase can result in phospholipase activation, which leads eventually to cell activation. Phosphorylation can have many other different effects on protein functions and fate.

□ Box 8-2 | Protein Phosphorylation

Central to most signaling is protein phosphorylation by receptor kinases. Phosphorylation is a form of reversible modification of proteins. All signal transduction systems involve the use of a high-energy phosphate-rich compound such as adenosine triphosphate (ATP) to modify a protein and send a signal to a cell. Cell growth, cell division, and other critical processes are all regulated by protein phosphorylation. Protein kinases enzymatically phosphorylate the amino acids serine, threonine, and tyrosine.

$$\text{Protein} + \text{ATP} \xrightarrow{\text{Protein kinase}} \text{protein-P} + \text{ADP}$$

In some proteins, only one amino acid is phosphorylated; in others, multiple amino acids are phosphorylated. Phosphorylated and nonphosphorylated proteins have different functional properties. For example, the phosphorylation of serine or threonine activates some enzymes, whereas dephosphorylation has the opposite effect. Phosphorylation of three key amino acids (serine, threonine, and tyrosine) plays a critical role in the regulation of many cellular functions. When phosphorylated proteins are examined, about 90% of the phosphate is linked to serine and about 10% to threonine. Only about 1/2000 of the phosphate is linked to tyrosine. Thus tyrosine phosphorylation is a rare event. Nevertheless it is a key mechanism in almost all the signal transduction pathways described in this book.

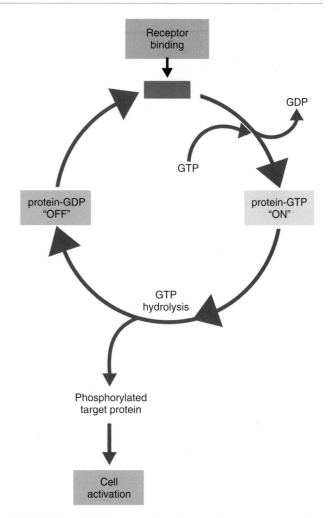

FIGURE 8-6 GTP-binding proteins (G-proteins) can act as signaling switches to turn cell functions on and off. They are often activated in the initial stages of signal transduction.

When activated by a G-protein, phospholipase C splits the membrane-bound lipid, phosphatidylinositol 4,5-bisphosphate (PIP_2), into two messenger molecules, inositol trisphosphate and diacylglycerol (Figure 8-7). Inositol trisphosphate binds to intracellular receptors releasing Ca^{2+} from internal stores and increases the concentration of intracellular Ca^{2+}. These calcium ions can activate many different proteins. The diacylglycerol remains in the plasma membrane and along with calcium activates an enzyme called protein kinase C. Immunological receptors that employ G-proteins include the receptors for C5a, chemokine receptors, leukotriene receptors, and the platelet-activating factor receptor. In neutrophils, G-proteins control responses to chemoattractants.

A fourth class of receptor acts in a totally different manner. It activates a sphingomyelinase that then hydrolyzes the cell membrane phospholipids sphingomyelin to form ceramide. The ceramide then activates a serine-threonine protein kinase that phosphorylates cellular proteins. This mechanism of signal transduction is used by the receptors for IL-1 and IFN-α.

Receptor Families

In general, most cytokines use receptors that act through tyrosine kinases. However, within this class, one can identify related families of receptors. For example, the IL-1/TLR receptor family participates in host responses to injury and infection. The family can be split into the molecules that are IL-1R-like (IL-1R1, IL-18R) and the molecules that are toll-like (TLR). Ligation of these receptors triggers activation of the transcription factor NF-κB (see Figure 2-4).

Another large receptor family, the group I cytokine receptor family, includes among its members the receptors for IL-2 (β chain), IL-4, IL-5, IL-6, IL-12, granulocyte colony-stimulating factor (G-CSF), and granulocyte-macrophage colony-stimulating factor (GM-CSF) (Figure 8-8). It also includes the common γ chain of IL-2, IL-4, IL-7, IL-9, and IL-15 receptors. These receptor chains dimerize in the presence of the ligand and form complexes with a separate kinase called a Janus kinase (JAK). JAK in turn phosphorylates a cytosolic protein called STAT (signal transducers and activators of transcription). STAT then dimerizes to form an active transcription factor.

The members of the group II cytokine receptor family have a very different structure. They bind interferons (α, β, γ, and λ) and members of the IL-10 cytokine family (IL-19, -20, -22,

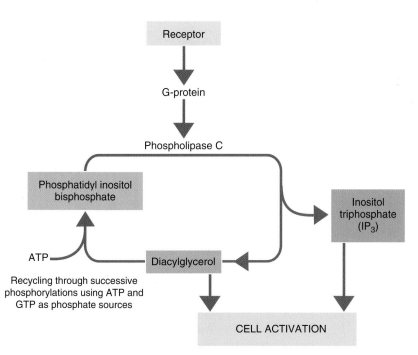

FIGURE 8-7 Activation of cell membrane phospholipase C generates both inositol triphosphate and diacylglycerol. These two molecules are messengers that initiate cell activation. The signaling molecules can then be recycled by phosphorylation.

-24, -26). These receptors also form heterodimers in the presence of the ligand and signal through the JAK-STAT pathway.

Cytokine Regulation

Cytokine signaling is regulated in three major ways: by changes in receptor expression, by specific binding proteins, and by cytokines that exert opposite effects. For example, IL-2 receptor expression largely determines the response of T cells to IL-2. Resting T cells express few receptors for IL-2 but many more once activated. In contrast, the activities of IL-1 are regulated by a receptor antagonist called IL-1RA. IL-1RA is an inactive form of the cytokine that binds to the IL-1 receptor but does not stimulate signal transduction. It therefore competes with and blocks the activities of active IL-1 (Figure 8-9). Other cytokines may bind to soluble receptors in body fluids. Examples include the soluble receptors for IL-1, IL-2, IL-4, IL-5, IL-6, IL-7, IL-9, TNF-α, and macrophage colony-stimulating factor (M-CSF). In most cases these soluble receptors compete for cytokine binding to cell surface receptors and hence inhibit cytokine activity. Cytokines such as IL-1, IL-12, and TGF-β may bind to glycosaminoglycans such as heparin or CD44 in connective tissue, where they form a reservoir of readily available molecules.

Some cytokine receptors act as decoys. They bind cytokines but do not transmit signals. The IL-1 type II receptor is such a receptor. Other decoy receptors have been identified for members of the IL1/IL-18 family as well as for the TNF, IL-10, and IL-13 receptor families. A receptor called D6 acts as a decoy for many different inflammatory chemokines.

Perhaps the most important way by which cytokine function is regulated is through the opposing effects of different cytokines. For example, IL-4 stimulates B cells to switch to IgE production, whereas IFN-γ suppresses IgE production (Chapter 28). Likewise IL-10 inhibits the activities of many other cytokines (see Figure 20-12).

It is also important to bear in mind that at any given time, a single cell may receive signals from multiple cytokine receptors. It must somehow integrate these multiple signals to produce a coherent response.

Signal Transduction

Cytokines are agonists for their cell surface receptors. Once a cytokine binds its receptor, the receptor transmits a signal to the cell to modify its behavior. This conversion of an extracellular signal into a series of intracellular events is called signal transduction. The key components of signal transduction include binding of an agonist to its receptor, possibly clustering of receptor chains, activation of kinases by the receptor, secondary activation of second messengers, generation of new transcription factors, and gene activation leading to altered protein synthesis and cell behavior (see Figure 8-4). Because cell signaling must be fast and precise, this is best accomplished by enzyme cascades. Since enzymes can produce or modify a large number of molecules very rapidly, a pathway that involves the use of several enzymes in sequence can amplify responses very rapidly.

Transduction Pathways

Although there are many different signal transduction pathways, three play key roles in the immune system. These involve the generation of the transcription factors: NF-κB, NF-AT, and JAK-STAT.

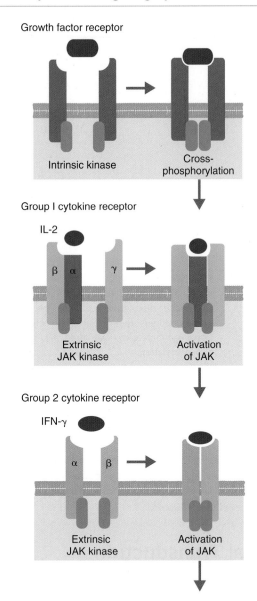

FIGURE 8-8 The major types of cytokine receptors. In all cases, protein kinases are activated by ligand binding. For example, growth factor receptors associate in the presence of their ligand to form a dimer. This brings the two tyrosine kinases on the cytoplasmic domains close together. The enzymes then activated each other by cross-phosphorylation. Group I cytokine receptors, so called because they bind the type 1 cytokines, associate in the presence of the ligand to form oligomers and form complexes with JAK kinases. When brought together, the JAK kinases are activated and in turn activate STAT proteins. The activated STAT proteins then dissociate and activate transcription factors. Group II cytokines such as the interferons and IL-10 bind receptors that have a similar mode of action to type I receptors. They differ, however, in their conserved sequences.

NF-κB Pathway The NF-κB pathway is probably the most significant signal transduction pathway in the immune system. It is the pathway that is activated when antigens bind to the T cell and B cell antigen receptors, TCR and BCR; when PAMPs bind to the pattern-recognition receptors (PRRs), such as the TLRs and nucleotide-binding oligomerization domains

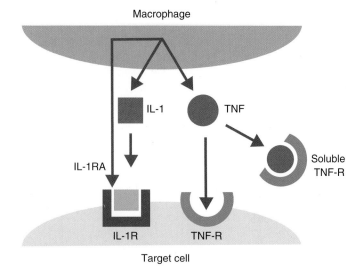

FIGURE 8-9 The control of cytokine activities as exemplified by IL-1 and TNF-α. IL-1 activity is regulated by the presence of IL-1RA, an inert isoform that binds and blocks the IL-1 receptor, preventing signal transduction. Soluble TNF-αR, in contrast, competes for TNF-α with the cell membrane receptor but also serves to inhibit cytokine signaling.

(NODs); and when TNF binds to its receptor. The term NF-κB refers to a family of five transcription factors that play a central role in both inflammation and immunity. More than 150 different stimuli can activate NF-κB, and more than 150 genes are expressed after NF-κB activation. NF-κB occurs in the cytosol in an inactive form associated with a protein called IκB. IκB inhibits NF-κB activity by masking its nuclear binding site. Thus in resting cells, NF-κB cannot move to the nucleus or activate genes.

Three major NF-κB activation pathways are recognized. The classical pathway is involved in proinflammatory signaling. It is triggered by inflammatory cytokines (IL-1 and TNF-α), TLRs, and antigen receptors and is essential for innate immunity. The signals induced by these stimuli converge on a central regulator of NF-κB, the IKK (IκB kinase) complex. This complex consists of multiple subunits with kinase activity. When activated, the IKK complex phosphorylates IκB. As a result, the IκB dissociates from the NF-κB and is destroyed. This permits the NF-κB to enter the nucleus, where it activates promoters on DNA molecules. As a result, many genes, including those encoding the cytokines IL-1β, IL-6, IL-18, IL-33, TNF-α, GM-CSF, and IL-4, are activated. NF-κB also activates the genes coding for several different chemokines, pro-angiogenic factors, adhesion molecules such as intercellular adhesion molecule 1 (ICAM-1), antiapoptotic proteins, inducible enzymes such as iNOS and cyclooxygenase-2 (COX-2), and IκB. This newly synthesized IκB will eventually bind and suppress NF-κB activation. Molecules or organisms that block the destruction of IκB have antiinflammatory and immunosuppressive effects. For example, corticosteroids stimulate the production of excess IκB, whereas some bacteria can block its degradation. Either way, the activation of cells and the development of inflammation and immune responses may be blocked. A second NF-κB pathway (sometimes called the alternative pathway) is triggered by some TNF receptors. This pathway is essential for lymphocyte development and activation. The third NF-κB pathway is activated by DNA-damaging drugs and ultraviolet light and does not involve IKK activation.

An example of the role of the NF-κB pathway is seen in TLR responses in macrophages (Figure 8-10). Thus occupation of a TLR by a PAMP from an invader causes the receptor to dimerize. As a result, it binds several adaptor molecules, of which one, MyD88 (myeloid differentiation primary response gene 88) is the most important. When MyD88 complexes with the TLR, it also binds two kinases called IRAK-1 and IRAK-4. IRAK-4 activates IRAK-1, and these in turn recruit TRAF6. TRAF6 and other proteins then activate the IKK complex. Activation of IKK phosphorylates IkB, causing its destruction and the release of active NF-κB. The NF-κB in turn enters the nucleus and activates the genes that encode the cytokines TNF-α, IL-1β, and caspase-1. Caspase-1 activates these newly produced cytokines that then trigger inflammation. Binding

of antigen to the TCR also activates NF-κB. Thus activation of the TCR activates a protein kinase C to form the CBM protein complex. (CARMA1, BCL10, and MALT1). This complex promotes the degradation of IKK. Another pathway involves stabilization of NF-κB–inducing kinase (NIK). This activates IKKα, which promotes the destruction of IkB by proteasomes. All NF-κB members affect TCR-induced T cell proliferation. Antigen dose and oscillations in calcium concentrations also play a key role in T cell differentiation by modulating the movement of transcription factors between the nucleus and cytoplasm.

NF-AT Pathway When an antigen binds to its receptor on a T cell, the signal is first transmitted from the antigen-binding receptor (TCR) to a signal transducing complex called CD3, where it causes the CD3 chains to cluster together in lipid rafts (Figure 8-11). Each CD3 protein has specific amino acid sequences in its cytoplasmic domains called immunoreceptor tyrosine–based, activation motifs (ITAMs). When the CD3

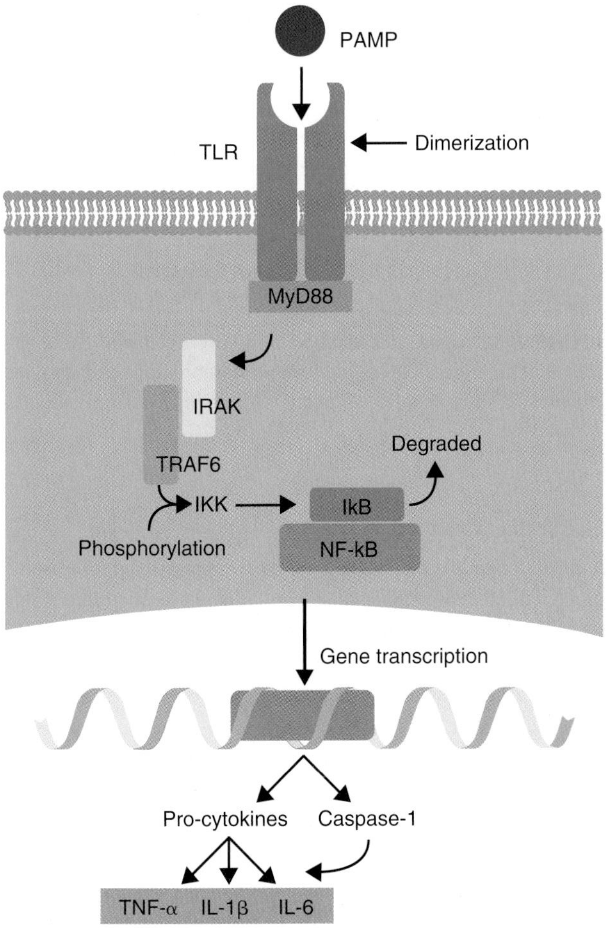

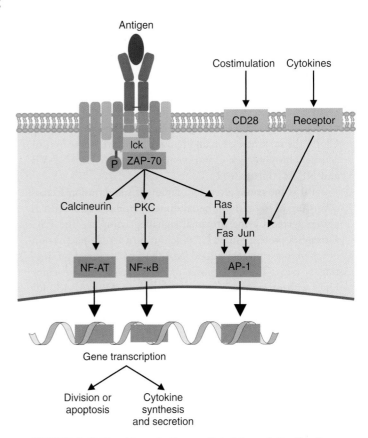

FIGURE 8-10 One major pathway of signal transduction is mediated by the transcription factor NF-κB. This is widely employed in immunologic signaling such as the response to sentinel cells to activation of their TLRs by PAMPs.

FIGURE 8-11 Signal transduction mediated through T cell antigen receptors generates three transcription factors: NF-AT, NF-κB, and AP-1. When TCRs cluster, they activate several protein kinases. The most important of these is called ZAP-70. This in turn triggers three signaling pathways and, with appropriate costimulation, generates multiple transduction factors. The jun-fos heterodimer (AP-1) is required to stimulate the genes for cytokines and their receptors. The final results of the stimulus include cell division or apoptosis as well as cytokine production.

chains cluster, their ITAMs bind and activate several tyrosine kinases (TKs). These tyrosine kinases are members of the Src-kinase family. They include lck and fyn in T cells and NK cells, and lyn and fyn in B cells and mast cells. In T cells, the first TK activated, called lck, phosphorylates the ITAMs. As a result, these sites then bind a second TK, called zeta-associated protein-70 (ZAP-70). The bound ZAP-70 is phosphorylated and after binding many other proteins forms a multimolecular proximal signaling complex (PSC). Signals generated by the PSC then activate at least three families of transcription factors. One pathway generates the second messengers, diacylglycerol and inositol trisphosphate. The inositol trisphosphate releases calcium ions from intracellular organelles and opens trans-membrane channels, allowing Ca^{2+} to enter the cell and raising intracellular calcium. This in turn activates a phosphatase called calcineurin. Calcineurin removes a phosphate from NF-AT. Dephosphorylated NF-AT enters the nucleus and with the help of another transcription factor called activator protein-1 (AP-1), binds to the promoters of at least 100 genes. The potent immunosuppressive drugs tacrolimus and cyclosporine bind to calcineurin and can block T cell–mediated responses (see Figures 39-4 and 39-5). If the T cell receives suppressive signals, such as those provided by IL-10 or TGF-β, this causes NF-AT to associate with a different transcription factor called Foxp3. Foxp3 activates a very different set of genes and converts the cell into a regulatory T cell (Treg) that suppresses immune responses (Chapter 20).

In B cells, the adaptor molecules Ig-α and Ig-β also have ITAMs. When aggregated by antigen and co-stimulated by CD19, the src kinases, lyn and fyn, are activated. These in turn activate phospholipase C and eventually generate both NF-VB and NF-AT (Figure 8-12).

AP-1 is the name given to a family of transcription factors consisting of fos and jun heterodimers. Production of AP-1 is also triggered by the proximal signaling complex. The PSC activates a protein kinase C, which in turn leads to activation of ras-mitogen protein kinase (MAPK) and increased production of c-fos. The c-fos moves to the nucleus, where it combines with preexisting jun proteins to form AP-1. AP-1 binds with NF-AT proteins integrating the calcium signaling with the ras-MPCK pathway. Collectively they stimulate the genes coding for IL-2, IFN-γ, GM-CSF, TNF-α, IL-3, IL-4, IL-13, IL-5, FasL, and CD25.

JAK-STAT Pathway Almost 40 different cytokines use the JAK-STAT pathway, including interleukins such as IL-4, -7, -11, -12, and -13, leptin, GM-CSF, and IFN-γ. They use group I cytokine receptors that consist of two identical transmembrane proteins. Ligand binding to the receptor causes its dimerization, which leads in turn to activation of the tightly associated JAK. These activated JAK molecules phosphorylate tyrosine residues on one of several STAT proteins. The phosphorylated STAT proteins then dimerize, dissociate from JAK, and move to the nucleus, where they act as transcription factors and modulate the expression of target genes. There are four JAK and seven STAT family members currently recognized. A

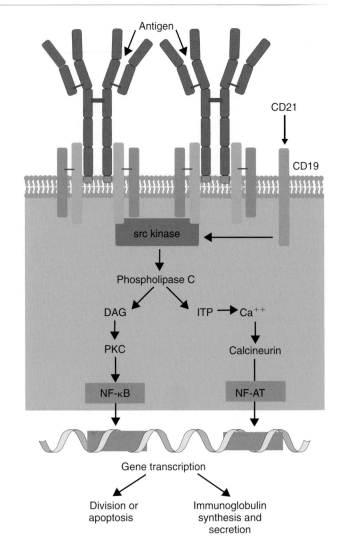

FIGURE 8-12 Signal transduction by two cross-linked BCRs activates B cells, triggering cell division, differentiation, and immunoglobulin synthesis. Both NF-κB and NF-AT are involved in B cell signal transduction.

specific JAK-STAT combination is paired with each cytokine receptor. For example, receptors for the growth factors usually use JAK2. Receptors with the common γ chain preferentially use JAK1 and JAK3. The IFN-γ receptor uses JAK 1 and JAK2. The IL-4R uses JAK1 and JAK3. Presumably the precise outcome of this signaling depends on which specific combination of JAK and STAT is activated.

Although the pathways described earlier are of greatest importance in cells of the immune system, many other transcription factors have been identified and on activation can trigger cell differentiation. This is especially important in the T cell system, where the cells are plastic and can readily transform from one subset to another. These transcription factors include T-bet, which controls transcription of IFN–γ in Th1 cells; GATA3, which controls cytokine transcription in Th2 cells; ROR γT, which that acts in Th17 cells; and FoxP3, which acts in Treg cells.

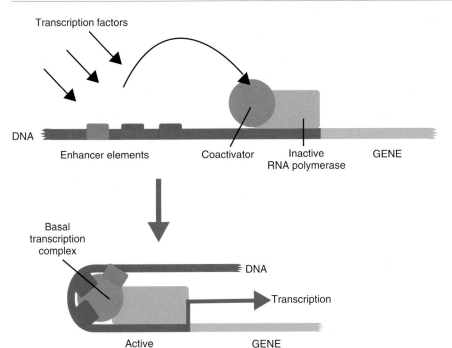

FIGURE 8-13 Transcription factors bind to enhancer elements on DNA located upstream of the genes they activate. Gene transcription is turned on by a carefully regulated RNA polymerase. However, the polymerase can only be turned on when transcription factors form a basal transcription complex and activate the basic transcriptional machinery.

Gene Transcription

The activity of each gene in a cell is carefully regulated. Central to gene control, however, are the transcription factors. Activation of genes depends on the presence of an appropriate mixture of transcription factors. As described earlier, these transcription factors are only generated when a cell receives an appropriate signal. The transcription factors then collectively activate the appropriate RNA polymerase, and gene transcription begins.

Transcription factors have two binding sites. One site binds DNA; the other binds regulatory proteins. When a transcription factor is generated, it enters the nucleus and binds to specific DNA control elements located between 50 and 200 bases upstream from the start site of the gene (Figure 8-13). Transcription factors may also bind to enhancer elements located thousands of bases upstream. These bound transcription factors then use their other binding site to bind either directly to basal transcription complexes or to coactivator molecules. This leads to assembly of the basal transcription complex. The basal transcription complex, together with attached coactivator molecules, then binds to the RNA polymerase and activates it. It is believed that the conformation of the polymerase changes when activated and that this permits transcription of the selected genes to begin.

For sources of additional information, please visit http://evolve.elsevier.com/tizard/immunology/

Antigens: Triggers of Adaptive Immunity

Key Points

- The adaptive immune system is optimized to recognize microbial macromolecules.
- The best antigens are therefore large, complex, stable, foreign proteins.
- Small molecules of less than 5000 Da are usually poor antigens.
- Small molecules may be made antigenic by linking them to large proteins. Small molecules used as antigens in this way are called haptens.
- The cells of the adaptive immune system use receptors that can recognize specific areas on the surface of foreign molecules. These areas are called antigenic determinants or epitopes.

Up to now we have considered only the body's innate reactions to microbial invasion. Innate responses are triggered by recognition of conserved microbial pathogen-associated molecular patterns (PAMPs) such as microbial nucleic acids or lipopolysaccharides. The triggering of inflammation and the mobilization of phagocytic cells such as neutrophils and macrophages by these molecules contributes to the rapid destruction of microbial invaders. Although this may be sufficient to protect the body, it cannot be guaranteed to provide complete resistance to infection. Nor does the body learn from the experience. Thus a more potent immune response should ideally recognize all the foreign molecules on an invading microbe. In addition, such a response would be able to learn from this experience and, given time, evolve more efficient procedures to combat subsequent invasions. This new and improved response is the function of the adaptive immune system.

During an adaptive immune response, molecules from invading organisms are captured, processed, and presented to the cells of the immune system. These cells have surface receptors that can bind appropriately presented molecules. These bound molecules or antigens then trigger a powerful immune response that ensures an animal's survival. In addition, the immune system "remembers" these antigens, makes minor adjustments, and by adapting, responds even more effectively when it encounters these organisms again.

Antigens

Since the function of the adaptive immune system is to defend the body against invading microorganisms, it is essential that these organisms be recognized as soon as they invade the body. The body must be able to recognize that these are foreign (and dangerous) if they are to stimulate an immune response. The innate immune system recognizes only a limited number of PAMPs—those that are characteristic of major groups of pathogens. The adaptive immune system, in contrast, can recognize and respond to almost all the foreign macromolecules present in an invading microorganism. These foreign macromolecules are called antigens.

Microbial Antigens

Bacterial Antigens

Bacteria are single-celled prokaryotic organisms consisting of a cytoplasm containing the essential elements of cell structure surrounded by a lipid-rich cytoplasmic membrane (Figure 9-1). Outside the cytoplasmic membrane is a thick, carbohydrate-rich cell wall. The major components of the bacterial surface thus include the cell wall and its associated protein structures, the capsule, the pili, and the flagella. The cell wall of Gram-positive organisms is largely composed of peptidoglycan (chains of alternating *N*-acetyl glucosamine and *N*-acetyl muramic acid cross-linked by short peptide side chains) (see Figure 2-2). Gram-positive cell walls also contain lipoteichoic acids that are involved in the transport of ions across the cell wall. The cell wall in Gram-negative organisms, in contrast,

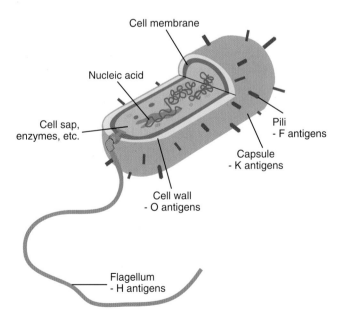

FIGURE 9-1 The structure of a typical bacterium and the location of its most important antigens.

consists of a thin layer of peptidoglycan covered by an outer membrane consisting of a lipopolysaccharide. Most of the antigenicity of Gram-negative bacteria is associated with the lipopolysaccharide. This consists of an oligosaccharide attached to a lipid (lipid A) and to a series of repeating trisaccharides. The structure of these trisaccharides determines the antigenicity of the organism. Many bacteria are classified according to this antigenic structure. For example, the genus *Salmonella* contains a major species, *Salmonella enterica*, that is classified into more than 2300 serovars based on antigenicity. These polysaccharide antigens are called O antigens. The outer cell wall lipopolysaccharides of Gram-negative bacteria bind to toll-like receptors (TLRs) and other pattern-recognition receptors and induce the production of inflammatory cytokines when an animal is infected. These cytokines cause a fever and sickness, so bacterial lipopolysaccharides are also called endotoxins.

Bacterial capsules consist mainly of polysaccharides that are usually good antigens. The capsules protect bacteria against phagocytosis and intracellular destruction, whereas anticapsular antibodies can overcome the effects of the capsule and protect an infected animal. Capsular antigens are collectively called K antigens.

Pili and fimbriae are short projections that cover the surfaces of some Gram-negative bacteria; they are classified as F or K antigens. Pili bind bacteria together and play a role in bacterial conjugation and movement. Fimbriae bind bacteria to cell surfaces. Antibodies to fimbrial proteins may be protective since they can prevent bacteria from sticking to body surfaces. Bacterial flagella are long filaments used for bacterial movement. They consist of a single protein called flagellin. Flagellar antigens are collectively called H antigens.

Other significant bacterial antigens include the porins, the heat-shock proteins, and the exotoxins. The porins are proteins that form pores on the surface of Gram-negative organisms. Heat-shock proteins are generated in large amounts in stressed bacteria. The exotoxins are toxic proteins secreted by bacteria or released into the surrounding environment when they die. Exotoxins are highly immunogenic proteins and stimulate the production of antibodies called antitoxins. Many exotoxins, when treated with a mild protein-denaturing agent such as formaldehyde, lose their toxicity but retain their antigenicity. Toxins modified in this way are called toxoids. Toxoids may be used as vaccines to prevent disease caused by toxigenic bacteria such as *Clostridium tetani*. Bacterial nucleic acids rich in unmethylated CpG sequences serve both as effective antigens for the adaptive immune system and as potent stimulators of innate immunity acting through TLRs.

Viral Antigens

Viruses are very small organisms that can grow only inside living cells. They are thus "obligate," intracellular parasites. Viruses usually have a relatively simple structure consisting of a nucleic acid core surrounded by a protein layer (Figure 9-2). This protein layer is termed the capsid, and it consists of

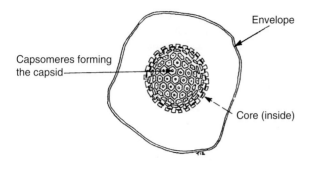

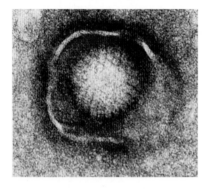

FIGURE 9-2 The structure of a virus. This is an electron micrograph of equine herpesvirus type 4 magnified 184,000 times. The virus is negatively stained; that is, the electron-dense "dye" has filled the low areas on the virion, leaving the higher areas unstained.

(Courtesy Dr. J. Thorsen.)

multiple subunits called capsomeres. Capsid proteins are good antigens, highly capable of stimulating antibody formation. Some viruses may also be surrounded by an envelope containing lipoproteins and glycoproteins. A complete viral particle is called a virion. When a virus infects an animal, the virion proteins are processed and trigger adaptive immune responses. Viruses, however, are not always found free in the circulation but live within cells, where they are protected from the unwelcome attentions of antibodies. Indeed, viral nucleic acid can be integrated into a cell's genome. In this situation, the viral genes code for new proteins, some of which are expressed on the surface of infected cells. These proteins, although they are synthesized inside an animal's own cells, can still bind to antigen receptors and provoke adaptive immunity. These newly synthesized foreign proteins are called endogenous antigens to distinguish them from the foreign antigens that enter from the outside and are called exogenous antigens.

Other Microbial Antigens

In addition to bacteria and viruses, animals may be invaded by fungi, protozoan parasites, arthropods, and even parasitic worms (helminths). Each of these organisms consists of many different structures composed of proteins, carbohydrates, lipids, and nucleic acids. Many of these can serve as antigens and trigger adaptive immunity. However, their antigenicity does vary, and the adaptive responses triggered by these

organisms are not always successful in protecting an animal or eliminating the invader.

Nonmicrobial Antigens

Invading microorganisms are not the only source of foreign material entering the body. Food contains many foreign molecules that under some circumstances may trigger immune responses and cause an allergic reaction. Likewise, inhaled dusts can contain antigenic particles such as pollen grains, and these may enter the body through the respiratory system. Foreign molecules may be injected directly into the body through a snake or mosquito bite, or by a veterinarian. Furthermore, foreign proteins may be injected into animals for experimental purposes. Organ grafts are an effective way of administering a large amount of foreign material to an animal.

Cell Surface Antigens

The outer membrane of every mammalian cell consists of a fluid lipid bilayer with a complex mixture of protein molecules embedded in it. Most of these proteins can act as antigens if they are injected into another species or even into a different individual of the same species. For example, glycoproteins known as blood-group antigens are found on the surface of red blood cells. Early attempts to transfuse blood between unrelated individuals usually met with disaster because the transfused cells were rapidly destroyed. Investigation revealed that the problem was due to the presence of naturally occurring antibodies against these foreign red cell glycoprotein antigens.

Nucleated cells, such as leukocytes, possess hundreds of different protein molecules on their surface. These proteins are good antigens and readily provoke an immune response when injected experimentally into a different species. These surface molecules are classified by the CD system (Chapter 4). Other cell surface proteins may provoke an immune response (such as graft rejection) if transferred into a genetically different individual of the same species. The cell surface proteins that trigger graft rejection are called histocompatibility antigens. Histocompatibility antigens are of such importance in immunology that they warrant a complete chapter of their own (Chapter 11).

Autoantigens

In some situations (and not always abnormal ones), an animal may mount immune responses against normal body components. These are called autoimmune responses. Antigens that induce autoimmunity are called autoantigens. They can include hormones, such as thyroglobulin; structural components, such as basement membranes; complex lipids, such as myelin; intracellular components, such as the mitochondrial proteins, nucleic acids, or nucleoproteins; and cell surface proteins, such as hormone receptors. The production of autoantibodies and the consequences of this are discussed in detail in Chapter 34.

What Makes a Good Antigen?

Molecules vary in their ability to act as antigens (their antigenicity) (Figure 9-3). In general, foreign proteins make the best antigens, especially if they are big (greater than 1000 Da is best). Many of the major antigens of microorganisms such as the clostridial toxins, bacterial flagella, virus capsids, and protozoan cell membranes are large proteins. Other important antigenic proteins include components of snake venoms, serum proteins, cell surface proteins, milk and food proteins, hormones, and even antibody molecules themselves.

Simple polysaccharides, such as starch or glycogen, are not good antigens simply because they are often degraded before the immune system has time to respond to them. More complex carbohydrates may be effective antigens, especially if bound to proteins. These include the major cell wall antigens of Gram-negative bacteria and the blood-group glycoproteins of red blood cells. Many of the so-called natural antibodies found in the serum of unimmunized animals are directed against polysaccharides and probably arise as a result of exposure to glycoproteins or carbohydrates from the intestinal microflora or from food. To this extent they can also be considered part of the innate immune system.

Lipids tend to be poor antigens because of their wide distribution, relative simplicity, structural instability, and rapid metabolism. Nevertheless, when linked to proteins or polysaccharides, lipids can trigger immune responses. Cells possess specific receptors used for the binding and processing of lipid, lipoprotein, and glycolipid antigens (Chapter 10).

Mammalian nucleic acids are very poor antigens because of their relative simplicity and flexibility and because they are very rapidly degraded. Microbial nucleic acids, on the other hand, have a structure very different from that found in eukaryotes with many unmethylated CpG sequences. As a result, they can stimulate potent immune responses. It is perhaps for this reason that autoantibodies to nucleic acids are produced in some important autoimmune diseases (Chapter 36).

Proteins are the most effective antigens because they have properties that best trigger an immune response. (More correctly, the adaptive immune system has evolved to trap, process, and then recognize foreign proteins). Thus large molecules are better antigens than small molecules, and proteins can be very large indeed (Figure 9-4). For example, hemocyanin, a very large protein from invertebrate blood (670 kDa) is a potent antigen. Serum albumin from other mammals (69 kDa) is a fairly good antigen but may also provoke tolerance. The small peptide hormone angiotensin (1031 Da) is a poor antigen.

Similarly, the more complex an antigen is, the better. For example, starch and other simple repeating polymers are poor antigens, but complex bacterial lipopolysaccharides are good. Complex proteins containing many different amino acids, especially aromatic ones, are better antigens than large, repeating polymers, such as lipids, carbohydrates, and nucleic acids.

Structural stability is an important feature of good antigens, especially those that trigger antibody responses. To bind to a foreign molecule, the cell surface receptors of the adaptive immune system must recognize its shape. Consequently, highly

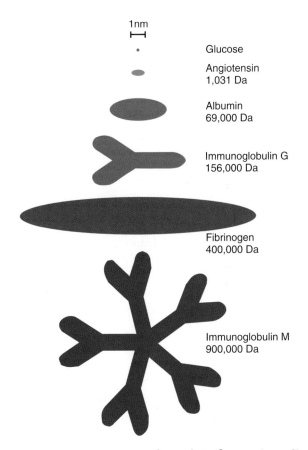

FIGURE 9-4 The relative sizes of several significant antigens. Size does matter! Big molecules are generally much more antigenic than small molecules. Molecules as small as angiotensin are poor antigens.

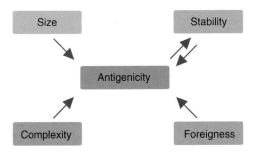

FIGURE 9-3 The factors that significantly influence the antigenicity of a molecule. Of these, either excessive or insufficient stability will reduce antigenicity. The best antigens are large, complex, and foreign. However, their ability to stimulate an immune response is also determined by their route of administration, by the amount of antigen administered, and by the genetic makeup of the immunized animal.

flexible molecules that have no fixed shape are poor antigens. For example, gelatin, a protein well known for its structural instability (which is why it can wobble), is a poor antigen unless it is stabilized by the incorporation of tyrosine or tryptophan molecules, which cross-link the peptide chains. Similarly, flagellin, the major protein of bacterial flagella, is a flexible, weak antigen. Its rigidity, and thus its antigenicity, is greatly enhanced by polymerization. Remember too that the route of antigen administration, its dose, and the genetics of the recipient animal also influence antigenicity.

Not all foreign molecules can stimulate an immune response. Stainless steel bone pins and plastic heart valves are commonly implanted in animals without triggering an immune response. The lack of antigenicity of large organic polymers, such as the plastics, is due not only to their molecular uniformity but also to their inertness. These polymers cannot be degraded and processed by cells to a form suitable for triggering an immune response. Conversely, since immune responses are antigen driven, foreign molecules that are unstable and destroyed very rapidly may not persist for a sufficient time to stimulate an immune response.

Foreignness

The cells that respond to antigens (antigen-sensitive cells) are selected so that their receptors do not normally bind to molecules originating within an animal (self-antigens). They will bind and respond, however, to foreign molecules that differ even in minor respects from those normally found within the body. This lack of reactivity of the adaptive immune system to normal body components occurs because cells whose receptors bind self-antigens are selectively killed or otherwise suppressed.

The immunogenicity of a molecule also depends on its degree of foreignness. The greater the difference in molecular structure between a foreign antigen and an animal's own antigens, the greater will be the intensity of the immune response. For example, a kidney graft from an identical twin will be readily accepted because its proteins are identical to those on the recipient's own kidney. A kidney graft from an unrelated animal of the same species will be rejected in about 10 days unless drugs are used to control the rejection. A kidney graft between different species such as from a pig to a dog will be rejected within a few hours despite the use of immunosuppressive drugs.

Epitopes

Foreign particles, such as bacteria, nucleated cells, and red blood cells, are a complex mixture of proteins, glycoproteins, polysaccharides, lipopolysaccharides, lipids, and nucleoproteins. The adaptive immune response against such a foreign particle is therefore a mixture of many simultaneous immune responses directed against each of the foreign molecules in the mixture.

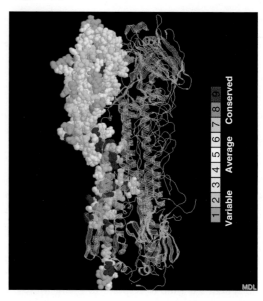

FIGURE 9-5 A molecular model of an antigen. This is an important influenza virus antigen called the hemagglutinin. It consists of two chains, one of which is lightly drawn so that the details of the other can be seen. The irregular surface forms characteristic shapes that can be recognized by the cells of the immune system. Influenza virus constantly changes the shape of this molecule, and this is denoted by the color coding.

(Courtesy Dr. Fabian Glaser.)

A single large molecule such as a protein can also be shown to stimulate multiple immune responses. Large molecules have specific regions against which immune responses are directed. These regions, usually on the surface of the molecule, are called epitopes, or antigenic determinants (Figure 9-5). In a large, complex protein molecule, many different epitopes may be recognized by the immune system, but some are much more immunogenic than others. Thus animals may respond to a few favored epitopes, and the remainder of the molecule may be ignored. Such favored epitopes are said to be immunodominant. In general, the number of epitopes on a molecule is directly related to its size and there is usually about one epitope for each 5 kDa of a protein. When we describe a molecule as "foreign," therefore, we are implying that it contains epitopes that are not found on self-antigens. The cells of the immune system recognize and respond to these foreign epitopes. A good example of a well-defined epitope is the peptide proline-glutamic acid-proline-lysine, which binds to antibodies against the bacterium *Streptococcus equi*. Presumably the shape of this peptide is identical to the major antigenic determinant on *S. equi*.

Haptens

Small molecules such as many drugs or hormones of less than 1000 Da are far too small to be appropriately processed and presented to the immune system. As a result, they are not immunogenic. If, however, these small molecules are

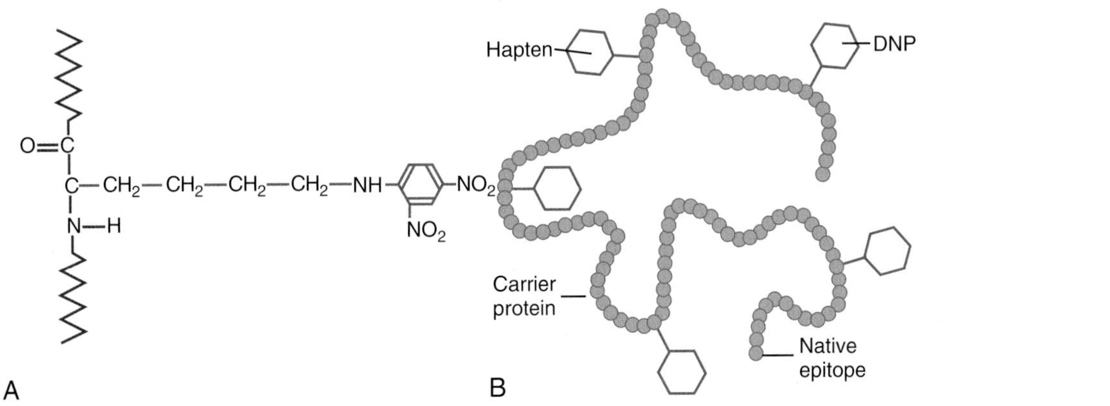

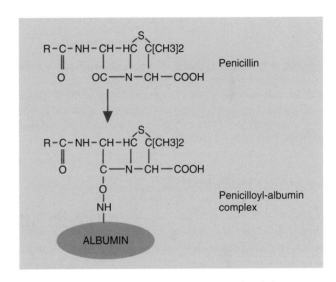

FIGURE 9-6 A, A typical hapten, in this case, dinitrophenol attached to a lysine side chain. **B,** When several haptens are attached to a peptide chain, they serve as new epitopes and will stimulate immune responses.

chemically linked to a large protein molecule, new epitopes will be formed on the surface of the larger molecule (Figure 9-6). If this molecular complex is injected into an animal, immune responses will be triggered against all its epitopes. Some of the antibodies made in response to the complex will be directed against new epitopes formed by the small molecule. Small molecules that can function as epitopes only when bound to other larger molecules are called haptens (in Greek, *haptein* means "to grasp or fasten"). The antigenic molecule to which the haptens are attached is called the carrier. Many drug allergies occur because the drug molecules, although small, can bind covalently to normal body proteins and so act as haptens.

By using haptens of known chemical structure, it is possible to study the interaction between antibodies and epitopes in great detail. For example, antibodies raised against one hapten can be tested for their ability to bind to other, structurally related molecules. Simple tests have shown that any alteration in the shape, size, or charge of a hapten alters its ability to bind to antibodies. Even very minor modifications to the shape of a hapten may influence its ability to be bound by an antigen receptor or by an antibody. Since there exists an enormous number of potential haptens, and since each hapten can provoke its own specific antibodies, it follows that animals must be able to generate an extremely large variety of antigen receptors and specific antibody molecules. It is this enormous diversity that enables animals to successfully fight the multitude of pathogenic microbes.

Some Examples of Haptens

Although the concept of haptens and carrier molecules provides the basis for much of our knowledge concerning the specificity of the antibody response, haptens may also be of clinical importance. For example, the antibiotic penicillin is a small nonimmunogenic molecule. Once degraded within the body, however, it forms a very reactive "penicilloyl" group, which can bind to serum proteins such as albumin to form penicilloyl-albumin complexes (Figure 9-7). The penicilloyl

FIGURE 9-7 Penicillin as a hapten. Penicillin can break down in vivo by several different pathways. The most important derivative is a penicillanic acid that combines with amino groups in a protein such as serum albumin to form a penicilloyl-protein complex. This complex may provoke an immune response and result in a penicillin allergy.

hapten can be recognized as a foreign epitope in some individuals and so provokes an immune response, resulting in penicillin allergy.

A second example of a naturally occurring reactive chemical that binds spontaneously to normal proteins and so acts as a hapten is the toxic component of the poison ivy plant (*Rhus radicans*). The resin of this plant, called urushiol, will bind to any protein with which it comes into contact, including the skin proteins of a person who rubs against the plant. The modified skin proteins are then regarded as foreign and attacked by lymphocytes in a manner similar to the rejection of a skin graft. The result is the uncomfortable skin rash called allergic contact dermatitis (Chapter 31).

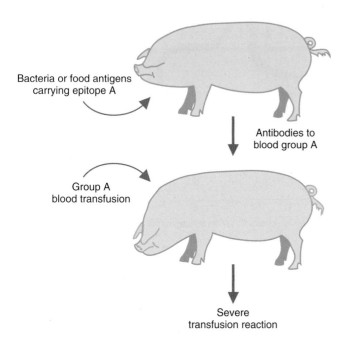

FIGURE 9-8 Food or bacterial antigens encountered in the diet carry epitopes that cross-react with blood group glycoprotein A. As a result, pigs of blood group O make antibodies to the A epitope despite never having received group A red cells. Should these animals be inadvertently transfused with group A blood, they will suffer an immediate and severe transfusion reaction.

□ Table 9-1	Degree of Cross-Reaction Between a Specific Antibody (Antibovine Light Chain Antibodies) and Related Proteins (Light Chains) from Other Mammals	
Cow	*Bos taurus*	100
Bison	*Bos bison*	100
Sheep	*Ovis aires*	100
Yak	*Pocphagus grunniens*	68
Goat	*Capra hircus*	68
Elk	*Cervus canadensis*	64
Buffalo	*Bubalus bubalus*	54
Reindeer	*Rangifer tarandus*	37
Human	*Homo sapiens*	17
Horse	*Equus caballus*	10
Rat	*Rattus rattus*	10
Mouse	*Mus musculus*	10
Pig	*Sus scrofa*	8
Camel	*Camelus dromedarius*	7

Data from Henning D, Nielsen K: Cross-reactivity of monoclonal antibodies to bovine immunoglobulins with immunoglobulins of other species, *Vet Immunol Immunopathol* 34:235–243, 1992.

Cross-Reactions

Identical or similar epitopes may sometimes be found on apparently unrelated molecules. As a result, antibodies directed against one antigen may react unexpectedly with an unrelated antigen. In another situation, the epitopes on a protein may differ in only minor respects from those on the same protein obtained from an animal of a related species. Consequently, antibodies directed against a protein in one species may also react in a detectable manner with the homologous or similar protein in another species. Both phenomena are called cross-reactions.

An example of a cross-reaction of the first type is seen when blood typing. Many bacteria possess cell wall glycoproteins with carbohydrate side chains that are identical to those found on mammalian red blood cell glycoproteins. For example, some intestinal bacteria possess glycoproteins with A or B side chains on their cell wall (Chapter 29). These glycoproteins are absorbed through the intestinal wall and trigger an antibody response. For example, blood-group glycoprotein side chain A is foreign to a pig of blood group O (Figure 9-8). Pigs of blood group O therefore develop antibodies that react with red cells from pigs of blood group A. These antibodies arise not as a response to previous immunization with group A red cells but following exposure to glycoproteins from the intestinal bacteria. Cross-reacting antibodies of this type are called heterophile antibodies. Another example of cross-reactivity occurs between *Brucella abortus* and some strains of *Yersinia enterocolitica*.

Y. enterocolitica, a relatively unimportant organism, may provoke cattle to make antibodies that cross-react with *B. abortus*. Since *Brucella*-infected animals are detected by testing for the presence of serum antibodies, a *Yersinia*-infected animal may be wrongly thought to carry *B. abortus* and so be killed. In another example, cross-reactivity occurs between the virus of feline infectious peritonitis (FIP) and the virus of pig transmissible gastroenteritis (TGE). It is very difficult to grow the FIP virus in the laboratory. TGE virus, on the other hand, is readily propagated. By detecting antibodies to TGE in cats, it is possible to diagnose FIP without having to culture the FIP virus.

The second type of cross-reactivity, which occurs between related proteins, may be demonstrated in many different biological systems. One example is the method used to determine relationships between mammalian species. Thus antisera to bovine serum albumin cross-react strongly with sheep and goat serum albumin but weakly with serum albumin from other mammals (Table 9-1). Presumably, this reflects the degree of structural similarity between the epitopes on serum proteins and is thus a useful tool in determining evolutionary relationships.

For sources of additional information, please visit http:// evolve.elsevier.com/tizard/immunology/

Dendritic Cells and Antigen Processing

Key Points

- Dendritic cells, macrophages, and B cells can capture and process foreign antigens so that they will trigger adaptive immune responses.
- Dendritic cells are the most efficient of these antigen-processing cells. Only dendritic cells can effectively stimulate naïve T cells.
- Immature dendritic cells are found throughout the body. They are especially equipped to capture and process antigens.
- Once stimulated by antigens, dendritic cells mature and become highly effective in presenting these processed antigens to T cells. They express high levels of antigen receptors called major histocompatibility complex (MHC) class II molecules on their surface.
- Dendritic cells ingest antigens, break them into small fragments, and then present them on their surface MHC molecules, where they can be recognized by T cells.
- Macrophages also act as antigen-presenting cells, but since they also destroy ingested antigens, they are much less efficient than dendritic cells.
- B cells can act as antigen-presenting cells and are especially effective during secondary immune responses.

The innate immune defenses have evolved to destroy microbes as soon as they enter the body. Most invaders, especially if they are of low virulence, are rapidly eliminated. However, in addition to being uncomfortable and damaging, inflammation is not a foolproof process. If the body is to be defended effectively, an animal must have defenses that detect and eliminate all microbial invaders without the damage and discomfort associated with inflammation. This is the task of the adaptive immune system.

In order to trigger adaptive immunity, a sample of foreign material must first be captured, processed, and presented in the correct fashion to cells that can recognize it. This is the responsibility of antigen-processing cells.

Antigen-processing cells are attracted by microbial products and tissue damage and are activated by the same stimuli that trigger inflammation. Indeed, dendritic cells and macrophages are both sentinel cells and antigen-processing cells. As a result, antigen processing can be initiated at the same time as the invader is being eliminated by the innate defenses. Once an invader has been eliminated, the body can proceed to develop adaptive immunity against a second attack by the same organism.

Processing involves breaking large protein molecules into small peptides within a cell. These peptides are then attached to specialized antigen-presenting receptors called major histocompatibility complex (MHC) molecules. The peptides bound to MHC molecules are then carried to the cell surface. Adaptive immunity is triggered when these MHC-bound peptides are recognized by specific receptors on lymphocytes. These lymphocytes (called T cells) bind and respond only to peptides that have been correctly processed and presented. This ensures that adaptive immune responses do not proceed indiscriminately.

The organisms that trigger adaptive immune responses are of two general types. One type is typified by the bacteria that invade the body from outside and then grow in the tissues and extracellular fluid. Their antigens are called exogenous antigens, and they are processed by specialized antigen-processing cells. A second type of invading organism is typified by viruses that invade a cell and force it to make viral proteins. These new proteins are called endogenous antigens. Endogenous antigens are processed by the cells in which they are produced. There are two classes of MHC molecules called MHC class I and MHC class II. MHC class I molecules are made by all nucleated cells and bind endogenous antigens. MHC class II molecules, in contrast, are restricted to specialized antigen-processing cells and bind exogenous antigens. The body mainly employs three cell types: dendritic cells, macrophages, and B cells to process exogenous antigens. The most important of these are dendritic cells (Figure 10-1).

Dendritic Cells

Dendritic cells perform three major functions. First, they serve as sentinel cells and activate innate defenses when they first encounter invaders. Second, they process exogenous antigens and thus initiate adaptive immune responses. Third, they can regulate adaptive immunity by determining whether an antigen will trigger an antibody-mediated or a cell-mediated response. Dendritic cells are at least 100 times more effective antigen-presenting cells than macrophages or B cells. Dendritic cells can take up many different antigens, including dead microorganisms, soluble antigens in tissue fluids, and antigens released by dying cells, and present them to T cells. Dendritic cells are the only antigen-processing cells that can activate those T cells that have never previously encountered an antigen (naïve cells)

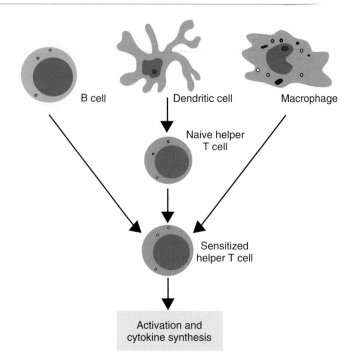

FIGURE 10-1 The three major populations of antigen-presenting cells: B cells, dendritic cells, and macrophages. Of these, only dendritic cells can activate naïve T cells and trigger a primary immune response.

and therefore are essential for initiating primary immune responses.

Origin

Dendritic cell precursors are derived from myeloid stem cells in the bone marrow. Under the influence of growth factors and cytokines, they differentiate into specialized subpopulations. Immature dendritic cells migrate throughout the body and form networks in virtually every tissue. Monocytes may also develop into dendritic cells when exposed to appropriate cytokines. (The precise relationship between dendritic cells and monocytes is currently being debated. Recent data are in conflict with the long-held belief that dendritic cells are simply specialized monocytes. This will take some time to sort out.) Dendritic cells are found in all organs except the brain, parts of the eye, and the testes. They are especially prominent in lymph nodes, skin, and mucosal surfaces—sites where invading microbes are most likely to be encountered.

Structure

The shape of dendritic cells depends on their state of activation. Typically, however, they are characterized by having a small cell body with many long cytoplasmic processes known as dendrites (Figure 10-2). The dendrites increase the efficiency of antigen trapping and maximize contact between dendritic cells and other cells.

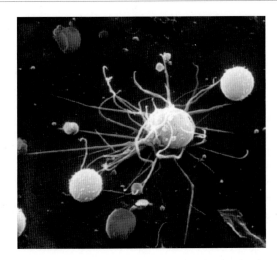

FIGURE 10-2 A scanning electron micrograph of a dendritic cell from a guinea pig lymph node. Note the relatively small cell body and the numerous long dendrites. Original magnification ×4000.

Subpopulations

Dendritic cells are a mixture of several different subpopulations. Thus they are divided into myeloid (M-DC) and plasmacytoid (P-DC) dendritic cells (Figure 10-3). These two subpopulations differ in morphology, in surface antigens, and in their functions, although they share adhesion molecules, co-stimulatory molecules, and activation markers. Other specialized dendritic cell subpopulations are found in the skin (Langerhans cells) and in lymphoid organs (follicular dendritic cells).

As pointed out earlier, the adaptive immune system has two major branches: the antibody-mediated and cell-mediated immune responses. The type of immune response mounted by an animal is determined by the type of helper T (Th) cells triggered in response to an antigen. Thus there are several types of Th cells (see Figure 14-2). One major type, Th1 cells, stimulates cell-mediated immune responses designed to protect animals against intracellular organisms. The other major type, Th2 cells, stimulates antibody-mediated immune responses designed to protect animals against extracellular invaders. Which Th cell type is activated depends on the use of different dendritic cell subpopulations.

Myeloid Dendritic Cells Blood monocytes are the immediate precursors of both tissue macrophages and M-DCs. Which of these cell types is produced depends on the mixture of cytokines and cells encountered by the monocyte as it differentiates. Each cell type can convert to the other until late in the differentiation process. M-DCs can therefore be considered part of the mononuclear phagocytic system being derived from a common stem cell, respond to the same growth factors, express the same surface markers, and in effect are in no specific way uniquely different from other macrophages. Thus macrophages may consist of a spectrum of cell types ranging from highly effective antigen presenters (dendritic cells) at one extreme to suppressors of T cell activation (M2 cells) at the other. Monocytes exposed to certain T cell cytokines differentiate into M-DCs, and functionally different dendritic cells can be induced according to the local cytokine environment. Bovine peripheral blood monocytes exposed to staphylococcal enterotoxin C1, a superantigen (Chapter 14), will convert to dendritic cells.

Plasmacytoid Dendritic Cells P-DCs are long-lived cells found in blood, bone marrow, and lymphoid organs. They are

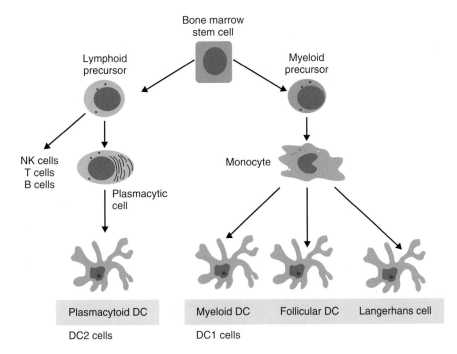

FIGURE 10-3 The origins of dendritic cells. One population, the plasmacytoid dendritic cells, originates from lymphoid precursors. These give rise to DC2-type cells. The second major population arises from myeloid precursors and is closely related to monocytes. These, together with follicular dendritic cells and Langerhans cells, constitute the DC1 type.

specialized to respond to viruses by producing massive amounts of the type I interferons (IFN-α and IFN-β). Their numbers increase during infection. It is possible that the P-DCs serve as an early warning system for viral infections since they are rapidly activated by viral nucleic acids. Plasmacytoid dendritic cells have a unique ability to link innate and adaptive immunity. After producing large amounts of type I interferon, they are still able to differentiate into mature DCs that can stimulate naïve T cells. Because P-DCs secrete large amounts of IFN-α, they also activate natural killer (NK) cells (Chapter 19).

Langerhans Cells Several dendritic cell subpopulations are found in skin. Langerhans cells, for example, are specialized, long-lived M-DCs found in the epidermis. Their long dendrites form an extensive network that is ideally situated to capture antigens (Figure 10-4). These antigens include not only invading microbes but also topically applied antigens, such as the resins of poison ivy, or intradermally injected antigens, such as those in mosquito saliva. Langerhans cells express multiple pattern-recognition receptors (PRRs), including the C-type lectins langerin and DC-SIGN that can bind bacteria, fungi, and some viruses. Langerhans cells influence the development of skin immune responses, such as delayed hypersensitivity and allergic contact dermatitis (Chapter 31). Langerhans cells contain characteristic rod- or racquet-shaped cytoplasmic granules called Birbeck granules whose function is unclear. Once antigens are captured, the Langerhans cells migrate to draining lymph nodes, where they present the antigen to T cells.

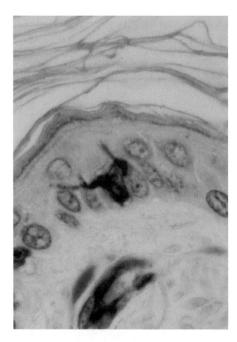

FIGURE 10-4 This dark red cell in the epidermis of a dog is a Langerhans cell stained for the protein vimentin. Note that its dendrites extend between the epidermal cells so that it can effectively trap antigens.

(Courtesy Dr. K.M. Credille.)

Follicular Dendritic Cells Specialized dendritic cells called follicular dendritic cells are found in secondary lymphoid organs (Chapter 12). They are a form of M-DC derived from stromal cell precursors. Follicular dendritic cells present antigens to B cells in two different ways. In an animal that has not previously been exposed to the antigen, antigen presentation is a passive process. The dendritic cells simply provide a surface on which antigen can be presented. In contrast, in animals that have previously been exposed to an antigen and possess antibodies, the antigen and antibody combine to form antibody-antigen complexes (also called immune complexes). Follicular dendritic cells take up these immune complexes on their surface and then shed them in membrane vesicles called exosomes. B cells can take up these exosomes and after processing the antigen present it to antigen-sensitive T cells. Follicular dendritic cells can retain antigens on their surface for more than 3 months. They integrate signals from toll-like receptors (TLRs) and other sources to support effective germinal center responses. Follicular dendritic cells play an important role in promoting immunoglobulin A (IgA) responses in Peyer's patches in the intestinal wall (Chapter 22). They respond to lipopolysaccharides, lipopeptides, and retinoic acid from the gut flora and support the recruitment and survival of IgA-producing B cells.

Dendritic Cell Maturation

Although many subpopulations of dendritic cells have been characterized, their most important division is based on their state of maturity (Figure 10-5). Thus immature dendritic cells are highly specialized and efficient antigen-trapping cells. As they mature, dendritic cells undergo cellular reorganization and become specialized and efficient antigen-presenting cells.

Immature Dendritic Cells Newly generated M-DCs migrate from the bone marrow through the blood to lymph nodes or tissues. Here they act as "sentinels" whose role is to capture invading microbes. With their short life span, they can be regarded as disposable antigen-trapping cells. If they do not encounter antigens, they die in a few days. If, however, they encounter antigens and are stimulated by tissue damage or inflammation, they become activated and mature rapidly. Immature dendritic cells have receptors that help them carry out their functions. These include cytokine receptors such as interleukin-1 receptor (IL-1R) and tumor necrosis factor receptor (TNFR), chemokine receptors; C-type lectins, Fc receptors (FcγR and FcεR), mannose receptors (CD206), heat-shock protein receptors, and TLRs.

Although the most important functions of dendritic cells are to trap, process, and present antigen to the cells of the immune system, they must also be able to kill any pathogens they encounter. Thus dendritic cells produce NADPH oxidase (NOX) and can kill invaders by mounting a respiratory burst. Activation of TLRs by pathogen-associated molecular patterns (PAMPs) enhances their production of superoxide.

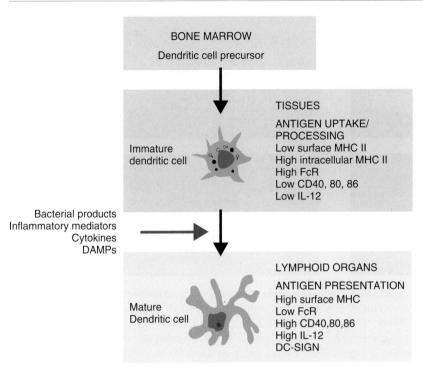

FIGURE 10-5 As dendritic cells mature, they change their function. Immature dendritic cells are specialized antigen-trapping cells. Mature dendritic cells, on the other hand, are specialized antigen-processing cells.

Dendritic cells mature in response to interleukin-1 (IL-1) and tumor necrosis factor-α (TNF-α) as well as to PAMPs and damage-associated molecular patterns (DAMPs). Injured and inflamed tissues release large amounts of soluble heparan sulfate that binds to TLR4 and activates dendritic cells. Breakdown of nucleic acids generates uric acid, another potent dendritic cell activator. One of the most important activators of immature dendritic cells is high mobility group box protein-1 (HMGB1). Immature dendritic cells are attracted to areas of inflammation by chemokines, defensins, and HMGB1.

Immature dendritic cells specialize in capturing antigens and cell fragments by phagocytosis, by pinocytosis (the uptake of fluid droplets—cell drinking), and by interaction with various cell surface receptors. They also capture apoptotic cell bodies. If they ingest bacteria, they can usually kill them. They can distinguish between normal tissue debris and foreign organisms by selectively sampling their environment. This differentiation depends on the ability of the foreign material to bind to TLRs. Activation of TLRs by PAMPs ensures that ingested material is processed in such a way that it triggers adaptive immunity. Material that does not activate TLRs is not processed and will not trigger an adaptive response.

The phagosomal contents of conventional phagocytic cells such as neutrophils and macrophages are very acidic and hence optimized for proteolytic destruction of foreign material. The pH within dendritic cell and B cell phagosomes is in contrast relatively alkaline since these phagosomes do not fuse with lysosomes. Cysteine and aspartyl proteases are inhibited at these high pH levels, and as a result, antigen is not completely degraded but rather is preserved for presentation on MHC class I molecules.

Mature Dendritic Cells After they have captured and processed antigens, immature dendritic cells carry these antigens to sites where they can be recognized by T cells. The activated DCs are attracted to lymphoid organs by the chemokine CCL20. Infection or tissue damage also promotes the migration of antigen-bearing dendritic cells to lymph nodes or the spleen. Once they enter a lymphoid organ, the cells mature rapidly.

Mature dendritic cells secrete the chemokine CCL22. This attracts T cells, which accumulate in clusters around the dendritic cell (Figure 10-6). The dendritic cells embrace the T cells in a net of dendrites as they interact. During this time, the T cells examine the mature dendritic cells for the presence of antigen fragments. If their antigen receptors can bind the presented fragments, the T cells will be triggered to respond.

As dendritic cells mature, their MHC molecules move from intracellular endosomes and lysosomes to the cell surface. Cell surface expression of their co-stimulatory molecules also increases. As a result, MHC molecules and MHC-peptide complexes are found at levels 100 times higher on mature dendritic cells than on other cell types such as B cells or macrophages. Their expression of co-stimulatory molecules such as CD86 (Chapter 14) may also rise 100-fold.

Mature dendritic cells are the only cells that can trigger a primary T cell response. One reason for this is that mature dendritic cells can assemble complete T cell activation complexes (antigen-loaded MHC plus co-stimulatory molecules) within the cell before they are carried to the cell surface. Mature dendritic cells also express DC-SIGN (CD209), a C-type lectin, that binds a ligand called intercellular adhesion

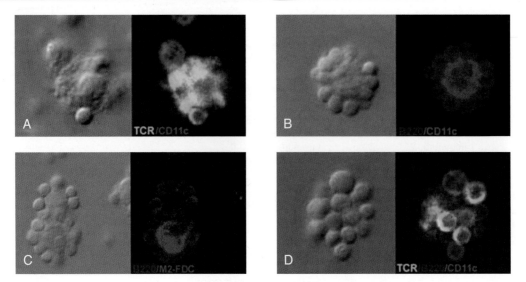

FIGURE 10-6 When dendritic cells and T cells interact, they form visible clusters as the cells converse among themselves. Thus, in these figures, dendritic cells are stained with a blue fluorescent dye (anti-CD11c), T cells are stained with a green dye (anti-CD3), and B cells are stained with a red dye (anti-B220). **A,** T cells are interacting with a dendritic cell. **B,** B cells are binding to a dendritic cell. **C,** B cells are binding to a follicular dendritic cell. **D,** There is a mixed B and T cell cluster. Note that some B cells appear to be attached to T cells.

(From Hommel M, Kyewski B: Dynamic changes during the immune response in T cell-antigen-presenting cell clusters isolated from lymph nodes, *J Exp Med* 197:269–280, 2003.)

molecule-3 (ICAM-3 or CD50) on naïve T cells. DC-SIGN thus permits transient binding between dendritic cells and T cells. It permits a single dendritic cell to rapidly screen thousands of T cells to find the few that are expressing a compatible antigen receptor. Because of their potency, only a few dendritic cells are needed to trigger a strong T cell response. Thus one dendritic cell may activate as many as 3000 T cells.

Tolerance Induction

Under steady-state conditions, in the absence of inflammation or infection, some immature dendritic cells will spontaneously mature and migrate to lymphoid tissues carrying normal tissue antigens on their MHC molecules. If a T cell recognizes this "normal" antigen, the T cell may undergo apoptosis and die. Alternatively, these DCs may trigger the production of IL-10, a suppressive cytokine that generates regulatory T cells. Either way, the processing of normal tissue antigens by dendritic cells leads to T cell deletion and immunological tolerance (Chapter 20).

DC1 and DC2 Cells

When dendritic cells stimulate Th cells, they provide three signals. The first signal is delivered when T cell antigen receptors bind antigen fragments attached to MHC molecules. The second signal provides the cells with additional critical stimuli (co-stimulation) through molecules such as CD40 and CD80/86. The third signal determines the way in which naïve Th cells will develop. The nature of this third signal is determined by the conditions under which the dendritic cells are

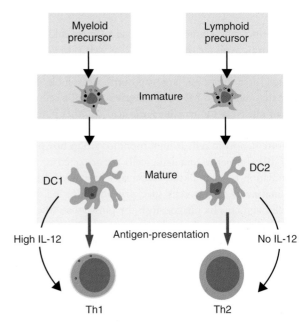

FIGURE 10-7 Two populations of dendritic cells appear to favor different helper T cell subpopulations. Th1 cells promote cell-mediated immunity, whereas Th2 cells promote antibody formation. The helper cell population employed depends on the cytokines produced by these dendritic cell subpopulations. These cells have different origins and secrete different costimulatory cytokines.

activated. For example, some microbial molecules promote dendritic cells to secrete a cytokine called IL-12 (Figure 10-7). These are called DC1 cells since their IL-12 activates Th1 cells. In contrast, other microbial molecules induce dendritic cells to secrete a mixture of IL-1 and IL-6. These cytokines stimulate Th2 cell production and are called DC2 cells. Other microbial molecules and DAMPs may induce dendritic cells to secrete IL-23 that provokes the Th cells to develop into Th17 cells.

Different PAMPs and DAMPs acting through different TLRs influence the development of these specific dendritic cell subpopulations. The stimuli that promote a DC1 response include double-stranded RNA acting through TLR3, lipopolysaccharide acting through TLR4, flagellin acting through TLR5, and nucleic acids acting through TLR7 and TLR9. On the other hand, inflammatory mediators, such as IL-10, transforming growth factor-α (TGF-α), prostaglandin E_2 (PGE$_2$), histamine, extracts of parasitic worms, or the toxin of *Vibrio cholerae*, promote DC2 responses. DC2 responses may also be triggered by bacterial lipopolysaccharides and proteoglycans acting through TLR2, TLR6, or TLR1. Ligands of TLR2 promote the production of IL-23 and thus promote Th17 cell responses. As pointed out previously, a similar functional division occurs in macrophages. Thus M1 and M2 cells, when acting as antigen-presenting cells, promote different Th cell responses.

It may also be that the same dendritic cell can promote a Th1, Th2, or Th17 response, depending on the dose and type of antigen it encounters. The response may also depend on its location. For example, dendritic cells from the intestine or airways seem to preferentially secrete IL-10 and IL-4 and thus promote Th2 responses. In those cases, bacteria in the intestinal microflora may provide the dendritic cell–polarizing signals.

Interleukin-12

IL-12 is a key cytokine that determines Th1/Th2 polarization. Th1 cells develop when it is present. Th2 cells develop when it is absent. IL-12 is produced by macrophages, dendritic cells, B cells, and neutrophils. Its targets are T cells and NK cells. It is a member of a family of related proteins, the IL-12 cytokine family, that also include IL-23, IL-27, and IL-35. These are all heterodimeric proteins. For example, IL-12 is formed by two chains, p35 and p40. Some of these chains are shared with other family members. All the members of the family regulate T cell function. Thus IL-12 and IL-27 generate Th1 cells, whereas IL-23 generates Th17 cells.

Dendritic Cells in Domestic Animals

Dendritic cells are found in all the major domestic mammals and do not appear to differ in any significant respect from dendritic cells in humans and mice. In domestic animals, M-DCs have been characterized in horses, ruminants, pigs, dogs and chickens, whereas Langerhans cells have been described in horses, ruminants, pigs, dogs, and cats. P-DCs have been identified in pigs.

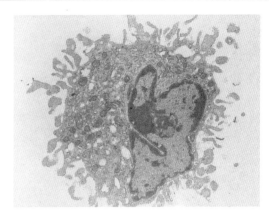

FIGURE 10-8 A transmission electron micrograph of a dendritic cell from bovine afferent lymph. It has been stained with a monoclonal antibody specific for bovine CD1b. (The antibody is linked to colloidal gold particles, which are visible as small, electron dense dots around the outside of the cell).

(Courtesy Dr. C.J. Howard and Dr. P. Bland, Institute for Animal Health, Compton, UK.)

For example, equine dendritic cells express MHC class II, CD11, EqWC1, and EqWC2. Bovine dendritic cells express MHC II, CD80, CD86, and CD40 (Figure 10-8). Cattle possess two dendritic cell subpopulations that differ in their ability to stimulate CD4 and CD8 T cells. One population synthesizes more IL-12, whereas the other population produces more IL-1 and IL-10; these may well represent DC1 and DC2 subpopulations. Dendritic cells derived from sheep peripheral blood monocytes express MHC class II, CD11c, and CD14−. Pigs have both M-DCs and P-DCs. Pig M-DCs are CD172a+, CD11R1+, CD1+/−, and CD80/86+/−, whereas their P-DCs are CD172a+, CD4+, CD1+/−, and CD80/86+/−. Both types secrete IL-10 and IL-12. (It is of interest to note that swine P-DCs produce IFN-α in response to several common viruses, including transmissible gastroenteritis, pseudorabies, and swine flu, but not porcine reproductive and respiratory syndrome virus (PRRSV). PRRSV causes persistent infection and weak immunity.) There are two main populations of canine dendritic cells. One is MHC class II+, CD34+, and CD14−; the other is MHC class II+, CD34+, and CD14+. CD40 is found on canine dendritic cells but not on monocytes. Feline Langerhans cells are CD18+, MHC class II+, CD1a+, and CD4+. Dendritic cells from feline blood mononuclear cells are CD1+, CD14+, and MHC class I and II+ (Figure 10-9).

Other Antigen-Processing Cells

Naïve T cells require prolonged close interaction with dendritic cells before they can respond to antigens. Once primed, however, these T cells may be further activated by relatively brief interactions with two other major cell types: antigen-presenting macrophages and B cells.

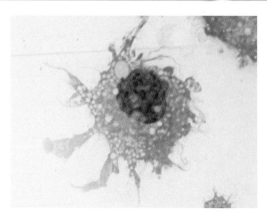

FIGURE 10-9 A feline dendritic cell cultured in the presence of recombinant human IL-4 and GM-CSF. Note the extensive dendrites so characteristic of these cells. Bright field illumination ×100.

(From Sprague WS, Pope M, Hoover EA: Culture and comparison of feline myeloid dendritic cells vs macrophages, *J Comp Pathol* 133:139, 2005.)

Macrophages

Macrophages are the most accessible and best understood of the antigen-processing cells. Their properties are described in Chapter 5. Once antigens are taken up by macrophages, a portion is processed and presented to sensitized T cells. Macrophages, however, are unable to engage in prolonged interactions with T cells. As a result, they cannot activate naïve T cells. In addition, antigen processing by macrophages is inefficient since much of the ingested antigen is destroyed by lysosomal proteases and oxidants. Indeed, macrophages and B cells can be considered cells with other priorities (some call them "semiprofessional" antigen-processing cells).

B Cells

B cells, like macrophages, cannot undertake prolonged interactions with T cells. They do, however, have antigen receptors that enable them to bind and process large amounts of specific antigen. They ingest and process antigens before presenting them, in association with MHC class II molecules, to sensitized T cells. B cells probably play a minor role in antigen processing in a primary immune response but a much more significant one in a secondary response when their numbers have greatly increased and T cells are easier to stimulate.

Other Cells

It has been generally believed that only the "professional" antigen-processing cells can stimulate T cell responses since only they can load antigen fragments onto their MHC molecules and provide the correct co-stimulatory signals. However, T cells may be activated by many different "nonprofessional" cell types. These include neutrophils, eosinophils, basophils, T cells, endothelial cells, fibroblasts, NK cells, smooth muscle cells, astrocytes, microglial cells, and some epithelial cells such as thymic epithelial cells and corneal cells. Their effectiveness may depend on the local environment. Thus fibroblasts may be very effective antigen-processing cells when located within granulomas. Presumably, co-stimulation can come from other nearby cells in this cytokine-rich environment. Vascular endothelial cells can also take up antigens, synthesize IL-1, and under the influence of IFN-γ, express MHC class II molecules. Even skin keratinocytes can secrete cytokines similar to IL-1, express MHC class II molecules, and present antigen to T cells. In pigs, a subpopulation of circulating γ/δ T cells may act as professional antigen-processing cells.

Antigen Processing

MHC Class II Pathway

The presentation of exogenous antigens is regulated by MHC class II molecules. MHC class II molecules are cell surface receptors that bind processed peptide fragments. Although many cells can phagocytose foreign antigens, only those that can express antigen fragments bound to MHC class II molecules can trigger an immune response. As described previously, the most efficient antigen-processing cells are thus mature MHC class II+ dendritic cells. Unlike macrophages, dendritic cell lysosomes have limited proteolytic activity and degrade internalized antigens slowly. As a result, these antigens may persist for a long time. MHC class II molecules can bind fragments of these ingested antigens and present them to Th cells (Figure 10-10). Th cells can recognize and respond to antigen fragments only when bound to MHC class II molecules. If an antigen is presented to T cells without being bound to an MHC class II molecule, the T cells will be turned off or die, and tolerance may result (Chapter 20).

Exogenous antigen processing involves multiple steps. First, the antigen must be endocytosed and taken into phagosomes. These phagosomes then fuse with lysosomes containing proteases. The ingested proteins are broken down by the lysosomal proteases into peptide fragments of varying length. The endosomes containing these peptide fragments then fuse with other endosomes carrying newly synthesized MHC class II molecules to generate the lysosome MHC class II compartment (MIIC). Endogenous antigens may also enter the MIIC through autophagy (Chapter 4).

Newly synthesized MHC class II chains are translocated to the endosomes, where, together with a peptide called the invariant chain (Ii), they form a protein complex. The invariant chain occupies the MHC antigen-binding site. This complex travels to the MIIC, where the invariant chain is digested, leaving a small peptide called the class II–associated Ii peptide (CLIP), filling the antigen-binding groove. When antigen-containing phagosomes fuse with the MHC-containing endosomes, the foreign peptide fragments are exchanged for the CLIP chain. An MHC class II antigen-binding groove can hold a peptide of 12 to 24 amino acids as a straight, extended chain that projects out of both ends of the binding site. Side

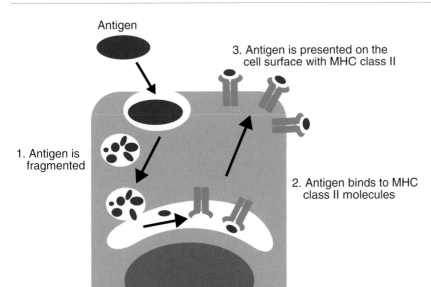

Antigen

3. Antigen is presented on the
cell surface with MHC class II

1. Antigen is
fragmented

2. Antigen binds to MHC
class II molecules

FIGURE 10-10 The processing of exogenous antigen by an antigen-presenting cell. Ingested antigens are taken into phagosomes where they are fragmented by proteases. Peptides are then carried to the endosomal compartments where the antigenic peptides are placed in the binding grooves of MHC class II molecules. The antigen-MHC complexes are then carried to the cell surface where they are presented to helper T cells.

chains from the peptide bind in pockets on the walls of the binding groove. The presence of the CLIP chain prevents endosomes containing MHC class II molecules from being prematurely transported to the cell surface Thus, unlike most new transmembrane proteins that are expressed minutes after assembly, MHC class II molecules are retained inside the cell for several hours until they are needed.

Once the antigen peptide is bound to an MHC molecule, the MIIC vesicles move toward the cell surface. When they reach the cell surface, the vesicle fuses with the cell membrane, and the MHC-peptide complex is exposed and available for inspection by any passing T cell.

It has been calculated that an antigen-processing cell carries about 2×10^5 MHC class II molecules that can present peptide fragments to T cells. If co-stimulation is provided, a single T cell can be activated by exposure to as few as 200 to 300 of these peptide-MHC complexes. It is therefore possible for a single antigen-processing cell to present many different antigens to different T cells simultaneously.

Since Th cells must recognize MHC-antigen complexes in order to respond to an antigen, the MHC class II molecules effectively determine whether an animal will mount an adaptive immune response to any antigen. Class II molecules can bind some, but not all, peptides created during antigen processing and in effect, select those antigen fragments that are to be presented to T cells. (Further coverage of MHC molecules is provided in Chapter 11.)

MHC Class I Pathway

One function of T cell–mediated immune responses is the identification and destruction of cells producing abnormal or foreign proteins. The best examples of such cells are those infected by viruses. Viruses take over the protein-synthesizing machinery of infected cells and use it to make new viral

proteins (Figure 10-11). To control virus infections, cytotoxic T cells must be able to recognize the viral proteins expressed on the surface of infected cells. T cells can indeed recognize and respond to these endogenous antigens but only if they are processed and bound to MHC class I molecules (Chapter 11). These T cells are thus said to be MHC restricted.

The MHC class I molecule is a cell surface receptor folded in such a way that a large antigen-binding site is formed on its surface (see Figures 11-5 and 11-6). This binding site, however, differs from that on MHC class II molecules in that it is closed at each end. As a result, long peptides cannot project out of the ends. Because of this, MHC class I molecules can only bind peptides containing about nine amino acids. Indeed, in order to do so, these peptides must bulge out in the middle. Overall, however, the antigen-binding sites on class II and class Ia molecules function in a similar manner.

The processing of endogenous peptides is very different from the processing of exogenous peptides. Living cells continually break down and recycle proteins. As a result, abnormal proteins are removed, regulatory peptides do not accumulate, and amino acids are made available for other purposes. As a first step, ubiquitin, a polypeptide found in all eukaryote cells, attaches to the lysine residues in target proteins. Additional ubiquitin molecules then attach to the protein-bound ubiquitin so that several ubiquitin molecules are added to the target protein, like beads on a string. A chain of four ubiquitin molecules appears to be optimal for processing. These polyubiquinated proteins are marked for destruction since they are recognized by enzyme complexes called proteasomes. Proteasomes are tubular molecular complexes consisting of an inner cylinder that contains the protease activity and two outer rings that regulate which proteins can enter and be destroyed. Ubiquitinated proteins bind to the outer rings, the target protein is unfolded, and the ubiquitin is released to be reused. The unfolded protein is inserted into the inner cylinder, where it

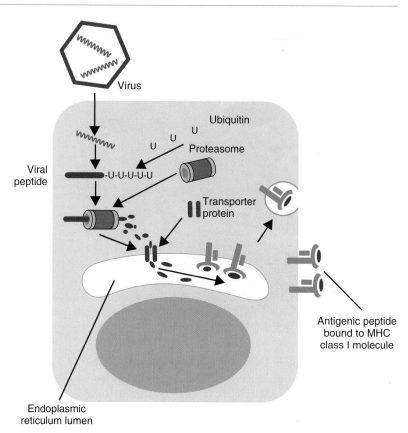

FIGURE 10-11 The processing of endogenous antigen. Samples of newly synthesized proteins are ubiquinated before being chopped into peptides by a proteasome. The peptides attach to a transporter protein located in the membrane of the endoplasmic reticulum. They are then carried into the lumen of the endoplasmic reticulum, where they are placed in the antigen-binding groove of MHC class I molecules. The MHC class I–peptide complexes are carried to the cell surface, where they encounter cytotoxic T cells.

is broken into 8- to 15-amino acid long peptides (like a meat grinder). Most of these peptide fragments are recycled into new proteins. For about 1 in 1 million molecules, however, the peptides are rescued from further breakdown by attachment to transporter proteins. Two transporter proteins have been identified: TAP-1 and TAP-2 (*TAP* stands for *t*ransporter for *a*ntigen *p*rocessing). TAP-1 and TAP-2 select peptide fragments and transport them into endosomes. Here the peptides are trimmed by an aminopeptidase, which shortens them, one amino acid at a time, until they are completely degraded—unless an intermediate, 8- to 10-amino acid peptide precisely fits the binding site on an empty MHC class I molecule. In this case, degradation stops, the peptide is loaded into the binding site, and the MHC-peptide complex is carried to the cell surface, where it is displayed for many hours.

A cell can express about 10^6 MHC-peptide complexes at any one time. A minimum of about 200 MHC class I molecules loaded with the same viral peptide is required to activate a cytotoxic T cell. Thus the MHC-peptide complexes can provide passing T cells with fairly complete information on virtually all the proteins being made by a cell. Cytotoxic T cells can then screen these peptides to determine whether any are "foreign" and bind to their TCRs.

Cross-Priming

It must not be assumed that the two antigen-processing pathways function in isolation. In fact, the pathways interact extensively. For example, under some circumstances, exogenous antigens may enter the cytoplasm, join the endogenous antigen pathway, and be presented on MHC class I molecules. Thus in antigen-presenting cells such as macrophages and dendritic cells, endocytosed viral antigen may not be degraded in lysosomes but by proteasomes and so is processed as an endogenous antigen. This antigen thus binds to MHC class I molecules and is recognized by cytotoxic T cells. This may be important in immunity to viruses since it implies that the antigens from dead virions may still be able to trigger a response by cytotoxic T cells (Chapter 26).

Histiocytosis and Histiocytomas

Domestic animals suffer from several diseases in which macrophage or dendritic cells proliferate excessively. These are called histiocytomas or histiocytosis. Canine cutaneous histiocytoma is a benign epidermal neoplasm of Langerhans cell origin that usually regresses spontaneously. Langerhans cell histiocytosis is a reactive lesion whose trigger is unknown but may be an infectious agent. This condition is not premalignant, and it may occur in cutaneous or systemic forms. Both forms of Langerhans cell histiocytosis present with lesions in the skin or subcutis, but systemic histiocytosis also involves other tissues. Cutaneous histiocytosis shows no breed predilection, occurs in adult dogs between 3 and 9 years old, and is characterized by the development of nonpainful solitary or multiple nodules in the skin or subcutis. These lesions tend to occur on the head, neck, extremities, perineum, and scrotum. In contrast, systemic histiocytosis tends to occur in large breeds such as Bernese Mountain dogs, Rottweilers, Golden Retrievers, and Labradors. The age of onset is between 4 and 7 years. The lesions develop in the skin, mucous membranes, eyes, nasal cavity, spleen, lung, liver, bone marrow, and spinal cord. Histologically these lesions are characterized as containing a mixture of cells. Phenotyping shows that the cells express CD1, CD11c, MHC class II, CD4, and CD90, a phenotype typical of Langerhans cells. The lesions also contain T cells and neutrophils and may be successfully treated with corticosteroids, cyclosporine, or leflunomide (Chapter 39). As many as 30% of cutaneous cases and 10% of systemic cases spontaneously regress following infiltration by CD4+ T cells and the production of Th1 cytokines such as IL-2, TNF-α, and IFN-γ, as well as NOS2, and subsequent recruitment of antitumor effector cells. Feline progressive histiocytosis is a skin disease presenting as solitary or multiple nonpruritic nodules on the feet, legs, and face. The histiocytes express CD1a, CD1c, CD18, and MHC class II molecules. Expression of E-cadherin, a characteristic of Langerhans cells, occurs in about 10% of cases. This is a slowly progressive disease that may involve internal organs in terminal cases.

For sources of additional information, please visit http://evolve.elsevier.com/tizard/immunology/

The Major Histocompatibility Complex

Key Points

- Antigen-presenting cells use receptors called MHC molecules to bind and present antigens.
- MHC molecules are encoded by genes located within the major histocompatibility complex.
- The classical MHC molecules are highly polymorphic. That is, they show an enormous variety of inherited structural variations that permit each individual animal to respond to a different set of antigens.
- Class I MHC molecules are found on all nucleated cells. Their function is to present endogenous antigens to CD8+ T cells.
- Class II MHC molecules are largely restricted to professional antigen-presenting cells such as dendritic cells, macrophages, and B cells. Their function is to present exogenous antigens to CD4+ T cells.
- The class III region of the MHC contains a mixture of genes, some of which encode complement components.

In order to trigger an adaptive immune response, antigen molecules must be broken up inside cells, and the fragments generated must then be bound to appropriate antigen-presenting receptors (Figure 11-1). These antigen-presenting receptors are glycoproteins encoded by genes located in a large gene cluster called the major histocompatibility complex (MHC). The receptors are therefore called MHC molecules. Antigen fragments can trigger an immune response only after they have bound to MHC molecules, and these antigen-MHC complexes have bound to T cell antigen receptors. Since the MHC molecules serve as specific antigen receptors, MHC genes determine which antigens can trigger adaptive immunity. Thus the MHC can be considered an organized cluster of genes that control antigen presentation and so determine an animal's susceptibility to infectious or autoimmune diseases.

Major Histocompatibility Complex

All vertebrates, from cartilaginous fish to mammals, possess cell-surface proteins coded for by genes clustered within an MHC. Each MHC has a fairly consistent structure consisting

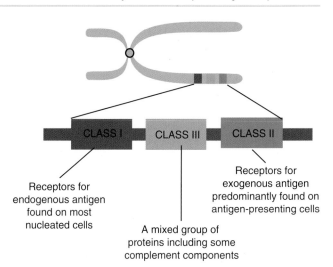

FIGURE 11-2 The three major classes of genes located within the major histocompatibility complex are grouped together in regions: their distribution and functions.

of about 200 expressed genes distributed over about 3 mb of DNA and divided into three regions containing different classes of MHC gene loci (I, II, and III) (Figure 11-2). Classical class I loci code for the MHC molecules expressed on most nucleated cells. Class I genes can be subdivided into those that are highly polymorphic (class Ia genes) and those that show very little polymorphism (class Ib, Ic, or Id genes). (Polymorphism refers to structural variations between proteins.) Class Id genes are located outside the MHC on a different chromosome. Genes in class II loci, on the other hand, encode polymorphic MHC molecules mainly restricted to professional antigen-presenting cells (dendritic cells, macrophages, and B cells) (Table 11-1). Genes in the class III region code for a diverse mixture of proteins, many of which are linked to innate immunity, such as complement proteins. Although each MHC contains all three gene regions, their gene content, and arrangement vary between species.

The collective name given to the proteins encoded by MHC genes depends on the species. In humans these molecules are

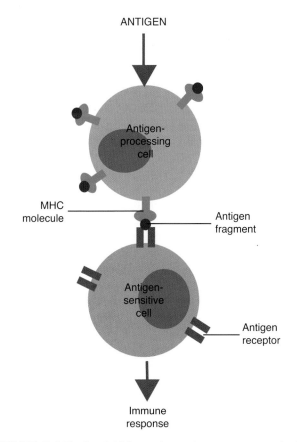

FIGURE 11-1 The key initial step in any immune response is the presentation of antigens by antigen-processing cells to antigen-sensitive cells. This step is mediated by MHC molecules located on the surface of antigen-processing cells.

□ Table 11-1	Comparison of MHC Class I and Class I Structure	
	CLASS I	**CLASS II**
Loci include	Typically A, B, and C	DP, DQ, and DR,
Distribution	Most nucleated cells	B cells, macrophages, and dendritic cells
Function	Present antigen to cytotoxic T cells	Present antigen to T helper cells
Result	T-cell–mediated toxicity	T-cell–mediated help

called human leukocyte antigen (HLA); in dogs they are called DLA; in rabbits, RLA; in cattle (bovines), BoLA; in horses, ELA; in swine, SLA; and so forth. In some species, MHC molecules were identified as transplantation antigens before their true function was recognized. In these cases, the nomenclature is anomalous. Thus, in the mouse the MHC is called H-2, and in chickens it is called B. The complete set of alleles found within an individual animal's MHC is called its MHC haplotype.

MHC Class Ia Molecules

Class Ia molecules are expressed on most nucleated cells. In pigs, for example, class I molecules have been detected on lymphocytes, platelets, granulocytes, hepatocytes, kidney cells, and sperm. They are not usually found on mammalian red cells, gametes, neurons, or trophoblast cells. Some cells, such as myocardium and skeletal muscle, may express very few class Ia molecules.

Structure

Class Ia molecules consist of two linked glycoprotein chains. An α chain (45 kDa) is associated with a much smaller chain called β_2-microglobulin (β_2M) (12 kDa). The α chain is inserted in the cell membrane (Figure 11-3). It consists of five domains: three extracellular domains called α_1, α_2, and α_3, each about 100 amino acids long; a transmembrane domain; and a cytoplasmic domain. The antigen-binding site on these molecules is formed by the α_1 and α_2 domains. β_2M consists of a single domain and serves to stabilize the structure.

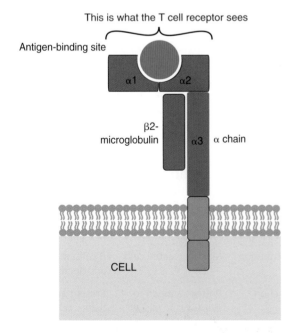

FIGURE 11-3 The structure of a class Ia MHC molecule on a cell membrane. Its antigen-binding site is formed by the folding of both its α_1 and α_2 domains.

Gene Arrangement

The size of the MHC class I region varies among mammals. Humans and rodents have the largest, and pigs have the smallest. The chicken class I region is very much smaller than in mammals (Chapter 40). The MHC class I region has a common framework of non-MHC genes, and size differences are mainly due to variations in the size and number of these framework genes.

The number of class Ia gene loci varies between mammals. For example, rats have more than 60, mice have about 30, humans have 20, cattle have 13 to 15, and pigs have 11. Not all these genes are functional. For example, in mice, only two or three class I genes are expressed. The remainder are pseudogenes (defective genes that cannot be expressed). In humans the functional polymorphic genes are called *A*, *B*, and *C*. In mice they are called *K* and *D* (and in some strains, *L*) (Figure 11-4). In other species they are usually numbered.

Polymorphism

Some class Ia loci encode proteins with very large numbers of alleles. These allelic differences cause variations in the amino acid sequences of the α_1 and α_2 domains. This variation is called polymorphism. The most extreme polymorphism is restricted to three to four small regions located within the α_1 and α_2 domains. In these variable regions, two or three different amino acids may occur at each position. The other domains of MHC class Ia molecules show little variation.

The α_1 and α_2 domains of MHC class I molecules fold together to form an open-ended groove (Figure 11-5). A flat β sheet forms the floor of this groove, and its walls are formed by two α helices (Figure 11-6). This groove binds antigenic peptides, 8 to 10 amino acids in size. The variable regions located along the walls of this groove determine its shape. The shape of the groove in turn determines which peptides can be bound and thus trigger immune responses.

The amino acid variability in the α_1 and α_2 domains results from variations in the nucleotide sequences between MHC alleles. These nucleotide variations result from point mutations, reciprocal recombination, and gene conversion. Point mutations are simply changes in individual nucleotides. Reciprocal recombination involves crossing over between two chromosomes. In gene conversion, small blocks of DNA are exchanged between different class I genes in a nonreciprocal fashion. The donated DNA blocks may come from nearby nonpolymorphic class I genes, from nonfunctional pseudogenes, or from other polymorphic class I genes. Class I MHC

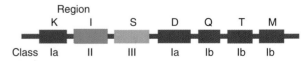

FIGURE 11-4 Arrangement of major loci within the MHC of the mouse—a typical mammalian MHC.

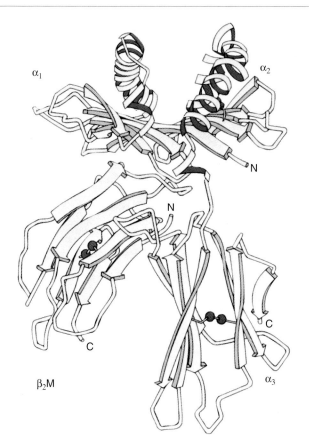

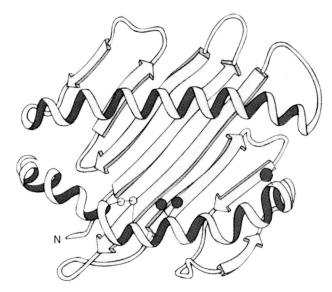

FIGURE 11-6 A view (from above) of the antigen-binding groove on an MHC class I molecule. The floor of the groove is formed by an extensive β-pleated sheet. The walls of the groove are formed by two parallel α helices. This structure is formed by the folding of the α_1 and α_2 domain of the α chain.

(From Bjorkman PJ, Saper MA, Samraoui B, Bennett WS, Strominger JL, Wiley DC: Structure of the human class I histocompatibility antigen, HLA-A2, *Nature* 329:506, 1987 Macmillan Magazines Ltd.)

FIGURE 11-5 Schematic three-dimensional view of the complete structure of HLA-A2 derived by x-ray crystallography. The antigen-binding groove at the top is formed by the α_1 and α_2 domains, whereas the α_3 domain binds to the cell membrane. The β chain (β₂-microglobulin) has no direct role in antigen binding.

(From Bjorkman PJ, Saper MA, Samraoui B, Bennett WS, Strominger JL, Wiley DC: Structure of the human class I histocompatibility antigen, HLA-A2, *Nature* 329:506, 1987 Macmillan Magazines Ltd.)

genes have the highest mutation rate of any germline genes yet studied (10^{-3} mutations per gene per generation in mice). This high mutation rate implies that there are significant advantages to be gained by having very polymorphic MHC genes.

Mammals use two distinct strategies for maintaining high levels of MHC class I diversity. Mice and humans simply use a small number of highly polymorphic genes. In other primates and rats, however, diversity is generated by varying the number and combinations of many different genes. Cattle use both strategies by employing various combinations of six or more classical class I genes, but three of these are also highly polymorphic.

Nonpolymorphic MHC Class I Molecules

Mammalian cells also express many nonpolymorphic class I molecules. Some are encoded by genes within the MHC class I region, others by genes on other chromosomes. They are classified according to their evolutionary origin.

Class Ib molecules show reduced expression and tissue distribution compared with class Ia molecules but are part of the MHC complex. They have limited polymorphism and their genes probably originated from class Ia precursors by gene duplication. For example, the class Ib genes in mice are found in three loci called *Q*, *T*, and *M* (see Figure 11-4). They code for proteins on the surface of regulatory and immature lymphocytes and on hematopoietic cells. These also consist of a membrane-bound α chain associated with β₂-microglobulin, so their overall shape and antigen-binding groove are similar to those in MHC class Ia molecules. Since they are not polymorphic, MHC class Ib molecules bind a limited range of ligands. Thus they are receptors for commonly encountered, microbial pathogen-associated molecular patterns (PAMPs).

Class Ic genes have limited polymorphism and are found within the MHC but probably originated before the radiation of the placental mammals. Their products include MICA and MICB, specialized proteins that are involved in signaling to natural killer (NK) cells but do not bind antigenic peptides (Chapter 19).

Class Id genes are nonpolymorphic class I–related genes not located on the MHC chromosome. Many of their products contribute to innate immunity since they bind PAMPs. For example, CD1 molecules bind bacterial lipids (Chapter 19). FcRn is a class Id MHC molecule that serves as an antibody (Fc) receptor on epithelial cells. It is expressed on mammary gland epithelium and on the enterocytes of newborn mammals (Chapter 21).

MHC Class II Molecules

Mammals differ in their expression of MHC class II molecules. In rodents, they are restricted to the professional antigen-presenting cells (dendritic cells, macrophages, and B cells) but can be induced on T cells, keratinocytes, and vascular endothelial cells. Resting mouse T cells do not express MHC class II molecules, but in pigs, dogs, cats, mink, and horses, the MHC class II molecules are constitutively expressed on nearly all resting adult T cells. In cattle, most MHC class II molecules are expressed only on B cells and activated T cells. In pigs, resting T cells express MHC class II molecules at about the same level as macrophages. In humans and pigs, MHC class II molecules are expressed on renal vascular endothelium and glomeruli—a fact of significance in kidney graft rejection. The expression of class II molecules is enhanced in rapidly dividing cells and in cells treated with interferon-γ (IFN-γ) (Chapter 14).

Structure

MHC class II molecules consist of two chains called α and β. Each chain has two extracellular domains (one constant and one variable), a connecting peptide, a transmembrane domain, and a cytoplasmic domain (Figure 11-7). A third chain, called the Ii or γ chain, is associated with the assembly of class II molecules within cells and was discussed in Chapter 10.

Gene Arrangement

A "complete" MHC class II region contains three paired loci. In primates, these are DPA and DPB, DQA and DQB, and DRA and DRB. (The genes for the α chains are designated A, and the genes for the β chains are called B.) Some of these genes are polymorphic. There may also be additional nonpolymorphic loci such as DM and DO in humans. The DO and DM gene products regulate the loading of antigen fragments into the MHC groove. Not all mammals possess a complete set of class II genes since nonprimates lack DPA and DPB. Not all loci contain genes for both chains, and some contain many pseudogenes. These pseudogenes serve as DNA donors that can be used to generate additional class II polymorphism by gene conversion.

Polymorphism

MHC class II proteins have an antigen-binding groove formed by their α_1 and β_1 domains. Its walls are formed by two parallel α helices, and its floor consists of a β sheet. Gene polymorphism results in variations in the amino acids forming the sides of the groove. These variations are generated in the same way as class Ia molecules. Other genes located in the class II region code for molecules involved in antigen-processing. These include the transporter proteins TAP1 and TAP2 and some proteasome components.

MHC Class III Molecules

The remaining genes within the MHC are located within the class III region (Figure 11-8). They code for proteins with many different functions. Some are important in the defense of the body such as the genes for the complement components C4, factor B, and C2 (Chapter 7). They also include genes that encode tumor necrosis factor-α (TNF-α), several lymphotoxins, and some NK cell receptors.

MHC of Domestic Animals

Every mammal studied has an MHC containing class I, class II, and class III regions. When the MHCs of different mammals are compared, some regions such as class III are conserved, whereas others are highly diverse. Likewise, the precise arrangement and number of loci varies among species (Figure 11-9). In general, genes within the class II and class III regions possess obvious orthologs in all species. That is, they are clearly derived from a single ancestor and have not usually been subjected to major rearrangements during evolution (ruminant class II genes are an exception). Class I genes, in contrast, have been reorganized so many different times by deletion and duplication that their amino acid sequences differ widely, and it is very difficult to compare class I genes in different species. They are said to be paralogous (Box 11-1).

Horses

In the horse, the ELA complex is of conventional structure, but its sequence is reversed in relation to the centromere, and it contains two large insertions between the gene regions

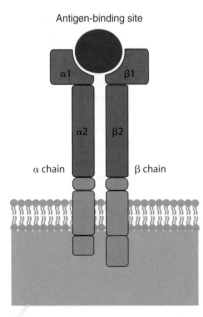

FIGURE 11-7 Diagram showing the structure of a MHC class II antigen located on a cell surface. Note that the antigen-binding site is formed by the variable domains from both peptide chains.

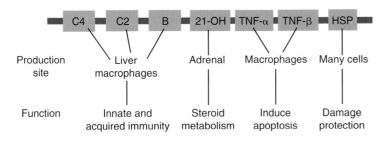

FIGURE 11-8 The arrangement of selected genes within the MHC class III region. These genes all play a role in innate and adaptive immunity. There are many other genes within this region that have no apparent role in immunity.

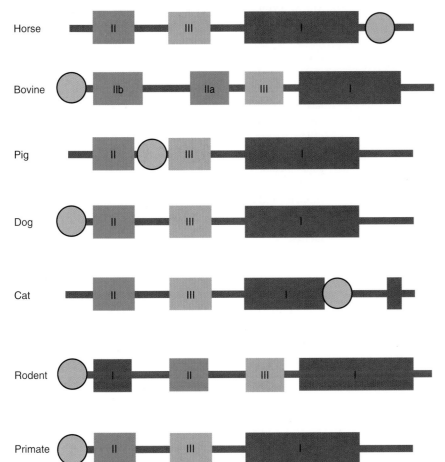

FIGURE 11-9 Arrangement of gene regions within the MHC in different species of domestic mammals.

(Figure 11-10). It is located on chromosome 20. Ten horse haplotypes have now been recognized, and at least 7 MHC class I loci are expressed among these haplotypes. They also have eight class I pseudogenes. Their haplotypes differ in the number of different class I genes expressed, ranging from two to five, so that the MHC haplotype organization of the horse is similar to that described for the cow and sheep rather than the human. There are extensive differences in haplotype structure within horse breeds. Unlike other mammals, the equine DRA locus is polymorphic, with at least 11 alleles.

Cattle

In cattle, the MHC is structurally unique in that inversion of a large chromosome segment has moved several class II genes close to the centromere of bovine chromosome 23. As a result,

the BoLA class II region is divided into two subregions called IIa and IIb. The class IIb genes are separated from the class IIa genes by a "gap" of 17 centimorgans (cM) (Figure 11-11).

Cattle have at least six class Ia loci but only one or combinations of two or three are expressed in different haplotypes (e.g., 1, 2, 4 or 3, 5 or 2, 3). Some combinations are more common than others. For example, there are three common, equally polymorphic genes that are only expressed in certain combinations. One of these (gene 2) is expressed on nearly all haplotypes. Genes 1 and 3 are never expressed together. Genes 4, 5, and 6 are expressed in a limited number of haplotypes. There is also some interlocus recombination, resulting in the production of "hybrid genes."

Cattle express only two class II proteins, DQ and DR, although in many cattle haplotypes, the DQ locus is duplicated. Because of this duplication, additional MHC diversity can be generated by interhaplotype pairing; that is, DQA and DQB gene products from different chromosomes can be paired. The DRA chain in cattle is not polymorphic, and polymorphism in the DRB chains is the only source of DR diversity. Both DQA and DQB are polymorphic. Cattle, sheep, and goats possess ruminant-specific class II genes (DYA, DYB, and DI) and lack a DP locus.

Sheep

The sheep MHC (*Ovar-Mhc*) has a basic structure similar to that of other mammals. It is located on chromosome 20. There are at least eight class I loci, but the number varies between haplotypes.

◻ **Box 11-1** ❘ **MHC Allele Nomenclature**

Recently there has been a move toward a standardized nomenclature system for MHC alleles based on gene sequences. Although minor differences in nomenclature occur between species, all are based on the human (HLA) system and on the amino acid sequence of the alleles. For example, in cattle MHC class II genes, alleles are described by a series of numbers separated by colons. For example: BoLA * 123:03:02:01. The first three digits represent the allele group, the second two are the number of changes in the coding region, the third two are the number of changes in the noncoding region, and the last pair are the number of changes in promoters or introns. In general the last four numbers are unknown or rarely used. A completely described locus will be nine digits long. A similar system is used for class I genes.

The class II region contains one DRA, four DRB (one coding and three pseudogenes), one DQA1, two DQA2, and one each of DQB1, DQB2, DNA, DOB, DYA, DYB, DMA, and DMB. The class IIa loci are arranged in the order DQB2, DQA2, DQB1, DQA,1 and DRB1. All five loci are transcribed. The class III region contains C4, C2, Bf, and TNF-α genes.

Pigs

The SLA complex is located on chromosome 7 and divided by the centromere. It contains class I, II, and III regions. The class I and III regions are therefore located on the short arm and the class II region is located on the long arm of this chromosome. The pig MHC is the smallest yet found among the mammals since it contains only about 2 million bases. Pigs have seven class Ia genes and three class Ib genes, but only three of the class Ia genes (SLA-1, -2, and -3) are functional, and the others are pseudogenes. As in cattle, the number of expressed class I genes varies between haplotypes. Pig class II expressed genes include the α and β chains of SLA-DR, -DQ, -DM, and -DO. There are no DP loci. The SLA class III region is centromeric and contiguous with the class I region.

Dogs

The DLA complex is located on chromosome 12. There are four transcribed class I genes (DLA-12, -79, -64, and -88), but only one, DLA-88, is polymorphic. DLA-DRA, DRB, DQA, and DQB class II loci have been identified, and many are highly polymorphic. For example, to date, 62 DRB1, 21 DQA1, and 48 DQB1 alleles have been identified. Some class II haplotypes appear to be characteristic of certain breeds, whereas

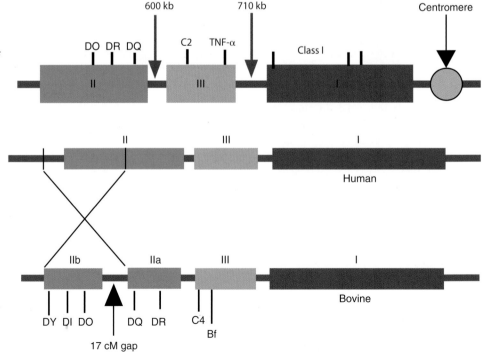

FIGURE 11-10 Schematic diagram showing the overall arrangement of the equine MHC (ELA).

(Courtesy Drs. AL Gustafson and L Skow.)

FIGURE 11-11 The arrangement of genes within the human and bovine MHC. The only major difference is the presence of a large inversion at the 5′ end of the bovine class II region that results in the development of a large gap within the bovine class II region.

variations between breeds are great. This high interbreed but low intrabreed variation likely accounts for the differences in breed susceptibility to infectious and autoimmune diseases.

Cats

The cat MHC is intermediate in size between mouse and human and is located on chromosome B2. The FeLA class I region is divided into two regions by the centromere and appears to contain only one functional polymorphic locus. Its class II region has no functional *DP* genes, and its DQ region has been deleted (a feature seen only in the cat). In compensation, it has a highly polymorphic DR locus with at least two *DRB* genes and 24 alleles and three *DRA* genes.

Primates

The human MHC, known as HLA, contains three class Ia loci, A, B, and C, and at least three functional class Ib loci, E, F, and G. Most Old World primates possess all of these except C, which is found only in humans, gorillas, and chimpanzees, and G, which is found only in humans. In orangutans and rhesus monkeys, the A and B loci are duplicated. In contrast, the New World primates, such as cotton-top tamarins, have MHC class I genes most closely related to HLA-G. They do not possess any genes related to HLA-A, -B, or -C. In view of the lack of class I MHC diversity in cotton-top tamarins, it is perhaps not surprising that they are susceptible to fatal infection with viruses that are not fatal in humans.

MHC Molecules and Disease

Since the function of MHC molecules is to present antigens to the cells of the immune system, MHC genes regulate immune responses. A foreign molecule that cannot bind to at least one MHC molecule will not trigger an adaptive immune response (Figure 11-12). Thus, expression of specific MHC alleles determines susceptibility to infectious and autoimmune diseases (Box 11-2).

Because class Ia and class II MHC molecules are structurally diverse, each MHC allele can bind and present a different set of antigenic peptides. The more diversity within an animal's MHC, the more antigens it can respond to. Thus an MHC heterozygous animal will express many more alleles and respond to a greater variety of antigenic peptides than can a homozygous animal (Figure 11-13).

MHC polymorphism is maintained in populations by a process called overdominant selection or heterozygote advantage. Simply put, MHC heterozygotes are at an advantage because they can respond to a greater range of antigens and so are best fitted to survive infectious diseases. The antigen-binding sites of MHC class Ia or II molecules are also very nonspecific (or degenerate), and it has been estimated that an average MHC molecule can bind about 2500 different peptides. This is because the MHC groove binds tightly to the peptide backbone rather than to its amino acid side chains. Nevertheless, structural constraints limit the efficiency of binding of each allele. As a result, it is likely that only one or two peptides from an average antigenic protein can bind to any given MHC molecule. The ability of MHC molecules to bind antigens must be a limiting factor in generating adaptive immunity and resistance to infectious agents. Increasing the diversity of MHC molecules increases the diversity of peptides that can be bound and so increases resistance to infections. Because most individuals are MHC heterozygotes, each individual normally expresses at most six different class Ia molecules (in humans, for example, two each are coded for by the HLA-A, -B, and C loci). The number of expressed MHC molecules is not greater because that would increase the risk that the MHC molecules could bind and present more self-antigens. This would require the elimination of many more

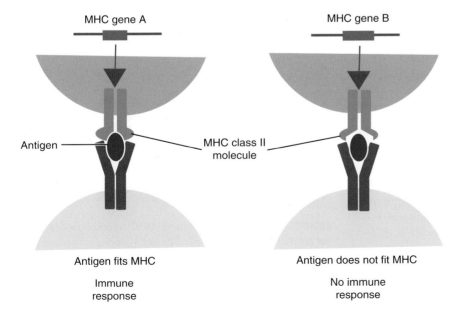

FIGURE 11-12 MHC molecules regulate the immune response. Only antigen fragments that can bind in the groove of a MHC molecule will trigger an immune response. This is called MHC restriction. Thus the genes that code for these MHC molecules will also regulate immune responsiveness.

□ Box 11-2 | **Why Are Infectious Diseases Still Important?**

It has often been asked why natural selection by infectious agents has not resulted in the selection of animals with very strong immunity and the consequent elimination of all susceptible animals? The answer lies in the relative benefits and costs of an effective immune response. Thus pressure from parasites and infectious agents should favor the development of resistance mechanisms and strong immunity. However, an effective immune system also incurs significant energy costs. Immune responses are expensive in terms of energy and protein use, and excessive investments in immunity may impair other key survival mechanisms such as reproductive ability. It is also theoretically possible that high-responding animals are more likely to develop autoimmunity.

This has been elegantly shown for Soay sheep living on the isolated island of Hirta near St. Kilda off the Scottish coast. Those sheep that mount the highest antibody response to parasites tended to be healthier and to survive the harsh winters more effectively. However, these sheep also tended to be less fertile and had not bred in the previous year. The advantages of increased survival were thus offset by decreased fertility. The costs of a high immune response are such that, on average, animals develop optimal rather than maximal immunity.

A similar phenomenon has been well recognized in birds whereby those male birds with the most developed breeding plumage tend to mount a poorer immune response and thus show impaired survival.

Graham AL, Hayward AD, Watt KA, et al: Fitness correlates of heritable variation in antibody responsiveness in a wild mammal, *Science* 330: 662–665, 2010.

HETEROZYGOUS

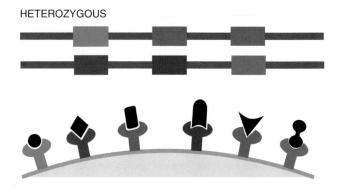

HOMOZYGOUS

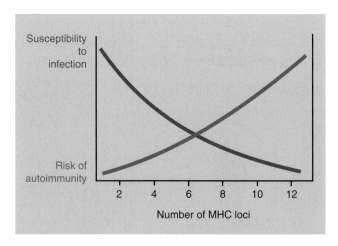

FIGURE 11-13 Heterozygous animals with two MHC alleles coded for at each locus express six different antigen-presenting molecules on the cell surface. Therefore, they generate a more diverse and effective immune response than homozygous animals with only one MHC a single allele coded for at each locus. An example of heterozygote advantage.

self-reactive T cells during development (Chapter 20). Thus the presence of six different MHC class Ia molecules appears to be a reasonable compromise between maximizing the recognition of foreign antigens while at the same time minimizing the chances of recognizing self-antigens (Figure 11-14).

MHC class Ia loci encode very polymorphic genes. For example, the H-2K locus in the mouse codes for more than 100 alleles. Since there can never be more than two alleles per locus in any individual animal, it appears that this number of alleles has evolved to maximize polymorphism in mice. This may protect the population as a whole from complete destruction. Because of MHC polymorphism, most individuals in a population carry a unique set of class Ia alleles, and each individual can therefore respond to a unique mixture of antigens. When a new infectious disease strikes such a population, it is likely that at least some individuals will possess MHC molecules that can bind the new microbial antigens and trigger immunity. Those that can respond will mount an immune response and live. Those that lack these molecules cannot respond and will die.

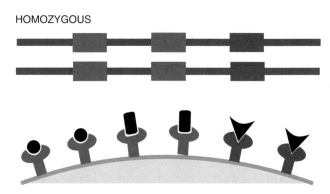

FIGURE 11-14 The optimal number of MHC loci is a balance between the need to respond to as many different microbial antigens as possible and the need to avoid autoimmune responses. Computer modeling suggests that the optimal number of MHC loci is six.

When large populations of humans or mice are examined, no single MHC haplotype predominates. In other words, no single MHC haplotype confers major survival advantages on individual animals. This reflects the futility of the host attempting to bind all the antigens in a population of invading microorganisms. Microbes will always be able to mutate and evade the immune response faster than mammals can develop resistance. Any changes in an MHC allele may increase resistance to one organism but at the same time decrease resistance to another. It is more advantageous therefore for the members of a population to possess many highly diverse MHC alleles so that any pathogen spreading through a population will have to adapt anew to each individual.

Highly adaptable social animals, such as humans or mice, with large populations through which disease can spread rapidly, usually show extensive MHC polymorphism (Figure 11-15). In contrast, low-density solitary species such as the marine mammals (whales and elephant seals), moose, Tasmanian devils, or Asiatic lions have much less polymorphism. It is also of interest to note the case of the cheetah, in which some captive populations have reduced polymorphism as a result of recent population bottlenecks. Because of this lack of MHC diversity, some cheetahs will accept allografts from other, unrelated cheetahs. Likewise an infectious disease such as feline infectious peritonitis causes 60% mortality in captive cheetahs compared with 1% to 2% mortality in domestic cats.

There are many examples of relationships between MHC haplotype and resistance to infectious disease. For example, in cattle there is an association between possession of certain BoLA alleles and resistance to bovine leukosis, squamous cell eye carcinoma, and trypanosomiasis; responsiveness to foot-and-mouth disease virus; and susceptibility to the tick *Boophilus microplus*. Cows with BoLA-Aw8 are more likely to be seropositive for leukosis, a disease caused by bovine leukemia virus (BLV). Resistance is associated with possession of BoLA-Aw7, and susceptibility is associated with possession of BoLA-Aw12. B cell proliferation and expression of BLV-induced B cell tumors are also controlled by BoLA. BoLA-Aw14 seems to influence age at seroconversion, whereas BoLA-Aw12 seems to

be associated with susceptibility to B cell proliferation. However, these associations with the BoLA-A locus are relatively weak compared with the association between susceptibility and certain BoLA-DRB alleles such as DRB3. BoLA-DRB3 polymorphism influences resistance or susceptibility to bovine leukemia virus. This resistance is associated with the presence of glu-arg in the antigen-binding site of DRB3 at positions 70 and 71, whereas the presence of val-asp-thr-tyr at positions 75 to 78, is associated with susceptibility.

BoLA-A*16 is associated with resistance to mastitis. BoLA-A*6 and BoLA-A*16 are associated with high, and BoLA-A*2 with low, antibody responses to human serum albumin. Disease associations are also seen with class II alleles. Thus possession of BoLA-DRB3.2*23 is associated with an increased incidence of severe coliform mastitis. The DRB3*3 allele is associated with a lower risk for retained placenta, whereas *6 and *22 are associated with a lower risk for cystic ovarian disease. Resistance to *Dermatophilus* species has also been mapped to the BoLA DR locus.

In sheep, there is an association of the class I allele SY1 with resistance to *Trichostrongylus colubriformis*. Ovar-DRB1 locus affects egg production in *Ostertagia* species infection. Resistance to scrapie and to caseous lymphadenitis appears to be associated with possession of certain MHC class I alleles.

In goats, the class I allele Be7 is associated with resistance, and Be1 and Be14 are associated with susceptibility to caprine arthritis-encephalitis (CAE). Genetic resistance or susceptibility to *Ehrlichia ruminantium* infection (heartwater) is associated with class I CLA and Be alleles.

In horses, an allergic response to the bites of *Culicoides* midges is linked to ELA-Aw7. There is also a strong association between ELA-A3, ELA-A15, and ELA-Dw13 and the development of sarcoid tumors (fibroblastic skin tumors likely induced by bovine papilloma viruses). An autoimmune disease, equine recurrent uveitis, is strongly associated with the haplotype ELA-A9.

In pigs, the SLA complex has an influence on major reproduction parameters such as ovulation rate, litter size, and piglet viability. This may be due to the role played by the enzyme 21-hydroxylase, whose gene is located in the class III region. Serum antibody levels are also influenced by SLA haplotype. Even the numbers of larvae of the parasite *Trichinella spiralis* in muscle are regulated by genes in the SLA complex. Quantitative trait loci for backfat thickness, average daily gain, weight, and reproductive traits have been mapped to the SLA complex. For example, low growth performance in large white pigs is associated with possession of SLA class I alleles 4, 5, and 20. High carcass fatness in Landrace pigs is associated with alleles 1, 15, and 18. The precise gene or genes responsible for these traits has not been identified. One possible candidate is the class III gene that codes for a 17β-hydroxysteroid dehydrogenase called *FABGL* since this enzyme oxidizes estradiol, testosterone, and dihydrotestosterone, and these hormones regulate adipose tissue formation.

Selection for specific MHC haplotypes has potential for use in developing disease-resistant strains of domestic animals.

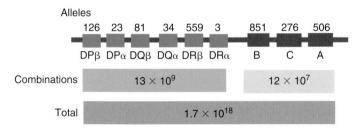

FIGURE 11-15 An example of how MHC polymorphism can generate an enormous number of different MHC haplotypes. The numbers above each locus are the number of identified alleles in the human MHC as of January 2007. The number of different combinations can be determined by multiplying all of them together. Thus there are 13 × 10⁹ class II combinations, 12 × 10⁷ class I combinations, and 1.7 × 10¹⁸ total possible combinations—more than sufficient to give every human a unique haplotype.

However, it must be pointed out that by selecting for a specific gene locus, one may also inadvertently select for susceptibility at closely linked loci. This may outweigh the benefits of a resistant allele at one locus. An animal cannot be resistant to all possible infectious diseases.

MHC and Body Odors

The vomeronasal organ in mammals is an olfactory organ that is used to detect information about another individual's gender, status, and individuality. The molecules that carry this information are small volatile peptides found in urine. These peptides can bind to the antigen-binding grooves of MHC class I molecules. Thus, peptides known to bind to two mouse MHC class I molecules of different haplotypes were shown to induce responses (field potentials) in mouse vomeronasal organs. The responses were not haplotype specific, but different peptides induced different activation patterns. This finding may well explain how mammals such as mice can recognize the MHC of other mice by smell.

The class I region of mice, cattle, and pigs contains numerous genes coding for pheromone olfactory receptors. As a result, the MHC haplotype affects the recognition of individual odors in an allele-specific fashion and thus influences the mating preferences of mammals. Under controlled conditions, mice (and humans!) prefer to mate with MHC-incompatible individuals. Such matings preferentially generate heterozygote advantage, resulting in optimized disease resistance. However, this type of mating could also prevent genome-wide inbreeding. Inbreeding avoidance may be the most important function of MHC-based mating preferences and therefore the fundamental selective force diversifying MHC genes in species with such mating patterns.

For sources of additional information, please visit http://evolve.elsevier.com/tizard/immunology/

Organs of the Immune System

Key Points

- Adaptive immunity is mediated by cells called lymphocytes that are found mainly within lymphoid organs.
- Lymphocytes arise from stem cells in the bone marrow.
- Lymphocytes mature within primary lymphoid organs. There are two types of lymphocyte: T cells and B cells.
- T cells mature within the thymus. B cells mature within gastrointestinal lymphoid tissues, the bone marrow, or the bursa of Fabricius, depending on species.
- If newly developed lymphocytes have receptors for self-antigens that could potentially cause tissue damage, they are killed before they can leave primary lymphoid organs.
- Mature lymphocytes leave the primary lymphoid organs to reside in secondary lymphoid organs, where their role is to encounter and respond to foreign antigens.
- The major secondary lymphoid organs include lymph nodes, spleen, bone marrow, and some Peyer's patches within the intestine.

Although antigens are captured and processed by dendritic cells, macrophages, and B cells, adaptive immune responses are actually mounted by cells called lymphocytes. Lymphocytes are the small round cells that predominate in organs such as the spleen, lymph nodes, and thymus (Figure 12-1). These are called lymphoid organs. Lymphocytes have antigen receptors on their surface and can therefore recognize and respond to foreign antigens. Lymphocytes are eventually responsible for the production of antibodies and for cell-mediated immune responses. The lymphoid organs must therefore provide an environment for efficient interaction among lymphocytes, antigen-presenting cells, and foreign antigens as well as sites where lymphocytes can respond optimally to processed antigens.

Immune responses must be carefully regulated. Lymphocytes must be selected so that their receptors will only bind foreign antigens, and the response of each lymphocyte must be regulated so that it is sufficient but not excessive for the body's requirements. The lymphoid organs may therefore be classified on the basis of their roles in generating lymphocytes, in regulating the production of lymphocytes, and in providing an environment for trapping foreign antigens, processing them, and maximizing the opportunity for processed antigens to encounter and interact with lymphocytes (Figure 12-2).

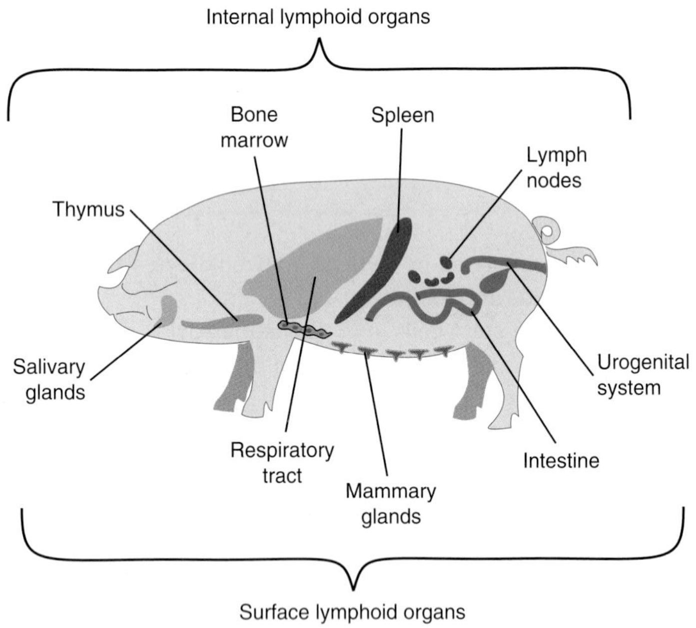

Sources of Lymphocytes

Lymphoid stem cells are first found in the fetal omentum, liver, and yolk sac. In older fetuses and in adults, these stem cells are mainly found in the bone marrow. The bone marrow has multiple functions in adult mammals. It is a hematopoietic organ containing the precursors of all blood cells, including lymphocytes. In some mammals, such as primates, it also acts as a primary lymphoid organ (a site where newly produced lymphocytes can mature). Like the spleen, liver, and lymph nodes, the bone marrow is also a secondary lymphoid organ. It contains many dendritic cells and macrophages and thus removes foreign material from the blood. It contains large numbers of antibody-producing cells and is therefore a major source of antibodies. Because of these multiple functions, the bone marrow is divided into a hematopoietic compartment and a vascular compartment. These compartments alternate, like slices of cake, in wedge-shaped areas within long bones. The hematopoietic compartment contains stem cells for all the blood cells as well as macrophages, dendritic cells, and lymphocytes and is enclosed by a layer of adventitial cells. In older animals these adventitial cells may become so loaded with fat

FIGURE 12-1 The major lymphoid tissues of the pig, a typical mammal.

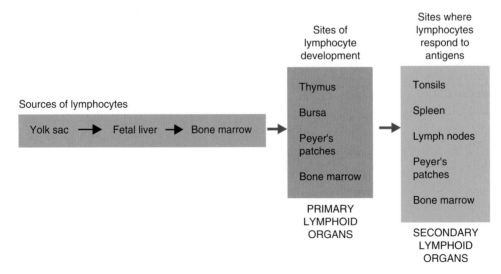

FIGURE 12-2 The lymphoid organs can conveniently be divided into three groups based on their role in the development and functioning of lymphocyte populations.

that the marrow may have a fatty yellow appearance. The vascular compartment, where antigens are mainly trapped, consists of blood sinuses lined by endothelial cells and crossed by a network of reticular cells and macrophages.

Primary Lymphoid Organs

The organs that regulate the development of lymphocytes are called primary lymphoid organs. Lymphocytes fall into two major populations called T cells and B cells, based on the primary organ in which they mature. Thus, all T cells mature in the thymus. B cells, in contrast, mature within different organs depending on species. These include the bursa of Fabricius in birds, the bone marrow in primates and rodents, and the intestinal lymphoid tissues in rabbits, ruminants, and pigs. The primary lymphoid organs all develop early in fetal life. As animals develop, newly produced, immature lymphocytes migrate from the bone marrow to the primary lymphoid organs, where they mature (Table 12-1). The primary lymphoid organs are not sites where lymphocytes encounter foreign antigens, and they do not enlarge in response to antigenic stimulation.

Thymus

The thymus is located in the thoracic cavity in front of and below the heart. In horses, cattle, sheep, pigs, and chickens, it also extends up the neck as far as the thyroid gland. The size of the thymus varies, its relative size being greatest in the newborn animal and its absolute size being greatest before puberty. It may be very small and difficult to find in adult animals.

Structure The thymus consists of lobules of loosely packed epithelial cells, each covered by a connective tissue capsule. The outer part of each lobule, the cortex, is densely infiltrated with lymphocytes (or thymocytes), but the inner medulla contains fewer lymphocytes, and the epithelial cells are clearly visible (Figure 12-3). Within the medulla are also found round, layered bodies called thymic or Hassall's corpuscles. These contain keratin, and the remains of a small blood vessel may be found at their center. In cattle these corpuscles may contain immunoglobulin A (Chapter 16). An abnormally thick basement membrane and a continuous layer of epithelial cells surround the capillaries that supply the thymic cortex. This barrier prevents circulating foreign antigens from entering the cortex. No lymphatic vessels leave the thymus. As an animal ages, the thymus shrinks and is gradually replaced by fat. However, the aged thymus still contains small amounts of lymphoid tissue and remains functionally active.

Function The functions of the thymus are best demonstrated by studying the effects of its removal in rodents. These effects depend on the age of the animal. For example, mice thymectomized within a day of birth become susceptible to infections and may fail to grow. These animals have very few circulating lymphocytes and cannot reject foreign organ grafts because they lose the ability to mount cell-mediated immune responses (Table 12-2). In contrast, adult thymectomy has no immediate obvious effect. But if these mice are monitored for several

▢ Table 12-1 ǀ Comparison of Primary and Secondary Lymphoid Organs		
	PRIMARY	**SECONDARY**
Origin	Ectoendodermal junction or endoderm	Mesoderm
Time of development	Early in embryonic life	Late in fetal life
Persistence	Involutes after puberty	Persists in adults
Effect of removal	Loss of lymphocytes	No or minor effects
Response to antigen	Unresponsive	Fully reactive
Examples	Thymus, bursa, some Peyer patches	Spleen, lymph nodes

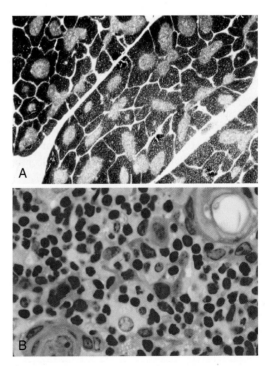

FIGURE 12-3 A, A section of a monkey thymus. Each lobule is divided into a cortex rich in lymphocytes, hence staining darkly, and a paler medulla consisting mainly of epithelial cells. Original magnification ×10. **B,** A high-power view of the medulla of a monkey thymus showing several pale-staining epithelial cells with cytoplasmic processes and many dark-staining, round lymphocytes. Original magnification ×1000.

☐ **Table 12-2** | **Effects of Neonatal Thymectomy and Bursectomy**

FUNCTION	THYMECTOMY	BURSECTOMY
Numbers of circulating lymphocytes	Disappear	No effect
Presence of lymphocytes in T-dependent areas	Disappear	No effect
Graft rejection	Suppressed	No effect
Presence of lymphocytes in T-independent areas	Minor depletion	Disappear
Plasma cells in lymphoid tissues	Minor drop	Disappear
Serum immunoglobulins	Minor drop	Major drop
Antibody formation	Minor effects	Major drop

months, the number of blood lymphocytes and their ability to mount cell-mediated immune responses gradually decline. This suggests that the thymus remains functional in adults, but there is a reservoir of long-lived thymus-derived cells that must be exhausted before the effects of adult thymectomy become apparent (Figure 12-4).

The results of thymectomy indicate that the neonatal thymus is the source of most blood lymphocytes and that these lymphocytes are mainly responsible for mounting cell-mediated immune responses. They are called thymus-derived lymphocytes or T cells. T-cell precursors originate in the bone marrow but then enter the thymus. Once within the thymus, the cells (called thymocytes) divide rapidly. Of the new cells produced, most die by apoptosis, whereas the survivors (about 5% of the total in rodents and about 25% in calves) remain in the thymus for 4 to 5 days before leaving and colonizing the secondary lymphoid organs.

T cells that enter the thymus have two conflicting tasks. They must recognize foreign antigens but at the same time must not respond strongly to normal body constituents (self-antigens). A two-stage selection process in the thymic medulla accomplishes this feat. Thus thymocytes with receptors that bind self-antigens strongly and that could therefore cause auto-immunity are killed by apoptosis. Thymocytes with receptors that cannot bind any major histocompatibility complex (MHC) class II molecules and thus cannot react to any processed antigen are also killed.

On the other hand, those thymocytes that survive this "negative selection" process but can still recognize specific MHC class II–antigen complexes with moderate affinity are stimulated to grow—a process called positive selection. These surviving cells eventually leave the thymus as mature T cells, circulate in the bloodstream, and colonize the secondary lymphoid organs.

Thymic epithelial cells are unusual since they express more than 400 antigens normally expressed in other tissues. In addition, these cells have a very high level of autophagy. As a result, their intracellular antigens are bound to MHC class II molecules and expressed in large amounts on the epithelial cell surfaces. This "promiscuous" antigen presentation ensures that developing T cells are exposed to an unusually diverse array of normal tissue antigens. Since T cells that respond to these antigens will die, the system ensures that those T cells leaving the thymus cannot respond to normal body components.

Thymic Hormones Within the thymus, cell functions are regulated by a complex mixture of cytokines and small peptides collectively known as thymic hormones. These include peptides variously called thymosins, thymopoietins, thymic humoral factor, thymulin, and the thymostimulins. Thymulin is especially interesting because it is a zinc-containing peptide secreted by the thymic epithelial cells, and it can partially restore T cell function in thymectomized animals. Zinc is an essential mineral for the development of T cells. Consequently, zinc-deficient animals have defective cell-mediated immune responses (Chapter 38). Hassall's corpuscles play a functional role in regulating thymic activity since they express a growth factor called thymic stromal lymphopoietin. This molecule activates thymic dendritic cells that can stimulate regulatory T cells and controls the positive selection process.

Bursa of Fabricius

The bursa of Fabricius is found only in birds. It is a round sac located just above the cloaca (Figure 12-5). Like the thymus, the bursa reaches its greatest size in the chick about 1 to 2 weeks after hatching and then shrinks as the bird ages. It is very difficult to identify in older birds.

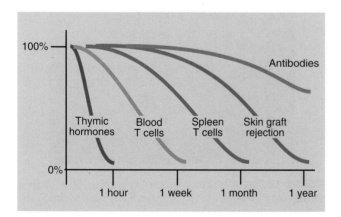

FIGURE 12-4 The effects of adult thymectomy on immune responses. Note that it takes up to a year for the full consequences to become apparent. This reflects the prolonged survival of circulating T cells.

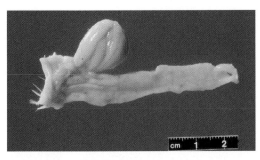

FIGURE 12-5 The bursa of Fabricius obtained from a 1-week-old chicken. It has been cut open to reveal the folds inside.

Structure Like the thymus, the bursa consists of lymphocytes embedded in epithelial tissue. This epithelial tissue lines a hollow sac connected to the cloaca by a duct. Inside the sac, folds of epithelium extend into the lumen, and scattered through the folds are round masses of lymphocytes called lymphoid follicles (Figure 12-6). Each follicle is divided into a cortex and a medulla. The cortex contains lymphocytes, plasma cells, and macrophages. At the corticomedullary junction there is a basement membrane and capillary network on the inside of which are epithelial cells. These medullary epithelial cells are replaced by lymphoblasts and lymphocytes in the center of the

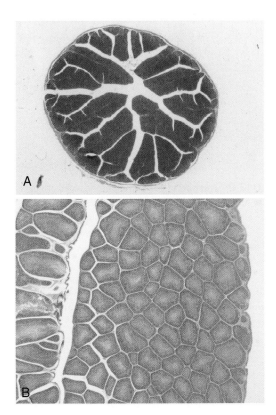

FIGURE 12-6 Photomicrographs showing the structure of the bursa of Fabricius. **A,** Low-power micrograph showing the bursa of a 13-day-old chick. Original magnification ×5. **B,** A high-power view. Original magnification ×360.

(From a specimen provided by Drs. N.H. McArthur and L.C. Abbott.)

follicle. Specialized neuroendocrine dendritic cells of unknown function surround each follicle.

Function The bursa may be removed either surgically or by infecting newborn chicks with a virus that destroys the bursa (infectious bursal disease virus). Since the bursa shrinks when chicks become sexually mature, bursal atrophy can also be provoked by administration of testosterone. Bursectomized birds have very low levels of antibodies in their blood, and antibody-producing cells disappear from lymphoid organs. However, they still possess circulating lymphocytes and can reject foreign skin grafts. Thus, bursectomy has little effect on the cell-mediated immune response. Bursectomized birds are more susceptible than normal to leptospirosis and salmonellosis but not to intracellular bacteria such as *Mycobacterium avium*.

Thus the bursa is a primary lymphoid organ that functions as a maturation and differentiation site for the cells of the antibody-forming system. Lymphocytes originating in the bursa are therefore called B cells. The bursa acts like the thymus insofar as immature cells produced in the bone marrow migrate to the bursa. These cells then proliferate rapidly, but 90% to 95% of these eventually die by apoptosis—the negative selection of self-reactive B cells. Once their maturation is completed, the surviving B cells emigrate to secondary lymphoid organs.

Close examination shows that the bursa is not a pure primary lymphoid organ because it can also trap antigens and undertake some antibody synthesis. It also contains a small focus of T cells just above the bursal duct opening. Several different hormones have been extracted from the bursa. The most important of these is a tripeptide (Lys- His-glycylamide) called bursin that activates B cells but not T cells.

Peyer's Patches

Structure Peyer's patches (PPs) are lymphoid organs located in the walls of the small intestine. Their structure and functions vary among species. Thus in ruminants, pigs, horses, dogs, and humans (group I), 80% to 90% of the PPs are found in the ileum, where they form a single continuous structure that extends forward from the ileocecal junction. In young ruminants and pigs, the ileal PPs may be as long as 2 m. Ileal PPs consist of densely packed lymphoid follicles, each separated by a connective tissue sheath, and contain only B cells (Figure 12-7).

The ileal PPs reach maximal size and maturity before birth at a time when they are shielded from foreign antigens and collectively form the largest lymphoid tissue in 6-week-old lambs. (They constitute about 1% of total body weight, like the thymus.) They disappear by 15 months of age and cannot be detected in adult sheep.

These group I species also have a second type of PP that consists of multiple discrete accumulations of follicles in the jejunum. These jejunal PPs persist for the life of the animal. They consist of pear-shaped follicles separated by extensive

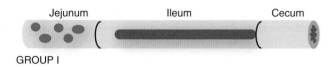

GROUP I

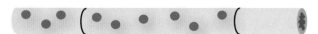

GROUP II

FIGURE 12-7 Schematic diagram showing the differences between the arrangement of Peyer's patches in group 1 and group II mammals. The large ileal Peyer's patch in some group I mammals is a primary lymphoid organ that regresses at about a year of age.

interfollicular tissue and contain mainly B cells with up to 30% T cells (Figure 12-8).

The pig is also a group I species. Pigs have about 30 jejunal PPs that are of conventional structure and a single, large ileal PP. Their ileal PP lacks T cells and has a structure similar to that seen in sheep. It regresses within the first year of life, but does not appear to be a primary lymphoid organ since it is not required for B cell development. Dogs also belong to group I. They have two types of PPs, including a single ileal PP that shows early involution and contains predominantly immature B cells.

In other mammals, such as primates, rabbits, and rodents (group II), PPs are located at random intervals in the ileum and jejunum. In these mammals, the PPs do not develop until 2 to 4 weeks after birth and persist into old age. The development of the PPs in some group II animals appears to depend entirely on stimulation by the normal intestinal microflora since they remain small and poorly developed in germ-free mice. The appendix also plays a key role in B cell development in rabbits.

Function The ileal PPs of some group I species function in a manner similar to the avian bursa. Thus, ileal PPs are sites of rapid B cell proliferation, although most cells then undergo apoptosis, and the survivors are released into the circulation. If their ileal PPs are surgically removed, lambs become B cell deficient and fail to produce antibodies. The bone marrow of lambs contains many fewer lymphocytes than the bone marrow of laboratory rodents, and their ileal PPs are therefore their most significant source of B cells.

Lymphoglandular Complexes

Lymphoglandular complexes are found in the wall of the large intestine and cecum in horses, ruminants, dogs, and pigs. They consist of submucosal masses of lymphoid tissue penetrated by radially branching extensions of mucosal glands. These glands penetrate both the submucosa and the lymphoid nodule. They are lined by intestinal columnar epithelium containing goblet cells, intraepithelial lymphocytes, and M cells (Chapter 22).

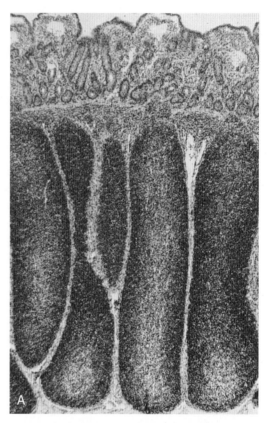

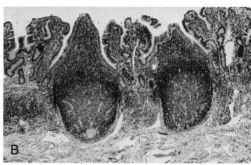

FIGURE 12-8 Structure of the two different types of Peyer's patch in sheep. **A,** An ileal Peyer's patch at age 8 weeks. **B,** A Peyer's patch from the jejunum, also at 8 weeks. Original magnification ×32.
(From Reynolds JD, Morris B: The evolution and involution of Peyer's patches in fetal and postnatal sheep, *Eur J Immunol* 13:631, 1983.)

Their function is unknown, but they contain many plasma cells, suggesting that they are sites of antibody production. Because of their structural similarity to the avian bursa and the presence of many M cells, they may be antigen-sampling sites.

Bone Marrow

The specialized ileal PP is the primary lymphoid organ for B cells only in group I mammals (ruminants, pigs, and dogs). In group II mammals the bone marrow probably serves this function. There is no exclusive B cell development site in the bone marrow, although it is suggested that precursor B cells develop at the outer edge of the marrow and migrate to the center as they mature and multiply. Negative selection occurs within the bone marrow so that, as in other primary lymphoid organs, most of the pre-B cells generated are destroyed.

Secondary Lymphoid Organs

The cells of the immune system must be able to respond to a huge diversity of pathogens that an animal may encounter. It is especially important that antigen-specific lymphocytes can encounter their target antigens. To maximize the probability of such encounters, the body employs secondary lymphoid organs. In contrast to the primary lymphoid organs, the secondary lymphoid organs arise late in fetal life and persist in adults. Unlike primary lymphoid organs, they enlarge in response to antigenic stimulation. Surgical removal of one of them does not significantly reduce immune capability. Examples of secondary lymphoid organs include the spleen, the lymph nodes, the tonsils, and other lymphoid tissues in the intestinal, respiratory, and urogenital tracts. These organs contain dendritic cells that trap and process antigens and lymphocytes that mediate the immune responses. The overall anatomical structure of these organs is therefore designed to facilitate antigen trapping and to provide the optimal environment for the initiation of immune responses. Secondary lymphoid organs are connected to both the blood and lymphoid systems, thus allowing them to continuously sample and concentrate circulating antigens.

Lymph Nodes

Structure Lymph nodes are round or bean-shaped filters strategically placed on lymphatic vessels in such a way that they can sample antigens carried in the lymph (Figure 12-9). Lymph nodes consist of a capsule beneath which is a reticular network filled with lymphocytes, macrophages, and dendritic cells and through which lymphatic sinuses penetrate (Figure 12-10). The lymph node thus acts as a filter for lymph fluid. A subcapsular sinus is located immediately under the connective tissue capsule. Other sinuses pass through the body of the node but are most prominent in the medulla. Afferent lymphatics enter the node around its circumference, and efferent lymphatics leave from a depression or hilus on one side. The blood vessels supplying a lymph node also enter and leave through the hilus.

The interior of lymph nodes is divided into three discrete regions: a peripheral cortex, a central medulla, and an ill-defined region in between, called the paracortex (Figure 12-11). B cells predominate in the cortex, where they are arranged in aggregates called follicles. In lymph nodes that have been stimulated by antigen, some of these follicles form specialized structures called germinal centers (Figure 12-12).

Germinal centers are sites where B cells grow undergo maturation. They are round, ovoid clusters of cells and can be divided into light and dark zones. They originate when a few antigen-specific B cells enter a follicle and then divide rapidly to become the centroblasts that form the dark zones. These are sites where B cells proliferate and undergo a process called

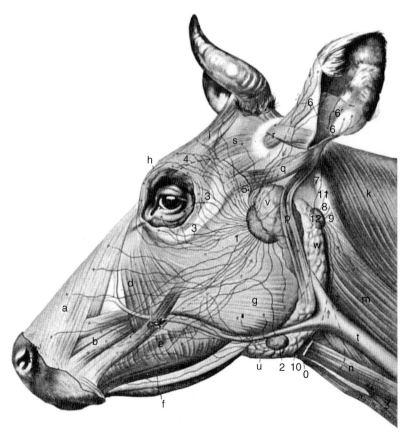

FIGURE 12-9 Lateral view of the head of a bovine showing the way in which the lymphatics drain to the parotid lymph node.

(From Sisson S [revised by Grossman JD]: *Anatomy of the domestic animals*, ed 4, Philadelphia, 1953, Saunders.)

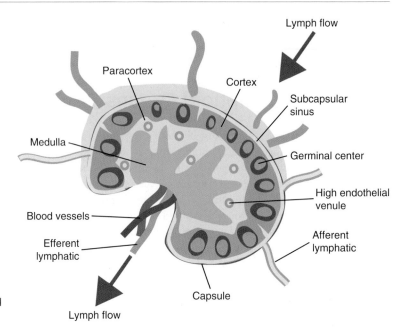

FIGURE 12-10 The major structural features of a typical lymph node.

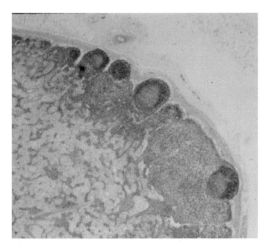

FIGURE 12-11 A section of bovine lymph node. Original magnification ×12.

(From a specimen provided by Dr. W.E. Haensly.)

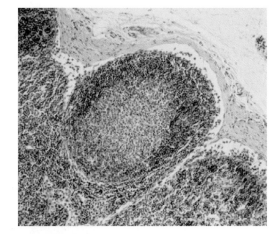

FIGURE 12-12 A germinal center in the cortex of a cat's lymph node. Note the obvious light zone in the center of the germinal center. Original magnification ×120.

(From a specimen provided by Dr. W.E. Haensly.)

somatic mutation (Chapter 17). The centroblasts eventually produce nondividing centrocytes that migrate to the light zones. The light zones are sites where immunoglobulin class switching and memory B cell formation occur (Chapter 15). They are rich in antigen-trapping follicular dendritic cells (fDCs) and CD4+ T cells (Figure 12-13).

T cells and dendritic cells predominate in the paracortex (Figure 12-14). The cells are arranged in cords between the lymphatic sinuses. At the center of each paracortical cord is a high endothelial venule (HEV). These vessels are lined with tall, rounded endothelial cells quite unlike the flattened endothelium found in other blood vessels (Figure 12-15). The HEVs are surrounded by concentric layers of fibroblastic reticular cells and a narrow space called the perivenular channel.

The lymph node medulla contains lymph-draining sinuses separated by medullary cords containing many plasma cells, macrophages, and memory T cells.

Lymph nodes are very busy places with cells coming and going in response to a multitude of chemical signals. These signals are delivered through the reticular fibers that provide the structural scaffolding of the lymph node. These fibers are hollow and serve as conduits for the rapid transmission of signaling molecules (Figure 12-16). The conduits consist of bundles of collagen fibers ensheathed by fibroreticular cells. The fibroreticular cell wall is not continuous, so that follicular B cells and dendritic cells can insert protrusions through tiny gaps and sample the antigens within the lymphatic fluid (Figure 12-17). A similar network of conduits occurs within the

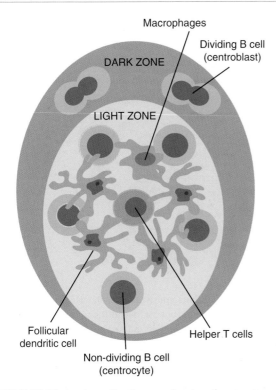

FIGURE 12-13 A schematic diagram showing the structure of a germinal center. The outer dark zone contains dividing B cells. The central pale zone is a location where antigen-presenting dendritic cells, helper T cells, and B cells interact.

T cell zones where antigens are sampled by dendritic cells. The conduits provide for the rapid delivery of soluble antigens from the afferent lymph to the lumen of HEVs and enable these antigens can reach deep into a node long before antigen-laden dendritic cells immigrate.

Function The principle function of secondary lymphoid organs such as lymph nodes is to facilitate the interactions between antigen-presenting cells and antigen-sensitive T and B cells. Each cell must be guided to its appropriate contacts with great precision. A complex mixture of chemokines directs these cells. Thus chemokines drive the emigration of lymphocytes from HEVs into the lymph node. Once they enter the lymph node, the T and B cells are guided to their respective regions by chemokines secreted by stromal cells and follicular dendritic cells. Immature dendritic cells, once they encounter antigen, are also guided into lymph nodes by chemokines. For example, dendritic cells are attracted to the paracortex, where they present their antigen to T cells. Once this is accomplished, the dendritic cells change their chemokine receptor phenotype and can leave the node.

An interesting feature of secondary lymphoid organs is the fact that both B and T cells are highly active and motile. The T cells in the paracortex and B cells in the cortex are guided by follicular dendritic cells. Chemokines control the relocation and recirculation of lymphocytes and ensure that lymphocytes end up in their correct positions. For example, T cells

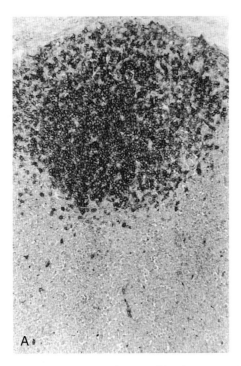
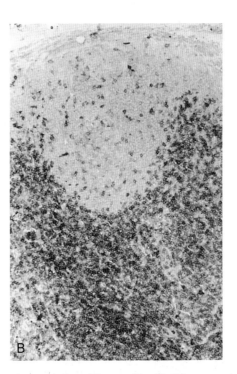

FIGURE 12-14 Normal bovine lymph node stained by the immunoperoxidase technique (Chapter 41) with **(A)** a monoclonal antibody that identifies B lymphocytes and **(B)** a monoclonal antibody that identifies T lymphocytes.

(Courtesy Drs. I. Morrison and N. MacHugh.)

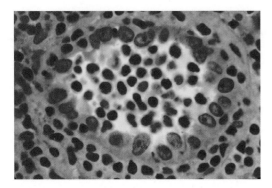

FIGURE 12-15 A section of human tonsil showing a high endothelial venule with its characteristic high, rounded endothelial cells. Note the lymphocytes emigrating between the endothelial cells.

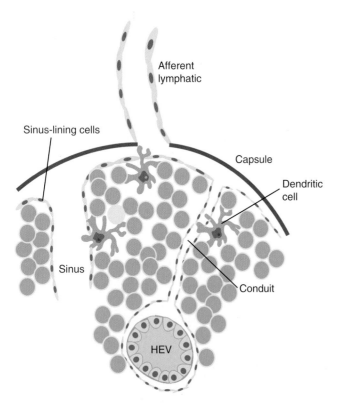

FIGURE 12-16 Conduits connect the subcapsular sinus directly to the perivenular space around high endothelial venules. As soluble antigens flow through these conduits, they can be sampled by dendritic cells.

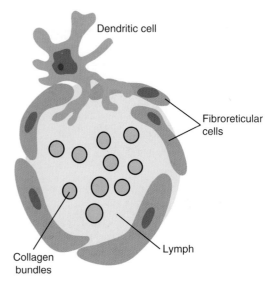

FIGURE 12-17 Conduits consist of loosely attached fibroreticular cells surrounding collagen bundles. Dendritic cell processes can reach into the conduits to sample their antigen content.

Soluble antigens (<70 kDa) entering the node through its afferent lymphatics first pass into the subcapsular sinus. From there they enter the conduit network and are carried into the cortex. Larger antigens such as viruses are captured by macrophages within the subcapsular sinus. These macrophages carry the viral particles through the sinus floor and directly present them to B cells in the underlying follicles. The B cells then migrate to the T cell–B cell boundary, where they receive specific T cell help. B cells can also enter the paracortex directly from HEVs. There is a specialized population of follicular dendritic cells clustered around these blood vessels so that immigrating B cells can survey any antigens they may be carrying. This is also a perfect location to receive T cell help.

When bacteria invade tissues, the resident dendritic cells are activated and migrate to the draining lymph node, where they accumulate in the paracortex and cortex. These dendritic cells form a web through which antigens must pass. Antigens that are captured are presented by the dendritic cells to T cells. T cells are initially activated in the paracortex, whereas the B cells remain randomly dispersed in the primary follicles. Both cell populations then migrate to the edges of the follicles where they interact. Once antibody production is stimulated, the progeny of these B cells move to the medulla and begin to secrete antibodies. Some of these antibody-producing cells may escape into the efferent lymph and colonize downstream lymph nodes. Several days after antibody production is first observed in the medulla, germinal centers appear in the cortex.

Some T cell–dendritic cell interactions are long lasting, and in the presence of antigen, T cells and dendritic cells form stable complexes for many hours. However, before selecting its partner a dendritic cell might sample as many as 500 different T cells/hour and can interact with up to 10 simultaneously (Figure 10-6).

expressing CCR7 are attracted to the perifollicular area of the cortex where the chemokines CCL19 and CCL21 are produced. B cells, on the other hand, express CXCR5 and are attracted to the interior of germinal centers where its ligand, the chemokine CXCL13, is produced. When T cells are activated, they too may express CXCR5 and thus enter germinal centers where they "help" B cells respond to antigens. Other secondary lymphoid organs employ different homing receptors. MAdCAM-1 is a homing receptor found in blood vessels in PPs. Lymphocytes that recirculate to the intestine express high levels of the integrin $\alpha_4\beta_7$, the ligand for MAdCAM-1.

Adherence to follicular dendritic cells is the predominant means of antigen trapping once an animal has been sensitized by previous exposure to an antigen. In a secondary response the germinal centers become less obvious as activated memory cells emigrate in the efferent lymph. Once this stage is completed, the germinal centers redevelop.

Antigen-stimulated lymph nodes also trap lymphocytes. Interactions between infectious agents and mast cells result in the production of tumor necrosis factor-α (TNF-α). The TNF-α blocks the passage of lymphocytes through these organs, the lymphocytes accumulate, and the lymph nodes swell. This trapping concentrates lymphocytes close to sites of antigen accumulation. After about 24 hours, the lymph nodes release their trapped cells. As a result, their cellular output is increased for several days.

Lymphocyte Circulation T cells constantly circulate around the body in the blood and tissue fluid and are the predominant lymphocytes in blood (Figure 12-18). As they travel, they survey the body for foreign antigens and preferentially home to sites of microbial invasion and inflammation. They also spend time in the secondary lymphoid organs such as lymph nodes. If they fail to encounter antigen, they leave the lymph node.

Circulating T cells leave the bloodstream by two routes. T cells that have not previously encountered antigens ("naïve" T cells) bind to HEV in lymph nodes. The high endothelial cells in these vessels are not joined by tight junctions but are linked by discontinuous "spot-welded" junctions. This means that lymphocytes can pass easily between the high endothelial cells. Circulating lymphocytes can adhere to these high endothelial cells and then migrate into the paracortex. The emigration of lymphocytes from HEVs resembles that of neutrophils in inflamed blood vessels. Thus, the cells first roll along the endothelial surface binding to selectins. For example, L-selectin (CD62L) on lymphocytes binds to GlyCAM-1 or CD34 (sialomucin) on endothelial cells (Figure 12-19). As they roll, the lymphocytes become activated and express integrins. This results in their complete arrest and emigration. The number and length of HEVs are variable and controlled by local activity. Thus, stimulation of a lymph node by the presence of antigens results in a rapid increase in the length of its HEVs. If, however, a lymph node is protected from antigens, its HEVs shorten. Recognizable HEVs are not normally found in ruminant lymph nodes, but paracortical venules serve the same function.

In contrast to naïve T cells, memory T cells leave the bloodstream through conventional blood vessels in tissues and are then carried to lymph nodes through afferent lymphatics. They leave the lymph nodes through the efferent lymphatics. Typically, afferent lymph in sheep contains 85% T cells, 5% B cells, and 10% dendritic cells. Efferent lymph contains greater than 98% lymphocytes, of which 75% are T cells and 25% are B cells. The efferent lymphatics eventually join together to form large lymph vessels. The largest of these lymph vessels is the thoracic duct, which drains the lymph from the lower body and intestine and empties it into the anterior vena cava.

Species Differences Domestic pigs and related swine, hippopotamuses, rhinoceroses, and some dolphins are different. Their lymph nodes consist of several lymphoid "nodules" oriented so that the cortex of each nodule is located toward the center of the node, and the medulla is at the periphery (Figure 12-20). Each nodule is served by a single afferent lymphatic that enters the central cortex as a lymph sinus. Thus afferent lymph is carried deep into the node. A cortex surrounds the lymph sinus. Outside this region are a paracortex and a medulla. This medulla may be shared by adjacent nodules

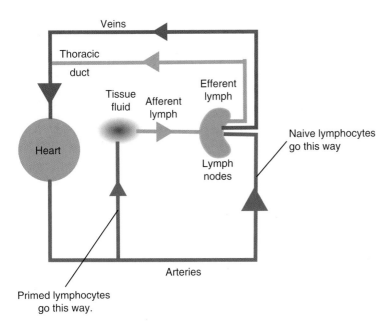

FIGURE 12-18 The circulation of lymphocytes. T cells circulate in both the bloodstream and the lymphatic fluid. Their precise route through a lymph node depends on whether they are naïve or primed. Thus naïve lymphocytes enter lymph nodes through the bloodstream and the high endothelial venules. Primed lymphocytes, in contrast, migrate through the tissues and enter through afferent lymphatics. They all leave through efferent lymphatics.

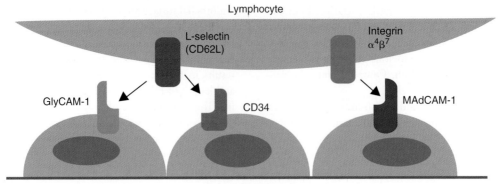

FIGURE 12-19 Binding of circulating lymphocytes to ligands on endothelial cells in high endothelial venules is brought about mainly by L-selectin binding to GlyCAM-1 and CD34. In the intestine, lymphocytes bearing the integrin $\alpha_4\beta_7$ bind to MAdCAM-1 endothelial cells.

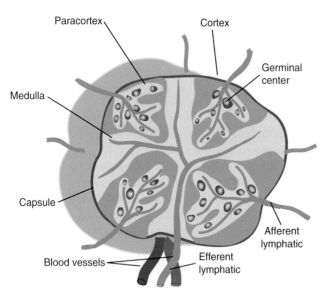

FIGURE 12-20 Structure of a pig lymph node. Compare this with Figure 12-10.

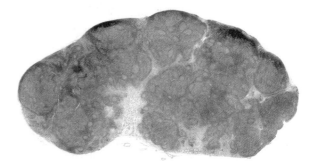

FIGURE 12-21 A section of a pig lymph node. Note how the germinal centers are located in the interior of the node. Original magnification ×12.

(From a specimen provided by Dr. Brian Porter.)

described previously. Thus both forms of lymph node may be present in a single individual.

Hemolymph Nodes

Hemolymph nodes are structures similar to lymph nodes found in association with some blood vessels of ruminants and other mammals. Their function is unclear. They differ from conventional lymph nodes in that their lymphatic sinuses contain numerous red cells. They have a cortex containing germinal centers and B cells. T cells predominate at the center in association with lymphatic sinuses. These cells differ, however, from those found in conventional lymph nodes (more γ/δ+, WC1+ T cells, fewer CD8+ T cells) (Chapter 14). Intravenously injected carbon particles are trapped in the sinusoids of hemolymph nodes, suggesting that they may combine features of both the spleen and lymph nodes.

Spleen

Just as lymph nodes filter antigens from lymph, so the spleen filters blood. Indeed, the spleen can be considered a specialized lymph node for blood-borne antigens. The filtering process

(Figure 12-21). Lymph passes from the cortex at the center of the node to the medulla at the periphery before leaving through the efferent vessels that drain the region between nodules. The cortex and paracortex have a similar structure to that seen in other mammals. The medulla has very few sinuses but consists of a dense mass of cells that is relatively impermeable to cells in the lymph. As a result, few cells migrate through the medulla. T cells in these species enter the lymph node in the conventional way through HEVs. However, they do not leave the lymph node through the lymphatics but migrate directly back to the bloodstream through the HEVs of the paracortex (Figure 12-22). Very few lymphocytes are found in pig lymph.

In marine mammals, lymph node structure is highly variable. Thus all the lymph nodes of bottlenose dolphins (*Tursiops truncatus*) are of conventional structure. In striped dolphins (*Stenella coeruleoalba*), on the other hand, some lymph nodes (mesenteric, for example) are of conventional structure, whereas others (mediastinal) have the inverted structure

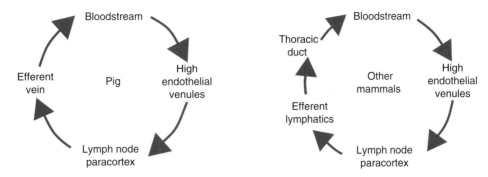

FIGURE 12-22 Comparison between the major route of circulation of T cells in the pig and that in other mammals. Note that pig lymphocytes are largely confined to the bloodstream.

removes antigenic particles such as blood-borne microorganisms, cellular debris, and aged blood cells. This filtering function, together with highly organized lymphoid tissue, makes the spleen an important component of the immune system. In addition to its immune functions, the spleen also stores red cells and platelets, recycles iron, and undertakes red cell production in the fetus. As a result, the spleen consists of two forms of tissue. One is used predominantly for blood filtering and for red cell storage, called the red pulp. It contains large numbers of antigen-presenting cells, lymphocytes, and plasma cells. The other is rich in both B and T cells where immune responses occur and is called the white pulp. The white pulp is separated from the red pulp by a region called the marginal zone. This zone contains numerous macrophages and dendritic cells and a large population of B cells. The spleen is not supplied with lymphatic fluid, although it does possess efferent lymphatics.

Structure of White Pulp Arteries entering the spleen pass through muscular trabeculae before entering the white pulp and branching into arterioles. Immediately on leaving the trabeculae, each arteriole is surrounded by a layer of lymphoid tissue called the periarteriolar lymphoid sheath (Figure 12-23). The arteriole eventually leaves this sheath and branches into penicillary arterioles. In some mammals, these penicillary arterioles are surrounded by ellipsoids (periarteriolar macrophage sheaths). These arterioles then open, either directly or indirectly, into venous sinuses that drain into the splenic venules. Ellipsoids are relatively large and prominent in pigs, mink, dogs, and cats; are small and indistinct in horses and cattle; and are absent in laboratory animals such as mice, rats, guinea pigs, and rabbits. In species that lack ellipsoids, particles are trapped primarily in the marginal zone of the white pulp.

The white pulp contains both B and T cells, which accumulate in their specific zones under the influence of chemokines. The periarteriolar lymphoid sheaths consist largely of T cells. Within these, the T cells interact with dendritic cells and

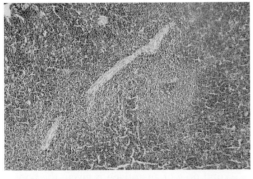

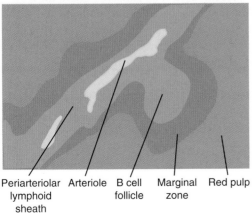

Periarteriolar Arteriole B cell Marginal Red pulp
lymphoid   follicle zone
sheath

FIGURE 12-23 Histological section and diagram showing the structure of the bovine spleen. Original magnification ×50.

(From a specimen provided by Dr. J.R. Duncan.)

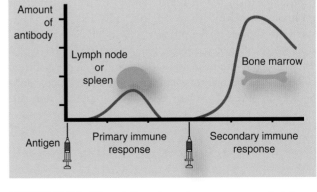

FIGURE 12-24 Although the primary immune response to intravenously injected antigen takes place in lymph nodes or spleen, the antibodies produced in a secondary response are largely produced in the bone marrow.

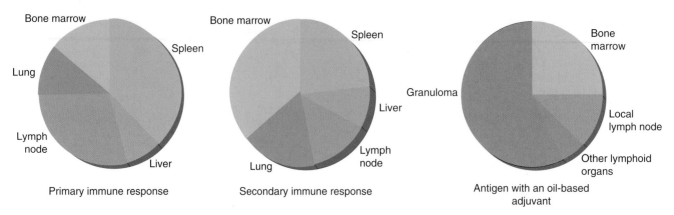

Primary immune response   Secondary immune response   Antigen with an oil-based adjuvant

FIGURE 12-25 Relative contribution of different organs or tissues to antibody production after administration of antigen either intravenously or intramuscularly with Freund's complete adjuvant. The adjuvant (Chapter 23) causes the accumulation of lymphocytes and antigen-processing cells. It thus forms a lymphoid nodule where antibodies are produced.

passing B cells. The B cell areas, in contrast, consist of round primary follicles scattered through the sheaths. These follicles are sites where germinal center formation, clonal expansion, isotype switching, and somatic hypermutation occur.

The white pulp is separated from the red pulp by a marginal sinus, a reticulum sheath, and a marginal zone of cells. This marginal zone is an important transit area for white cells moving between the blood and the white pulp. It is also rich in macrophages, dendritic cells, and B cells. Most of the blood that enters the spleen flows into the marginal sinus and through the marginal zone before returning to the circulation through venous sinuses. This flow pattern ensures that these antigen-presenting cells can capture any blood-borne antigens and deliver them to the B cells in the marginal zone. The white pulp is involved in adaptive immune responses, whereas the cells of the marginal zone can participate in both innate and adaptive responses. White pulp does not contain HEVs. Instead, lymphocytes enter the white pulp through the marginal zone, although the route by which they leave is unclear.

Function Intravenously administered antigens are trapped in the spleen. Depending on the species, they are taken up by dendritic cells in the marginal zone or in the periarteriolar macrophage sheaths. These dendritic cells and macrophages carry the antigen to the primary follicles of the white pulp, from which, after a few days, antibody-producing cells migrate. These antibody-producing cells (plasma cells and plasmablasts) colonize the marginal zone and move into the red pulp. Antibodies produced by these cells diffuse rapidly into the

bloodstream. Germinal center formation also occurs in the primary follicles. In an animal possessing circulating antibodies, trapping by dendritic cells within the follicles becomes significant. As in a primary immune response, the antibody-producing cells migrate from these follicles into the red pulp and the marginal zone where antibody production occurs.

Other Secondary Lymphoid Organs

Secondary lymphoid organs include not only the spleen and lymph nodes but also the bone marrow, tonsils, and lymphoid tissues scattered throughout the body, most notably in the digestive, respiratory, and urogenital tracts. The lymphoid tissues of the intestinal tract constitute the largest pool of lymphocytes in the body, but the bone marrow also contains very large numbers of lymphocytes. If antigen is given intravenously, much will be trapped not only in the liver and spleen but also in the bone marrow. During a primary immune response, antibodies are mainly produced in the spleen and lymph nodes (Figure 12-24). Toward the end of that response, memory cells leave the spleen and colonize the bone marrow. When a second dose of an antigen is given, the bone marrow produces very large quantities of antibody and is the major source of antibodies in adult rodents. Up to 70% of the antibody to some antigens may be produced by cells in the bone marrow (Figure 12-25).

For sources of additional information, please visit http://evolve.elsevier.com/tizard/immunology/

13

Lymphocytes

Key Points

- Lymphocytes are the cells that can recognize and respond to foreign antigens.
- Lymphocytes all look the same but can be differentiated by their characteristic cell surface molecules.
- These cell surface molecules are classified by the CD (cluster of differentiation) system.
- Lymphocytes possess antigen receptors plus the signal transducing molecules required to activate the cell.
- They also possess receptors for cytokines, immunoglobulins, and complement.
- In domestic animal species, some cell surface molecules are unique to each species. These are classified by the WC (workshop cluster) system.
- The collection of cell surface molecules on a lymphocyte is called its immunophenotype.

Lymphocytes are central to the adaptive immune system and the defense of the body. There are three major types of lymphocyte. These are natural killer (NK) cells that play a role in innate immunity; T cells that regulate adaptive immunity and are responsible for cell-mediated immune responses; and B cells that are responsible for antibody production. Within these major types are many subpopulations, each with different characteristics and functions. This chapter reviews the structure and properties of these lymphocytes and some important subpopulations.

Lymphocyte Structure

Lymphocytes are small, round cells, 7 to 15 μm in diameter. Each contains a large, round nucleus that stains intensely and evenly with hematoxylin (Figure 13-1). The nucleus is surrounded by a thin rim of cytoplasm containing some mitochondria, free ribosomes, and a small Golgi apparatus (Figure 13-2). Scanning electron microscopy shows that some lymphocytes are smooth surfaced, whereas others are covered by many

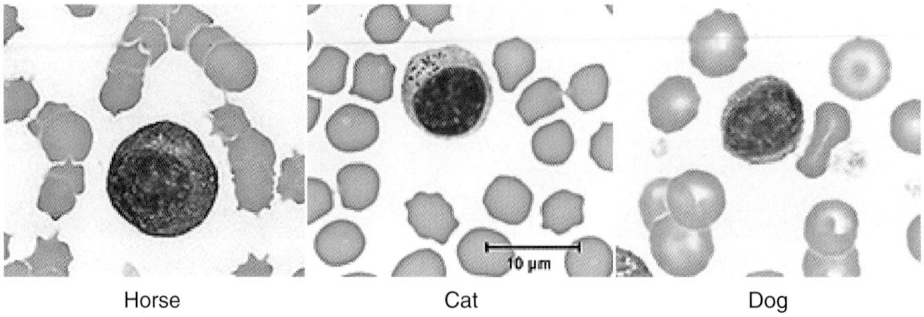

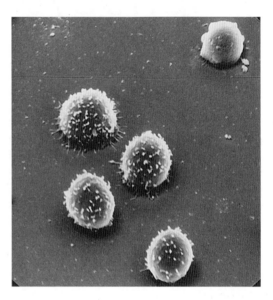

FIGURE 13-1 Photomicrographs showing lymphocytes in stained blood smears from horse, cat, and dog. Giemsa stain.

(Courtesy Dr. M.C. Johnson.)

Horse   Cat   Dog

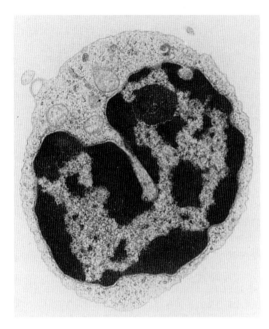

FIGURE 13-2 Transmission electron micrograph of a blood lympho-cyte from a rabbit.

(Courtesy Dr. S. Linthicum.)

FIGURE 13-3 Scanning electron micrograph of lymphocytes from a mouse lymph node. Original magnification ×1500.

small projections (Figure 13-3). NK cells are usually larger than T or B cells and may contain obvious cytoplasmic granules. With this exception, lymphocyte structure provides no clue as to their function or complexity (Figure 13-4).

Lymphocyte Populations

Lymphocytes are found throughout the body in lymphoid organs, in blood, and scattered under mucosal surfaces (Figure 13-5). Despite their uniform appearance, they are a diverse mixture of subpopulations. Although these subpopulations cannot be identified by their structure, they can be identified by their characteristic cell surface molecules and by their behavior (Table 13-1). The pattern of cell surface molecules expressed on a cell is called its phenotype. By analyzing cell phenotypes, it is possible to identify many lymphocyte subpopulations.

The loss of cell-mediated immunity as a result of neonatal thymectomy first demonstrated the existence of T lymphocytes

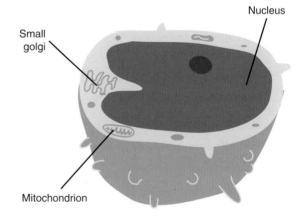

FIGURE 13-4 Essential structural features of a lymphocyte. There are actually very few characteristic structural features.

(Figure 13-6). After T cells leave the thymus, they accumulate in the paracortex of lymph nodes, the periarteriolar lymphoid sheaths of the spleen, and the interfollicular areas of the Peyer's patches. T cells also account for 60% to 80% of the lympho-cytes in blood (Table 13-2).

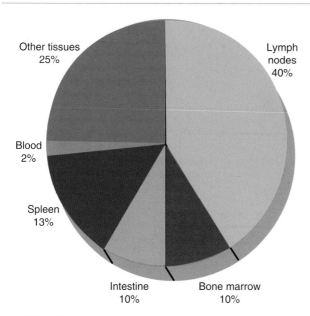

Other tissues
25%

Lymph
nodes
40%

Blood
2%

Spleen
13%

Intestine
10%

Bone marrow
10%

FIGURE 13-5 Locations of lymphocytes within the body.

Similar experiments involving bursectomy in chickens pointed to the existence of B lymphocytes. In mammals, B cells originate in the bone marrow but mature within Peyer's patches or in the bone marrow before migrating to the secondary lymphoid organs. B cells predominate in the cortex of lymph nodes, in follicles within the Peyer's patches and spleen, and in the marginal zone of the white pulp of the spleen. B cells account for 10% to 40% of blood lymphocytes (see Table 13-2).

NK cells were identified as a result of the presence of cytotoxic activity in lymphocytes from unsensitized animals. NK cells probably originate from the same stem cells as T cells but do not undergo thymic processing. They are widely distributed throughout the lymphoid organs. They account for 5% to 10% of blood lymphocytes.

Lymphocyte Surface Molecules

Many lymphocyte surface molecules have been characterized, especially in humans and mice (Box 13-1). Each molecule usually has a functional or chemical name as well as a cluster of differentiation (CD) designation (Figures 13-7 and 13-8). Currently, the CD nomenclature system gives sequential numbers to each molecule: CD4, CD8, CD16, and so on, up to CD360. Since arbitrary numbers are difficult to remember, the basic principle used in this text is that if the molecule's common name is well accepted or describes its function, that name will be used. Examples include FcαR (CD89), interleukin-6R (CD126), and L-selectin (CD62L). CD nomenclature is also used for molecules for which the designation is well accepted, such as CD8 and CD4. A list of the most relevant CD molecules and their functions can be found in Appendix 1.

CD molecules expressed on the cells of the domestic mammals fall into two categories. The great majority are also found in humans and mice (homologs) and thus have the same CD number. There are, however, several cell surface molecules in domestic mammals that have no recognized homolog in human or mouse. These unattributable molecules are given a species abbreviation and the prefix WC (workshop cluster), for example, BoWC1 and BoWC2, which are found in cattle.

□ Table 13-1 | Identifying Features of T and B Cells

PROPERTY	B CELLS	T CELLS
Develop within	Bone marrow, bursa, Peyer's patches	Thymus
Distribution	Lymph node cortex Splenic follicles	Lymph node paracortex Spleen periarteriolar sheath
Circulate	No	Yes
Antigen receptors	BCR—immunoglobulin	TCR—protein heterodimer Associated with CD3, CD4, or CD8
Important surface antigens	Immunoglobulins	CD2, CD3, CD4, or CD8
Mitogens	Pokeweed, lipopolysaccharide	Phytohemagglutinin, concanavalin A, BCG vaccine, pokeweed
Antigens recognized	Free foreign proteins	Processed foreign proteins in MHC antigens
Tolerance induction	Difficult	Easy
Progeny cells	Plasma cells, memory cells	Effector T cells, memory T cells
Secreted products	Immunoglobulins	Cytokines

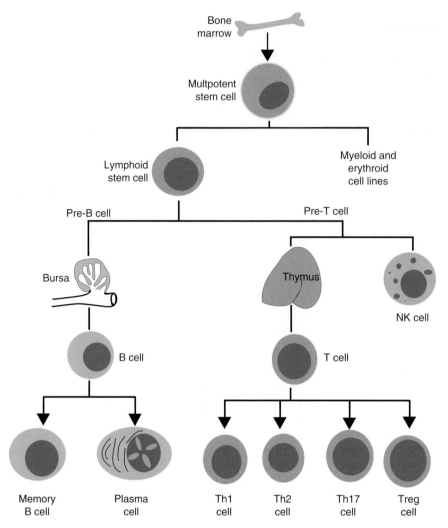

FIGURE 13-6 Development of T and B lymphocytes. Both arise from bone marrow precursors. B cells develop in the bursa, Peyer patches, or bone marrow. T cells develop in the thymus. Natural killer cells are a third population of lymphocytes that are distinct from T and B cells.

Cell surface receptors are characterized through the use of an instrument called a flow cytometer. This is described in Chapter 41.

Antigen Receptor Complex

The most important structures on the surface of lymphocytes are their antigen receptors. These are abbreviated TCR (T cell antigen receptor) or BCR (B cell antigen receptor). Both are complex structures containing many different proteins. Some of these proteins bind antigen, whereas others are used for signal transduction. There are two populations of T cells differentiated by their TCR antigen-binding chains. One uses paired α and β peptide chains (TCR α/β) and the other uses paired γ and δ chains (TCR γ/δ) (Chapter 14). There are also subpopulations of B cells that use one of five different heavy chains (γ, μ, α, ε, and δ) in their BCR antigen-binding chains. BCRs also differ from TCRs in that they are shed in large amounts into tissue fluid and the blood, where they are

called antibodies. Thus antibodies are simply soluble BCRs (Chapter 15).

NK cells do not have antigen receptors like T and B cells. In contrast, they have receptors that can bind molecules expressed on healthy normal cells but not on diseased, abnormal cells. NK cells thus recognize and kill target cells that fail to express these surface molecules (Chapter 19).

CD3 is the collective name given to the signal transducing proteins in the TCR. CD3 is therefore found on all T cells. Another protein, CD4, is found only on helper T cells. CD4 molecules are receptors for major histocompatibility complex (MHC) class II molecules on antigen-presenting cells. A third protein, CD8, is, in contrast, only expressed on T cells that attack and kill abnormal cells, the cytotoxic T cells. CD8 molecules are receptors for MHC class I molecules. Most human and mouse T cells express either CD4 or CD8, but rarely both. For example, about 65% of human T cells are CD4+, CD8−, and 30% are CD4−, CD8+. The remaining T cells express neither (CD4−, CD8−) and are said to be double

◻ Table 13-2 | Major Peripheral Blood Lymphocyte Populations in Mammals as Percentages of the Total Population

	T CELLS	B CELLS	CD4+	CD8+	CD4/CD8
Horses	38-66	17-38[g]	56[h]	20-37[g]	4.75[h]
Bovine	45-53[a]	16-21[a]	8-31	10-30	1.53[a]
Sheep	56-64[b]	11-50[c]	8-22[c]	4-22[c]	1.55[b]
Pigs	45-57[d]	13-38[e]	23-43	17-39	1.4[f]
Dogs	46-72	7-30	27-33[i]	17-18[i]	1.7[i]
Cats	31-89[j]	6-50[j]	19-49[j]	6-39[j]	1.9[j]
Humans	70-75	10-15	43-48[k]	22-24[k]	1.9-2.4[k]

[a]Park YH, Fox LK, Hamilton MJ, Davis WC: Bovine mononuclear leukocyte subpopulations in peripheral blood and mammary gland secretions during lactation, *J Dairy Sci* 75:998–1006, 1992.

[b]Thorp BH, Seneque S, Staute K, Kimpton WG: Characterization and distribution of lymphocyte subsets in sheep hemal nodes, *Dev Comp Immunol* 15:393–400, 1991.

[c]Smith HE, Jacobs RM, Smith C: Flow cytometric analysis of ovine peripheral blood lymphocytes, *Can J Vet Res* 58:152–155, 1994.

[d]Pescovitz MD, Sakopoulos AB, Gaddy JA, et al: Porcine peripheral blood CD4+/CD8+ dual expressing T-cells, *Vet Immunol Immunopathol* 43:53–62, 1994.

[e]Saalmüller A, Bryant J: Characteristics of porcine T lymphocytes and T-cell lines, *Vet Immunol Immunopathol* 43:45–52, 1994.

[f]Joling P, Bianchi AT, Kappe AL, Zwart RJ: Distribution of lymphocyte subpopulations in thymus, spleen, and peripheral blood of specific pathogen free pigs from 1 to 40 weeks of age, *Vet Immunol Immunopathol* 40:105–118, 1994.

[g]McGorum BC, Dixon PM, Halliwell RE: Phenotypic analysis of peripheral blood and bronchoalveolar lavage fluid lymphocytes in control and chronic obstructive pulmonary disease affected horses, before and after "natural (hay and straw) challenges," *Vet Immunol Immunopathol* 36:207–222, 1993.

[h]Grunig G, Barbis DP, Zhang CH, et al: Correlation between monoclonal antibody reactivity and expression of CD4 and CD8 alpha genes in the horse, *Vet Immunol Immunopathol* 42:61–69, 1994.

[i]Rivas AL, Kimball ES, Quimby FW, Gebhard D: Functional and phenotypic analysis of in vitro stimulated canine peripheral blood mononuclear cells, *Vet Immunol Immunopathol* 45:55–71, 1995.

[j]Walker R, Malik R, Canfield PJ: Analysis of leucocytes and lymphocyte subsets in cats with naturally-occurring cryptococcosis but differing feline immunodeficiency virus status, *Aust Vet J* 72:93–97, 1995.

[k]Bleavins MR, Brott DA, Alvey JD, de la Iglesia FA: Flow cytometric characterization of lymphocyte subpopulations in the cynomolgus monkey (Macaca fascicularis), *Vet Immunol Immunopathol* 37:1–13, 1993.

◻ Box 13-1 | A Note on Cell Phenotypes

All the cells of the body arise from a single precursor cell, the fertilized ovum. As the embryo develops and grows, cells differentiate both structurally and biochemically. They do this by activating required genes while turning off unneeded ones. One obvious result is that cells acquire a characteristic morphology. Histologic examination shows these structural differences and has provided much useful guidance regarding a cell's function. Structural differences are limited, however, in what they can tell us. For example, T and B cells look identical but differ significantly in their biochemistry and their function. As a result, biochemical differences must be determined to identify functional cell types. One of the best ways to do this is to examine the proteins expressed on the cell surface. Cells express hundreds of different proteins on their surface, and their identification provides a powerful tool to characterize cells. The CD system of identifying cell surface proteins is an organized attempt to catalog these cell surface proteins.

Two otherwise identical cell populations may be distinguished by the set of cell surface molecules they express. In identifying cells in this way, it is possible not only to identify cell subpopulations but also to follow cell development and differentiation as cells differentiate. Different genes are turned on and off depending on changes in the cell's function.

In many cases it has proved possible to identify cell subpopulations or changes in a cell's phenotype without determining the cell's functional significance. Different phenotypes occur in different domestic animal species. Students will therefore find much of the literature in this area confusing, especially if large numbers of CD molecules are reported for a specific cell phenotype.

The signal transducing components of the B cell antigen receptor complex are protein heterodimers formed by pairing CD79a (Ig-α) with CD79b (Ig-β). These are discussed in detail in Chapter 15.

Molecules That Regulate Lymphocyte Function

Proteins on cell surfaces serve physiological functions. Some are enzymes, some are transport proteins, and many are receptors. All cells use receptors to receive signals from their environment, including nearby cells. They also need receptors to bind other cells and to receive signals from cytokines, antibodies, and complement components.

Cytokine Receptors Lymphocytes express many different cytokine receptors. Examples include CD25, a part of the interleukin-2 (IL-2) receptor; CD118, an interferon (IFN) receptor; CD120, the tumor necrosis factor (TNF) receptor; and CD210, the IL-10 receptor. (These are discussed in Chapter 8.)

negative. The ratio of CD4+ to CD8+ cells in blood may be used to estimate lymphocyte function. An elevated CD4 count implies increased lymphocyte reactivity because helper cells predominate, whereas a high CD8 count implies depressed lymphocyte reactivity. The relative proportions of CD4 and CD8 cells differ between humans and other mammals (Table 13-3). Neither CD4 nor CD8 are expressed on B cells or NK cells.

CD45 is expressed in large amounts on all three lymphocyte populations. For example, about 10% of the T cell surface is covered by CD45 molecules. Different forms of CD45 have been identified. Thus naïve T cells express one form of CD45, whereas stimulated and memory T cells express another.

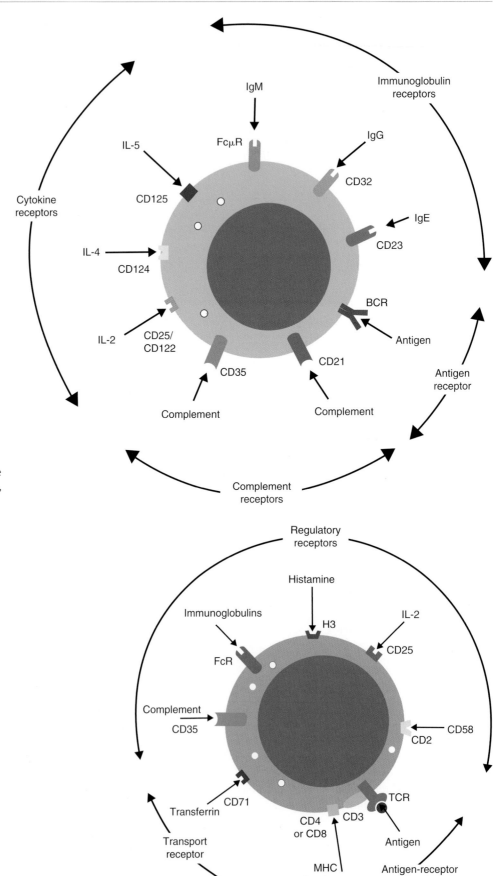

FIGURE 13-7 Major surface receptors of B cells, their ligands, and their functions.

FIGURE 13-8 Major surface receptors of T cells, their ligands, and their functions.

□ Table 13-3 | Surface Molecules on Peripheral Blood T Cells

MARKER	CELL PERCENTAGE			
	MOUSE	BOVINE	SWINE	SHEEP
TCRα/β	85-95	5-30	14-34	5-30
TCRγ/δ	5-15	45-50	31-66	22-68
CD2	95	41-60	58-72	10-36
CD4	24	8-28	23-43	8-22
CD8	11	10-30	17-39	4-22
WC1	—	5-44	40	15-70

Antibody Receptors Lymphocytes receive signals from and hence must have receptors for antibodies. Since these receptors bind to the Fc regions of antibody molecules, they are called Fc receptors (FcR). (The meaning of the term Fc can be found in Chapter 16.) The Fc receptors for immunoglobulin G (IgG) are designated FcγR since they bind the γ chain of IgG. Likewise those for IgA are designated FcαR and those for IgE are FcεR. Receptors for IgM have been identified on both B and T cells but are not well characterized.

Four different IgG receptors have been described on mouse leukocytes (Table 13-4). They are called FcγRI (CD64), FcγRII (CD32), FcγRIII (CD16), and FcγRIV. All are multichain glycoproteins. One chain usually binds the antibody, whereas the other chains are used for signal transduction. CD64 (FcγRI) is found on dendritic cells, monocytes, and macrophages and to a much lesser extent on neutrophils. (It is not found on lymphocytes but is mentioned here for the sake of completeness.) CD64 binds IgG with high affinity. CD32 (FcγRII) is found on B cells, dendritic cells, and macrophages. It has a moderate affinity for IgG and will therefore only bind immune complexes (antibody molecules attached to an antigen). There are three subtypes of CD32 called a, b, and c. CD32a is expressed on macrophages and neutrophils, where it is an activating receptor. It promotes phagocytosis and

stimulates the release of cytokines. CD32b is found on B cells, where it is an inhibitory receptor and regulates antibody production. The function of CD32c is unclear. All three subtypes are expressed on dendritic cells and stimulate dendritic cell maturation and antigen presentation. CD16 (FcγRIII) binds IgG with low affinity and will therefore only bind immune complexes. It is found on granulocytes, NK cells, and macrophages but not on B cells. Signaling through CD16 can trigger NK cell activation.

Mice have an additional receptor for IgG called FcγRIV, and related proteins are found in humans, chimpanzees, rats, dogs, cats, pigs, and cattle. This receptor binds IgG2 antibodies with moderate affinity, but it does not bind IgG1 or IgG3. It is expressed exclusively on neutrophils, macrophages, and dendritic cells.

Cattle and sheep also have a unique FcR called Fcγ2R. It is not related to other mammalian FcγRs but belongs to a novel gene family that includes FcαRI (CD89) and the KIRs (Chapter 19). It is expressed on myeloid cells and binds only aggregated bovine IgG2. It is important in promoting phagocytosis of antibody-opsonized bacteria in these species.

FcαRI (CD89) is expressed on neutrophils, eosinophils, monocyte-macrophages, and dendritic cells. It binds IgA and mediates its endocytosis and recycling. FcεRI is a high-affinity IgE receptor found on mast cells and discussed in Chapter 28. It plays an important role in allergies. CD23, or FcεRII, in contrast, is a low-affinity IgE receptor expressed on activated B cells, platelets, eosinophils, macrophages, NK cells, dendritic cells, and possibly even T cells. Activated B cells can secrete soluble CD23, which then regulates allergic responses.

PIgR and FcRn are Fc receptors involved in immunoglobulin transport across epithelial surfaces. They are described in Chapters 21 and 22.

Complement Receptors There are four major complement receptors on lymphocytes (CR1 to CR4). B cells and activated T cells express CR1 (CD35), which binds C3b and C4b, and CR2 (CD21), which binds C3d and C3bi. CR2 is closely associated with the BCR and regulates B cell responses to antigen. NK cells express CR3 and CR4.

□ Table 13-4 | Receptors for Immunoglobulin G (FcγR)

PROPERTY	FcγRI	FcγRII	FcγRIII	FcγRIV
CD designation	CD64	CD32	CD16	
Molecular weight	75 kDa	39-48 kDa	50-65 kDa	
Cells	Monocytes, macrophages	B cells, macrophages granulocytes eosinophils	NK cells, granulocytes, macrophages	Neutrophils, macrophages, dendritic cells
Affinity	High	Moderate	Low	Intermediate/high
Function	Phagocytosis	B cells: inhibition Macrophages: phagocytosis	NK cells: ADCC Granulocytes: phagocytosis	Proinflammatory

Adherence Molecules

As discussed in Chapter 4, some cell surface molecules bind cells together. They regulate signal network transmission between the cells of the immune system and control the movement of leukocytes in tissues. The cell adhesion molecules found on lymphocytes include integrins, selectins, and members of the immunoglobulin superfamily.

Integrins Integrins are heterodimeric proteins with an α and a β chain. The $β_1$-integrins consist of a $β_1$ chain (CD29) paired with one of several different α chains (CD49). The $β_1$-integrins bind cells to extracellular matrix proteins such as fibronectin, laminin, and collagen. The $β_2$-integrins consist of a $β_2$ chain (CD18) paired with one of several α chains (CD11). These $β_2$-integrins control the binding of leukocytes to vascular endothelium and bind T cells to antigen-presenting cells. For example, LFA-1 (CD11a/CD18) on a T cell binds to its ligand, intercellular adhesion molecule-1 (ICAM-1), on the antigen-presenting cell. By prolonging and stabilizing cell interactions, this binding permits successful antigen recognition (Figure 13-9).

Selectins The emigration of lymphocytes from the bloodstream into tissues is regulated by P-selectin (CD62P), L-selectin (CD62L), and E-selectin (CD62E). P- and E-selectins are found on vascular endothelial cells. When these cells are activated by inflammation, they express selectins that bind neutrophils, activated T cells, and monocytes. L-selectin binds lymphocytes to high endothelial venules in lymphoid organs (Chapter 12).

Immunoglobulin Superfamily Some members of the immunoglobulin superfamily (IgSF) are lymphocyte adhesion molecules. For example, ICAM-1 (CD54) binds to the integrin, CD11a/CD18 (see Figure 13-9). ICAM-1 is normally expressed on dendritic cells and B cells. Inflammation induces ICAM-1 expression on vascular endothelium and permits phagocytic cells to bind and move into inflamed tissues. ICAM-1 is also responsible for the migration of T cells into areas of inflammation (so-called delayed hypersensitivity reactions; Chapter 31). Another IgSF adherence molecule is vascular cell adhesion molecule-1 (VCAM-1), or CD106. VCAM-1 is expressed on inflamed vascular endothelial cells. It binds the $β_1$-integrin, CD49d/CD29, on lymphocytes and monocytes.

CD58 and CD2 CD58 is the ligand for CD2. CD2 is found only on T cells, whereas CD58 is widely distributed on many cell types. When cytotoxic T cells encounter their target cells, CD2 and CD58 bind them together. It is likely that CD58 facilitates T cell binding to any cell undergoing surveillance (Chapter 33). CD58 is also found on antigen-presenting cells such as dendritic cells and macrophages. When it binds to T cell CD2, CD58 enhances the recognition of antigen by the T cell and at the same time stimulates the antigen-presenting cell to secrete cytokines.

Other Major Surface Molecules

B cells can function as antigen-presenting cells and express MHC class II molecules on their surface. In contrast, T cell expression of MHC class II varies between species. Both types of lymphocytes express MHC class Ia and class Ib molecules.

WC1 Lymphocytes of the major domestic mammals express several cell surface proteins not found in either humans or

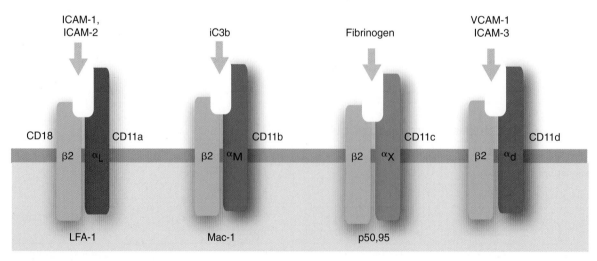

FIGURE 13-9 The integrin families are based on the pairing of many different α chains with a limited number of β chains. This example shows the structure of the very important $β_2$-integrins that act as cell surface adhesion molecules to link cells together so that they can communicate privately.

mice. The best defined of these is WC1. WC1 is a family of single-chain type 1 glycoproteins of 220 kDa belonging to the "scavenger receptor cysteine-rich" (SRCR) protein superfamily. They are expressed exclusively on γ/δ T cells. These WC1+ T cells are found in high numbers in the skin and mucous membranes as well as in hemal nodes and the thymus. WC1 belongs to a protein family found in many different mammals, amphibians, and invertebrates. About 13 *WC1* gene family members occur in cattle, whereas 50 to 100 are found in sheep. Three subsets have been defined by serological testing. Homologs of WC1 have been identified in pigs, camels, llamas, deer, elk, platypuses, and chicken. Although their natural ligand is unknown, WC1 proteins probably bind to macrophages and dendritic cells and act as co-stimulatory molecules. Some members of the family may bind directly to bacteria such as *Leptospira* and *Anaplasma*.

Changes in Immunophenotype

Lymphocytes do not express the same immunophenotype at all stages in their life cycle. Thus a cell's phenotype depends on its maturity and activation status. For example, immature human T cells carry both CD9 and CD10. As the T cells mature within the thymus, CD9 is lost, and the cells gain CD4 and CD8. Mature thymocytes can then split into two subpopulations; one population becomes CD4+, the other becomes CD8+. In addition, the phenotype of lymphocytes changes after exposure to antigen. For example, naïve T cells express high levels of CD45R and L-selectin and low levels of CD44. Memory T cells show the reverse of this: low levels of CD45R and L-selectin and high levels of CD44.

Species Differences

Horses

Horse lymphocytes express two species-specific proteins. EqWC1 is found on 70% of equine T cells, 30% of B cells, and 50% of granulocytes and may be a homolog of CD90. EqWC2 is found on granulocytes and most T cells.

Bovine

Cattle lymphocytes express the species-specific cell surface molecules BoWC1 through BoWC15. (BoWC3 is now known to be CD21; BoWC6 is CD205, a C-type lectin expressed on dendritic cells; and BoWC10 is CD26).

In adult cattle about 10% to 15% of circulating T cells are γ/δ positive, whereas the remainder are α/β positive. In young calves the proportion of γ/δ T cells may rise to 40%. However, this proportion fluctuates in response to management and stress. The majority of bovine γ/δ T cells also express WC1. Indeed, these cells can be activated either through their TCR or through WC1. In response they produce TNF-α, IL-1, IL-12, and IFN-γ. This mixture suggests that they contribute to both inflammation and a Th1 bias in the bovine immune response and thus link the innate and adaptive immune systems.

CD4 is expressed on 20% to 30% of blood lymphocytes in adult ruminants. Double-negative T cells constitute 15% to 30% of the blood T cells in young ruminants, but this may reach 80% in newborn calves. Most of these double-negative cells are γ/δ+ and WC1+. Thus the major circulating T cells in ruminants (γ/δ+, WC1+, CD4−, CD8−) are different from the predominant T cells in the humans and mice (α/β+, WC1−, CD4+, CD8−).

Sheep

Sheep T cells express OvWC1 (also called T19). The isoform of this molecule expressed on α/β T cells is different from the isoform on γ/δ T cells. When lambs are born, γ/δ T cells account for 60% of blood T cells, but this drops to 30% by 1 year of age and to 5% by 5 years.

Pigs

Pig leukocytes express nine unique surface proteins (SWC1 to SWC9). SWC1 is expressed on resting T cells, monocytes, and granulocytes but not on B cells. SWC3 is found on monocytes and macrophages. SWC9 is expressed only by mature macrophages. In young pigs, up to 66% of blood T cells are γ/δ positive, but this drops to 25% to 50% in adults. Pigs have two subpopulations of γ/δ T cells. One is CD2+ and the other is CD2− and has not been identified in other species. Some pig γ/δ T cells can function as antigen-presenting cells using MHC class II molecules. Up to 60% of T cells in pig blood are double positive CD4+, CD8+. The rest are predominantly double negative (CD4−,CD8−).

Dogs and Cats

In dogs, CD4 is expressed on neutrophils and macrophages but not on monocytes, whereas in cats, CD4 is found on only a subset of T cells and their precursors.

Lymphocyte Mitogens

In addition to their surface proteins, lymphocytes can be characterized by the stimulants that make them divide. The most important of these are the lectins that bind to cell surface glycoproteins and so trigger cell division (Box 13-2). These lectins are commonly isolated from plants. Examples include phytohemagglutinin (PHA) obtained from the red kidney bean (*Phaseolus vulgaris*), concanavalin A (Con A) obtained from the jack bean (*Canavalis ensiformis*), and pokeweed mitogen (PWM) obtained from the pokeweed plant (*Phytolacca americana*). Lectins specifically bind sugar residues on glycoprotein side chains. For example, PHA binds *N*-acetylgalactosamine, and Con A binds α-mannose and

□ Box 13-2 | **How to Measure Mitogenicity**

To measure the effect of mitogens, lymphocytes are grown in tissue culture. Lymphocytes can be obtained directly from blood. The lymphocytes are cultured for at least 24 hours before the mitogen is added. Once this is done they begin to divide, synthesize new DNA, and take up any available nucleotides from the medium. It is usual to incorporate a small quantity of thymidine labeled with the radioactive isotope of hydrogen, tritium (^{3}H), in the tissue culture fluid. The thymidine is only incorporated into the DNA of cells that are dividing. After about 24 hours, the cultured cells are separated from the tissue culture fluid, either by centrifugation or filtration, and their radioactivity is counted. The amount of radioactivity in the mitogen-treated cells may be compared with that in an untreated lymphocyte culture. This ratio is called the stimulation index (see Figure 31-7). As an alternative to the use of tritiated thymidine, a radiolabeled amino acid such as ^{14}C-leucine can be used. Uptake of this compound indicates increased protein synthesis by the cells.

α-glucose. Not all lymphocytes respond equally well to all lectins. Thus PHA primarily stimulates T cells, although it has a slight effect on B cells. Con A is also a T cell mitogen, whereas PWM acts on both T and B cells.

Although the plant lectins are the most efficient lymphocyte mitogens, mitogens may also be found in other unexpected sources. For example, an extract from the snail *Helix pomata* stimulates T cells, whereas lipopolysaccharide from Gram-negative bacteria stimulates B cells. Other important B cell mitogens include proteases, such as trypsin, and Fc fragments of immunoglobulins. Bacille Calmette-Guérin (BCG) vaccine, an avirulent strain of *Mycobacterium bovis* that is used as a vaccine against tuberculosis, is a T cell mitogen. These mitogens can assist in the differentiation of T and B cells and, by measurement of the response provoked, provide an estimate of the responsiveness of T and B cells.

For sources of additional information, please visit http://evolve.elsevier.com/tizard/immunology/

14

Helper T Cells and Their Response to Antigen

Chapter Outline

Key Points

- Helper T cells express antigen receptors (TCRs) consisting of paired peptide chains, either α and β or γ and δ.
- These paired chains form antigen-binding receptors whose ligands are peptides linked to major histocompatibility complex (MHC) molecules on antigen-presenting cells.
- The antigen-binding chains of the TCR connect to a complex signal transducing component called CD3.
- Each TCR is also associated with either CD4 or CD8. CD4 binds to MHC class II molecules on antigen-presenting cells. CD8 binds to MHC class I molecules expressed on all nucleated cells.
- To respond to antigens, T cells must bind to antigenic peptides linked to MHC molecules. They must also receive co-stimulation from cytokines and other molecules.
- The multiple signals sent by an antigen-presenting cell are communicated to a T cell through an immunological synapse.
- There are three major subpopulations of helper T cells. Th1 cells are stimulated by interleukin-12 (IL-12) and secrete interferon-γ (IFN-γ) in response. They generally promote cell-mediated responses.
- Th2 cells secrete IL-4, 1L-13, and IL-10. They generally promote antibody responses.
- Th17 cell development is stimulated by IL-6, TGF-β, and IL-23. They secrete IL-17 and promote neutrophil-mediated inflammation.
- α/β Helper T cells are the predominant T cells in most mammals. γ/δ Helper T cells are mainly confined to the intestinal wall in humans but are the predominant circulating T cells in young ruminants and pigs.

Unlike the innate immune responses that are triggered by a limited number of molecular patterns restricted to the major groups of microorganisms, the lymphocytes of the adaptive immune system are able to recognize and respond to "everything," or at least to a large number of very diverse foreign antigens. These lymphocytes have receptors that bind specific antigens and, under the right conditions, respond by mounting cell-mediated or antibody-mediated immune responses.

There are four major populations of lymphocytes with antigen-binding receptors. These include helper T cells that regulate immune responses; effector or cytotoxic T cells that destroy cells expressing endogenous antigens; regulatory T cells that control everything, and B cells that produce antibodies. Each of these cell populations can trigger an immune response only when antigens bind to their specific receptors. This chapter discusses the first of these major lymphocyte populations, the helper T cells.

Exogenous antigen is trapped and processed by dendritic and other antigen-presenting cells and then presented to helper T cells. Each T cell is covered by thousands of identical antigen receptors. If these receptors bind antigen in the correct manner, the helper T cell is activated and initiates an immune response by secreting cytokines, dividing, and differentiating. As you will see later, the other antigen-responsive cell populations, the B cells and the cytotoxic T cells, cannot respond to antigens unless they too are stimulated by helper T cells. Because of the central role of helper T cells, they must be carefully regulated through cell-cell interactions and by the activities of many different cytokines.

It is important to point out at this stage that the antigen receptors on T cells do not develop in order to bind to specific foreign antigens. On the contrary, these antigen receptors are generated randomly. As a result, the antigen receptors on all the T cells in the body form a large diverse repertoire. It may be expected that any foreign antigen that enters the body will encounter and bind to at least one T cell. Because each T cell has a single receptor specificity, the repertoire of receptors is, in effect, the repertoire of the T cells. T cell antigen receptors recognize the complexes formed between antigens and MHC molecules. They cannot recognize or respond to free antigen molecules.

Given the random nature of receptor binding, the strength of binding (or affinity) between an antigen and its receptors will vary. Thus an antigen may be bound strongly by some receptors and weakly by others. If this binding strength is very weak, the encounter between the antigen and its receptor may be insufficient to activate the T cell.

In a newborn animal that has never previously encountered antigens, the number of T cells that can bind any specific antigen may be very low. To increase the probability of an antigen encountering a T cell with the correct receptor, the T cells are concentrated in secondary lymphoid organs such as lymph nodes, where their chances of a successful interaction with antigen-bearing dendritic cells are maximized. In primed animals in which mature T cells are plentiful, they can migrate into the tissues, where they can encounter other antigen-presenting cells, such as macrophages, and B cells.

Immunoglobulin Superfamily

Proteins are constructed by linking together multiple peptide modules or domains. Each domain usually has a specialized function. For example, in proteins located on a cell surface, the membrane-binding domain contains hydrophobic amino acids that can penetrate cell membrane lipid bilayer. Other domains may be responsible for the structural stability of a protein or for its biological activities. In antibody (immunoglobulin) molecules, one domain is used to bind antigen, and other domains are responsible for cell binding. The presence of similar domains in dissimilar proteins suggests that they have a common origin, and proteins may be classified into families or superfamilies based on their domain structure.

Proteins belonging to the immunoglobulin superfamily play key roles in immunity. The members of this superfamily all contain at least one immunoglobulin domain. In a typical immunoglobulin domain, the peptide chains weave back and forth to form a pleated sheet that folds into a sandwich-like structure. Immunoglobulin domains were first identified in antibody molecules (immunoglobulins). They have since been found in many other proteins, and collectively these proteins form the immunoglobulin superfamily. The superfamily includes some proteins with multiple immunoglobulin domains and some with only a single domain. Important proteins with multiple domains include the B cell antigen receptors (BCRs), the T cell antigen receptors (TCRs), and the MHC class I and II molecules (Figure 14-1). All of the members of this superfamily are receptors, most are found on cell surfaces, and none has enzymatic activity. Many cellular responses are triggered by interactions between two different members of the superfamily as, for example, between TCR and MHC molecules.

T Cell Antigen Receptor

Antigen-Binding Component

Each T cell has about 30,000 identical antigen receptors (TCRs) on its surface. Each TCR is a complex structure containing multiple glycoprotein chains. Two of these chains are paired to form the antigen-binding site; the other chains transmit the signal generated by antigen binding to the cell. Two different types of TCR have been identified based on the paired peptide chains used for antigen binding (Figure 14-2). One type employs γ and δ (γ/δ) chains. The other employs α and β (α/β) chains. In humans, mice, and probably most nonruminants, 90% to 99% of T cells use α/β receptors. In calves, lambs, and piglets in contrast, up to 66% of T cells may use γ/δ receptors.

The four antigen-binding chains (α, β, γ, δ) are similar in structure, although they differ in size. Thus the α chain is 43 to 49 kDa, the β chain is 38 to 44 kDa, the γ chain is 36 to 46 kDa, and the δ chain is 40 kDa. Size differences are due to variations in glycosylation. Each of these chains is formed from four domains (Figure 14-3). The N-terminal domain contains about 100 amino acids whose sequence varies greatly among

cells. This is therefore called the variable (V) domain. The second domain contains about 150 amino acids. Its amino acid sequence does not vary, so it is called the constant (C) domain. The third, very small domain consists of 20 hydrophobic amino acids passing through the T cell membrane. The C-terminal domain within the cytoplasm of the T cell is only 5 to 15 amino acids long. The paired chains are joined by a disulfide bond between their constant domains to form a stable heterodimer. As a result, the two V domains form a groove in which antigens and MHC molecules bind. The precise shape

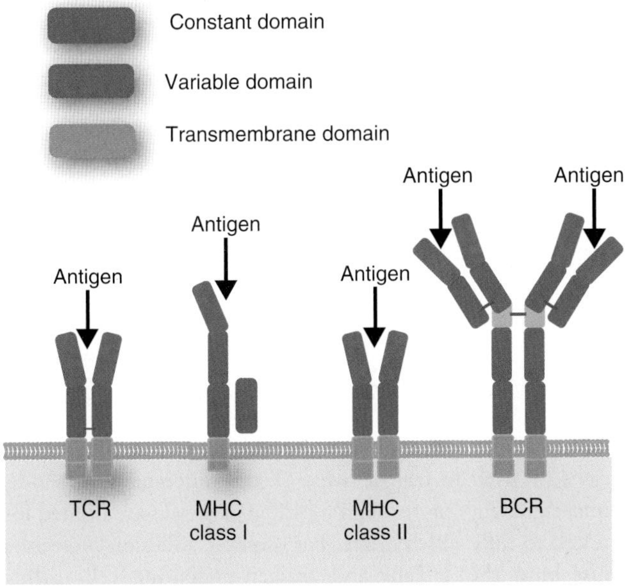

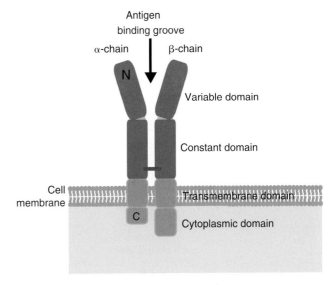

FIGURE 14-3 Schematic diagram showing the domain structure of the two peptide chains that make up the antigen-binding component of an α/β TCR.

FIGURE 14-1 The four key antigen receptors of the immune system—TCR, MHC class I, MHC class II, BCR—are each constructed using immunoglobulin domains as building blocks. Each binds antigen through the use of variable domains. All are members of the immunoglobulin superfamily.

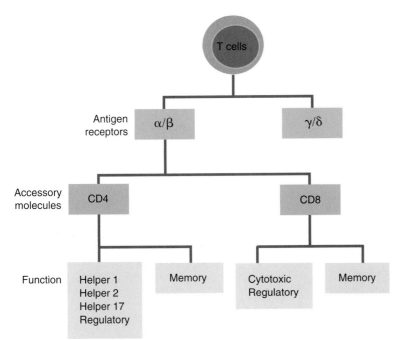

FIGURE 14-2 T cells can be divided into many different subpopulations based on the antigen receptors they employ, on the accessory molecules that support their activity, and ultimately on their functions.

of this antigen-binding groove varies among different TCRs because of the variable amino acid sequences in the V domains. The specificity of the binding between a TCR and an antigen is determined by the shape of the groove formed by the V domains.

When the V domains are examined closely, it is found that within each V domain is a region where the amino acid sequence is especially highly variable. This is the region that actually comes into contact with the antigen. For this reason, it is called the hypervariable or the complementarity determining region (CDR). The antigen-binding site of the TCR is formed by the paired CDRs that line the groove. The rest of each V domain outside the CDRs has a constant sequence and is called the framework region.

Signal Transduction Component

CD3 Complex The binding of antigen to the TCR sends a signal to trigger the T cell response. The two antigen-binding chains of each TCR are associated with a cluster of signal transducing proteins called the CD3 complex (Figure 14-4). The CD3 complex consists of five chains (γ, δ, ε, ζ, and η) (Table 14-1) arranged as three dimers γ-ε, δ-ε, and either ζ-ζ or ζ-η. The TCR β chain is linked to the γ-ε dimer, and the TCR α chain is linked to the δ-ε dimer. About 80% of α/β

TCRs contain a ζ-ζ homodimer, so that the complete complex consists of αβ-γε-δε-ζζ. The remaining 20% contain ζ-η heterodimers (they therefore consist of αβ-γε-δε-ζη).

CD4 and CD8 Two other proteins closely associated with the TCR are CD4 and CD8. CD4 is a single-chain glycoprotein of 55 kDa, and CD8 is a dimer of 68 kDa. (One chain of CD8 is called α, the other is β. In humans, pigs, mice, and cats, CD8 is an α-β heterodimer or, less commonly, an α-α homodimer.) Both CD4 and CD8 are members of the immunoglobulin superfamily. The presence of CD4 or CD8 determines the class of MHC molecule that is recognized by the T cell (Figure 14-5). For example, CD4, found only on helper T cells, binds MHC class II molecules on antigen-presenting cells. CD8, in contrast, is found only on cytotoxic T cells and binds MHC class Ia molecules on virus-infected or other abnormal cells. CD4 and CD8 enhance TCR signal transduction 100-fold when they cross-link to an MHC molecule on an antigen-presenting cell.

Co-stimulators

The binding of a TCR to a peptide-MHC complex is not sufficient by itself to trigger helper T cell differentiation. Additional signals acting through multiple pathways are needed for the cell to fully differentiate. For example adhesion molecules must bind the T cells and antigen-presenting cells firmly together and thus permit prolonged, strong signaling between the cells. TCR-antigen binding then triggers the initial steps. Ligands such as CD40 on antigen-presenting cells bind to T cells and amplify their responses. T cells are also stimulated by

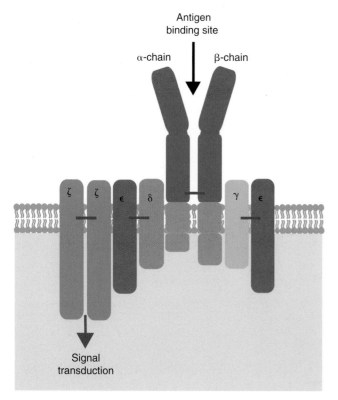

FIGURE 14-4 Overall structure of the TCR/CD3 complex. The signal transduction proteins are collectively classified as CD3. About 80% of α/β TCRs use ζζ dimers. The remaining 20% use ηζ heterodimers. Most γ/δ TCRs probably use a completely different signal transduction complex.

▫ Table 14-1 | TCR-CD3 Receptor Complex

PEPTIDE CHAIN	FUNCTION	MOLECULAR WEIGHT (kDa)
TCR α	Recognition of antigen and MHC	45-60
TCR β		40-55
TCR γ	Recognition of antigen	36-46
TCR δ		40-60
CD3 γ	Signal transducer	21-28
CD3 δ	Signal transducer	20-28
CD3 ε	Signal transducer	20-25
CD3 ζ	Signal transducer	16
CD3 η	Signal transducer	22
CD4	MHC II receptor	55
CD8	MHC I receptor	34

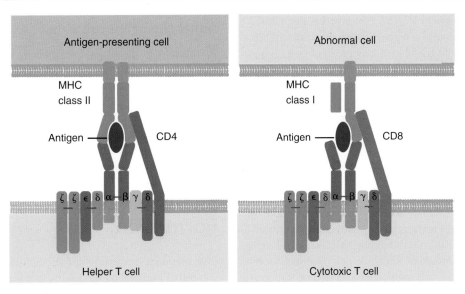

FIGURE 14-5 Role of CD4 and CD8 in promoting T cell responses. These molecules link the T cell to the antigen-presenting cell, binding the two cells together and ensuring that an effective signal is transmitted between them. CD4 binds to MHC class I molecules. This interaction is seen in Figure 10-6, A.

cytokines secreted by the antigen-presenting cells. These determine the way in which a T cell responds to antigen, turning on some pathways and turning off others.

Co-stimulatory Receptors

Several additional receptors must be stimulated in order to activate T cells.

CD40-CD154 Signaling CD40 is a receptor expressed on antigen-presenting cells. Its ligand is CD154, a protein expressed on helper T cells several hours after their TCRs have bound antigen (Figure 14-6). When CD154 and CD40 bind, signals are sent in both directions. The signal from the antigen-presenting cell to the T cell causes it to express a receptor called CD28. The signal from the T cell to the antigen-presenting cell stimulates it to express either CD80, or CD86. CD40-CD154 signaling also stimulate the antigen-presenting cell to secrete multiple cytokines, including interleukin-1 (IL-1), IL-6, IL-8, IL-12, CCL3, and tumor necrosis factor-α (TNF-α).

CD28-CD80/CD86 Signaling CD28, a T cell receptor induced by CD40-CD154 signaling, has two alternative ligands: either CD80 on dendritic cells, macrophages, and activated B cells, or CD86 on B cells. When CD80 or CD86 binds CD28, signals are generated that stimulate the T cell, in turn, to express yet another receptor, CD152 (also called CTLA-4). CD152 may also bind to CD80 or CD86. The binding of CD28 to its ligands is required for complete helper T cell activation since the engagement of CD28 amplifies the stimulus to the T cell eight-fold. CD28 stimulation enhances the production of IL-2 and other cytokines, upregulates cell survival genes, promotes energy metabolism, and facilitates T cell division. On the other hand, when CD152 binds to CD80

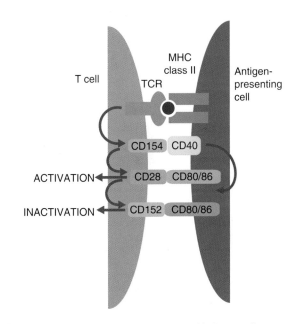

FIGURE 14-6 Antigen-presenting cells and helper T cells engage in a dialog. Thus binding of antigen to the TCR causes the T cell to express CD40 ligand (CD154). This engages CD40 on the antigen-presenting cell. As a result, CD28 and CD152 are expressed on the T cell, and CD80 or CD86 is expressed on the antigen-presenting cell. Depending on which receptors are engaged, the T cell may be stimulated or suppressed.

or 86, T cell activation is suppressed. The opposing signals delivered to T cells through these two receptors, CD28 and CD152, regulate the intensity of T cell responses.

Resting antigen-presenting cells express neither CD80 nor CD86. It takes 48 to 72 hours after T cell CD154 binds to CD40 before the antigen-presenting cells begin to express CD80/86 and the T cells express CD152. CD80 and CD86 can bind to either CD28 or CD152. However, because CD152 binds these molecules with a higher affinity than does CD28, the inhibitory effect of CD152 gradually predominates. When CD152 binds to CD80 on antigen-presenting cells, it induces the production of indoleamine dioxygenase (IDO), an enzyme that destroys tryptophan. In the absence of this amino acid, T cells cannot respond to antigen, and so the T cell response is terminated.

Co-stimulatory Cytokines

Cytokines, as described in Chapter 8, are signaling proteins that regulate immune cell functions. Cytokine secretion by antigen-presenting cells is triggered by many different stimuli. These include microbial PAMPs binding to TLRs, and T cells signaling through CD40 and CD154. As described in Chapter 10, different dendritic cell subpopulations secrete different cytokine mixtures. These mixtures in turn influence the nature of the helper T cell response. For example, IL-12 from DC1 cells promotes the differentiation of Th1 cells. Further differentiation is promoted by IFN-γ and IL-18. In the absence of IL-12, immature T cells differentiate into Th2 cells and their further differentiation is promoted by IL-4 and IL-13. Dendritic cells and macrophages stimulated through TLR2 secrete IL-23. This cytokine, together with IL-6 and transforming growth factor-β (TGF-β), results in the differentiation of Th17 cells (Figure 14-7).

Adherence Molecules

In addition to the dialog mediated by co-stimulatory molecules, T cells and antigen-presenting cells stimulate each other most effectively if they are bound together by adhesive molecules such as the integrins. For example, CD2 and CD11a/CD18 on T cells bind to their ligands CD58 and CD54 on antigen-presenting cells and lock the cells together. Once locked together an immunological synapse forms.

Immunological Synapse Formation

Cell membranes consist of fluid lipid bilayers that contain segregated areas called lipid rafts, where patches in the membrane are enriched in sphingolipids, cholesterol, and proteins. Small rafts are distributed evenly over the surface of resting T cells. When a T cell and an antigen-presenting cell come into contact, their cell membrane rafts aggregate so that the TCR-peptide-MHC complexes and the co-stimulatory receptors cluster together in the area of contact to form an immunological synapse (Figure 14-8). This synapse consists of concentric

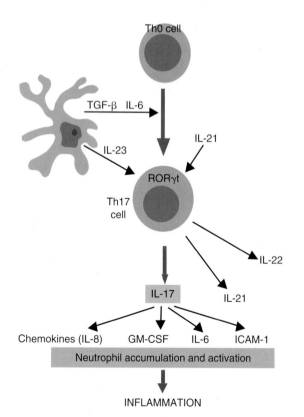

FIGURE 14-7 The induction of Th17 cells by exposure to a cytokine mixture containing TGF-β and IL-6. Differentiation is promoted by IL-21 and maintained by IL-23. Th17 cells promote inflammation.

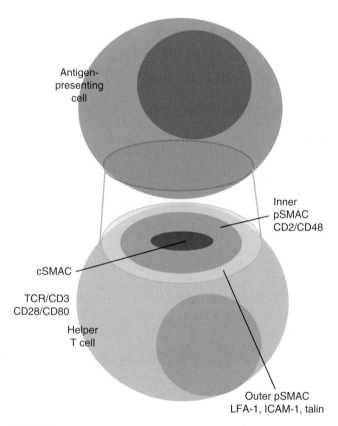

FIGURE 14-8 Interaction between a T cell and an antigen-presenting cell generates the supramolecular structure called an immunological synapse. Thus a series of concentric rings form around the interacting TCR-MHC complex. These rings contain different co-stimulating molecules.

rings of molecular complexes called supramolecular activation clusters (SMACs). They form a characteristic "bull's eye structure" consisting of a central (c) SMAC surrounded by a peripheral (p) SMAC and an outer ring. The cSMAC of Th1 cells contains the MHC and TCR molecules as well as CD4, CD3, CD2, CD28, CD80/86, and CD40/154. The pSMAC contains CD45 and the adhesion molecules ICAM-1 and leukocyte function-associated antigen-1 (LFA-1). The third, outer ring contains proteins excluded from the central synapse such as CD43. CD43 is a very large antiadhesive molecule that could interfere with the functioning of the synapse.

Th2 cells, in contrast, do not form a "bull's eye" synapse. They form multifocal immunological synapses at high antigen concentrations. Whereas the immunological synapse is on the cell surface, mitochondria in the cytosol migrate beneath the synapse and reduce the local concentration of Ca^{2+}. This inactivates Ca channels in the plasma membrane, resulting in a sustained Ca influx and activation of transcription factors such as NF-AT.

It is important to note that T cells may initially form synapses with multiple antigen-presenting cells but then polarize toward the cell providing the strongest stimulus. Thus, in effect, the T cell seeks the antigen that binds most strongly to its TCR. Once signaling is complete, the components of immunological synapses are endocytosed and degraded, terminating cell interactions.

Signal Transduction

Once a TCR binds to antigen on a presenting cell and an immunological synapse forms, the receptor signals to the T cell. The first signal is transmitted from the antigen-binding TCR α and β chains to the CD3 complex. This is probably the result of the clustering of several TCRs together. When the chains are clustered, the immunoreceptor tyrosine-based activation motifs (ITAMs) on the CD3 chains can activate several Src family tyrosine kinases (Chapter 8). These then cause the formation of a multimolecular proximal signaling complex. This complex in turn causes Ca signaling through calcineurin to activate NF-AT. It activates the Ras-mitogen-activated protein kinase (MAPK) pathway that triggers AP-1 production. It also activates a protein kinase C–dependent pathway that activates NF-κB. These three transcription factors activate multiple cytokine genes (Figure 8-11). As a result, T cells enlarge, enter the cell cycle, and synthesize and secrete a mixture of cytokines (Figure 14-9). The newly produced cytokines trigger the next stages of the immune responses.

Overall Considerations

T cells are highly mobile cells. As described in Chapter 12, they migrate rapidly through lymph nodes while continuously scanning the surfaces of dendritic cells for antigens. When it recognizes a foreign antigen, a T cell changes its behavior. It slows

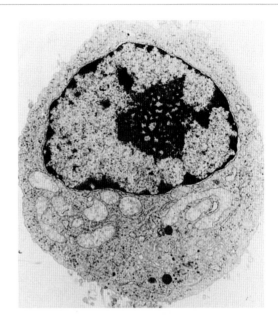

FIGURE 14-9 Transmission electron micrograph of a lymphoblast. Compare this with an unstimulated lymphocyte in Figure 13-2. Note the extensive cytoplasm, ribosomes, and large mitochondria.

(Courtesy Dr. S. Linthicum.)

down, stops, and eventually binds strongly to the antigen-presenting cell. This contact eventually leads to the formation of an immunological synapse. Whether or not a T cell stops depends on how strongly it binds to the target antigen. It will not stop for weakly binding antigens.

Once the immunological synapse forms, TCRs and co-stimulatory molecules signal to the T cell. However, the TCR does not function simply as a binary (on/off) switch. Instead differences in the strength of binding, in the amount of co-stimulation, and in the duration of the cell interaction affect T cell responses.

Because MHC molecules can bind many different antigenic peptides, any individual peptide will only be displayed in small amounts. T cells must be able to recognize these few specific peptide-MHC complexes among a vast excess of MHC molecules carrying irrelevant peptides. The number of MHC-peptide complexes signaling to the T cell is also important since the stimulus needed to trigger a T cell response varies. For example, only one MHC-peptide complex is needed to trigger a CD8+ T cell response, whereas about 1000 such complexes are required to trigger CD4+ T cells. T cell activation, in general, appears to involve tunable thresholds. Each threshold for signaling depends on the level of co-stimulation (Figure 14-10). For example, a minimum of 8000 TCRs must bind antigen for a CD4+ T cell to become activated in the absence of CD28, but only about 1000 TCRs need to be engaged if CD28 is present. The duration of signaling also determines a T cell's response. Sustained signaling is required for T cell activation and is maintained by serial triggering of its TCRs. Thus, during the prolonged cell interaction process, each MHC-peptide complex may trigger up to 200 TCRs. This serial triggering depends on the kinetics of TCR-ligand

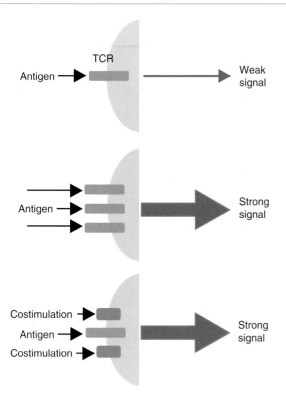

FIGURE 14-10 Successful stimulation of a T cell requires multiple signals. Depending on the antigen, the T cell may be activated by signals from multiple TCRs or by appropriate costimulation.

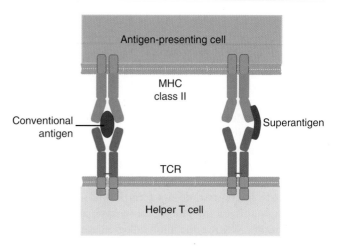

FIGURE 14-11 Differences in binding to a TCR between a conventional antigenic peptide that fills the groove between the α and β chains as opposed to a superantigen that binds only to the β chain.

interaction. CD28, for example, reduces the time needed to trigger a T cell and lowers the threshold for TCR triggering. Adhesion molecules stabilize the binding of T cells to antigen–processing cells and allow the signal to be sustained for hours.

The fate of a helper T cell is determined by the type of antigen-presenting cell used and by the nature of the signal received from it. Thus naïve T cells have strict requirements for activation. They must receive a sustained signal for at least 10 hours in the presence of co-stimulation or for up to 30 hours in its absence. This level of co-stimulation can only be provided by dendritic cells, which supply high levels of co-stimulatory and adhesion molecules. In contrast, other antigen-presenting cells act only transiently. Although macrophages and B cells can briefly trigger a TCR, they are unable to complete the process and thus fail to activate naïve T cells. Once primed, however, T cells require about an hour to reach commitment. Only then can they be activated by macrophages and B cells.

In the absence of effective costimulation, a T cell will undergo abortive activation. It will not divide or produce cytokines but either becomes unresponsive to antigen (anergic) or undergoes apoptosis and dies.

Superantigens

Fewer than 1 in 10,000 T cells can bind and respond to any specific foreign antigen. However, some microbial molecules called superantigens are unique in that they may stimulate as many as one in five T cells to divide. It was originally thought that these proteins were simply nonspecific mitogens. This is not the case. Superantigens only activate T cells whose TCR β chains contain certain V domains to which they can bind. Unlike conventional antigens that must bind within the grooves of both an MHC molecule and a TCR, superantigens directly link a TCR V_β domain to an MHC class II molecule on the antigen-presenting cell. All superantigens come from microbial sources such as streptococci, staphylococci, and mycoplasmas and from viruses such as rabies virus. The responses to superantigens are not MHC restricted (i.e., they do not depend on specific MHC haplotypes), but the presence of MHC antigens is required for an effective response since superantigens do not bind to the antigen-binding groove of the MHC class II molecule but attach elsewhere on its surface (Figure 14-11). As a result, they bind the T cell and the antigen-presenting cell together. Because of this strong binding, superantigens trigger a powerful T cell response. Some superantigens may stimulate the secretion of such large amounts of cytokines that they trigger a toxic shock syndrome (Chapter 6).

Helper T Cell Subpopulations

Naïve CD4+ T cells can express low levels of interferon-γ (IFN-γ) and IL-4. As they differentiate, however, they become polarized and produce only one of these. Three major subpopulations of CD4+ helper T cells have been identified. They are called helper 1 (Th1), helper 2 (Th2), and helper 17 (Th17) T cells and are distinguished by the mixture of cytokines that they secrete (Figure 14-12). As always, many of the details of their function have been investigated in mice and humans, and it must not be assumed that they function in a completely identical manner in other mammals.

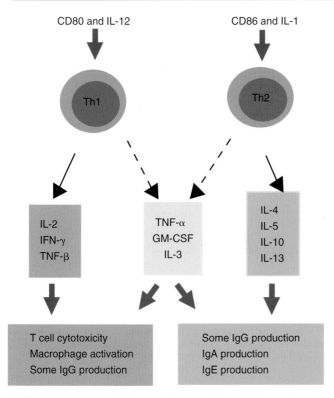

FIGURE 14-12 Major differences between Th1 and Th2 populations. Note that the co-stimuli that trigger them are different as are the set of cytokines they secrete.

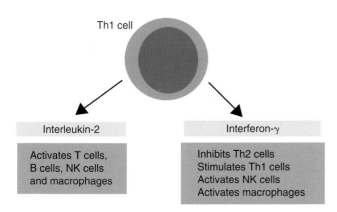

FIGURE 14-13 The cytokines produced by Th1 cells and their major properties.

Th1 Cells

The differentiation of Th1 cells is driven by IL-12 produced by antigen-presenting myeloid dendritic cells (DC1), macrophages (M1), and B cells plus co-stimulation by CD80. Complete Th1 cell activation, proliferation, and maximal IFN-γ production is achieved by additional stimulation with IL-18. IL-18 and IFN-γ thus reinforce each other's activities. This signaling activates the transcription factor T-bet. T-bet is the master regulator of Th1 cell differentiation. Once activated, Th1 cells produce IL-2, IFN-γ, TNF-α, and lymphotoxin (TNF-β) (Figure 14-13). Activated helper T cells secrete IL-2 and IFN-γ in a highly directed manner through the

immunological synapse. They secrete TNF-α in all directions. Presumably the cytokines secreted through the synapse are for specific communication with other cells; those secreted multi-directionally promote inflammation and systemic responses. Th1 cells promote cell-mediated immune responses such as the delayed hypersensitivity reaction and macrophage activation. They thus generate immunity to intracellular organisms such as mycobacteria and to viruses (Figure 14-14).

Interferon-γ

This cytokine is a glycoprotein of 17 kDa. As an interferon it has some antiviral activity, but its major role is the regulation of Th1 cell responses (Figure 14-15). It also upregulates antigen-processing pathways in dendritic cells and other antigen-presenting cells. IFN-γ is mainly produced by Th1 cells, CD8+ cytotoxic T cells, and natural killer (NK) cells, with lesser amounts from antigen-presenting cells, B cells, and NKT cells. It activates cells through the JAK-STAT pathway. It promotes macrophage activation, suppresses Th2 cells, and promotes NK cell activity.

Interleukin-2

IL-2 is a glycoprotein of 15 kDa produced by activated Th1 cells; its targets are T, B, and NK cells and macrophages. It stimulates cell proliferation, IFN-γ production, and antibody production and it enhances cytotoxicity (Figure 14-16). IL-2 supports the survival of regulatory T cells. As a result, it is an essential regulator of immune responses.

Th2 Cells

Dendritic cells that do not secrete IL-12 preferentially promote Th2 cell differentiation. These Th2 cells respond optimally to antigen presented by plasmacytoid dendritic cells (DC2 cells) and macrophages, and less well to antigen presented by B cells (Figure 10-3). DC2 cells provide co-stimulation through CD86. Th2 cells may require additional co-stimulation by IL-1 from macrophages or dendritic cells. Once produced, IL-4 acts in a paracrine manner to promote additional IL-4 production and suppress IFN-γ production.

Activated Th2 cells secrete IL-4, IL-5, IL-10, and IL-13 (Figure 14-17). These cytokines stimulate B cell proliferation and immunoglobulin secretion but have no effect on delayed hypersensitivity or other cell-mediated reactions. The cytokines from Th2 cells enhance B cell production of immunoglobulin G (IgG) and IgA up to 20-fold and production of IgE up to 1000-fold. Th2 responses are associated with enhanced immunity to parasitic worms but with decreased resistance to mycobacteria and other intracellular organisms.

Interleukin-4

IL-4 is a glycoprotein of 20 kDa produced by activated Th2 cells and mast cells. The targets of IL-4 are T cells, B cells, and macrophages. Signaling through STAT6, it activates cytokine

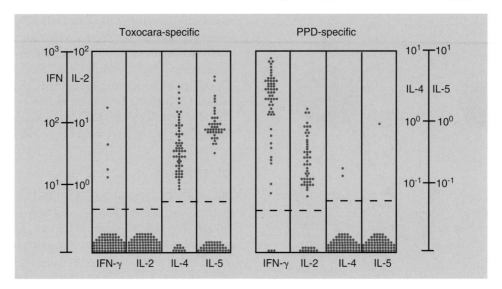

FIGURE 14-14 Different antigens can trigger distinctly different Th cell subpopulations. For example, T cells exposed to a parasite antigen from the roundworm *Toxocara canis* mount a Th2 response and secrete primarily IL-4 and IL-5. In contrast, T cells exposed to PPD, an antigen from *Mycobacterium tuberculosis*, mount a Th1 response characterized by secretion of IFN-γ and IL-2.

(From Del Prete G, De Carli M, Mastromauro C, et al: Purified protein derivative of Mycobacterium tuberculosis and excretory-secretory antigen(s) of Toxocara canis expand in vitro human T cells with stable and opposite (type 1 T helper or type 2 T helper) profile of cytokine production, *J Clin Invest* 88:346–350, 1991.)

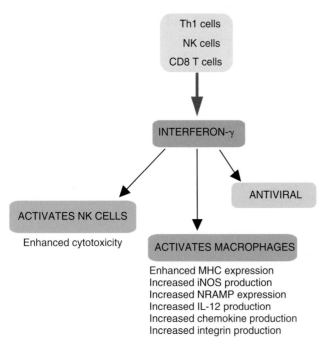

FIGURE 14-15 The origins and some properties of IFN-γ.

genes and the Th2-specific transcription factor GATA3. GATA3 is the master regulator of Th2 differentiation. IL-4 promotes IgG and IgE production, inhibits IFN-γ expression and Th17 cell production. In humans and rodents, IL-4 is essential for antibody production because it stimulates B cell activity (Figure 14-18). In pigs, however, IL-4 is not a B cell stimulant. Indeed, it blocks antibody and IL-6 production and suppresses antigen-induced B cell proliferation. Thus IL-4 may

play a very different role in pigs than it does in mice or humans. IL-4 shares overlapping intracellular signaling pathways and biological functions with IL-13.

Th0 Cells

Although the T cell subpopulations described earlier are usually considered to be discrete subsets, it has been argued that T cell cytokine profiles form a continuous spectrum with Th1 and Th2 cells as the extreme phenotypes. Thus some cells secrete a mixture of Th1 and Th2 cytokines. These cells, called Th0 cells, may be precursors of Th1 and Th2 or cells that are in transition between the two populations. Some IL-2-secreting T cells may switch to become IL-4–secreting cells after exposure to antigen, implying a change in phenotype from Th1 to Th2. The principal molecules that control this switch are IL-4 and IL-12. When cultured in the presence of IL-4, Th0 cells become Th2 cells. When cultured in the presence of IL-12, they become Th1 cells. Mixed (Th0) cell populations are most obvious early after initiation of an immune response, whereas Th1 and Th2 subsets are more obvious in chronic diseases where the antigens are persistent and cannot be easily removed.

Th17 Cells

The third population of CD4+ T cells characteristically secrete IL-17 (see Figure 14-7). The differentiation of Th17 cells is promoted by a cytokine mixture containing IL-6, TGF-β, IL-23, and IL-21. Of these, IL-23 appears to be of greatest importance since it enhances IL-17 expression. Th17 cells use a unique transcription factor, ROR-γt, which in association with other transcription factors causes Th17 cells to produce a

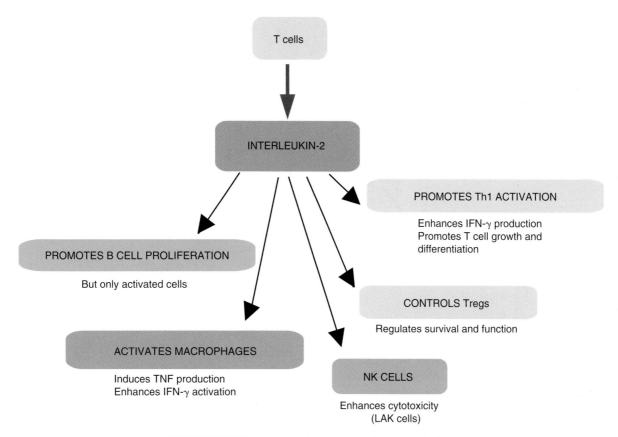

FIGURE 14-16 The origins and some properties of interleukin-2.

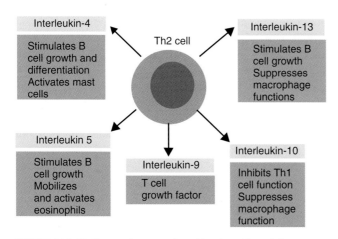

FIGURE 14-17 The cytokines produced by Th2 cells and their major properties.

distinctive mixture of cytokines, namely IL-17A, IL-17F, IL-21, and IL-22. They do not produce either IFN-γ or IL-4.

Th17 cells have two major functions: they regulate inflammation and they are potent B-cell helpers. Th17 cells promote inflammation because their cytokine products are proinflammatory. IL-17 recruits granulocytes through its actions on stem cells. It promotes the recruitment and survival of macrophages, and it stimulates the production of proinflammatory cytokines

and antibacterial peptides from many cell types. Cytokines of the IL-17 family regulate immune responses adapted to clearing extracellular bacteria and fungi. Thus Th17 cells play a key role in protective responses to extracellular Gram-negative bacteria and assist in the clearance of fungi. Th17 cells also can convert quite readily to Th1 cells. It is possible that Th17 cells may be a transient stage in T cell development and eventually convert into IFN-γ-producing Th1 cells.

Species Differences

The details of helper T cell subpopulation function described above have largely been derived from studies in laboratory mice. Cattle most certainly possess Th1 and Th2 cells and can mount polarized immune responses. Bovine IgG1 expression is positively regulated by IL-4 and IgG2 expression by IFN-γ. Many bovine CD4+ cells produce IL-2, IL-4, IL-10, and IFN-γ and thus appear to be Th0 cells.

γ/δ T Cells

The function of T cells bearing γ/δ TCRs remains an enigma as a result of major species differences (Figure 14-19). For example, only 5% to 15% of blood lymphocytes in humans and mice but up to 66% of young ruminants and pigs have

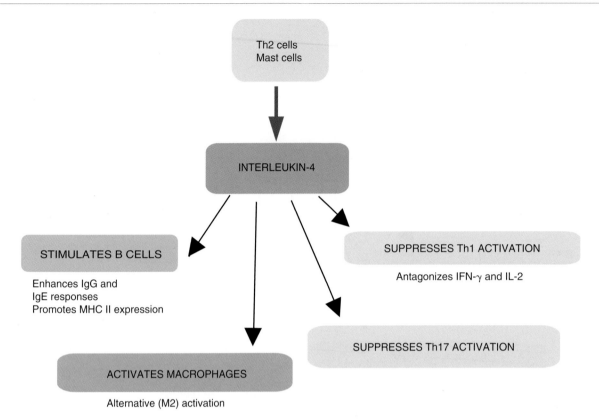

FIGURE 14-18 The origins and some properties of interleukin-4.

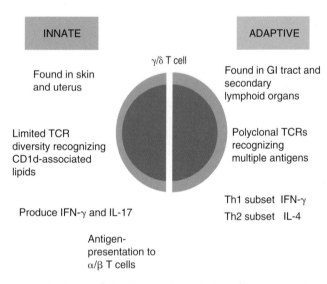

FIGURE 14-19 γ/δ T cells may, depending on the species, act as innate immune cells with an invariant antigen receptor. Others may act as classic helper T cells with diverse TCRs of polyclonal origin.

γ/δ TCRs. It is probable that this cell population has different functions in the two groups of mammals. In humans and mice in which γ/δ T cells are a minor lymphocyte subpopulation, they are subdivided into two subsets. One subset is engaged in innate immunity, has limited γ/δ receptor diversity, and is mainly found in the skin and genital tract. These skin T cells preferentially bind to common microbial PAMPs, especially

heat-shock proteins and phospholigands (carbohydrates or nucleotides with a phosphate group). Other γ/δ T cells preferentially respond to the class Ib MHC molecules, MICA and MICB, both of which are produced by stressed cells, cancer cells, and virus-infected cells (Chapter 19). When stimulated, these γ/δ T cells secrete large amounts of IL-17 and IFN-γ. Like Th17 cells, these γ/δ T cells are activated by IL-23. The functions of skin γ/δ T cells may differ according to the stages of infection. Thus, early in infection, the cells with restricted antigen binding may serve an innate immune function and help resist intracellular bacteria such as *Mycobacterium* or *Listeria* species. Later in infections, they may serve an anti-inflammatory or wound healing role.

In contrast, the second subset has extensive receptor diversity and is mainly found in secondary lymphoid organs and intestinal mucosa. These cells can recognize antigens directly without the need for a MHC molecule. These γ/δ T cells with diverse antigen-binding receptors form at least two subpopulations. One subpopulation can be further divided into Th1 and Th2 subsets based on their secreted cytokines. The other subpopulation is cytotoxic and can destroy target cells, such as cells infected with mycobacteria and some leukemic cells. Since the vast majority of these cells are located on body surfaces, presumably they have a major defensive function. In humans, γ/δ T cells can also act as professional antigen-presenting cells.

In young ruminants and pigs, γ/δ T cells can bind a wide variety of antigens, suggesting that they have a role in adaptive immunity. These cells colonize the skin, the mammary gland, the reproductive organs, and the intestinal wall where they form the major T cell population. In pigs, γ/δ T cells are polyclonal at birth, but their T cell diversity becomes increasingly restricted with age. In addition, γ/δ T cells located in different organs or even different parts of the gastrointestinal tract have different repertoires.

Up to 90% of ruminant γ/δ T cells express WC1 and are engaged in innate immunity, whereas the remaining WC1– cells are regulatory. The two subpopulations have a different tissue distribution. In mycobacterial and schistosomal infections, granulomas form around the invading organisms. In both cases the initial T cell infiltration is dominated by γ/δ T cells and is followed later by α/β T cells. A second wave of γ/δ T cells may terminate the response. These WC1+ γ/δ T cells secrete IL-12 and IFN-γ and may thus promote a Th1 bias in the immune response. There is also evidence that they play a key role in immunity to *Leptospira* species.

Human and bovine γ/δ T cells respond to microbial PAMPs by increasing the expression of lymphotactin (XCL1), MIP-1β, TNFα, and granulocyte-macrophage colony-stimulating factor. The responding γ/δ T cells express TLR3, TLR9, mannose-binding lectin, and CD36. These γ/δ T cells may well be major contributors to innate immunity. Many γ/δ T cells have nonpolymorphic TCRs that recognize microbial glycolipids presented by CD1-positive antigen-presenting cells and release cytokines and lyse target cells just like conventional α/β T cells. The role of γ/δ T cells on mucosal surfaces is discussed further in Chapter 22. Porcine γ/δ T cells can be divided into two subpopulations based on the presence or absence of CD2.

Memory T Cells

When naïve T cells differentiate into Th1 cells, two types of cell develop. One cell type secretes IFN-γ and acts as helper cells. These cells are short-lived because they are eliminated either by autocrine IFN-γ and IL-2 that trigger Fas-mediated apoptosis or by nitric oxide produced by macrophages. Cells of the second type do not secrete IFN-γ, are resistant to apoptosis, and develop into long-lived memory cells. This differentiation into two distinct populations may result from asymmetrical T cell division (Figure 14-20). As described earlier, T cells interact with antigen-presenting cells for several hours through an immunological synapse. Once it receives sufficient stimulation the T cell undergoes mitosis and begins to divide even before it separates from the antigen-presenting cell. The dividing T cell is polarized since one pole of the cell contains the immunological synapse and associated structures. The other pole contains molecules excluded from the synapse. Thus when the T cell divides, it forms two distinctly different daughter cells. The daughter cell adjacent to the synapse is the precursor of effector cells. The daughter cell formed at the opposite pole is the precursor of the memory cells. Memory T

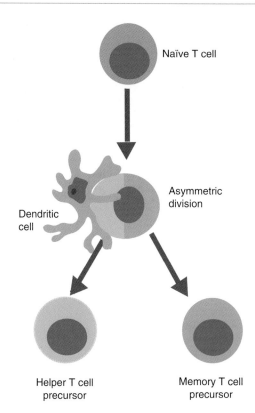

FIGURE 14-20 Following T cell-DC interactions, the T cell divides asymmetrically. The cell at the contact pole becomes a helper T cell. The cell at the opposite pole becomes a memory T cell.

cells are themselves functionally heterogeneous. Thus central memory T cells remain in the secondary lymphoid tissues, such as lymph nodes, awaiting the arrival of invaders, whereas other effector memory T cells are found in inflamed tissues, where they immediately attack invaders. Memory CD4+ and CD8+ T cells persist in the absence of antigen. These cells slowly divide and replenish their numbers. IL-7 and IL-15 are required for the survival of memory CD8+ T cells, whereas only IL-7 is needed for the survival of CD4+ T cells. These maintain the cells in a state of slow proliferation. In humans, memory CD4+ T cells have a half-life of 8 to 12 years, whereas memory CD8+ T cells have a half-life of 8 to 15 years. On the other hand, some individuals may lose their memory CD8+ T cells very rapidly for unknown reasons. The size of the immune system is fixed somewhat, but the effector memory CD8 T cell pool can double without loss of preexisting memory cells.

Human memory T cells express TLR2. If exposed to its ligand lipopeptide in the presence of either IL-2 or IL-15, they will proliferate. Thus it is possible that bacterial PAMPs such as lipopeptides may promote the long-term survival of memory T cells even in the absence of persistent antigen.

For sources of additional information, please visit http:// evolve.elsevier.com/tizard/immunology/

B Cells and Their Response to Antigen

Key Points

- B cells express multiple identical antigen binding receptors (BCRs) on their surface.
- When BCRs are shed into body fluids, they are called immunoglobulins or antibodies.
- BCRs consist of two heavy and two light chains bound together by disulfide bonds.
- B cells can recognize most antigens without prior processing. However, an optimal B cell response normally requires additional stimulation by helper T cells.
- Helper T cells stimulate B cells through an immunologic synapse containing costimulatory molecules and interactive receptors.
- B cells require co-stimulation by cytokines.
- Responding B cells may become either memory cells or antibody-secreting plasma cells.
- Plasma cells are the progeny of B cells that have differentiated to secrete very large amounts of antibodies.
- The differentiation of B cells into plasma cells takes place in the germinal centers of lymph nodes and other secondary lymphoid organs.
- Cancerous plasma cells, called myeloma cells, produce large quantities of very pure immunoglobulin. If fused with a normal plasma cell, the resulting hybridomas can produce large quantities of pure monoclonal antibodies.

The division of the adaptive immune system into two major components is based on the need to recognize two distinctly different forms of foreign invaders. Some invaders enter the body openly and grow in extracellular fluids. These exogenous antigens are destroyed by antibodies. Other invaders grow inside cells, where antibodies cannot reach. These are destroyed by T cell–mediated responses. Antibodies are produced by the lymphocytes called B cells. This chapter discusses B cells and their response to antigens.

B cells are mainly found in the cortex of lymph nodes, in the marginal zone in the spleen, in the bone marrow, throughout the intestine and in Peyer's patches. Few B cells circulate in the blood. Like T cells, B cells have a large number of identical antigen-binding receptors on their surface. Each B cell, therefore, can only bind and respond to a single antigen. Antigen receptors are generated at random during B cell development in a process described in Chapter 17. If a B cell encounters an antigen that can bind its receptors, it will, with appropriate co-stimulation, respond by secreting its receptors into body fluids, where they are called antibodies. Each B cell thus makes antibodies of the same binding specificity as its receptors.

B Cell Antigen Receptors

Each B cell is covered with about 200,000 to 500,000 identical antigen receptors (BCRs), many more than the 30,000 antigen receptors (TCRs) expressed on each T cell. Each BCR is constructed from multiple peptide chains and, like the TCR, can be divided into antigen-binding and signaling components. Unlike the TCR, however, the BCR can also bind antigens when in solution. Antibodies are simply soluble BCRs secreted into body fluids; they all belong to the family of proteins called immunoglobulins (Chapter 16).

Antigen-Binding Component

The antigen-binding component of the BCR (or immunoglobulin) is a glycoprotein of 160 to 180 kDa consisting of four linked peptide chains. These chains consist of two identical pairs—a pair of heavy chains, each 60 kDa in size, and a pair of light chains, about 25 kDa each (Figure 15-1). The light chains are linked by disulfide bonds to the heavy chains so that the complete molecule is shaped like the letter Y. The tail of the Y (called the Fc region) is formed from paired heavy chains and is attached to the B cell surface. The arms of the Y (called the Fab regions) are formed by paired light and heavy chains, and they bind antigens (Figure 15-2). The antigen-binding sites are formed by the grooves between the light and heavy chains. Thus each BCR has two identical antigen-binding sites.

Light Chains Light chains are constructed from two domains each containing about 110 amino acids. The amino acid sequences in the C-terminal domains from different B cells are identical and form a constant domain (C_L). In contrast, the

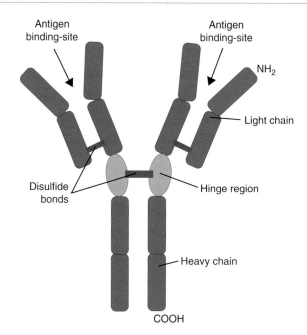

FIGURE 15-1 The overall structure of an immunoglobulin molecule. When bound to a B cell surface, this molecule acts as an antigen receptor (BCR). When released by the B cell and free in the circulation, it acts as an antibody. Note that unlike a TCR, it has two antigen-binding sites.

sequences in the N-terminal domains differ in each cell examined and so form variable domains (V_L). Mammals make two types of light chains, called κ (kappa) and λ (lambda). Although their amino acid sequences are different, they are functionally identical. The ratio of κ to λ chains in BCRs varies among mammals, ranging from mice and rats, which have more than 95% κ chains, to cattle and horses, which have 95% λ chains. Primates such as the rhesus monkey and the baboon have 50% of each, whereas humans have 70% κ chains. Carnivores such as cats and dogs have 90% λ chains.

Heavy Chains Immunoglobulin heavy chains contain 400 to 500 amino acids. They consist of four or five domains each of

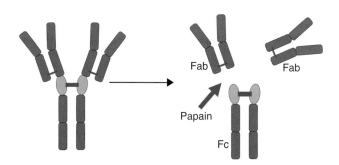

FIGURE 15-2 The effect of treating an immunoglobulin molecule with the proteolytic enzymes, pepsin, or papain. Papain cleaves the molecule into three large fragments. Pepsin cleaves the molecule into one large fragment and many small ones. The names of these fragments denote the nomenclature of different regions of an immunoglobulin molecule.

about 110 amino acids. The N-terminal domain has a highly variable sequence and is the variable (V_H) domain. The remaining three or four domains show few sequence differences and form constant (C_H) domains.

B cells make five different classes of heavy chain that differ in their sequence and domain structure. As a result, each of these classes has a different biological activity. The five different immunoglobulin heavy chains are called α, γ, δ, ε, and μ. These heavy chains determine the immunoglobulin class (or isotype). Thus immunoglobulin molecules that use α heavy chains are called immunoglobulin A (IgA), and those that use γ chains are called IgG; μ chains are used in IgM, δ chains in IgD, and ε chains in IgE.

Variable Regions When the amino acid sequences of V domains from light and heavy chains are examined in detail, two features become apparent. First, their sequence variation is largely confined to three regions, each consisting of 6 to 10 amino acids, within the variable domain (Figure 15-3). These regions are said to be hypervariable. Between the three hypervariable regions are relatively constant sequences called framework regions. The hypervariable regions on paired light and heavy chains determine the shape of the antigen-binding site and thus the specificity of antigen binding. Since the shape of the antibody-binding site is complementary to the conformation of the antigenic determinant, the hypervariable sequences are also called complementarity determining regions (CDRs). Each V-domain is folded in such a way that its three CDRs come into close contact with the antigen (Figure 15-4).

Constant Regions The number of constant domains differs between immunoglobulin classes. For example, there are three constant domains in a γ heavy chain; they are labeled, from the N-terminal end, as C_H1, C_H2, and C_H3. A similar arrangement is found in α and most δ chains, whereas μ and ε chains have an additional constant domain called C_H4.

Since heavy chains are paired, the domains in each chain come together to form structures by which antibody molecules can exert their biological functions. Thus V_H and V_L together form an antigen-binding site, and C_H1 and C_L together stabilize the antigen-binding site. The paired C_H2 domains of IgG

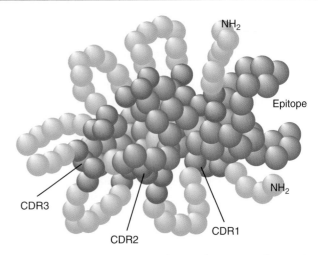

FIGURE 15-4 The way in which the complementarity-determining regions are folded to form the antigen binding site on an immunoglobulin molecule. A similar folding occurs in the peptide chains of the TCR.

contain a site that activates the classical pathway of the complement system (Chapter 7) and a site that binds to Fc receptors on phagocytic cells (Figure 15-5). The heavy chain also regulates the transfer of IgG into colostrum (Chapter 21) and antibody-mediated cellular cytotoxicity (Chapter 18). When immunoglobulin molecules act as BCRs, part of their Fc region is embedded in the B cell surface membrane. These cell-bound immunoglobulins differ from the secreted form in that they have a small transmembrane domain located at their C-terminus. This contains hydrophobic amino acids that associate with the cell-membrane lipids.

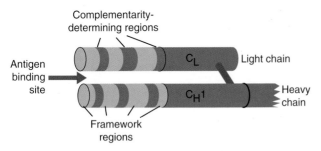

FIGURE 15-3 The variable regions of the light and heavy chains of an immunoglobulin molecule are divided into three highly variable complementarity-determining regions separated by relatively constant framework regions.

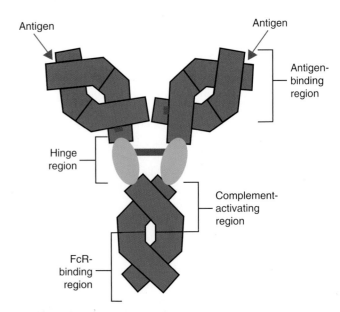

FIGURE 15-5 The structure of an IgG molecule, showing how the light and heavy chains intertwine to form clearly defined regions of the molecule. Each region has defined biological functions.

Hinge Region One important feature of the immunoglobulins is that the Fab regions, which contain the antigen-binding sites, can swing freely around the center of the molecule as if hinged. This hinge consists of a short domain of about 12 amino acids located between the C_H1 and C_H2 domains. The hinge region contains many hydrophilic and proline residues that cause the peptide chain to unfold and make this region readily accessible to proteases (Figure 16-10). This region also contains all the interchain disulfide bonds. Proline, because of its configuration, produces a 90-degree bend when inserted in a polypeptide chain. Because amino acids can rotate around peptide bonds, the effect of closely spaced proline residues is to produce a universal joint around which the immunoglobulin chains can swing freely. The μ chains of IgM do not possess a hinge region.

Signal Transducing Component

BCR immunoglobulins cannot signal directly to their B cell since their cytoplasmic domains contain only three amino acids. However, their C_H4 and transmembrane domains associate with glycoprotein heterodimers formed by pairing CD79a (Ig-α) with CD79b (Ig-β). These heterodimers act as signal transducers (Figure 15-6). The CD79b chains are identical in all BCRs. The CD79a chains differ depending on their associated heavy chains and employ different signaling pathways. BCR signaling is initiated by antigen binding. This leads to receptor clustering and subsequent phosphorylation of the immunoreceptor tyrosine-based activation motifs (ITAMs) on

CD79a and CD79b. Phosphorylation of the tyrosines in these ITAMs by src family kinases activates downstream signaling cascades (see Figure 8-12).

Co-stimulation of B Cells

Although the binding of antigen to a BCR is an essential first step in triggering a B cell response, it is usually insufficient to trigger antibody formation. Complete activation of a B cell requires additional stimulation by helper T cells and cytokines (Figure 15-7). In order to do this, however, the helper T cells must themselves be presented with antigen. This antigen can be presented by one of the professional antigen-presenting cells, a dendritic cell, a macrophage, or even from a B cell. Thus a B cell can capture and process antigen, present it to a T cell, and then receive co-stimulation from the same T cell. B cells thus play two roles. They respond to antigen by making antibodies while at the same acting as antigen-processing cells. The helper T cells provide the B cell with co-stimulatory signals from cytokines as well as through interacting receptor pairs.

Antigen Presentation by B Cells

B cells are effective antigen-presenting cells. Following antigen binding, the BCR may be internalized and degraded or transported to an intracellular compartment, where major histocompatibility (MHC) class II molecules and antigen fragments combine. These antigen-MHC class II complexes are carried to the B cell surface, where they are presented to helper T cells (Figure 15-8). This activates the T cells that then provide co-stimulation to the B cell and permit its full activation. Since all the antigen receptors on a single B cell are identical, each B cell can bind only one antigen. This makes them much more efficient antigen-presenting cells than macrophages that must present any foreign material that comes their way. This is especially true in a primed animal, in which large numbers of B cells can bind and present a specific antigen. As a result, B cells can activate Th cells with $\frac{1}{1000}$ of the antigen concentration required to activate macrophages.

Cytokine Secretion

Th2 cells secrete cytokines that activate B cells and trigger their differentiation. The four most important are interleukin-4 (IL-4), IL-5, IL-6 and IL-13.

IL-4 is mainly produced by activated Th2 cells and mast cells. It stimulates the growth and differentiation of B cells. It also enhances their expression of MHC class II and Fc receptors. IL-4 also induces immunoglobulin class switching in B cells. For example, it stimulates IgA and IgE production (Table 15-1). The actions of IL-4 are neutralized by IFN-γ, which inhibits both IgA and IgE synthesis as well as B cell proliferation.

IL-5 promotes the differentiation of activated B cells into plasma cells. It stimulates IgG and IgM production and

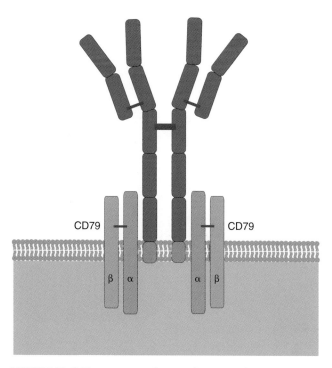

FIGURE 15-6 The structure of a complete BCR, showing both the antigen-binding component (immunoglobulin) and the signal transducing components (CD79). Note the small transmembrane domain at the end of each heavy chain.

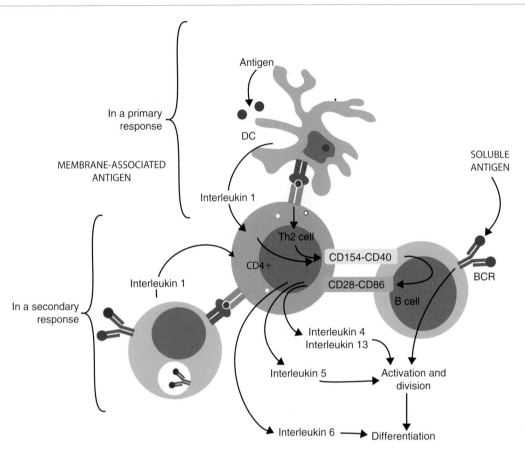

FIGURE 15-7 The sequence of events that must occur for a B cell to respond to antigen. Not only must the B cell be stimulated by antigen, but it must also receive costimulation from helper T cells and their cytokines. This complex interaction can be seen in Figure 10-6, *D*.

FIGURE 15-8 The sequence of events that occurs when an antigen-processing B cell interacts with a helper T cell. During a primary immune response, antigen is processed by a dendritic cell and presented to the helper T cell. During a secondary immune response, the B cell itself can act as an antigen-presenting cell. Co-stimulators, such as CD154 and CD28, engage serially to trigger IL-4 secretion by the T cell and IL-4R production by the B cell.

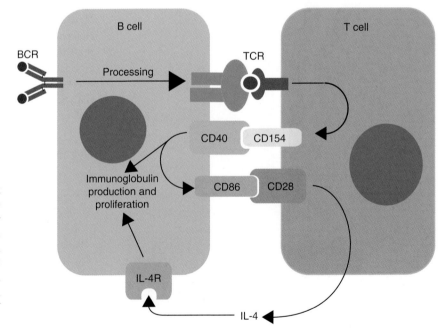

□ Table 15-1 | Immunoglobulins Produced by B cells in the Presence of Th1 and Th2 Antigen-Specific helper T Cell Clones in Mice

CLASS	Th1 CELLS (ng/mL)	Th2 CELLS (ng/mL)
IgG1	<8	21,600
IgG2a	14	39
IgG2b	<8	189
IgG3	<8	354
IgM	248	98,000
IgA	<1	484
IgE	<1	187

Adapted from Coffmann RL, Seymour BW, Lebman DA, et al: The role of helper T cell products in mouse B cell differentiation and isotype regulation, *Immunol Rev* 102:5, 1988.

enhances IL-4-induced IgE production. IL-5 selectively stimulates IgA production in mucosal B cells.

IL-6 is needed for the final differentiation of activated B cells into plasma cells. It acts together with IL-5 to promote IgA production and with IL-1 to promote IgM production.

IL-13 has biological activities similar to those of IL-4 because it acts through a receptor (IL-13R) that shares a common α chain with the IL-4R. It has similar effects to IL-4 on B cells, stimulating their proliferation and increasing immunoglobulin secretion. IL-13 is required for optimal induction of IgE, especially if IL-4 is low or absent.

CD40 and CD154

Cytokines alone cannot fully activate B cells. Complete activation also requires signaling through receptor pairs such as CD40 and CD154. For example, the co-stimulatory molecule CD40 is expressed on resting B cells, whereas its ligand, CD154, is expressed on activated helper T cells. CD40 must receive a signal from CD154 in order for a B cell to begin its cell cycle and upregulate its expression of IL-4 and IL-5 receptors (Figure 15-9; see Figure 15-8). The signals from CD40 synergize with those from IL-4 and IL-5 receptors to drive B cell activation, memory cell development, and immunoglobulin class switching. CD28 on T cells must also signal to CD86 on activated B cells for optimal costimulation to occur.

CD21/CD19 Complex

Effective co-stimulation also requires that B cells receive signals from complement transmitted through a CD21-CD19 complex on the B cell surface. CD21 is a complement receptor (CR2) whose ligand is C3d. CD19 is its accompanying signaling component. If an antigen molecule with C3d attached binds to CD21, a signal is transmitted through CD19 to the B cell (Figure 15-10). These signals synergize so that stimulation of a BCR plus CD19/CD21 lowers the threshold for B cell activation 100-fold. The importance of complement in stimulating B cells is emphasized by the observation that mice deficient in the complement components C3, C4, or CR2 cannot mount effective antibody responses to T-dependent antigens.

The B cell Fc receptor, FcγRIIb, is a negative regulator of B cell function. When an IgG molecule binds and links this receptor to a BCR through antigen, it inhibits antibody formation. This has important practical consequences when vaccinating young animals (Chapter 21).

Toll-like Receptors and Pathogen-Associated Molecular Patterns

Although BCR-antigen binding and T cell–derived co-stimulation trigger initial B cell division, they cannot induce a prolonged, self-sustaining B cell response. In fact, complete activation of B cells requires signals from their toll-like receptors (TLRs). The B cell–stimulating ligands include flagellins,

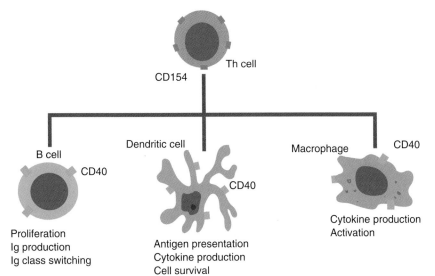

FIGURE 15-9 CD40 and CD154 participate in a dialog between T cells and the professional antigen-presenting cells. As a result, both cell types are stimulated. In the case of B cells, T cell stimulation permits B cell proliferation and immunoglobulin production.

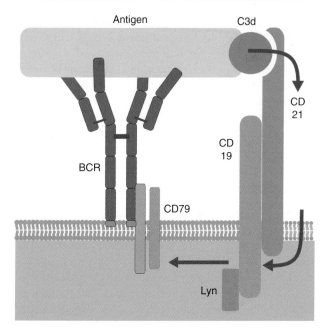

FIGURE 15-10 The stimulation of B cells through the CD21/CD19 complex. CD21 binds to C3d on the antigen. Signaling through CD19, it generates a potent costimulatory signal to enhance B cell responses.

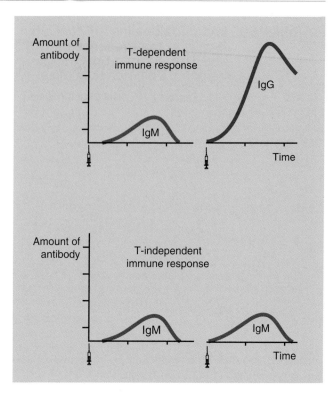

FIGURE 15-11 The differences in the time course of a T-dependent and T-independent antibody response. T-independent antigens cannot induce an immunoglobulin switch or immunological memory, as demonstrated by a secondary antibody response.

lipopolysaccharides, and CpG DNA. Signaling from TLR4 enhances B cell antigen presentation, promotes germinal center formation, and is required for optimal antibody production against T-dependent antigens (at least for some IgG subclasses). TLR signaling to memory B cells increases antibody production but it does not appear to be required for IgA and IgE production. Thus TLR signaling can substitute in part for T cell help and explains why antibody production still occurs in patients with AIDS despite their lack of T cells.

B Cell Response

Binding of antigen to the BCR, especially if two receptors are cross-linked, exposes ITAMs, triggers activation of several different tyrosine kinases, and results in phosphorylation of a phospholipase C and a G-protein (see Figure 8-12). As with the TCR, these reactions are dynamically regulated by CD45 tyrosine phosphatases. Subsequent hydrolysis of phosphatidylinositol and calcium mobilization leads to activation of a protein kinase C and calcineurin and activation of the transcription factors NF-κB and NF-AT.

Differential Signaling

Like the TCR, the BCR probably produces a tunable signal. That is, it generates signals that depend on the properties of the antigen and the amount of co-stimulation received. BCR affinity for its antigen influences B cell proliferation and antibody secretion. On the other hand, receptor occupancy influences MHC class II expression and signal transduction. The

direction of the immunoglobulin class switch also depends on signals received from Th1 or Th2 cytokines.

Certain antigens can provoke antibody formation in the absence of helper T cells. These so-called T-independent antigens are usually simple repeating polymers (and pathogen-associated molecular patterns [PAMPs]), such as *Escherichia coli* lipopolysaccharide, polymerized salmonella flagellin, and pneumococcal polysaccharide. T-independent antigens bind directly to B cell TLRs and cross-link several BCRs, providing a sufficient signal for B cell proliferation. Characteristically, T-independent antigens only trigger IgM responses and fail to generate memory cells (Figure 15-11). This is because they do not induce T cell co-stimulation and thus cannot trigger the class switch.

It is appropriate to emphasize at this stage that the BCR has the same antigen-binding ability as antibody molecules. Thus, antibodies can bind free intact antigens in solution. This is very different from the α/β TCR that can respond only to processed antigen bound to an MHC molecule (Figure 15-12). This difference in the antigen-recognizing ability of B and T cells is significant in that B cells can respond to a greater variety of antigens than T cells. Likewise, antibodies are directed, not against breakdown products of antigens, but against intact antigen molecules. As a result, antigen-antibody interactions usually depend on maintenance of the conformation of an antigen. A good example of this is seen with tetanus toxoid. Antibodies raised against the intact molecule will bind only to

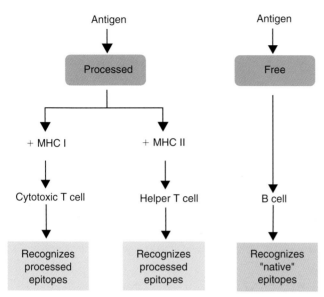

FIGURE 15-12 TCRs and BCRs recognize antigen in a very different fashion. Thus a BCR can bind to free, soluble antigen. A TCR, in contrast, can recognize only antigen processed and presented on a MHC molecule.

the intact molecule and may be unable to bind proteolytic fragments such as those produced by macrophage processing.

Cellular Responses

The term clonotype is used to describe a clone of B cells expressing a BCR capable of responding to a single epitope. A newborn animal has available only a limited number of different clonotypes, but this number increases with age as a result of increased use of alternative sets of V genes and somatic hypermutation in these V genes (Chapter 17). In an adult animal the number of B cells within a given clonotype varies as a result of exposure to different antigens over the animal's lifetime. Thus as an individual ages, the most used clonotypes will increase greatly in number. Conversely, for some rarely encountered antigens, their clonotypes will remain very small, and an individual may have as few as 10 responsive cells in the spleen or bone marrow. For commonly encountered antigens, in contrast, there may be as many as 10^4 responsive B cells (Box 15-1).

In mice and probably most other mammals, each B cell initially expresses both IgM and IgD BCRs on its surface, with about 10 times as many IgD molecules as IgM. These unstimulated B cells may secrete small amounts of monomeric IgM. When antigen binds to their BCR in the presence of helper T cells with appropriate costimulation, the signals generated result in increased expression of IgM BCR and MHC class II, as well as receptors for IL-4, IL-5, IL-6, tumor necrosis factor-α (TNF-α), and transforming growth factor-β (TGF-β), and start the process that leads to B cell division.

An appropriately stimulated B cell will therefore divide repeatedly, and its progeny will differentiate along one of two

> **□ Box 15-1 | Cell Membrane Exchange**
>
> It has generally been assumed that individual cells conserve their major structural components and do not share them with other cells. In recent years, however, it has become abundantly clear that different cells may exchange cell surface membranes and their associated receptors. Thus macrophages may accept fragments of neutrophil membranes. Activated B cells can also donate their antigen receptors to nearby bystander cells. This process is mediated by membrane transfer between adjacent B cells and is amplified by the interaction of the BCR with specific antigen. The net effect is to permit a dramatic expansion of the number of antigen-binding B cells in vivo. The B cells with their newly acquired receptors can act as antigen-presenting cells for CD4+ T cells. This is yet another example of the remarkable efficiency of the adaptive immune system in responding to a specific antigen once an animal is primed.

pathways. One population develops a rough endoplasmic reticulum, increases its rate of synthesis, and secretes large quantities of immunoglobulins and develops into plasma cells. These are essential for rapid antibody production and early protection. Within a few days, the responding cells switch from making IgM to making another immunoglobulin class. This switch occurs while B cells are in the germinal center and leads to production of IgG, IgA, or IgE. The class switch results from deletion of unwanted heavy chain genes and the joining of variable-region genes to the next available heavy chain genes (Chapter 16). The specificity of the antibody produced remains unchanged. Class switching is controlled by IL-4, IFN-γ, and TGF-β. Thus IL-4 from Th2 cells directs mouse B cells to produce IgG1 and IgE, whereas it directs human B cells to produce IgG4 and IgE (see Table 15-1). IL-4 alone is insufficient for class switching, and additional signals are required to complete the process. In humans, the additional signals are provided through CD40 and CD154. IFN-γ from Th1 cells stimulates a switch to IgG2a and IgG3 in mouse B cells and effectively suppresses the effects of IL-4. IFN-γ acts by promoting the production of the B cell–stimulating cytokines BAFF and APRIL (Box 15-2). TGF-β promotes the switch to IgA production on body surfaces. As described previously, signals from IL-5 and IL-6 also contribute to class switching.

Plasma Cells

Plasma cells develop from antigen-stimulated B cells (Figure 15-13). Cells that are structurally intermediate between lymphocytes and plasma cells (plasmablasts) can be identified in the lymph node cortex and paracortex and in the marginal zone in the spleen. Fully developed plasma cells emigrate from these areas. They are found in greatest numbers in the spleen, the medulla of lymph nodes, and the bone marrow.

□ Box 15-2 | **BAFF/APRIL System**

B cell activating factor (BAFF) (CD257) and "a proliferation-inducing ligand" (APRIL) (CD256) are two related cytokines. BAFF is produced by monocytes, dendritic cells, T cells, and neutrophils. APRIL is produced by monocytes, dendritic cells, T cells, and intestinal epithelial cells. They bind to the same or related receptors on B cells. BAFF is expressed on the cell membranes of producing cells but can be cleaved off as a soluble cytokine. It functions in both situations. APRIL only functions as a soluble cytokine. They both promote B cell division and inhibit their apoptosis. Both BAFF and APRIL are crucial survival factors for B cells and essential for their production and differentiation. Overexpression of BAFF results in severe autoimmune disease.

Data from Ng LG, Mackay CR, Mackay F: The BAFF/APRIL system: life beyond B lymphocytes, *Mol Immunol* 42:763–772, 2005.

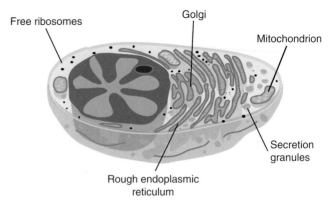

FIGURE 15-14 The structure of a typical plasma cell. The possession of an extensive rough endoplasmic reticulum is typical of a cell dedicated to the rapid production of large amounts of immunoglobulin.

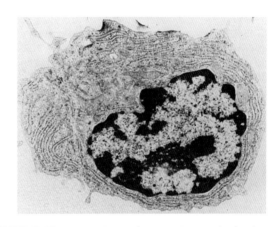

FIGURE 15-15 A transmission electron micrograph of a plasma cell from a rabbit.

(Courtesy Dr. S. Linthicum.)

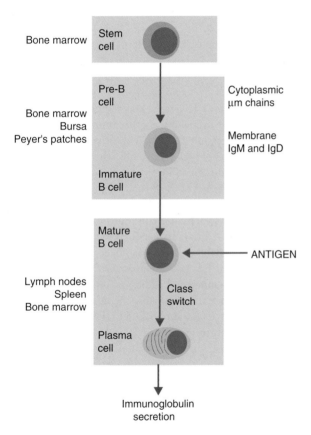

FIGURE 15-13 B cells originate in the bone marrow and proceed through a series of differentiation stages before becoming able to respond to antigen. When B cells respond to antigen, they respond by division and differentiation of their progeny into plasma cells.

Plasma cells are ovoid cells, 8 to 9 μm in diameter (Figure 15-14). They have a round, eccentrically placed nucleus with unevenly distributed chromatin. As a result, the nucleus may resemble a clock face or cartwheel. Plasma cells have an extensive cytoplasm that is rich in rough endoplasmic reticulum and stains strongly with basic dyes and pyronin. They have a large, pale-staining Golgi apparatus (Figures 15-15 and 15-16). Plasma cells can make and secrete up to 10,000 molecules of immunoglobulin per second. The immunoglobulin produced by a plasma cell is of identical specificity to the BCRs on its parent B cell.

Memory B Cells

One reason that the primary immune response ends is that the responding B cells and plasma cells are simply removed by apoptosis. If all these cells died, however, immunological memory could not develop. Clearly some B cells must survive as memory cells. B cells are activated by antigen and helper T cells in the paracortex of lymph nodes. Most of these B cells differentiate into plasma cells and migrate to the bone marrow, spleen, and other organs, but some memory precursors remain in the cortex, proliferate, and form germinal centers. These cells persist under the influence of programming and rescue signals. Thus, memory cells are first screened for their ability

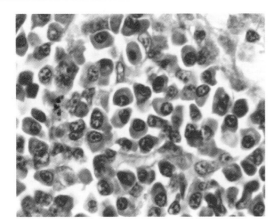

FIGURE 15-16 Plasma cells in the medulla of a dog lymph node. Their cytoplasm is rich in ribosomes and so stains intensely with pyronin, giving a dark red appearance. Original magnification ×450.

(From a specimen kindly provided by Drs. N. McArthur and L.C. Abbott.)

to bind antigen. This induces CD154 on nearby T cells, which in turn promotes expression of *bcl*-2. *Bcl*-2 protects against apoptosis and allows B cells to differentiate into memory cells (Chapter 18).

Memory cells form a reserve of antigen-sensitive cells to be called on following subsequent exposure to an antigen. There are probably several types of memory cells. One population consists of small, long-lived resting cells with IgG BCR. These cells, unlike plasma cells, do not have a characteristic morphology but resemble other lymphocytes. Their prolonged survival does not depend on antigen contact. On exposure to antigen, they proliferate and differentiate into plasma cells without

undergoing further mutation. It has been calculated that in a secondary immune response, the clonal expansion of memory B cells results in 8- to 10-fold more plasma cells than does a primary immune response. A second type of memory cell population consists of large, dividing cells with IgM BCR. These cells persist within germinal centers, where their continued survival depends on exposure to antigen on follicular dendritic cells. In humans, memory B cell levels appear to be stable for up to 60 years after vaccination.

There are at least two populations of plasma cells: a short-lived population that lives for 1 to 2 weeks and produces large amounts of antibodies shortly after antigen exposure, and a long-lived population that can survive for months or years. (In humans these plasma cells have a half-life of 8 to 15 years.) These antibodies provide immediate immunity to microbial pathogens. The short-lived cells are found in the spleen and lymph nodes soon after immunization. The long-lived plasma cells, in contrast, accumulate in the bone marrow. These long-lived plasma cells probably develop from a population of self-renewing, long-lived, slowly dividing memory B cells. These memory B cells require a functional BCR to survive, suggesting that constant low-affinity antigen binding keeps them alive. Thus cats immunized with killed panleukopenia virus will continue to produce antibodies at low levels for many years. The source of these antibodies is believed to be the long-lived plasma cells stimulated to secrete antibodies by exposure to PAMPs and by T cell help.

If a second dose of antigen is given to a primed animal, it will encounter large numbers of memory B cells, which respond in the manner described previously for antigen-sensitive B cells (Figure 15-17). As a result, a secondary immune response is

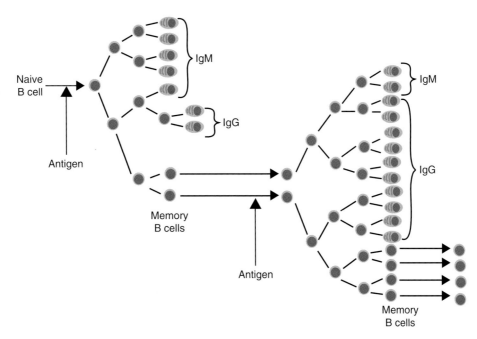

FIGURE 15-17 The time course of a B cell response and the cellular events that accompany it. Note how some IgG is made in the primary immune response, whereas a small amount of IgM is made in a secondary immune response.

much greater than a primary immune response. The lag period is shorter since more antibodies are produced, and they can be detected earlier. IgG is also produced in preference to the IgM characteristic of the primary response.

Germinal Centers

As described in Chapter 12, the development of germinal centers in the lymph nodes and spleen parallels the development of memory B cells (Figure 15-18). Thus germinal centers are sites where antigen-driven cell proliferation, somatic hypermutation, and positive and negative selection of B cell populations occur. B cells stimulated by antigen and helper T cells migrate to a germinal center about 6 days after the response begins. There they divide rapidly. During this rapid B cell division, the BCR V region genes mutate at a rate of about one mutation per division. This somatic mutation generates large numbers of B cells whose BCRs differ from those of the parent cell. Once these cells have been clonally expanded, a process that takes 10 to 20 days, they migrate to the periphery of the germinal center, where they encounter antigen on dendritic cells. Follicular dendritic cells in germinal centers trap antigen very effectively. Because of mutation, some of the germinal

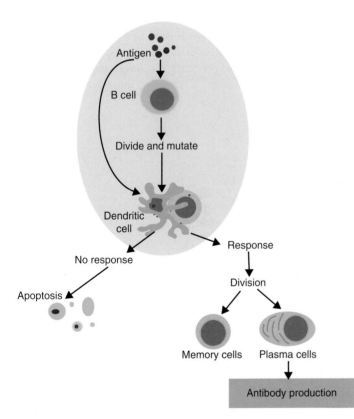

FIGURE 15-18 B cells in the germinal center undergo somatic mutation as they respond to antigen presented by dendritic cells. If the mutation enables them to bind antigen more strongly, they will be stimulated to grow still further. If, on the other hand, the mutation reduces their antigen-binding ability, they will undergo apoptosis.

center B cells bind this antigen with greater affinity, but many, perhaps the great majority, bind the antigen less strongly. If mutation has resulted in greater affinity of the BCR for the antigen, B cells with these receptors will divide further and leave the center to form either plasma cells or memory cells. However, the majority of mutated BCRs show reduced antigen binding. The cells with these receptors undergo apoptosis, and their remains are removed by macrophages. Thus the B cell population that emerges from a germinal center is very different from the population of cells that entered it. In addition to mutation of BCR V genes, BCRs undergo class switching within germinal centers.

B Cell Subpopulations

There are two subpopulations of B cells that develop from different precursor stem cells. They are called B1 and B2 cells. B2 cells are the conventional B cells that are central to adaptive antibody responses and are discussed in this chapter and throughout the book. These B2 cells appear late in neonatal life and are the predominant population in adult bone marrow. They produce most of the body's IgG.

B1 cells, in contrast, originate from stem cells in the fetal liver or omentum rather than the bone marrow. In mice, there are two subpopulations of B1 cells termed B1a and B1b. B1a cells develop exclusively in the neonate, are self-replenishing, and are responsible for most "natural" IgM in serum. They participate in innate immunity. B1a cells express CD5, an adhesion and receptor molecule. (CD5 is the receptor for CD72.) They recognize common bacterial molecules such as phosphoryl-choline as well molecules such as immunoglobulins and DNA. They produce antibodies in a T-independent manner. B1a cells also differ from conventional B2 cells in that they are found in the peritoneal and pleural cavities of rodents and have the potential to renew themselves. B1b cells are distinguished from B1a cells by lacking CD5. They are, however, required for protection against several parasites and bacteria. B1b cells are produced throughout adult life. Many of the IgA-producing cells in the intestine originate from B1 cells. B1 cells have been identified in humans, mice, rabbits, guinea pigs, pigs, sheep, and cattle. It is unclear, however, whether the B1-B2 classification applies to all these species.

Myelomas

If a B cell turns cancerous, it may generate a clone of immunoglobulin-producing tumor cells. The structure of these cells varies, but they are usually recognizable as plasma cells (Figure 15-19). Plasma cell tumors are called myelomas or plasmacytomas. Because myelomas arise from a single precursor cell or clone, they secrete a homogeneous immunoglobulin called a myeloma protein. On serum electrophoresis, this homogeneous myeloma protein will appear as a sharp, well-defined peak. This is called a monoclonal gammopathy (Figure 15-20).

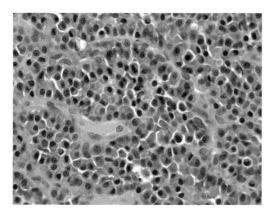

FIGURE 15-19 A section of a myeloma tumor mass in a dog. Original magnification ×600. These cells are clearly plasma cells.
(Courtesy Dr. Brian Porter.)

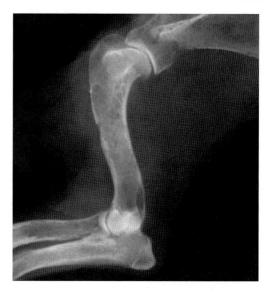

FIGURE 15-21 A radiograph of a dog, showing the round, radiolucent areas where bone has been eroded by the presence of a myeloma.
(Courtesy Dr. Claudia Barton.)

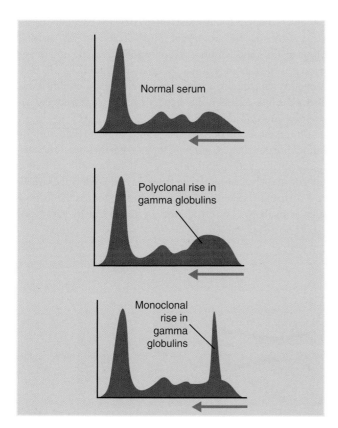

FIGURE 15-20 Serum electrophoretic patterns showing the normal pattern and the characteristic features of monoclonal and polyclonal gammopathies. The monoclonal antibody spike reflects the production of large amounts of homogenous immunoglobulins. Monoclonal gammopathies commonly result from the presence of a myeloma. The arrow denotes the direction of migration.

Myeloma proteins may belong to any immunoglobulin class. For example, IgG, IgA, and IgM myelomas have been reported in dogs. In humans, in addition to myelomas of the major immunoglobulin classes, rare cases of IgD and IgE myelomas have also been described. The prevalence of myelomas expressing the various immunoglobulin classes in myeloma

proteins correlates well with their relative quantities in normal serum. Light chain disease is a myeloma in which light chains alone are produced or the production of light chains is greatly in excess of the production of heavy chains. Similarly, there is a very rare form of myeloma in which Fc fragments alone are produced. This condition is erroneously termed heavy chain disease.

Myelomas have been described in humans, mice, dogs, cats, horses, cows, pigs, ferrets, and rabbits. They account for less than 1% of all canine tumors, and they are considerably rarer in the other domestic species. The clinical presentation of myelomas differs between species. There are, however, several key manifestations, including bleeding disorders, hyperviscosity, renal failure, and hypercalcemia. Other symptoms include lethargy, recurrent infections, anemia, lameness, bone fracture, and neurological signs, including dementia and peripheral neuropathy. The most common clinical manifestation in dogs is excessive bleeding as a result of a thrombocytopenia and a loss of clotting components as they bind to myeloma proteins. The presence in serum of abnormally large quantities of immunoglobulins results in a hyperviscosity syndrome, which is especially severe in animals with IgM myelomas (macroglobulinemia). As a result of the increase in blood viscosity, the heart must work harder, and congestive heart failure, retinopathy, and neurological signs may result. Because myeloma cells stimulate osteoclast activity, the presence of tumors in bone marrow may lead to severe bone destruction. Multiple radiolucent osteolytic lesions and diffuse osteoporosis develop and are readily seen by radiography (Figure 15-21). These lesions result in pathological fractures. Light chains, being relatively small, are excreted in the urine. Unfortunately, they are toxic for renal tubular cells and, as a result, may cause renal failure. The light chains may be detected by electrophoresis of concentrated urine or, in some cases, by heating the urine. Light chains precipitate when heated to 60° C but redissolve as the temperature is raised to 80° C. Proteins possessing this curious property are called Bence-Jones proteins, and their presence in urine suggests a myeloma. They occur in about 40% of canine cases. Nonsecretory myelomas are occasionally diagnosed in dogs.

Because of the overwhelming commitment of the body's immune resources to the production of neoplastic plasma cells, as well as the replacement of normal marrow tissue by tumor cells and the negative feedback induced by elevated serum immunoglobulins, animals with myelomas are often immunosuppressed and anemic. In humans, renal failure and overwhelming infection are the most common causes of death in myeloma patients.

Animals with myelomas characteristically have a monoclonal gammopathy that can be identified by serum electrophoresis. The class of immunoglobulin involved can be identified by immunoelectrophoresis (Figure 15-22), and it may be measured by radial immunodiffusion (Chapter 41).

Affected animals should receive supportive therapy to relieve their immediate clinical problems. Antibiotics can be used to control secondary infections, and fluid therapy should be administered to combat the dehydration resulting from renal failure. Steroids and diuretics may assist in promoting calcium excretion. The serum hyperviscosity may be reduced by plasmapheresis to remove the myeloma protein. The tumor itself can be treated with specific chemotherapy. The drug of choice is melphalan, an alkylating agent. Prednisone may be used in association with melphalan. In unresponsive cases, cyclophosphamide or thalidomide may be employed.

Sometimes, in clinically normal humans, dogs, and horses, a monoclonal gammopathy may develop that is not due to a myeloma. These monoclonal antibodies are usually an accidental finding on serum electrophoresis, and their origin is unclear. They may disappear spontaneously within a short period, or they may persist for many years. Affected animals may show abnormally large numbers of plasma cells in their internal organs on necropsy.

Polyclonal Gammopathies

In contrast to monoclonal gammopathies, which are usually produced by a myeloma, polyclonal gammopathies are observed in many different diseases. Polyclonal gammopathies are characterized by an increase in all immunoglobulins as a result of excessive activity of many different clones of plasma cells. The condition that most resembles a myeloma is Aleutian disease in mink (Chapter 26). Animals infected by the Aleutian disease virus show, in the progressive form of the disease, marked plasmacytosis and lymphocyte infiltration of many organs and tissue, as well as polyclonal (occasionally monoclonal) gammopathy. As a result of the elevated immunoglobulin levels, affected mink experience a hyperviscosity syndrome and are severely immunosuppressed.

Other causes of polyclonal gammopathy include autoimmune diseases such as systemic lupus erythematosus, rheumatoid arthritis, and myasthenia gravis (Chapter 36), as well as infections such as tropical pancytopenia of dogs due to *Ehrlichia canis*, African trypanosomiasis, and chronic bacterial infections such as pyometra and pyoderma. In horses heavily parasitized

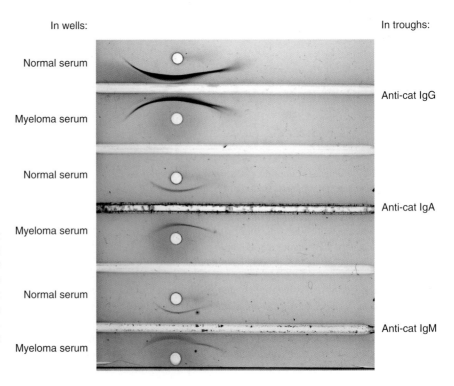

FIGURE 15-22 Immunoelectrophoresis of cat serum. Note that the line of precipitate formed by the reaction between anti-cat IgM and the myeloma serum is distorted (*bottom well*). The line is much thicker than the control, and it forms two distinct joined arcs as a result of the presence of a monoclonal IgM myeloma protein. (Details of this technique can be found in Chapter 41.)

(Courtesy Dr. G. Elissalde.)

with *Strongylus vulgaris*, polyclonal IgG3 levels rise significantly. Polyclonal gammopathy also occurs in virus diseases such as feline infectious peritonitis and African swine fever and in diseases in which there is extensive liver damage.

Hybridomas

The plasma cells in myelomas become neoplastic in an entirely random manner, so the immunoglobulins that they secrete are not usually directed against any antigen of practical importance. Nevertheless, myeloma cells can be grown in tissue culture, where they survive indefinitely. It is highly desirable to be able to establish a system to obtain large quantities of absolutely pure, specific immunoglobulins directed against an antigen of interest. This can be done by fusing normal plasma cells making the antibody of interest with myeloma cells that can grow in tissue culture. The resulting mixed cell is called a hybridoma.

The first stage in making a hybridoma is to generate antibody-producing plasma cells (Figure 15-23). This is done by immunizing a mouse against the antigen of interest and repeating the process several times to ensure that a good antibody response is mounted. Two to 4 days after the antigen is administered, the spleen is removed and broken up to form a cell suspension. These spleen cells are suspended in culture medium, together with cultured mouse myeloma cells. Generally, myeloma cells that do not secrete immunoglobulins are used since this simplifies purification later on. Polyethylene glycol is added to the mixture. This compound induces many of the cells to fuse (although it takes about 200,000 spleen cells on average to form a viable hybrid with one myeloma cell). If the fused cell mixture is cultured for several days, any unfused spleen cells will die. The myeloma cells would normally survive, but they are eliminated by blocking their nucleic acid synthesis.

There are three pathways by which cells can synthesize nucleotides and therefore nucleic acids. The myeloma cells are selected so that they lack two enzymes: hypoxanthine phosphoribosyl transferase and thymidine kinase. As a result, they cannot use either thymidine or hypoxanthine and are obliged to use an alternative biosynthetic pathway to convert uridine to nucleotides. The fused cell mixture is therefore grown in a culture containing three compounds: hypoxanthine, aminopterin, and thymidine (known as HAT medium). Aminopterin is a drug that prevents cells from making their own nucleotides from uridine. Since the myeloma cells cannot use hypoxanthine or thymidine and the aminopterin stops them from using the alternative synthetic pathway, they cannot make nucleic acids and soon die (Figure 15-24). Hybrid cells made from a myeloma and a normal cell are able to survive and grow since they possess the critical enzymes. The hybridomas divide rapidly in the HAT medium, doubling their numbers every 24 to 48 hours. On average, about 300 to 500 different hybrids can be isolated from a mouse spleen, although not all will make antibodies of interest.

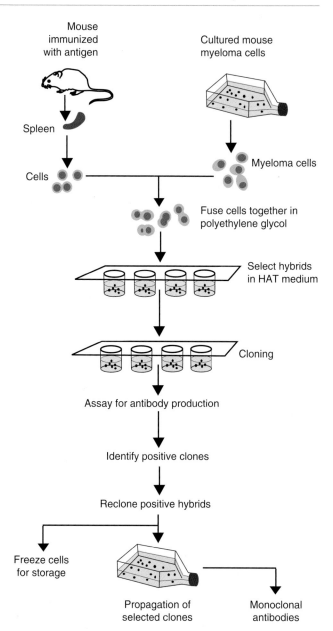

FIGURE 15-23 A schematic diagram showing the method of production of monoclonal antibodies. Antibody-producing plasma cells are fused with myeloma cells. The resulting hybridoma cells are cultured, cloned, and selected so that they produce antibodies against the antigen of interest.

If a mixture of cells from a fusion experiment is cultured in wells on a plate with about 50,000 myeloma cells per well, it is usual to obtain about one hybrid in every three wells. After culturing for 2 to 4 weeks, the growing cells can be seen, and the supernatant fluid can be screened for the presence of antibodies. It is essential to use a sensitive assay at this time. Radioimmunoassays or enzyme-linked immunosorbent assays are preferred (Chapter 41). Clones that produce the desired antibody are grown in mass culture and recloned to eliminate non–antibody-producing hybrids.

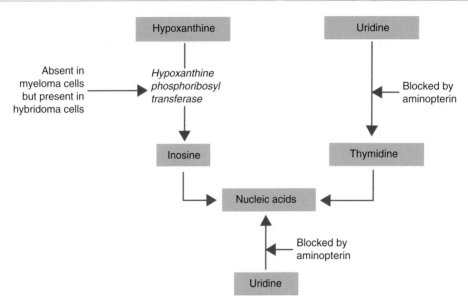

FIGURE 15-24 The pathways of purine synthesis and the mechanism of action of HAT medium.

Unfortunately, antibody-producing clones tend to lose this ability after being cultured for several months. Thus it is usual to make large stocks of hybridoma cells and store them frozen in small aliquots. These can then be thawed as required and grown up in bulk culture. Alternatively, the hybridoma cells can be injected intraperitoneally into mice. Since they are tumor cells, the hybridomas grow rapidly and provoke the effusion of a large volume of fluid into the mouse peritoneal cavity. This fluid is rich in monoclonal antibody and can be readily harvested.

Although the classical methods of making hybridomas produce only mouse immunoglobulins, it is possible to produce monoclonal antibodies from cells of other mammalian species. For example, it is possible to make bovine hybridomas by fusing bovine B cells with a cultured bovine lymphoblastoid cell line. It is generally easier, however, to make hybridomas by fusing B cells from the species under study with mouse myeloma cells. These xenohybridomas or heterohybridomas are made as described previously, but the source of the antibody-producing cells is a species other than a mouse. Thus equine xenohybridomas can be produced by fusing antibody-producing equine spleen cells with mouse myeloma cells. The resulting interspecific hybridomas may secrete equine monoclonal antibodies. Unfortunately, these xenohybridoma cells are unstable and tend to lose the nonmurine chromosomes as

they divide. As a result, they may cease immunoglobulin synthesis prematurely. Improved stability can be achieved by first growing the xenohybridoma cells in the presence of 8-azaguanine to select for aminopterin sensitivity. These xenohybridomas are then used as fusion partners with lymphocytes from immunized animals of the correct species. The resulting secondary xenohybridomas may be further selected and used as fusion partners to produce tertiary xenohybridomas.

Monoclonal antibodies are the preferred source of antibodies for much immunological research. They are absolutely specific for single epitopes and are available in large amounts. Because of their purity, they can function as standard chemical reagents. Monoclonal antibodies are used in clinical diagnostic tests in which large quantities of antibodies of consistent quality are required. Although mouse cells have been the preferred source, studies have shown that cattle and goats can be genetically engineered to produce monoclonal antibodies in their milk. It has even proved possible to incorporate antibody genes into plants such as soy, corn, and tobacco. These "plantibodies" are produced in very large quantities and appear to be functional.

For sources of additional information, please visit http:// evolve.elsevier.com/tizard/immunology/

Antibodies: Soluble Antigen Receptors

Chapter Outline

Key Points

- Mammals make five classes of immunoglobulins: immunoglobulin G (IgG), IgM, IgA, IgE, and IgD. All originate as B cell antigen receptors (BCRs) shed into body fluids.
- IgG is the predominant immunoglobulin in serum and is mainly responsible for systemic defense.
- IgM is a very large immunoglobulin mainly produced during a primary immune response.
- IgA is the immunoglobulin produced on body surfaces. It is responsible for the defense of the intestinal and respiratory tracts.
- IgE is found in very small quantities in serum and is responsible for immunity to parasitic worms and for allergies.
- IgD is found on the surface of immature lymphocytes. Its function is unknown.

The properties of the B cell antigen receptors (BCRs) are discussed in Chapter 15. These receptors are, however, not restricted to the B cell surface. Once a B cell response is triggered, its antigen receptors are produced in huge amounts and shed into the surrounding fluid, where they act as antibodies. These antibodies bind to foreign antigens and mark them for destruction or elimination. Antibodies are found in many body fluids but are present in highest concentrations and are most easily obtained from blood serum. Antibodies have to defend an animal against a variety of microbes, including bacteria, viruses, and protozoa. They also must act in several different environments, for example, in blood and milk and on body surfaces. It is not surprising, therefore, that multiple immunoglobulin classes exist. Each class is optimized for action in a specific environment; for instance, IgA protects body surfaces. Immunoglobulins may also be optimized for activity against a specific group of pathogens. For example, IgE is important in the defense against parasitic worms.

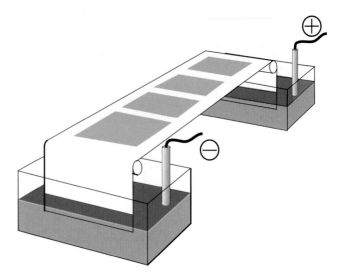

FIGURE 16-1 The electrophoresis of a protein mixture on a strip of paper or other support. The support bridges two buffer baths, and an electrical potential is applied across them.

Immunoglobulins

Antibody molecules are glycoproteins called immunoglobulins (abbreviated as Ig). The term immunoglobulin is used to describe all soluble BCRs. There are five different classes (or isotypes) of immunoglobulins, which differ in their use of heavy chains. The class found in highest concentrations in serum is called immunoglobulin G (abbreviated IgG). The class with the second highest serum concentration (in most mammals) is immunoglobulin M (IgM). The third highest concentration in most mammals is immunoglobulin A (IgA). IgA is, however, the predominant immunoglobulin in secretions such as saliva, milk, and intestinal fluid. Immunoglobulin D (IgD) is primarily a BCR and is rarely encountered in body fluids. Immunoglobulin E (IgE) is found in very low concentrations in serum and mediates allergic reactions. The characteristics of each of these classes are shown in Table 16-1.

When serum is subjected to electrophoresis, its proteins separate into four major fractions (Figure 16-1). The most

negatively charged fraction consists of a single homogeneous protein called serum albumin. The other three major fractions contain protein mixtures classified as α, β, and γ globulins, according to their electrophoretic mobility (Figure 16-2). Most immunoglobulins are found in the γ globulins, although IgM migrates with the β globulins.

Immunoglobulin molecules are bilaterally symmetrical with two identical Fab regions linked to a stem consisting of an Fc region. It has generally been assumed that once an antibody molecule has formed, its structure remains unchanged until it is destroyed by catabolic processes. That assumption now appears to be incorrect. The IgG4 subclass in humans can exchange subunits with other antibody molecules to generate a hybrid antibody with two different Fab arms. As a result, this antibody can cross-link two different antigens. IgG4 is the least abundant human IgG subclass. This exchange of Fab arms between IgG4 molecules is dynamic. Thus a homogeneous IgG4 antibody, when administered to a human, will rapidly

▫ Table 16-1 | Major Immunoglobulin Classes in the Domestic Mammals

	IMMUNOGLOBULIN CLASS				
PROPERTY	**IgM**	**IgG**	**IgA**	**IgE**	**IgD**
Molecular weight	900,000	180,000	360,000	200,000	180,000
Subunits	5	1	2	1	1
Heavy chain	μ	γ	α	ε	δ
Largely synthesized in:	Spleen and lymph nodes	Spleen and lymph nodes	Intestinal and respiratory tracts	Intestinal and respiratory tracts	Spleen and lymph nodes

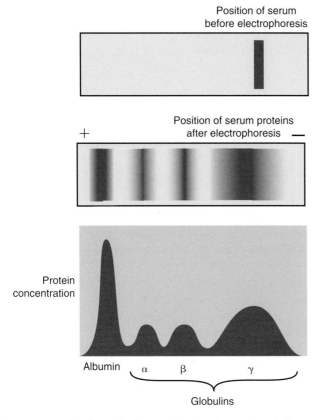

Position of serum
before electrophoresis

Position of serum proteins
after electrophoresis

+   —

Protein
concentration

Albumin   α   β   γ

Globulins

FIGURE 16-2 Schematic diagram showing the results of electrophoresis of whole serum. Four major peaks develop consistently: the albumin and three globulin peaks.

	IMMUNOGLOBULIN LEVELS (mg/dL)			
SPECIES	**IGG**	**IGM**	**IGA**	**IGE**
Horses	1000-1500	100-200	60-350	4-106
Cattle*	1700-2700	250-400	10-50	
Sheep	1700-2000	150-250	10-50	
Pigs	1700-2900	100-500	50-500	
Dogs	1000-2000	70-270	20-150	2.3-4.2
Cats†	400-2000	30-150	30-150	
Chickens	300-700	120-250	30-60	
Humans	800-1600	50-200	150-400	0.002-0.05

□ **Table 16-2 | Serum Immunoglobulin Levels in the Domestic Animals and Human**

*Cattle show significant seasonal differences in serum immunoglobulin levels.
†Immunoglobulin levels in pathogen-free cats are about half those in pet cats.

begin to swap arms. It is not known whether this occurs in the domestic mammals.

Immunoglobulin Classes

Immunoglobulin G

IgG is produced by plasma cells in the spleen, lymph nodes, and bone marrow. It is the immunoglobulin found in highest concentration in the blood (Table 16-2) and plays the major role in antibody-mediated defenses. It has a molecular weight of about 180 kDa and a typical BCR structure with two identical light chains and two identical γ heavy chains (Figure 16-3). Its light chains may be of the κ or λ type. Because it is the smallest of the immunoglobulin molecules, IgG can escape from blood vessels more easily than can the others. This is especially important in inflammation, in which increased vascular permeability allows IgG to participate in the defense of tissues and body surfaces. IgG binds to specific antigens such as those found on bacterial surfaces. Binding of these antibody molecules to bacterial surfaces can cause clumping (agglutination) and opsonization. IgG antibodies activate the classical complement pathway only when sufficient molecules have

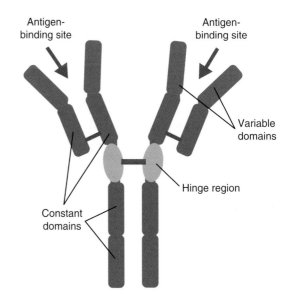

Antigen-
binding site   Antigen-
binding site

Variable
domains

Hinge region

Constant
domains

FIGURE 16-3 The structure of IgG, the prototypical immunoglobulin molecule. Compare this with Figure 15-6, a typical BCR.

clustered in a correct configuration on the antigenic surface (Chapter 7).

Immunoglobulin M

IgM is also produced by plasma cells in the secondary lymphoid organs. It occurs in the second highest concentration after IgG in most mammalian serum. When attached to the B cell surface and acting as a BCR, IgM is a 180-kDa immunoglobulin monomer. However, the secreted form of IgM consists of five (occasionally six) 180-kDa units linked by disulfide

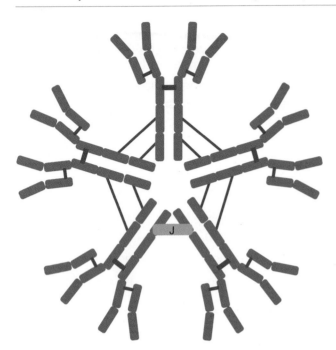

FIGURE 16-4 The structure of IgM. This diagram shows a pentameric structure with 5 subunits which is the most abundant form of the molecule. Some IgM molecules may however contain 6 subunits.

(Courtesy Drs. K. Neilsen and B. Stemshorn.)

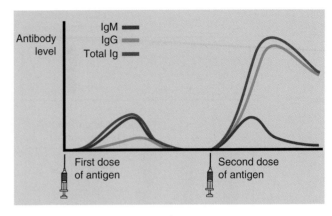

FIGURE 16-5 The relative amounts of each immunoglobulin class produced during the primary and secondary immune responses. Note that IgM predominates in a primary immune response, whereas IgG predominates in a later response.

bonds in a circular fashion. Its total molecular weight is 900 kDa (Figure 16-4). A small polypeptide called the J chain (15 kDa) joins two of the units to complete the circle. Each IgM monomer is of conventional immunoglobulin structure and consists of two κ or λ light chains and two μ heavy chains; μ chains differ from γ chains in that they have an additional, fourth constant domain (C_H4), as well as an additional 20-amino acid segment on their C-terminus but have no hinge region. The complement activation site on IgM is located on the C_H4 domain.

IgM is the major immunoglobulin produced during a primary immune response (Figure 16-5). It is also produced in secondary responses, but this tends to be masked by the predominance of IgG. Although produced in small amounts, IgM is more efficient (on a molar basis) than IgG at complement activation, opsonization, neutralization of viruses, and agglutination. Because of their very large size, IgM molecules rarely enter tissue fluids even at sites of acute inflammation.

Immunoglobulin A

IgA is secreted by plasma cells located under body surfaces. Thus it is made in the walls of the intestine, respiratory tract, urinary system, skin, and mammary gland. Its serum concentration in most mammals is usually lower than that of IgM. IgA monomers have a molecular weight of 150 kDa, but they are normally secreted as dimers. Each IgA monomer consists of two light chains and two α heavy chains containing three

constant domains. In dimeric IgA, two molecules are joined by a J chain (Figure 16-6). Higher polymers of IgA are occasionally found in serum.

IgA produced in body surfaces is transported through epithelial cells into external secretions. Thus most of the IgA made in the intestinal wall is carried into the intestinal fluid. This IgA is transported through intestinal epithelial cells bound to the polymeric immunoglobulin receptor (pIgR) or secretory component (Figure 22-13). Secretory component binds IgA dimers to form a complex molecule called secretory IgA (SIgA). It protects the IgA from digestion by intestinal proteases.

Secretory IgA is the major immunoglobulin in the external secretions of nonruminants. As such, it is of critical importance in protecting the intestinal, respiratory, and urogenital tracts,

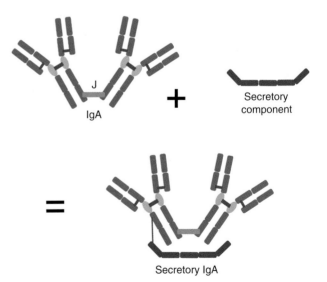

FIGURE 16-6 The structure of IgA and secretory IgA. The secretory component consists of five linked immunoglobulin domains. It is found on the surface of certain epithelial cells, where it acts as a receptor for polymeric immunoglobulins (pIgR). It can also bind to IgM.

the mammary gland, and the eyes against microbial invasion. IgA does not activate the classical complement pathway, nor can it act as an opsonin. It can, however, agglutinate particulate antigens and neutralize viruses. IgA prevents the adherence of invading microbes to body surfaces. Because of its importance, IgA is examined in more detail in Chapter 22.

Immunoglobulin E

IgE, like IgA, is mainly made by plasma cells located beneath body surfaces. It is a typical Y-shaped, four-chain immunoglobulin with four constant domains in its ε heavy chains and a molecular weight of 190 kDa (Figure 16-7). IgE is, however, present in extremely low concentrations in serum. Because of this, it cannot act simply by binding and coating antigens, as the other immunoglobulins do. IgE triggers acute inflammation by acting as a signal transducing molecule. Thus IgE molecules bind tightly to FcεRI receptors on mast cells and

basophils. When antigen binds to this IgE, it triggers the rapid release of inflammatory molecules from the mast cells. The resulting acute inflammation enhances local defenses and helps eliminate the invader. IgE mediates type I hypersensitivity reactions and is responsible in part for immunity to parasitic worms. IgE has the shortest half-life of all immunoglobulins (2 to 3 days) and is readily destroyed by mild heat treatment. IgE is described in more detail in Chapter 28.

Immunoglobulin D

IgD has been found in horses, cattle, sheep, pigs, dogs, rodents, and primates but has not yet been detected in rabbits or cats. It has been identified in many different bony fish (catfish, flounder, halibut, carp, salmon, rainbow trout, fugu, zebra fish, and cod) but has not been found in chickens. IgD is a BCR mainly found attached to B cells, and very little is secreted into the blood. IgD molecules consist of two δ heavy chains and two light chains. In contrast to the other immunoglobulin classes, IgD is evolutionarily labile and shows many variations in structure. For example, mouse IgD lacks a Cδ2 domain and thus has only two constant domains in its heavy chains. It has a molecular weight of about 170 kDa (Figure 16-8). Horse, cow, sheep, dog, monkey, and human IgD, in contrast, has three heavy chain constant domains and a very long hinge domain coded for by two exons (Figure 16-9). Pig IgD has a short hinge coded for by a single exon. In cattle, sheep, and pigs, but not horses or dogs, the Cδ1 domain is almost identical to the Cμ1 domain of IgM, whereas the other constant domains are distinctly different. In mice, the two constant region domains (Cδ1 and Cδ3) are separated by a very long exposed hinge region. Because of this long hinge region and the fact that it has no interchain disulfide bonds, mouse IgD is unusually susceptible to destruction by proteases and cannot be detected in serum, although it may be detected in plasma. Like IgE, IgD is destroyed by mild heat treatment.

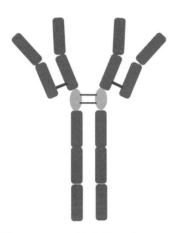

FIGURE 16-7 The structure of IgE. Note the presence of four constant domains in addition to a hinge in the heavy chain.

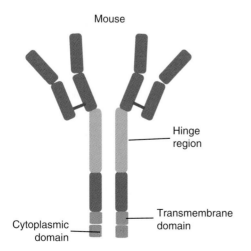

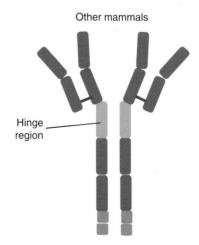

FIGURE 16-8 The structure of IgD in mice and other mammals. Note the long exposed hinge region in mouse IgD that makes this molecule very unstable.

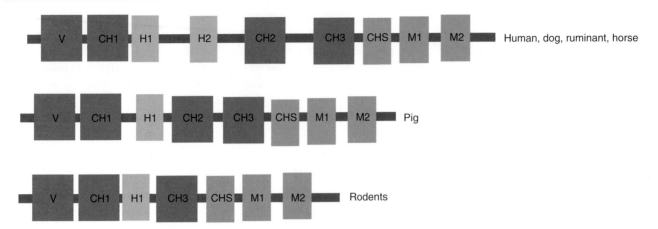

FIGURE 16-9 The gene structure of IgD differs greatly among mammals. This diagram shows the exon structure of IgD heavy chains in different species. No other immunoglobulin class shows such variation, and its significance is unknown.

The role of IgD has so far defied explanation. IgM to IgD class switching, however, has been described in the upper respiratory mucosa of humans. This generates IgD-producing plasma cells that react with respiratory bacteria. The circulating IgD binds to basophils and induces the basophils to produce cathelicidins, IL-1, IL-4, and B cell–activating factor (BAFF) (Chapter 22). Thus in humans, IgD orchestrates a defense system at the interface between innate and adaptive immunity.

Three-Dimensional Structure of Immunoglobulins

Immunoglobulin peptide chains fold in such a way that an IgG molecule consists of three globular regions (two Fab regions and one Fc region) linked by a flexible hinge (Figure 16-10). Each of these globular regions is made up of paired domains. Thus, the Fab regions each consist of two interacting domains (V_H-V_L and C_H1-C_L), whereas the Fc region contains either two or three paired domains, depending on the immunoglobulin class (i.e., C_H2-C_H2, C_H3-C_H3, and in IgE or IgM, C_H4-C_H4). The peptide chains within each domain are closely intertwined. In the Fab regions, a groove is located between the two variable domains, V_H and V_L. The amino acids of the complementarity determining regions (CDRs) line this groove, and as a result, the surface of the groove has a highly variable shape. This groove forms the antigen-binding site. The CDRs from both light and heavy chains contribute to the binding of an antigen, although the heavy chain usually contributes most to the process. Because immunoglobulins are bilaterally identical, the CDRs on each of the Fab regions are also identical. Thus, the molecule has two identical antigen-binding sites and binds two identical epitopes.

The presence of a hinge region in the middle of their heavy chains makes immunoglobulins such as IgG very flexible. Since the two antigen-binding sites on each Fab region are identical,

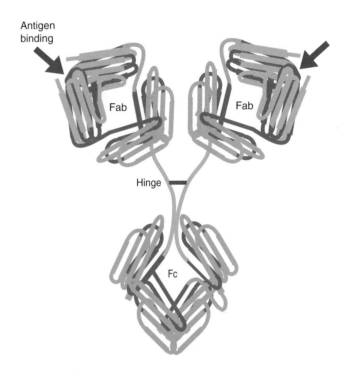

FIGURE 16-10 A ribbon diagram showing the folding of the peptide chains in IgG. Compare this with the very schematic diagrams of IgG structure seen elsewhere in the text. The globular domain structure is very obvious. It is also clear that the peptide chains in the hinge region are very exposed to breakage by proteases.

immunoglobulins are able to cross-link two antigens at the same time.

Immunoglobulin Variants

Subclasses

All immunoglobulin molecules are made of two heavy and two light chains. Several different heavy chains are employed in making these molecules. Thus when γ chains are used, the resulting immunoglobulin is IgG. IgM contains μ chains; IgA contains α chains, and so on. However, closer examination shows that even these immunoglobulin classes consist of mixtures of molecules using structurally different heavy chains known as subclasses.

Immunoglobulin subclasses have arisen as a result of gene duplication. Thus during the course of evolution, heavy chain (*IGH*) genes have been duplicated, and the new gene then is gradually changed through mutation. The amino acid sequences coded by these new genes may differ from the original in only minor respects. For example, bovine IgG is a mixture of three subclasses—IgG1, IgG2, and IgG3—coded for by the heavy chain genes *IGHG1, IGHG2,* and *IGHG3,* respectively. They differ in amino acid sequence and in physical properties such as electrophoretic mobility. These immunoglobulin subclasses may also have different biological activities; for example, bovine IgG2 agglutinates antigenic particles, whereas IgG1 does not. All animals of a species possess all these subclasses.

The number and properties of immunoglobulin subclasses vary among species. For example, most mammals have only one or two IgA subclasses, but rabbits have as many as 13. These variations among species are probably not of major biological significance; they simply reflect the number of immunoglobulin gene duplications a species has undergone.

Allotypes

In addition to subclass differences, individual animals show inherited variations in immunoglobulin amino acid sequences. Thus the immunoglobulins of one individual may differ from those of another individual of the same species (Figure 16-11). These allelic sequence variations in heavy chain genes are reflected in structural differences called allotypes.

All cattle possess a complete set of classes and subclasses (ISOTYPES)

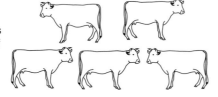

Within a population individual cattle possess different ALLOTYPES. For example, some possess IgG2(A1), others possess IgG2(A2)

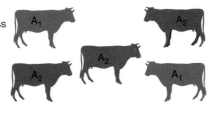

Each individual animal has a very large number of different IDIOTYPES

FIGURE 16-11 A schematic diagram showing the differences among the inheritance of the major immunoglobulin variants.

Idiotypes

The third group of structural variants found in immunoglobulins results from the variations in the amino acid sequences within the variable domains on light and heavy chains. These variants are called idiotopes. The collection of idiotopes on an immunoglobulin is called its idiotype. Some idiotopes may be located within the antigen-binding site. Others are located on nonantigen binding areas of the V domain.

Production of Immunoglobulin Heavy Chains

Two genes code for each immunoglobulin heavy chain. One gene codes for the variable domain (and thus the antigen-binding site), whereas a separate gene codes for the constant domains. The way in which genes code for the variable domains is discussed in Chapter 17. The genes that code for the constant regions of immunoglobulin heavy chain (*IGH* genes) each consist of several expressed sequences or exons. One exon codes for each constant domain, and one codes for the hinge region (Figure 16-12). A complete IgM constant region gene (*IGHM*) therefore consists of five exons, whereas an IgA constant region gene (*IGHA*) contains four exons. All the heavy chain constant region genes are clustered on one chromosome. They are generally arranged in the order 5′-*IGHM-IGHD-IGHG-IGHE-IGHA*-3′. Thus the gene for the μ chain is followed by the gene for the δ chain, and these are followed by the γ chain genes and so on.

As they mature, B cells undergo two different DNA recombination events. The first, called V(D)J recombination, creates the antigen binding site of the B cells while they develop within the bone marrow. Later, when antigens activate the B cells, a second phase of DNA recombination occurs. This second phase coincides with a switch in the class of antibody

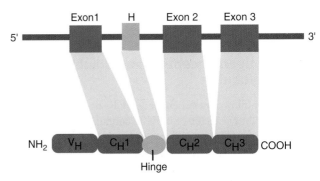

FIGURE 16-12 A peptide chain such as an immunoglobulin heavy chain is coded for by a series of expressed sequences (exons) separated by intervening sequences or introns. Usually each exon codes for a single domain. When transcription occurs, the introns are spliced out and the exon sequences joined together in RNA.

produced by a B cell. This class switch recombination does not affect the antigen-binding specificity of a cell but results in the production of different heavy chain constant chains.

Class Switch Recombination

During the course of a B cell response, the class of immunoglobulin produced changes, although their antigen-binding specificity does not. This "class switch" can be explained by the way in which heavy chain genes are assembled.

During an antibody response, the immunoglobulin classes are synthesized in a standard sequence. Thus, a B cell first uses the *IGHM* gene to make IgM BCRs. The remaining genes located 3′ to *IGHM* are ignored. In species that make IgD, the B cell also transcribes the *IGHD* gene and then expresses both IgM and IgD. Eventually, however, as the immune response progresses, a responding B cell switches to using *IGHG, IGHA,* or *IGHE* genes and becomes committed to synthesizing BCRs and immunoglobulins of one of the other major classes—namely, IgG, IgA, or IgE. The unwanted, unused *IGH* genes are excised as a DNA circle and are lost from the cell, whereas the required *IGH* gene is spliced directly to the *IGHV* gene.

For example, if IgM is to be synthesized, an *IGHV* gene is spliced directly to the *IGHM* gene (Figure 16-13). On the other hand, if IgA is to be synthesized, the genes coding for Cμ to Cε inclusive are deleted, and the *IGHV* gene is then spliced directly to the *IGHA* gene. There are several ways by which these intervening genes can be excised. The simplest is called looping out-deletion. In this case, the V region and C genes come together by looping out and then excising the intervening DNA using an enzyme called a recombinase. Two signals are needed to initiate class switching in a B cell. First, the B cell must receive an activation signal. This is generated when CD40 on the B cell binds CD154 on a helper T cell. Second, the specific class switch must be determined. This choice is regulated by cytokines, especially by IL-4, transforming growth factor-β (TGF-β), and interferon-γ (IFN-γ). Signals from CD40 and the antigen activate the recombinase in the B cell while signals from the cytokine receptors, by activating specific promoter regions, target the recombinase to a specific immunoglobulin gene.

B Cell Antigen Receptors and Soluble Immunoglobulins

Immunoglobulins can exist either as BCRs or as secreted antibodies. The heavy chain of a BCR contains a hydrophobic transmembrane C-terminal domain that attaches it to a B cell. This domain is absent from the secreted antibody. The switch between the two forms results from the differential splicing of exons. For example, in the *IGHM* gene, there are two short exons: CμS and CμM located 3′ to Cμ4 (Figure 16-14). CμS codes for the C-terminal domain of the secreted form, whereas CμM codes for the hydrophobic domain of the cell-bound form. When IgM is made, all the Cμ exons are first transcribed

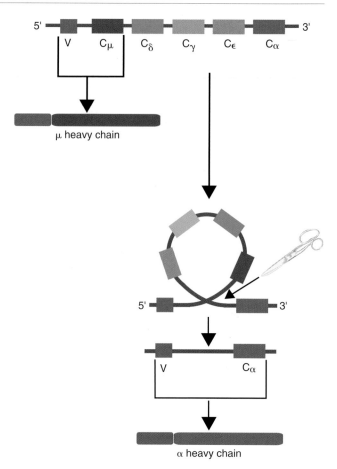

FIGURE 16-13 The mechanism of class switching. In this example, a switch is made from IgM production to IgA production by deleting intervening heavy chain genes and joining the V genes to the appropriate heavy chain gene.

to messenger RNA (mRNA). To produce cell-bound IgM, the mRNA is cleaved so that the CμS exon is deleted, and the Cμ4 exon is spliced directly to the CμM exon. To produce secreted IgM, the exon coding for the CμM domain is deleted, and translation is stopped after Cμ4 and CμS are read.

Immunoglobulins of Domestic Mammals

All mammals possess genes for and express four or five major immunoglobulin classes (IgG, IgM, IgA, IgE, IgD), although these may not have been formally identified in all species (Table 16-3). The basic characteristics of each of these classes are as described previously. However, during the course of evolution, as pointed out earlier, the immunoglobulin heavy chain (*IGH*) genes have duplicated, sometimes several times. These duplicated genes can then mutate so that mammals may produce several different subclasses of a specific immunoglobulin. If a duplicated gene mutates in such a way that it is no

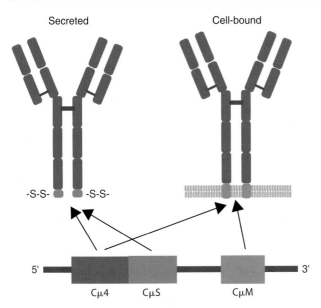

Secreted   Cell-bound

-S-S-   -S-S-

5'   3'

Cμ4   CμS   CμM

FIGURE 16-14 IgM immunoglobulins serving as BCRs have a choice as to which C terminal domain they will use. The membrane-bound form uses a hydrophobic transmembrane domain (CμM). In contrast, the secreted form deletes this sequence and uses the CμS gene. The difference between the two forms is determined by RNA splicing following transcription.

□ Table 16-3 | **Immunoglobulin Classes and Subclasses in Selected Mammals**

| | IMMUNOGLOBULIN CLASSES | | | | |
SPECIES	IgG	IgA	IgM	IgE	IgD
Horses	G1, G2, G3, G4, G5, G6, G7	A	M	E	D
Cattle	G1, G2, G3	A	M	E	D
Sheep	G1, G2, G3	A1, A2	M	E	D
Pigs	G1, G2a, G2b, G3, G4	A	M	E	D
Dogs	G1, G2, G3, G4	A	M	E1, E2	D
Cats	G1, G2, G3, (G4?)	A	M	(E1, E2?)	?
Mice	G1, G2a, G2b, G3	A1, A2	M	E	D
Chimpanzees	G1, G2, G3,	A	M	E	D
Humans	G1, G2, G3, G4	A1, A2	M1, M2	E	D

longer functional, it becomes a pseudogene. The number of duplications and hence the number of immunoglobulin subclasses and pseudogenes varies among species. In looking at these species differences, the reader might gain additional insight by examining the phylogeny of domestic animal species (see Figure 40-14).

Horses

The horse has seven *IGHG* genes, and all are expressed. Thus there are seven IgG subclasses: IgG1 thru IgG7. (The previous nomenclature for IgG1 thru IgG4 was IgGa, IgGc, IgG[T], and IgGb. IgG6 was previously called IgG[B]. The designation IgG[T] was originally derived from the observation that this subclass predominates in the serum of horses used for tetanus immune globulin production.) IgG3 does not activate guinea pig complement and reacts in a precipitation reaction by a rather characteristic flocculation. The order of the Ig heavy chain genes in the horse is 5'-M-D-G1-G2-G3-G7-G4-G6-G5-E-A-3'. The gene, coding for IgG7, is closely related to IGHG4 and likely resulted from a recent duplication of the *IGHG4* gene. The horse heavy chain gene locus is located on chromosome 24qtr. This corresponds to human chromosome 14 where the human IGH locus is located. Horses also express IgM, IgD, IgA, and IgE. The horse *IGHD* gene is located downstream from *IGHM*. It appears to be expressed at least at the mRNA level. Horses have two IgG4 alleles (IgG4[a] and IgG4[b]) and four IgE alleles (IgE[1-4]).

Cattle

Cattle have three *IGHG* genes and thus three subclasses: IgG1, IgG2, and IgG3. IgG1 constitutes about 50% of the serum IgG and is remarkable for being the predominant immunoglobulin in cows' milk rather than IgA. IgG2 levels are highly heritable; thus concentrations vary greatly among cattle. Cattle possess a unique Fc receptor on their macrophages and neutrophils that is structurally unlike any other Fc receptor and binds only IgG2. Since bovine IgG2 has a very small hinge region, this receptor might represent a special adaptation to the structure of this immunoglobulin. Some cattle IgM antibodies are unusually large because they make use of an exceptionally long third hypervariable polypeptide loop that may contain up to 61 amino acids. The benefits of this are unclear. Two heavy chain allotypes (a and b) have been identified in all three classes. Allotype B1 is found on light chains of some cattle but is relatively uncommon. IgA, IgM, and IgE also occur in cattle. Cattle have a functional *IGHD* gene, and IgD may be expressed on the B cell surface. Cattle are also unique in that they have two *IGHM* genes, although one, the *IGHML* gene, is a pseudogene located on chromosome 9. The functional

IGHM gene is located on chromosome 21 together with the other heavy chain genes.

Sheep

The immunoglobulin subclasses of sheep are similar to those of cattle with three *IGHG* genes coding for IgG1, IgG2, and IgG3. Some sheep have an IgG1a allotype. An *IGHD* gene has been detected in sheep. Three IgA heavy chain allotypes have been identified, as have three IgE allotypes.

Pigs

The pig IgG subclasses have been examined in greater detail than those of other domestic mammals. It has been shown that pig IgG diversified into its subclasses after speciation. Thus it is not possible to extrapolate the effector functions of the "same name" subclass to other species. Eleven pig Cγ gene sequences have been described. These code for six IgG subclasses named IgG1 thru IgG6. There are two allelic forms of all of these subclasses except IgG3. The differences between the alleles may be minor. For example, IgG2^a and IgG2^b differ by only three amino acids. IgG3 has an extended hinge, is structurally unique, and appears to be the most evolutionarily conserved porcine IgG. IgG5^b differs most from its allele, and its C_H1 domain shares sequence homology with the C_H1 of IgG3. Some healthy animals may lack IgG4 or IgG6. IgG is the predominant serum immunoglobulin, accounting for about 85% of the total. IgM accounts for about 12% and dimeric IgA for about 3% of serum immunoglobulins. Pigs have a single *IGHA* gene with two alleles. IgA^b differs from IgA^a by a 12-nucleotide deletion in the hinge region owing to a mutation in its splice acceptor site. The consequences of this are unclear. An *IGHD* gene has been identified in pigs. The first heavy chain constant domain may be coded by either a C_H1 δ gene or by a C_H1 μ gene! Thus pig IgD heavy chain transcripts may contain either VDJ-CH1μ-CH2δ-CH3δ or VDJ-CH1δ-CH2δ-CH3δ. This pattern has not been reported in other mammals. These two genes, however, show almost 99% similarity, so the biological consequences are probably not great. IgD has not been identified as a protein and may not be expressed in pigs. Pig IgE has also been identified. One IgM allotype has been reported (Box 16-1).

Dogs and Cats

Dogs have four *IGHG* genes and hence four IgG subclasses, named IgG1, IgG2, IgG3, and IgG4 in order of abundance. (These were previously called IgG-A through IgG-D). In addition, dogs have IgA, IgM, IgD, and IgE. Preliminary evidence also suggests that they may have two IgE subclasses, IgE1 and

---

☐ **Box 16-1** | **Curious Case of the Camel**

Members of the camel family from both the Old and New Worlds (camels and llamas) have three IgG subclasses: IgG1, IgG2, and IgG3. IgG1 has a conventional four-chain structure and therefore has a molecular weight of 170 kDa. In contrast, IgG2 and IgG3, which together account for 75% of camel immunoglobulins, are 100-kDa heavy-chain dimers that have no light chains! In addition, camel IgG2 heavy chains lack a CH1 domain but compensate for this by having a very long hinge region. Despite lacking light chains, these molecules can still bind to many antigens. It has been noted that these antibodies bind effectively to the substrate pockets of enzymes. Studies have also shown that the antigen-binding site on these heavy chains is very convex. This enables it to fit snugly into the concave active site on an enzyme. Thus these single-chain antibodies may have a structural advantage over conventional immunoglobulins in neutralizing enzyme activity.

IgE2. Four alleles have been identified in the dog *IGHA* gene. All are restricted to the hinge region.

Cats have at least three, and possibly four, *IGHG* genes (IgG1, IgG2, IgG3, IgG4), one IgM subclass, and possibly two IgA subclasses (IgA1 and IgA2), as well as two possible IgE subclasses. An IgM allotype has been described in the dog.

Primates

Humans have four *IGHG* genes coding for IgG1 to IgG4. Chimpanzees and rhesus macaques possess three *IGHG* genes coding for IgG1, IgG2, and IgG3. The chimpanzee IgG2 molecule contains epitopes also found on both human IgG2 and IgG4, suggesting that the *IGHG*2 and *IGHG*4 genes split after humans separated from chimpanzees. Baboons (*Papio cynocephalus*) have four *IGHG* genes, but they differ significantly from human IgG in their hinge region. Rhesus macaques may have two IgM subclasses. All the great apes, with the exception of the orangutan, have two IgA subclasses.

Other Mammals

Rats and mice have four or five functional *IGHG* genes. In contrast, rabbits have only one *IGHG* gene despite having 13 *IGHA* genes, at least 12 of which are functional! They appear to lack IgD. The expression of these IgA subclasses varies among different tissues.

For sources of additional information, please visit http:// evolve.elsevier.com/tizard/immunology/

How Antigen-Binding Receptors Are Made

Key Points

- Antigen molecules bind to a T cell receptor (TCR) or B cell receptor (BCR) when their shape matches the conformation of the groove in the antigen-binding receptor.

- The shape of the antigen-binding groove depends on the sequence of the amino acids that line the groove. The sequence of these amino acids depends on the genes encoding the variable domains of the receptor.

- Because of the ways by which nucleotide sequences can be rearranged in these genes, an enormous number of different BCRs and TCRs can be generated.

- In some mammals, variable regions may be constructed by means of gene recombination. Different genes selected at random from a large library are joined to generate great sequence diversity.

- In other mammals, receptor diversity is generated by gene conversion. Small blocks of donor nucleotides are inserted into V-region genes to generate sequence changes.

- The genes coding for antigen-binding sites in BCRs, but not TCRs, also undergo random somatic mutation, resulting in even more sequence changes.

- These mechanisms collectively enable an animal to make the millions of different receptors that can bind to almost all foreign antigens.

One of the central problems encountered in understanding adaptive immunity is to explain how lymphocytes recognize the enormous diversity of microbes that may invade the body. Given that microorganisms change rapidly, the immune system must be able to respond not only to existing organisms but also, within reason, to newly evolved organisms. The ability of the adaptive immune responses to respond specifically to an enormous number of foreign antigens implies the existence of an enormous number of different lymphocytes, each with its own specific antigen receptors. This then raises the question, How do lymphocytes generate such an enormous diversity of antigen-specific receptors?

The ability of a receptor to bind an antigen is determined by the shape of its binding site. This shape depends on the folding of its peptide chains, which is governed, in turn, by their amino acid sequences. Each amino acid in a peptide chain exerts an influence on its neighboring amino acids, which determines their relative configuration. The shape of a peptide chain therefore represents the contributions of all amino acids in the chain as the peptide assumes its most energetically favorable conformation. The folding of a protein is determined by its amino acid sequence, and that sequence is determined by the sequence of bases in the DNA coding for that protein. The diversity of antigen receptors implies either a corresponding diversity in the genes coding for these receptors or a mechanism that generates diversity from a limited pool of receptor genes. This second mechanism is now known to be the method employed by the adaptive immune system.

Receptor-Antigen Binding

When an antigen and its receptor bind, they interact through the chemical groups on the surface of the antigen and on the complementarity determining regions (CDRs) of the receptor. In classic chemical reactions, molecules are assembled through the establishment of firm, covalent bonds. These bonds can be broken only by the input of a large amount of energy, energy that is not readily available in the body. In contrast, the formation of noncovalent bonds provides a rapid and reversible way of forming complexes and permits reuse of molecules in a way that covalent bonding would not allow. However, noncovalent bonds act over short intermolecular distances and, as a result, form only when two molecules approach each other very closely. The binding of an antigen to a BCR or TCR is exclusively noncovalent, so the strongest binding occurs when the shape of the antigen and the shape of the receptor conform to each other. This requirement for a close conformational fit has been likened to the specificity of a key for its lock.

The major bonds formed between an antigen and its receptor are hydrophobic (Figure 17-1). When antigen and antibody molecules come together, they exclude water molecules from the area of contact. This frees some water molecules from constraints imposed by the proteins and is therefore energetically stable. (The bond can be likened to two wet glass microscope slides stuck together. Anyone who has tried to separate two wet glass slides can confirm the effectiveness of this type of bonding.)

A second type of binding between an antigen and its receptor is through hydrogen bonds. When a hydrogen atom covalently bound to one electronegative atom (e.g., an–OH group) approaches another electronegative atom (e.g., an O=C— group), the hydrogen is shared between the two electronegative atoms. This situation is energetically favorable and is called a hydrogen bond. The major hydrogen bonds formed in

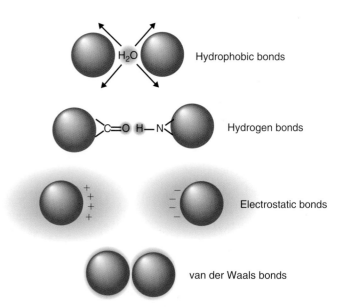

FIGURE 17-1 Noncovalent bonds that link an antigen with its receptor arranged in order of relative importance. All these bonds are effective only over a very short distance. It is therefore essential that the shape of the antigen and its receptor site match very well if strong binding is to be achieved.

antigen-receptor interaction are O–H–O, N–H–N, and O–H–N. Hydrogen bonds are already present between proteins and water molecules in aqueous solution, so the binding of an antigen to its receptor by hydrogen bonds requires relatively little net energy change.

Electrostatic bonds formed between oppositely charged amino acids may contribute to antigen-receptor binding, but the charge on many protein groups is commonly neutralized by electrolytes in solution. As a result, the importance of electrostatic bonding is unclear.

When two atoms approach very closely, a nonspecific attractive force, called a van der Waals force, becomes operative. It occurs as a result of a minor asymmetry in the charge of an atom because of the position of its electrons. This force, although very weak, may become collectively important when two large molecules come into contact. It can therefore contribute to antigen-receptor binding.

The binding of a receptor to its antigen is therefore mediated by multiple noncovalent bonds. Each bond is relatively weak in itself, but collectively the bonds may have a significant binding strength. All these bonds act only across short distances and weaken rapidly as that distance increases. Electrostatic bond and hydrogen bond strengths are inversely proportional to the square of the distance between the interacting molecules; the van der Waals forces and hydrophobic bonds are inversely proportional to the seventh power of that distance. Thus the strongest binding between an antigen and its receptors occurs when their shapes match perfectly and

multiple noncovalent bonds form. Antigens can bind to receptors when they fit less than perfectly, although the strength of this binding will be much reduced.

Antigen Receptor Genes

The information needed to make all proteins, including antigen receptors, is stored in an animal's genome. All that is required for the production of these molecules is that the necessary genes be turned on. Once the appropriate genes are activated, they can be transcribed into RNA and translated into the appropriate receptor protein on B or T cells. It has been estimated that mammals can produce up to 10^{15} different antigen receptors to be expressed on B and T cells. In order to produce this enormous diversity, they use fewer than 500 genes!

Multiple genes code for each receptor peptide chain. Several genes code for each variable region, whereas only one codes for a constant region. As a result, the single constant-region gene can be combined with any one of several different variable-region genes to make a complete receptor chain (Figure 17-2). Instead of having genes for all possible receptor chains, it is only necessary to have genes for all the variable regions and to join these to an appropriate constant-region gene as required. In addition, antigen receptor chains may be paired in different combinations to yield even greater diversity, a process called combinatorial association.

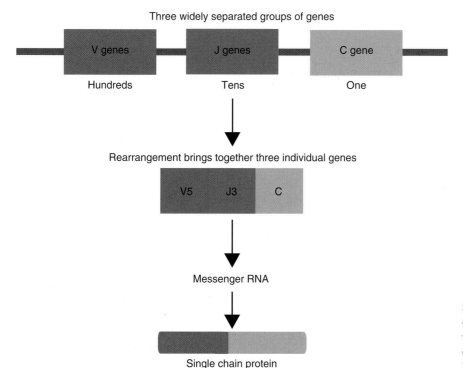

FIGURE 17-2 Antigen receptor chains are coded for by three genes originating in three widely separated groups. The genes for a complete receptor chain are assembled by joining one gene selected from each group.

Immunoglobulin/B Cell Receptor Diversity

To make as many different antibodies as possible, it is necessary to diversify the amino acid sequences of the variable domains in both light and heavy chains. Since these amino acid sequences are determined by the nucleotide sequences in the genes coding for these variable regions, mechanisms must exist for generating this nucleotide sequence diversity. In practice, gene diversity is generated through three distinct mechanisms: gene recombination, somatic mutation, and gene conversion. All three mechanisms alter and diversify antibody gene sequences in such a way that an incredibly diverse array of antigen receptors is generated. The relative importance of each of these mechanisms differs among species, and the diversity-generating mechanisms that operate in humans and mice are not the same as those that operate in domestic mammals. The assembly of these diverse antigen receptors is carefully controlled during lymphocyte development by such factors as DNA methylation, chromatin structure, and location within the nucleus.

Gene Recombination

Gene recombination results from the random selection of one gene from each of several groups of genes followed by recombining these selected genes to generate sequence diversity. It is well seen in the genes that code for immunoglobulins.

Three gene loci code for immunoglobulin peptide chains, and each is found on a different chromosome (Figure 17-3). One locus, called *IGK*, codes for κ light chains; one, called *IGL*, codes for λ light chains; and one, called *IGH*, codes for heavy chains.

IGL Locus

Each λ light chain is coded for by three genes. These are called *IGLV, IGLJ,* and *IGLC*. The *IGLV* gene codes for most of the variable region up to position 95 from the N-terminus. The *IGLC* gene codes for the constant region starting at position 110. The intervening 15 amino acids are coded for by *IGLJ*. In humans each *IGL* locus contains about 100 different *IGLV*, 6 *IGLJ*, and 3 *IGLC* genes. (The three *IGLC* genes code for three λ-chain subtypes).

IGK Locus

κ Light chains are also coded for by three genes, *IGKV, IGKJ,* and *IGKC*. In the human *IGK* locus, for example, there are 40 different *IGKV* genes, five different *IGKJ* genes, and a single *IGLC* gene.

IGH Locus

In humans, heavy chain V regions are coded for by three genes, *IGHV, IGHD,* and *IGHJ*. The *IGH* locus contains about 90 different *IGHV* genes. Mouse *IGH* may have as many as 1500 different *IGHV* genes, but up to 40% of these are pseudogenes. The *IGH* locus also contains several *IGHJ* genes situated 3′ to the *IGHV* genes. Several short genes, called *IGHD* genes (D for diversity), are located between the *IGHV* and *IGHJ* genes (see Figure 17-3). In mice there are about 12 *IGHD* genes, and in humans there are at least 30. A large noncoding region separates the *IGHJ* genes from the *IGHC* genes. The *IGHC* genes consist of a series of constant-region genes, one for each heavy chain class and subclass, arranged in the order 5′-Cμ-Cδ-Cγ-Cε-Cα-3′ along the chromosome.

Generation of Junctional Diversity

Gene Rearrangement

The most obvious way to generate V-region diversity is to randomly select one V gene from the available pool and join it to one randomly selected J gene—a process called recombination. Since many different V and J genes are available, the number of possible combinations can be very large. For example, if there are 100 V genes and 10 J genes, then 100 × 10 = 1000 different V regions can be constructed.

Light chain assembly requires the combination of one V, one J, and one C gene. During B cell development, the intervening

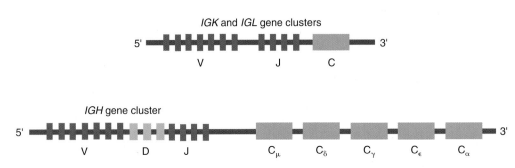

FIGURE 17-3 Genes coding for immunoglobulin light chains and heavy chains. Note that there are two distinct light chain loci, one coding for kappa chains and one coding for lambda chains. These are located on different chromosomes. The precise number of V, D, and J genes varies among species.

genes are looped out, excised, and discarded. The V and J genes have sites at each end that guide the cutting enzymes (Figure 17-4). The looped-out genes are chopped off, and the free ends of the DNA are rejoined so that the V and J genes form a continuous sequence. Two sets of enzymes are used in this process. Recombinases cut the DNA at two points, thus excising unwanted genes. Following this, DNA repair enzymes join the two free ends to reform a continuous sequence. If these enzymes are defective, antibodies (and TCRs) cannot be made. In foals with severe combined immunodeficiency, for example, there is a defect in the DNA repair enzyme that joins the cut ends. As a result, these foals cannot make either TCRs or BCRs and thus have no functional B or T cells (Chapter 37).

Light chain gene recombination occurs in two stages. Randomly selected V and J genes are first joined to form a complete V-region gene. The joined V-J genes remain separated from the C gene until messenger RNA (mRNA) is generated. At that time the unwanted J genes are excised, and the complete V-J-C mRNA is then translated to form a light chain (Figure 17-5).

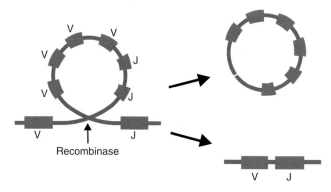

FIGURE 17-4 One of the most important mechanisms of deleting unwanted genes is by looping out. In this case, unwanted V genes form a loop that is then cut off by a recombinase enzyme and the cut ends joined together. As a result, the desired V gene is linked directly to a J gene. The excised loop is destroyed.

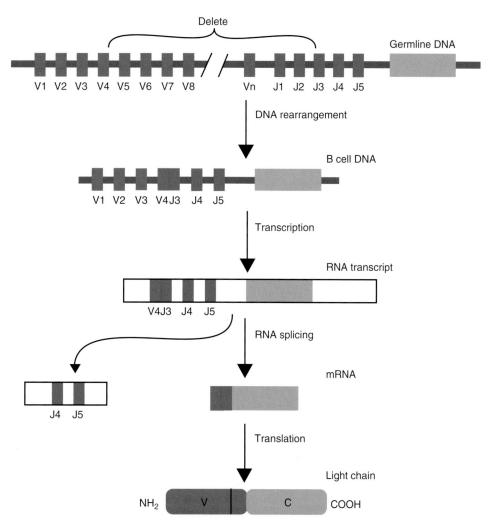

FIGURE 17-5 Construction of an immunoglobulin light chain. Selected V and J genes are first joined as the intervening genes are deleted. The VJ and C genes remain separated until RNA splicing occurs. At that time the intervening RNA segments are deleted leaving the V, J, and C genes together in the mRNA. DNA rearrangement occurs during early B cell development so that each individual B cell is committed to making a single form of light chain for its antigen receptor.

When a heavy chain V region is assembled, its construction requires the splicing together of *IGHV, IGHD,* and *IGHJ* genes (Figure 17-6). This use of three randomly selected genes enormously increases the amount of variability. For example, if a pool of 100 V, 10 J, and 10 D genes are recombined, then 100 × 10 × 10 = 10,000 different V regions can be constructed. The recombination of these genes also occurs in a specific order. Thus *IGHD* is first joined to *IGHJ,* then V genes are attached to make a complete V-region gene. After transcription, any unwanted J genes are deleted, the C gene mRNA is attached, and the completely assembled V-D-J-C mRNA is translated to form a heavy chain.

Base Deletion

Although random recombination of genes generates much V-region diversity, additional mechanisms increase this diversity still further. For example, endonucleases can remove nucleotides randomly from the cut ends of the genes. As a result, the precise nucleotide at which V and J genes join can vary, leading to changes in the nucleotide sequence at the splice site and variations in the amino acid sequence in the V region.

Base Insertion

In immunoglobulin heavy chain gene processing, additional nucleotides may be inserted at the V-D and D-J splice sites. Some of these nucleotides (N-nucleotides) are added randomly by an enzyme called terminal deoxynucleotidyltransferase (TdT). Up to 10 N-nucleotides may be inserted between V and D and between D and J.

Although the random selection of genes from two or three different pools generates a large number of different combinations, not all of these combinations will produce usable antibodies. Some combinations may result in a nucleotide sequence that cannot be translated into protein. These are called nonproductive rearrangements. For example, nucleotides are read as triplets called codons, each of which codes for a specific amino acid. If the codons are to be read correctly, then the sequence must be in the correct reading frame. If nucleotides are inserted or deleted so that the codon reading frame is changed, the resulting gene may code for a totally different amino acid sequence. If this frameshift results in inappropriate splicing, translation is prematurely terminated. It is probable that nonproductive rearrangements are produced in two of

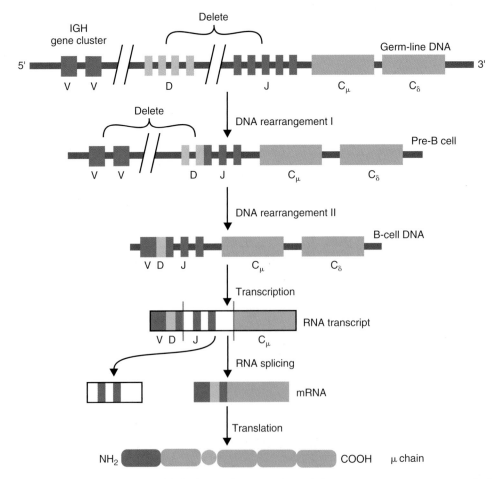

FIGURE 17-6 Production of a complete immunoglobulin heavy chain gene. Two DNA rearrangement events are required to link V, D, and J genes together. The first event joins selected D and J genes; the second event adds a selected V gene. Finally, unwanted J genes are excised and VDJ joined to C in the mRNA.

three attempts during B cell development. When this happens, the B cell has several additional opportunities to produce a functional antibody. For example, immature B cells initially rearrange one of the *IGK* genes (Figure 17-7). If this fails to produce a functional light chain, they switch to the other *IGK* allele for a second attempt. If this does not work, the B cell will use one of the *IGL* alleles, and if this fails, the second *IGL* allele represents the last resort. If all these efforts fail to produce a functional light chain, the B cell cannot make a functional immunoglobulin. It will undergo apoptosis without participating in an immune response.

The sequence of events described previously has been worked out in mice and humans and may not apply to domestic mammals. One obvious difference lies in the use of κ and λ light chains. In mice, rabbits, pigs, and humans, κ chains are preferentially used (95% in mice, 90% in rabbits, 60% in pigs, 60% in humans). In the other domestic species, λ light chains predominate (98% in ruminants, 60% to 90% in horses). The reasons for these differences are unknown.

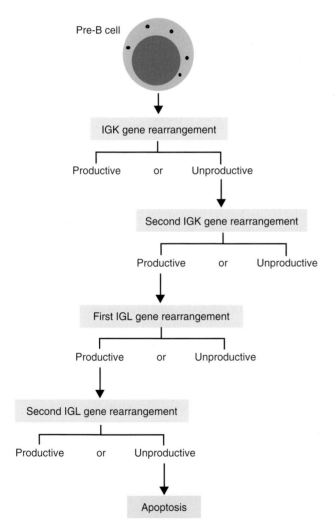

FIGURE 17-7 During its development, each B cell has four attempts to make a productive gene rearrangement coding for a functional immunoglobulin. If it fails in all four attempts, the cell undergoes apoptosis.

It should also be pointed out that immunoglobulin gene rearrangement is not entirely random. For example, in rabbits, mice, and humans the most 3′ *IGHV* genes tend to be used most often. This preferential use of certain genes results from a combination of factors, including the recombination signal sequences, the accessibility of the genes to the recombinase enzyme, sequences at the splicing sites, and way in which DNA can fold.

Receptor Editing

Although each new B cell expresses a specific antigen receptor, developing B cells may continue to rearrange their V, D, and J genes even after exposure to antigen. Thus a B cell expressing a specific κ chain may restart V gene rearrangement by switching to the other *IGKV* genes or even switching to either of the *IGLV* genes. The cell can continue to rearrange upstream nonrearranged V genes or downstream non-rearranged J genes. This receptor editing, which occurs within germinal centers, may be a method of eliminating receptors that bind to self-antigens (Chapter 34).

Somatic Mutation

Although gene recombination can generate many diverse antigen receptors in immature B cells, their antigen-binding specificity is a matter of chance. Thus antibodies, especially those produced early in an immune response, may bind antigens relatively weakly. In addition, recombination cannot account for all the sequence variability found in immunoglobulin V regions. For example, there are three hypervariable areas (CDRs) within a V region (Figure 17-8). One of these, CDR3, is located around position 96 and clearly results from recombination between V and J genes. However, CDR1 and CDR2 are located far from V-J or V-D-J splice sites. Other mechanisms of generating antibody variability must therefore exist (Box 17-1). In fact, gene recombination is only the first step in generating antibody diversity. It is followed by adaptive mechanisms that can generate antibodies that bind much more strongly and specifically to antigens. Thus the antibody response adapts to the antigens it encounters. This is driven by a process called somatic mutation.

□ Box 17-1 | **Methods of Generating Antibody Diversity**

VJ and *VDJ* gene recombination
Base deletion
Base insertion
Somatic mutation
Combinatorial association
Gene conversion
Receptor editing

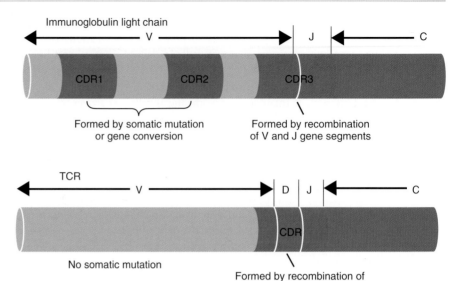

FIGURE 17-8 The major difference between the variable regions of the TCR and immunoglobulins is in the formation of CDRs. Immunoglobulins have three CDRs. CDR1 and CDR2 are generated by somatic mutation. CDR3 is generated by gene conversion. This option is not available to the TCR, in which somatic mutation is stringently avoided to prevent self-reactivity.

Following initial exposure to an antigen, B cells form germinal centers (Chapter 12). The B cells proliferate and undergo antigen-driven selection in the dark zones of germinal centers. As a result, if antibodies are obtained at intervals after immunization and their V-region sequences determined, progressive changes in these sequences are seen to occur. These changes result from random mutations occurring within the recombined *IGHV* genes.

The generation of mutations in immunoglobulin V genes is triggered by antigen cross-linking of two BCRs, by the binding of CD40 to CD154 and by the binding of CD80 to CD28. These signals activate a B cell enzyme called cytidine deaminase. This enzyme deaminates the cytidines in V gene DNA and converts them to uracils. These uracils are recognized as errors (after all, uracil is not normally found in DNA), and their presence therefore triggers repair processes. One of these repair processes uses a DNA polymerase that mistakenly replaces the uracils with thymines during transcription. Other enzymes delete the uracils and leave a gap that is repaired by DNA polymerases using randomly selected nucleotides. The gaps are "patched" by short nucleotide sequences. As a result of this "repair," V gene sequences gradually change as the B cells respond to antigens. On average, one amino acid changes each time a B cell divides.

The degree to which a B cell responds to antigen is directly related to the strength (affinity) with which its receptors binds that antigen. The better the fit between antigen and receptor, the greater will be the stimulus sent to the B cell. If a BCR cannot bind an antigen, the B cell will not be stimulated and will die. In contrast, those B cells whose receptors bind antigen with a high affinity will survive and proliferate (Figure 17-9). Thus as B cells respond to an antigen, successive cycles of mutation and selection of the highest affinity receptors lead progressively to the generation of populations of B cells producing very-high- affinity antibodies.

Somatic mutation does not begin until after B cells have switched from making immunoglobulin M (IgM) to making either IgG or IgA. This suggests that the mutation mechanism is not activated until after a responding B cell had committed to utilizing a specific heavy chain V gene. As a result, the affinity of IgM antibodies for antigen does not increase during an immune response, whereas the affinity of IgG antibodies does.

Gene Conversion

In mammals other than the human and mouse, there may not be a lot of V gene diversity. As a result, gene recombination cannot explain immunoglobulin diversification. In these species, V gene diversity is generated by gene conversion (Figure 17-10). Species that employ gene conversion must have available a supply of multiple V genes or pseudogenes. (Pseudogenes are segments of DNA that are defective and so cannot be transcribed.) During gene conversion, B cell cytidine deaminase inserts a uracil, which is then removed, leaving a gap in the nearest V gene. This gap is then filled by randomly selected short segments of DNA obtained from an upstream V-region gene or pseudogene. The "repaired" V gene will therefore have a different sequence than its precursor. Some of these gene conversion events produce an "inactive" V gene that cannot make a functional V region. In these cases, affected B cells are eliminated. B cells with functional V genes, on the other hand, can bind antigen, divide, and differentiate.

Receptor Assembly

When B cell antigen receptors are generated, the assembly process occurs in a consistent order. The first chain to be assembled is the chain that splices V, D, and J genes together. This chain is capable of generating much more junctional and combinatorial diversity than the other and is the major contributor to antigen binding. In B cells, this is the immunoglobulin heavy chain. This heavy chain is linked to signal transduction molecules, and a surrogate partner chain is

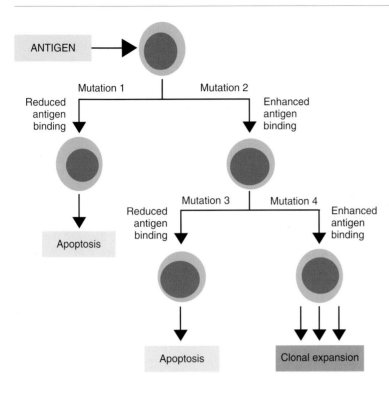

FIGURE 17-9 The selection of somatic mutants. Spontaneous mutation during the expansion of a B cell clone results in the development of cells with antigen receptors that differ in their affinity for antigen. Cells that bind antigen strongly will be more intensely stimulated than cells that bind it weakly. As a result of this selection pressure, the B cell population gradually increases its binding affinity during the course of an antibody response.

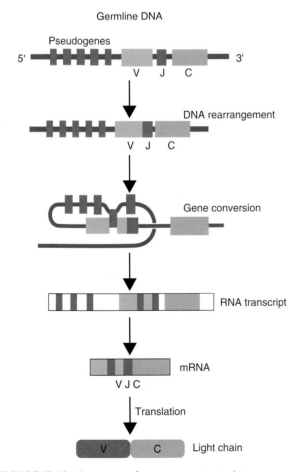

FIGURE 17-10 The process of gene conversion. In this process, segments of upstream genes or pseudogenes are inserted into a single V region to generate sequence diversity.

provided so that the pre-B cell can respond in a limited way to antigens. As a result, a small clone of B cells expressing only the heavy chain is formed. Signaling through this prereceptor triggers limited proliferation. This is followed by the assembly of a partner chain. In B cells this is the light chain. The partner chain is the one that uses only the single splice site between V and J and thus contributes much less diversity to the antigen receptor. Once assembled a complete BCR is formed. Once a complete first chain is formed using V, D, and J genes, signaling mechanisms tend to prevent further recombination and rearrangement of its genes and do not permit assembly of the second heavy chain allele. The presence of the first chain also influences the generation of diversity in the partner chain so that diversity generation in the second chain tends to fine-tune the antigen-binding abilities of the receptor.

Potential Immunoglobulin Diversity

Gene rearrangement generates enormous V-region diversity and antigenic specificity in several ways. First, as occurs in the case of the human *IGKV* family, only 1 of a possible 80 V genes is selected for transcription, as is only 1 of the 5 *IGKJ* genes. This random joining of genes will provide significant variability since there are 400 (80 × 5) possible *IGKV-IGKJ* combinations. The use of a third randomly selected gene will increase sequence diversity still further. With 300 *IGHV*, 5 *IGHD*, and 2 *IGHJ* genes employed, as many as 3000 (300 × 5 × 2) different heavy chain V regions can be generated in humans. Since paired heavy and light chains are used to form the antigen-binding site, the total number of possible combinations in humans is 1.2 million (400 × 3000). In addition, the presence of two splice sites multiplies the potential for diversity generated as a result of base deletion and insertion. However, as pointed out previously, many of the gene combinations so formed may be of little functional use.

Taking all possible mechanisms into account, the number of different antigen-binding sites and hence binding specificities generated is about 1.8×10^{16} without accounting for somatic mutation. (This figure may be compared with the estimated 1×10^7 different antigens that the immune system may recognize.)

Species Differences

Antigen receptor diversity is generated in two different ways depending on species. Some mammals rely on gene recombination followed by somatic mutation. In these species, immunoglobulin diversity is continuously generated from B cell precursors throughout an animal's life. Other mammals, in contrast, use gene conversion for a short period early in life. After initial B cell diversity is generated, this pool of B cells expands by a self-renewing mechanism with little somatic mutation.

Horses

The horse IGH locus contains 40 D genes, 8 J genes, and 59 V genes. The IGK locus contains a single C gene, 5 J genes, and 80 V genes. The IGL locus contains 7 C genes, each preceded by a single J gene and 34 V genes located downstream of the J-C cluster. Horses therefore predominantly employ gene recombination.

Cattle

Cattle likely employ recombination for their light chains and a combination of recombination and conversion for their heavy chains. Initial diversification occurs in lymphoid organs followed by somatic mutation in ileal Peyer's patches. They

have 15 closely related *IGHV* genes, all of which belong to a single family (Table 17-1). Cattle also have many V pseudogenes and 10 long and short *IGHD* genes. As a result, their heavy chain CDR3 regions are variable in size. In addition, conserved short nucleotide sequences of 13 to 18 nucleotides may be inserted at V-D junctions, so that the CDR3 loop is exceptionally long and may contain as many as 61 amino acids.

The bovine IGL locus contains 25 V genes, of which 17 are functional, organized in three subclusters 5′ to four J-C genes. The predominantly expressed *IGLV1* genes are found in two 5′ subclusters, whereas the rarely expressed *IGLV2* and *IGLV3* genes are proximal to the J-C genes. Cattle have more than one *IGLJ* gene, but only one is expressed. Many of the pseudogenes are fused to *IGLJ* in the germline. Cattle also have four *IGLC* genes. Two of these (*IGLC2* and *IGLC3*) are functional, whereas the other two (*IGLC1* and *IGLC4*) are pseudogenes. *IGLC3* is preferentially expressed.

Sheep

Sheep also use both recombination and conversion. Immature B cells first diversify their V (D) and J genes in lymphoid tissues such as the spleen or bone marrow. The immature cells then migrate to follicles in the ileal Peyer's patch, where somatic mutation occurs (Figure 17-11). The initial diversification step is mediated by several mechanisms. Sheep light chain genes have more than 90 *IGLV* genes and a single *IGLJ* gene, so these are diversified by recombination. On the other hand, sheep have only a limited number of *IGHV* genes and therefore use conversion to diversify their heavy chains. They have 6 *IGHJ* genes, 2 of which are pseudogenes. One of the active genes, *IGHJ1*, is used in 90% of heavy chains, suggesting that recombination is minimal. More than 98% of all rearrangement events are in frame, and there are few N- or P-nucleotides. Unlike in the rabbit, human, or mouse, stimulation by intestinal commensal bacteria is not absolutely necessary for V gene diversification in sheep.

☐ Table 17-1 | Examples of Different Gene Use in Mammals

SPECIES	IGKV	IGKJ	IGLV	IGLJ	IGHV	IGHJ	IGHD
Horses	20	5	25	4	>7	5	10
Bovine			20	4	15	2	10
Sheep	10	3	>100	1	7	2	>1
Pigs	250	>5	100	3	20	1	2
Mice	111	9	14	3	200	7	18
Humans	48	9	69	8	215	27	30
Rats					353	5	21

Pigs

Pigs have about 20 *IGHV* genes, two *IGHD* genes, and a single germline *IGHJ* gene. Early in fetal life, the pig uses only four or five *IGHV* genes, and their early repertoire consists of only 8 to 10 combinations. Later in fetal life, this restricted repertoire is compensated for by early TdT activity and extensive, in frame, N-region addition leading to significant junctional diversity. Pig B cells do not undergo receptor editing because they have only one *IGHJ* gene. Pigs possess only two functional *IGHD* genes. V_H use is independent of gene position, but three *IGHV* genes account for 40% of the preimmune repertoire and six genes for 70%. The neonatal piglet has very little combinatorial diversity available at birth.

The presence of the intestinal microbiota significantly assists the development of pig B cells, whose numbers increase greatly during the first 2 weeks of age, although receptor diversity may not increase significantly until 4 to 6 weeks of age. Germ-free

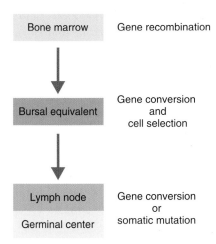

FIGURE 17-11 Lymphoid organs where gene recombination, gene conversion, and somatic mutation occur.

pigs have serum immunoglobulin levels 20- to 100-fold less than conventional pigs. Conventional pigs exhibit much greater diversity in their mucosal IgM and IgA V genes (but not splenic IgG V genes) than germ-free pigs.

Rabbits

Rabbits generate antibody diversity by gene conversion. Immature rabbit B cells first join a small number of V (D) and J genes and then migrate to the appendix. These *IGHV* genes are subsequently diversified by gene conversion and somatic mutation within the germinal centers. The presence of commensal bacteria is necessary for this diversification to occur. Glycans and other pathogen-associated molecular patterns (PAMPs) produced by these bacteria are required to stimulate both antibody diversification and B cell growth. Rabbits actually have more than 200 *IGHV* genes, but almost 90% of V-region rearrangements employ the *IGHV* gene closest to the D genes. The other V genes presumably serve as donors for gene conversion.

Humans and Mice

Humans and mice with many *IGHV* genes use multiple gene recombination to generate most of their antibody diversity (Table 17-2). Additional diversity is generated by base deletion and insertion. Additional diversity is generated in these species by somatic mutation. In these species, B cells with diverse antigen receptors are produced throughout an animal's life.

Intestinal Bacteria and Expansion of the B Cell Repertoire

As pointed out previously, some mammals, including the large domestic herbivores, develop their B cell antibody repertoire in two stages. The first stage involves diversification involving

□ Table 17-2 | Immunoglobulin Diversity Among Mammals

SPECIES	C_H GENES					C_L GENES		V_H AND V_L FAMILIES		
	IGM	IGD	IGG	IGE	IGA	λ	κ	H	λ	κ
Horses	1	1	7	1	1	4	1	7	1	?
Bovine	2	1	3	1	1	4	1	1	2	?
Sheep	1	1	3	1	2	>1	1	1	6	3
Pigs	1	1	8-12	1	1	1?	1	1	?	?
Dogs	1	1	4	2?	1					
Rabbits	1	0	1	1	13	8	2	1	?	?
Mice	1	1	4	1	1	3	1	14	3	4
Humans	1	1	4	1	2	7	1	7	7	7

From Butler JE: Immunoglobulin gene organization and the mechanism of repertoire development, *Scand J Immunol* 45:455–462, 1997, and other sources.

rearrangements of a small number of V, D, and J genes. These B cells then migrate to the gut-associated lymphoid tissue (GALT), where they greatly increase their numbers of B cells as well as the diversification of their B cell repertoire. This second phase of B cell diversification takes place in intestinal lymphoid organs that are in direct content with the intestinal microflora. The importance of the microflora is supported by the failure of germ-free pigs to develop significant B cell diversity. Intestinal bacteria play an especially critical role in this process. For example, in rabbits, normal GALT development can take place in the presence of both *Bacteroides fragilis* and *Bacillus subtilis* but not with either alone. Other bacterial combinations are also effective, suggesting that some form of bacterial interaction is needed for optimal effect. It has been demonstrated that a glycan from *B. fragilis* is processed by antigen-presenting cells and stimulates the growth, maturation, and cytokine production of CD4+ T cells. These T cells in turn stimulate the complete development and maturation of B cells.

Analysis of the expansion of intestinal B cells by commensal bacteria also shows that it tends to affect B cells with certain V_H domains. This expansion is not simply a specific response to microbial antigens but rather a polyclonal, non–antigen-specific response. It may be directed through pattern recognition receptors such as the toll-like receptors (TLRs) or as a result of microbial superantigens binding to the BCR, or some combination thereof.

T Cell Receptor Diversity

TCR and immunoglobulin gene rearrangements are specific in that immunoglobulin genes are not rearranged in T cells and TCR genes are not rearranged in B cells. Like immunoglobulins, the four peptide chains, α, β, γ, and δ, that make up the two types of TCR can bind many different specific antigens. They are able to do this because they each consist of a variable region attached to a constant region. The diversity of TCR V

regions is generated only by gene recombination. This is significantly different from the diverse mechanisms employed by B cells. Our understanding of the numbers of TCR V-region genes is still evolving. There have been many such genes identified within the germline of each species. Not all these genes are expressed, and many are pseudogenes or gene fragments. Estimates of the numbers of these genes may be expected to rise as these genomes are studied in greater detail.

T Cell Receptor Gene Structure

The four TCR peptide chains are coded for by three gene loci. The TRA/D locus codes for both α and β chains since the *TRD* genes are embedded within the TRA locus. The TRB locus codes only for ß chains, and the TRG locus codes only for γ chains. All four TCR loci contain V, J, and C genes, whereas the TRB and TRD loci also contain D genes (Figure 17-12).

Each TCR locus contains two or more C genes. In the TRA/D locus one C gene codes for *TRAC* and the other for *TRDC*. The TRB and TRG loci, in contrast, may contain multiple C genes. For example there are two identical *TRBC* genes and two *TRGC* genes in humans. The number of *TRGC* genes is especially high in domestic mammals. There are eight different *TRGC* genes in dogs. α/β T cells rearrange and express *TRA* and *TRB* genes, whereas γ/δ T cells express *TRG* and *TRD* genes. α/β T cells and γ/δ T cells arise from a common precursor cell. It is not known how the TCR class switch is determined, but it probably results from signals generated within the thymic microenvironment. Developing T cells committed to the α/β TCR lineage delete their *TRD* genes by looping out and switch to using the *TRA* genes. Some of the V genes in the TRA/D locus may be used by either α or δ TCR chains.

α Chain The number of *TRAV* genes varies between species ranging from 4 and 5 in the horse and sheep and 33 in the pig to more than 300 in the bovine. Likewise, *TRAJ* gene

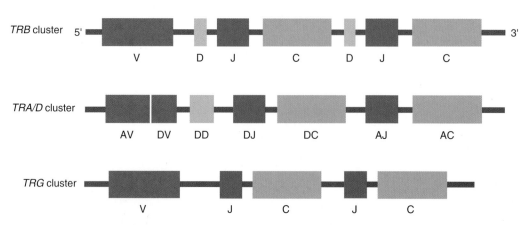

FIGURE 17-12 The basic structure of the three gene loci that code for the four different TCR chains.. The genes for β chains are embedded within the α-chain genes to form a single locus.

availability ranges from 5 in the horse to 61 in pig, mouse, and human. Only one *TRAC* gene has been identified in the mammals investigated so far. In addition, some *TRA/D* V genes may lack a second CDR but still appear to be functional. In these cases the CDR1 region is extended. Perhaps they employ a novel way of interacting with antigen!

β Chain The TRB locus commonly contains a cluster of V genes located upstream of two nearly identical D-J-C casettes, each containing several functional J genes. The D genes are all similar in sequence and length and their use is optional. Any of the V genes may be joined to either of the two D-J-C casettes, and the V gene may join to either a D or a J gene. Dogs have about 38 *TRBV* genes, but about one third of these make up 90% of the T cell repertoire. *TRBV* gene use may in fact be restricted to a single V gene family in the dog. In the pig, 10 *TRBV* genes and 3 D-J-C casettes have been identified. Other species may have many more V genes, ranging from 10 in the pig to 134 in cattle.

δ Chain The TRD locus contains between 8 and 100 V genes depending on species, 2 to 10 J genes, 2 to 6 D genes, and only 1 C gene in all species examined. As mentioned previously, D gene use is optional.

γ Chain The TRG locus contains 4 to 17 V genes, from 4 to 16 J genes, and from 2 to 8 C genes depending on species. In the dog, the TRG locus is organized into eight cassettes, each containing a basic V-J-J-C unit, except for a J-J-C cassette at the 3′ end. It contains a total of 40 genes (16 V, 16 J, and 8 C). Eight of the 16 canine *TRGV* genes, 7 of 16 *TRGJ* genes, and 6 of 8 *TRGC* genes are functional. The existence of these multiple *TRGC* genes suggests that the TCRs they generate may have different biological properties.

Generation of T Cell Receptor V-Region Diversity

There are three hypervariable regions (CDRs) in each TCR V region. The first two, located within the V genes, have probably arisen through selection. The third is by far the most variable and is located in the region where V, D, and J genes recombine (Table 17-3). Neither somatic mutation nor gene conversion occurs in TCR genes. The genes that are separate in the germline are brought together by DNA rearrangement and are then modified by base insertion or deletion as T cells differentiate (Figure 17-13).

Gene Rearrangement TCR α and γ chains are constructed with V, J, and C genes. TCR β and δ chains use V, D, J, and C genes. Both β and δ chains usually contain and use multiple D genes. As a result, V-D-D-J or larger constructs can be formed. This amount of recombination means that the reading frame of the D genes may change and can yield productive rearrangements. This is a rare event in immunoglobulins. Looping out and deletion account for more than 75% of TCR rearrangements. The remainder of these rearrangements are due to either unequal sister chromatid exchange or inversion, that is, moving an inverted segment of gene into a position beside a segment in the opposite orientation. Looping out and deletion of TCR genes are mediated by the same processes employed by BCRs. Thus the same joining enzyme (a recombinase) probably acts on both immunoglobulin and TCR genes.

Base Insertion and Deletion Although in general TCRs are constructed from fewer V-, D-, and J-region genes than immunoglobulins, their diversity is greater as a result of junctional diversity (Box 17-2). Random N-nucleotides may be inserted at

◻ Table 17-3 | TCR Diversity Among Mammal Germlines*

SPECIES	TCRA			TCRD				TCRB				TCRG		
	V	J	C	V	J	D	C	V	D	J	C	V	J	C
Horses	5	5	1	8	3		1	16	1	14	2			2
Bovine	>300	52	1	>100	3	5	1	134	3	21	3	17	8	6
Sheep	4			28				120	3	18	3	13	13	5
Pigs	33	61	1	31	10	6	1	10	3	21	3			6
Dogs								38	1	6	1	16	16	8
Cats												4	8	6
Mice	100	61	1	10	2	2	1	52	2	13	2	7	4	4
Humans	54	61	1	8	4	3	1	88	2	14	2	15	5	2

*The numbers in this table have been drawn from multiple references. They represent the number of germline genes reported at each locus. Not all these genes will be expressed, and many are pseudogenes. When sources differ, I have chosen the highest number of genes reported since as genetic analysis proceeds, more and more genes are being identified, and these numbers may be expected to rise.

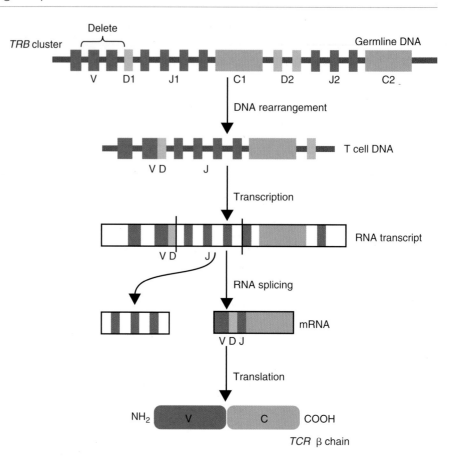

FIGURE 17-13 The production of a complete TCR peptide chain. Note the similarities between this and Figure 17-6.

□ Box 17-2 | **Methods of Generating TCR Diversity**

VJ, VJJ, VDJ, and *VDDJ* gene recombination
Base deletion
Base insertion
Combinatorial association

the V, D, and J junctions as a result of the action of TdT. As many as five nucleotides may be added between V and D and four between D and J genes. Likewise random nucleotides may be removed by nucleases. This insertion of N-nucleotides and base deletion is much more extensive than in immunoglobulin genes and is probably the most significant component of TCR junctional diversity.

Somatic Mutation Somatic mutation does not occur in TCR V genes. Although T cells must be able to recognize a foreign antigen in association with the presenting major histocompatibility complex (MHC) molecule, it is essential that they do not respond to self-antigens. If random somatic mutation were to occur, it would carry the unacceptable risk of altering MHC restriction and rendering the foreign antigen unrecognizable. It might also lead to the production of TCRs able to bind self-antigens and thus trigger autoimmunity.

Where Does This Happen?

TCR genes are rearranged and expressed in the thymus. Although both types of T cell arise from a common precursor stem cell, the decision as to which type of TCR to express probably depends on the signals received by the developing T cell within the thymus. Immature thymocytes begin to rearrange *TRB, TRG,* and *TRD.* If *TRB* is productively rearranged, *TRG* is silenced and *TRD* is deleted so that the cell commits to using *TRA* and expressing α/β TCR. Because of the geometry of the TRA/D locus, joining of a *TRAV* gene to *TRAJ* inevitably deletes the *TRD* genes on that allele. Thus α-chain rearrangements eliminate any possibility of δ-chain expression. Alternatively the cell may successfully rearrange *TRG* and *TRD* and express γ/δ TCR.

T Cell Receptor Diversity

In the human TRA locus there are at least 61 *TRAJ* genes and 54 *TRAV* genes, giving more than 3000 possible combinations. There is, in addition, N-region addition and base deletion resulting in great junctional diversity. After correction for codon redundancy and correct reading frame, the number of potentially different TCR α chains is about 10^6. In the human TRB locus, there are at least 88 *TRBV* genes, 2 *TRBD* genes, and 14 *TRBJ* genes giving $88 \times 2 \times 14 = 2464$ possible combinations. In addition, there is junctional diversity and the use of many different *TRBD* combinations. After corrections there are about 5×10^9 possible *VDJ* ß sequences. Thus, the number of possible different TCR α/β combinations is about 5×10^{15}. (A somewhat similar figure can be arrived at for the mouse. However, a mouse has only 5×10^7 T cells, so this is much more potential diversity than a mouse would ever be able to use.)

In the human *TRD* locus, a combination of V-region diversity, two *TRDD* genes, three sites where N addition and deletion can occur, and diversity in V-J joining position can generate about 10^{14} possible amino acid sequences, whereas in *TRGV*, 7×10^6 different sequences are possible. There is no difficulty, therefore, in accounting for the enormous diversity seen in the TCRs.

γ/δ T Cell Diversity

The function of γ/δ T cells differs among mammals. For example, in humans and mice there are relatively few V genes in the TRD and TRG loci, and the combinational repertoire is therefore relatively small. In addition, the γ/δ TCR repertoire tends to be restricted since the cells bearing these receptors use only a few V gene combinations. For example, 70% to 90% of human γ/δ T cells express the *TRGV9* and *TRDV2* gene products. In contrast, human α/β T cells show a much wider range of binding specificities. Thus, in humans and mice, there is a marked difference between the size of the α/β and γ/δ TCR repertoires. Their γ/δ T cells probably have a limited role in adaptive defense but recognize conserved PAMPs.

The situation in artiodactyls is very different. In these mammals, γ/δ T cells form a much larger proportion of total T cells. As discussed in Chapter 14, in young lambs or calves, they account for up to 60% of T cells. In addition, ruminant γ/δ T cells show a considerably greater receptor diversity. In the sheep, γ/δ V-region diversity results from the use of 28 *TRDV* genes and 13 *TRGV* genes that contain two distinct hypervariable segments similar to the CDRs seen in immunoglobulin V genes. In addition, there are multiple TCR γ/δ isoforms generated by the association of a single C δ chain with up to six or eight Cγ chains. All this suggests that γ/δ T cells in domestic mammals may recognize a very wide diversity of antigens and mount adaptive rather than innate responses.

For sources of additional information, please visit http:// evolve.elsevier.com/tizard/immunology/

18

T Cell Function and the Destruction of Cell-Associated Invaders

Key Points

- Apoptosis is a mechanism whereby the body rids itself of unwanted cells. There are two major apoptotic pathways: one originates within the cell (intrinsic); the other is triggered by extracellular signals (extrinsic). Both result in the activation of an intracellular caspase cascade and eventual disassembly of cellular components.
- Cell-mediated immune responses eliminate abnormal cells and intracellular organisms.
- The elimination of abnormal cells involves the forced apoptosis of virus-infected target cells by cytotoxic T cells.
- Cytotoxic T cells use two mechanisms to kill targets. They may trigger the extrinsic pathway using perforins and granzymes. Alternatively, they may trigger the intrinsic pathway using the death receptor Fas and its ligand.
- Some bacteria and parasites may evade destruction by living within the endosomes of phagocytic cells, especially macrophages.
- The elimination of these intracellular organisms is mediated by activation of M1 macrophages by interferon-γ (IFN-γ) produced by Th1 cells

Antibodies bind to invading organisms in the circulation or tissue fluids, hastening their destruction. However, not all foreign organisms are found outside cells. All viruses and some bacteria can grow inside cells at sites inaccessible to antibodies. Antibodies are therefore of limited use in defending the body against these invaders. Viruses and other intracellular organisms must be eliminated by other mechanisms. For this, the body uses two different cell-mediated techniques. Either infected cells are killed rapidly so that the invader has no time to grow, or infected cells develop the ability to destroy the intracellular organism. In general, organisms such as viruses that enter the cell cytosol or nucleus are killed by cell destruction, whereas organisms such as bacteria or parasites that reside within endosomes are destroyed through cell activation. T cells mediate both processes. The antigens that trigger these responses arise from intracellular locations and are called endogenous antigens.

Endogenous Antigens

As described in Chapter 10, every time a cell makes a protein, a sample is processed and peptides are carried to the cell surface bound to major histocompatibility complex (MHC) class I molecules (Figure 18-1). If these peptides are not recognized by T cells, no response is triggered. If, however, the peptide-MHC complex binds T cell antigen receptors (TCR), then T cells will be triggered to respond. For example, when a virus infects a cell, T cells may recognize many of the peptides derived from the viral proteins. The T cells that respond to these endogenous antigens are CD8+. They use this CD8 to bind to MHC class

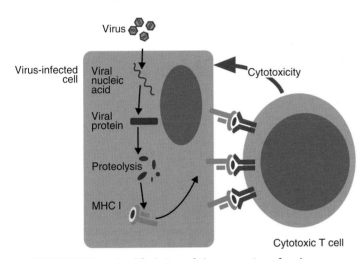

FIGURE 18-1 A simplified view of the processing of endogenous antigen. Endogenous antigen is first broken down into small peptides and inserted into the antigen-binding groove of MHC class I molecules. When presented on a cell surface, antigen bound to MHC class I molecules triggers a cytotoxic T-cell response.

I molecules on the target cells, thus promoting intercellular signaling and eventually killing the target cells.

Apoptosis

Cells can kill themselves. Old, surplus, damaged, or abnormal cells that would otherwise interfere with normal tissue functions can be persuaded to die as necessary. This cell suicide is called apoptosis. Apoptosis is carefully regulated and must only be activated when a cell must die. Structurally, apoptosis is characterized by membrane blebbing, nuclear fragmentation, and phagocytosis of the dying cell.

There are two major pathways of apoptosis. The extrinsic or death receptor pathway and the intrinsic or mitochondrial pathway. The death receptor pathway is triggered by cytokines such as tumor necrosis factor-α (TNF-α) acting through specific death receptors such as CD95 (Fas). Death receptors are a family of type 1 cell surface receptors that when activated trigger apoptosis. They all possess an 80-amino acid cytoplasmic sequence called a death domain. The most important of these death receptors are Fas (CD95) and the receptors for tumor necrosis factor (TNFR). Death receptors are activated by ligands commonly expressed on cytotoxic cells. The ligands bind to the death receptors and as a result assemble multiple adaptor proteins into a signaling complex. Once assembled, this complex activates initiator caspases-8 and -10 (Figure 18-2).

The mitochondrial pathway, in contrast, is triggered by noxious stimuli that cause mitochondrial injury. The damaging stimuli (e.g., oxidants, radiation) activate proapoptotic bcl-2 proteins, which then cause the release of cytochrome C from mitochondria (Figure 18-3). The cytochrome C triggers the formation of a large multiprotein complex called an apoptosome. The apoptosome then activates initiator caspase-9.

The initiator caspases activated by either pathway then trigger a cascade of "effector caspases" (caspase-3, -6, and-7) that degrade numerous proteins, activate endonucleases, break down organelles, and result in cell death and disassembly. The

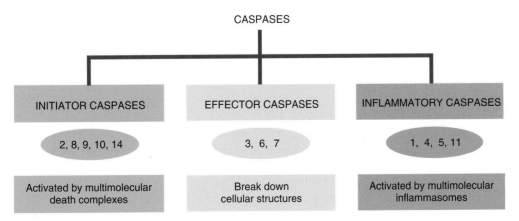

FIGURE 18-2 The role of the three different types of caspase in inflammation and apoptosis. The inflammatory caspases are described in Chapter 2.

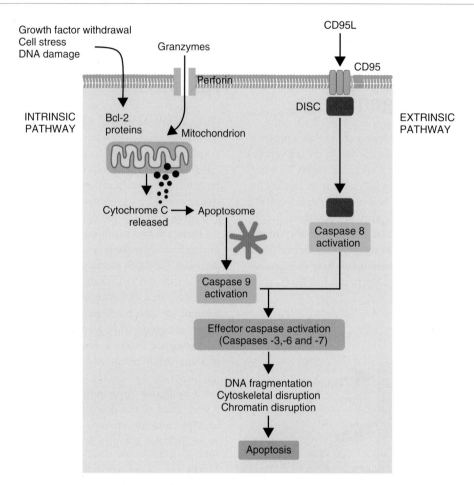

FIGURE 18-3 The two pathways, intrinsic and extrinsic, by which apoptosis may be triggered. Both lead to caspase activation, DNA fragmentation, and cell death. The extrinsic pathway is activated by ligation of death receptors such as CD95 and formation of the death-inducing signaling complex (DISC). The intrinsic pathway is initiated by multiple damage signals, including injection of granzymes, and leads to the release of cytochrome C from mitochondria, the formation of an apoptosome, and activation of caspase 9.

DNA of apoptotic cells characteristically breaks into many low-molecular-weight fragments. This fragmentation may be responsible for the characteristic way in which the nuclear chromatin condenses against the nuclear membrane (Figure 18-4). Affected cells shrink and detach from the surrounding cells. Eventually nuclear break-up and cytoplasmic budding form cell fragments called apoptotic bodies (Figure 18-5).

As cells undergo apoptosis, their cell membrane "flips" so that the lipid phosphatidylserine is exposed on their surface. This lipid binds to receptors on macrophages and dendritic cells and triggers phagocytosis of the dying cell. It also triggers the release of anti-inflammatory cytokines such as transforming growth factor-β (TGF-β) while inhibiting the release of proinflammatory cytokines such as TNF-α.

If cells are severely damaged as a result of trauma, toxicity, or microbial invasion, they may die as a result of necrosis. This has been believed to be a largely unregulated process, although a molecular signaling network regulating the process (necroptosis) has been partially defined. Cells killed by necrosis will trigger inflammation. Thus HMGB-1 escaping from necrotic cell nuclei is a potent inflammatory mediator. Likewise, when

dendritic cells engulf necrotic cells, they not only process their proteins into MHC-antigen complexes but also express co-stimulatory molecules. T cells that recognize this antigen therefore are activated. Thus a cell killed by a virus through necrosis can trigger inflammation and provoke a T cell response to the viral antigens.

Cell Cooperation

During a primary immune response, CD8+ cytotoxic T cells cannot respond to infected cells alone. There are about 10^{13} nucleated cells in a human-sized body and possibly several hundred naïve T cells with receptors for each individual viral antigen. Clearly it would be almost impossible for these T cells to find all the cells expressing corresponding viral antigens by themselves. Naïve cytotoxic T cells tend to remain within lymphoid organs, and dendritic cells can carry antigens to them. A subset of dendritic cells processes these endogenous antigens, links them to their MHC class I molecules, and carries them to secondary lymphoid organs where they are

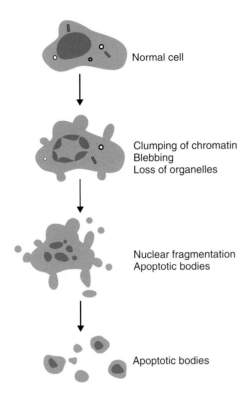

FIGURE 18-4 Major morphological features of cell death by apoptosis.

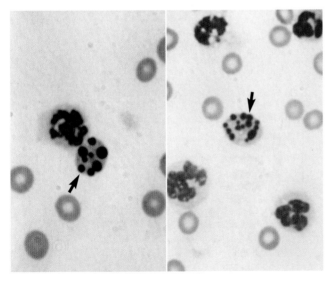

FIGURE 18-5 Two rat neutrophils showing nuclear condensation and fragmentation characteristic of apoptosis.

(Courtesy Ms. K. Kennon.)

of MHC and co-stimulatory molecules and are thus poor T cell stimulators. Helper T cells, however, activate these dendritic cells, upregulate their expression of MHC, and stimulate their production of interleukin-12 (IL-12) and the T cell chemotactic chemokine CCL22. Only when it is fully activated in this way can a dendritic cell successfully trigger a cytotoxic T cell response.

Once activated, dendritic cells present MHC class I–linked peptides to CD8$^+$ T cells. They do this readily if the dendritic cells are themselves infected. However, they can also present peptides from nonreplicating organisms or from dying infected cells. Thus by processing dying cells, dendritic cells can present T cells with endogenous antigens. The cytotoxic T cells require three key signals. The first is IL-12 from activated dendritic cells. The second signal comes from the antigen–MHC class I complex on an abnormal cell. The third signal comes from IL-2 and IFN-γ secreted by the Th1 cells. After all three signals are received, the CD8 T cells can respond.

Different levels of stimulation trigger different responses in CD8 T cells. As with Th cells, the duration of the stimulus is also important. Thus although activated cytotoxic T cells can be triggered by brief exposure to antigen, naïve T cells must be stimulated for several hours before responding. The required stimulation time may be shortened by increasing TCR occupancy or by providing additional co-stimulation. Once activated, cytotoxic T cells divide rapidly.

Cytotoxic T Cell Responses

Once fully activated, CD8+ T cells leave lymphoid organs and seek out infected cells by themselves. When they recognize an antigen expressed on another cell, the T cells will kill their target. Although most cells only undergo apoptosis after receiving very specific signals, cytotoxic T cells can induce apoptosis in any cell they recognize (Figure 18-6).

The density of peptide-MHC complexes on a target cell required to stimulate T cell cytotoxicity is much lower than that needed to stimulate cytokine production. Thus T cell binding to a single peptide-MHC complex may be sufficient to kill a target, whereas binding to 100 to 1000 complexes is required to stimulate cytokine production and clonal expansion. Presumably cytotoxic T cells need to be highly sensitive to viral peptides so that they can kill infected cells as soon as possible. These differences in signal thresholds are probably due to the structure of the immunological synapses formed when a cytotoxic T cell encounters another cell.

When T cells encounter a target, an immunological synapse forms at the point of contact (Figure 18-7). This synapse has two "centers." One part of the central zone contains the TCR-CD8 complex. The other serves as the portal of entry of T cell cytotoxic molecules into the target cell. Both are surrounded by a pSMAC rich in adhesion molecules that forms a "gasket," preventing the accidental spill of cytotoxic molecules. Once a synapse forms, cytotoxic T cell killing is highly efficient. Within seconds after contacting a T cell, the

presented to CD8+ T cells. To respond fully, these CD8+ cells must also be co-stimulated by CD4+ Th1 cells. Co-stimulation is only effective if both the CD8+ and CD4+ T cells recognize antigen on the same antigen-presenting cell. This happens in a defined sequence. Thus a helper T cell first interacts with an antigen-presenting dendritic cell in the normal way through CD40 and CD154. Immature dendritic cells express low levels

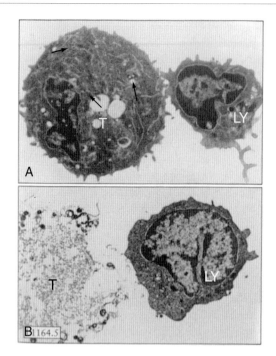

FIGURE 18-6 Destruction of target cells by cytotoxic T cells. **A,** Conjugation between a peritoneal exudate lymphocyte (the small cell on the right) and a target cell. Note the lysosome-like bodies *(LY)* and the nuclear fragmentation of the target cell *(T)*. **B,** A lymphocyte with the remains of a lysed target cell.

(From Zagury D Bernard J, Thierness N, Feldman M, Berke G. Isolation and characterization of individual functionally reactive cytotoxic T lymphocytes, conjugation, killing and recycling at the single cell level. *Eur J Immunol* 5:881–822, 1975.)

organelles and the nucleus of the target show apoptotic changes, and the target is dead in less than 10 minutes. Cytotoxic T cells are also serial killers that can disengage and move on to kill other targets within 5 to 6 minutes.

Cytotoxic T cells kill their targets through two pathways. One pathway involves the secretion of perforins and granzymes from secretory lysosomes (the perforin pathway) (Figure 18-8). This kills cells through intrinsic apoptotic mechanisms. The other pathway kills cells by signaling through the CD95 death receptor. The perforin pathway is used to destroy virus-infected cells, whereas the CD95 pathway is mainly used to kill unwanted surplus T cells.

Perforin Pathway

The killing process can be divided into three phases: adhesion, lethal hit, and cell death (see Figure 18-8).

Adhesion Phase When CD8-TCR complexes on cytotoxic T cells bind to MHC class I molecules on the target cell, an immunological synapse rapidly forms around the area of contact. The TCRs and other signaling molecules cluster at one of the centers of the complex, where they are surrounded by rings of adhesion molecules. The CD8 molecules bind target cell MHC class I and enhance T cell—target binding. If the

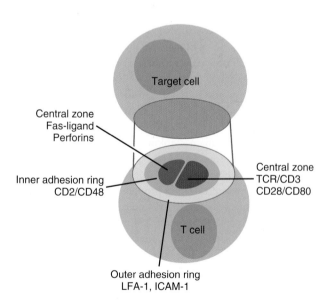

FIGURE 18-7 Structure of the immunological synapse that forms between a cytotoxic T cell and its target. The outer ring of adhesive proteins forms an effective "gasket" that prevents leakage of cytotoxic molecules into tissue fluid. There are, however, two central SMACs. One is dedicated to signaling and contains the TCR together with accessory molecules and co-stimulators. The other is dedicated to cytotoxic mechanisms. It is through this cSMAC that perforins, granzymes, and the Fas-FasL signals are transmitted.

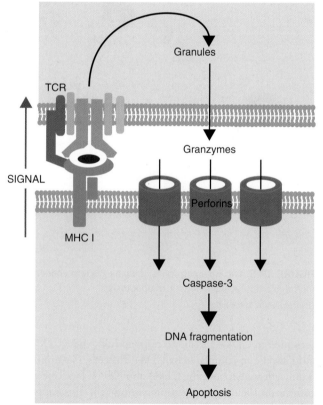

FIGURE 18-8 The perforin pathway by which T cells kill targets.

TCR has a very high affinity for the target antigen, co-stimulation through CD8 may not be necessary.

In addition to receiving signals from antigen-MHC-CD8 complexes, cytotoxic T cells need co-stimulation. As with CD4 helper T cells, CD8 cytotoxic cells require signals from CD28 bound to CD86 on the target cell. Additional adhesion between cytotoxic T cells and their targets is mediated by T cell CD2 binding to target cell CD58 (in nonrodents) or CD48 (in rodents) and T cell CD11a/CD18 (LFA-1) binding to target cell CD54 (ICAM-1).

Lethal Hit Within a few minutes of binding to a target, the T cells orient their microtubule organizing center, their Golgi complex, and their granules toward the target cell. The cytoplasmic granules migrate to the center of the immunological synapse. Here they fuse with the T cell membrane in such a way that the toxic granule contents are sent directly into the target. Cytotoxic T cell granules contain several lethal molecules, of which the most important are perforins, granzymes, and granulysin.

Perforins are membrane-perturbing glycoproteins produced by cytotoxic T cells and natural killer (NK) cells. Perforins can insert themselves into the target cell membrane and oligomerize to form tubular transmembrane channels (Figure 18-9).

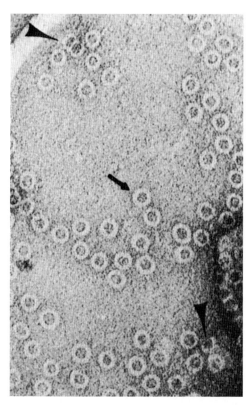

FIGURE 18-9 Perforins from human natural killer cells on the surface of a rabbit erythrocyte target. The arrowheads point to incomplete rings and double rings.

(From Podack ER, Dennert G, Assembly of two types of tubules with putative cytolytic function by cloned natural killer cells, *Nature* 302(5907):442–445, 1983.)

Between 19 and 24 perforin monomers aggregate to form a circular membrane attack complex that forms large (13-20 nM) pores in target cell membranes. The perforins are related to and act in a similar manner to C9, the molecule that forms the terminal complement complex. Although the size of the central pore of the polyperforin permits granzyme monomers and dimers to enter target cells, killing also occurs at low perforin concentrations. It is believed that perforins release granzymes from target cell endosomes. Perforin activity in cytotoxic T cells is increased significantly by IL-2, IL-3, IL-4, and IL-6 and to a lesser degree by TNF-α and IFN-γ.

Granzymes are serine proteases found in T cells, where they account for about 90% of the total granule contents. Granzyme A is the most abundant and triggers apoptosis of target cells. It destroys histones and releases a nuclear DNase from repression, and it is this enzyme that causes the DNA damage. Granzyme B then enters the target cell, either by injection through the central pore of the perforin complex or by endocytosis. It activates proapoptotic bcl-2 proteins, triggering the release of mitochondrial cytochrome C. As described previously, the cytochrome C activates an apoptosome that in turn activates caspase 9 and the effector caspase cascade. Once activated, the effector caspases activate endonucleases, leading to DNA fragmentation and cell death.

Granulysin is an antibacterial peptide found in the granules of both cytotoxic T cells and NK cells. A related molecule (Bo-lysin) is expressed in bovine T cells. Granulysin can kill target cells as well as a wide variety of extracellular bacteria, fungi, and parasites. It shares homology with other proteins that attack lipid membranes called saposins. Saposins do not form pores but activate lipid-degrading enzymes such as sphingomyelinases. An increase in saposins therefore increases ceramide content, and ceramide can induce apoptosis. For example, cytotoxic T cells can control *Listeria monocytogenes* and *Mycobacterium tuberculosis* infections simply by killing infected cells. It is possible that living bacteria released from these killed cells might infect healthy cells. To avoid this, the T cell–derived granulysin kills not only infected macrophages but also any intracellular bacteria.

TNF-β (also called lymphotoxin-α [LT-α]), is secreted by some cytotoxic T cells and has a similar mode of action to CD95L. TNF-β either binds to LT-β in the T cell membrane to form a complex that kills target cells on contact or, alternatively, binds to receptors on target cells and triggers their apoptosis. Structural changes are seen by 2 to 3 hours, and by 16 hours more than 90% of target cells exposed to TNF-β are dead.

CD95 Pathway

The second mechanism of T cell–mediated cytotoxicity involves the binding of a T cell surface protein called CD95L (Fas ligand or CD178) to a target cell death receptor called CD95 (Fas) (Figure 18-10). CD95L is expressed on activated CD8+ T cells and NK cells. It binds to CD95 on target cells. When the cells touch, CD95L binds to CD95, and the CD95 trimerizes. This leads to the formation of a death-inducing signaling complex (DISC) that activates initiator caspases-8 and -10 (see Figure 18-2). These in turn activate the effector caspase-3 and trigger the apoptosis cascade. The CD95L-CD95 system regulates T-cell survival. Unwanted surplus or self-reactive T cells are conveniently eliminated once they have served their functions. For example, when activated T cells have completed their task of killing their targets, they themselves undergo CD95-mediated apoptosis.

In mice, *lpr* (lymphoproliferation) and *gld* (generalized lymphoproliferative disease) are loss-of-function mutations in the genes encoding CD95 and CD95L, respectively. Both mutations permit activated T cells to accumulate and accelerate autoimmune diseases. For example, *lpr* mice do not express CD95 on their thymocytes. As a result their thymocytes do not undergo apoptosis (negative selection) and they escape into the secondary lymphoid organs. Here they proliferate, resulting in a gross increase in the size of their lymphoid organs (lymphadenopathy). Many of these cells respond to self-antigens and *lpr* mice develop an autoimmune disease similar to systemic lupus erythematosus (Chapter 36).

Cytotoxic T Cell Subsets

Subsets of CD8+ T cells have been identified in rodents, where they are called Tc1 and Tc2. Tc1 cells secrete IL-2 and IFN-γ, whereas Tc2 cells secrete IL-4 and IL-5. A third subset, Tc0, has an unrestricted cytokine profile. Unlike helper cells that can differentiate readily into Th1 or Th2 cells, CD8+ T cells show a strong preference for the Tc1 phenotype. Differentiation into Tc2 requires exposure to large amounts of IL-4. All three subsets are cytotoxic.

Other Mechanisms of Cellular Cytotoxicity

T cell–mediated cytotoxicity is not the only way by which the immune system can destroy abnormal cells (Table 18-1; Figure 18-11). For example, cells that possess the antibody receptors FcγRI or FcγRII may bind target cells or bacteria through specific antibodies and then kill them. These cytotoxic cells may include monocytes, eosinophils, neutrophils, B cells, and NK cells (Chapter 19). The mechanism of this antibody-dependent cell-mediated cytotoxicity (ADCC) is unclear. However, neutrophils and eosinophils probably release oxidants. ADCC is slower and less efficient than direct T cell–mediated cytotoxicity, taking 6 to 18 hours to occur.

Whether a macrophage participates in ADCC depends on its expression of Fc receptors and its degree of activation. Macrophage-activating cytokines such as IFN-γ or granulocyte-macrophage colony-stimulating factor (GM-CSF) promote ADCC. Macrophages may also destroy target cells in an antibody-independent process. For example, when they ingest bacteria or parasites, macrophages release nitric oxide, proteases, and TNF-α. The nitric oxide will kill nearby bacteria and cells, whereas the TNF-α is cytotoxic for some tumor cells.

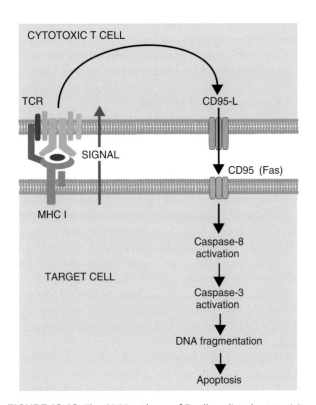

FIGURE 18-10 The CD95 pathway of T cell mediated cytotoxicity.

☐ Table 18-1 | Comparison of the Three Major Mechanisms of Cell-Mediated Cytotoxicity

CYTOTOXIC CELLS	TIME	MECHANISM	MHC RESTRICTED	ANTIGEN SPECIFIC
NK cells	24 hr	NK-mediated cytotoxicity	No	No
Normal lymphocytes or macrophages with FcγRIII with specific antibody	6 hr	ADCC activity	No	Yes
Primed T cells	10 min	T-cell mediated cytotoxicity	Yes	Yes

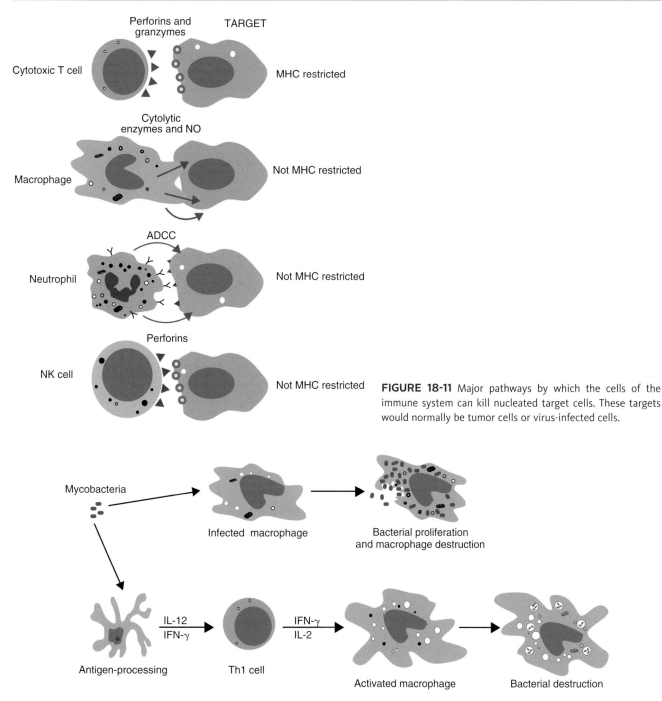

FIGURE 18-11 Major pathways by which the cells of the immune system can kill nucleated target cells. These targets would normally be tumor cells or virus-infected cells.

FIGURE 18-12 Normal macrophages are killed by growing intracellular bacteria. IFN-γ and IL-2 released by Th1 cells can activate macrophages and enable them to kill otherwise resistant intracellular bacteria.

Macrophage Activation

When macrophages attack and ingest invading bacteria, they produce many different molecules that assist in the killing process. For example, they produce cytokines such as TNF-α, IL-1β, IL-6, and IL-12, as well as many new chemokines, and they upregulate production of nitric oxide synthase. This response, however, may be insufficient to kill some invaders. For example, bacteria such as *L. monocytogenes, M. tuberculosis,* and *Brucella abortus*, and protozoa such as *Toxoplasma gondii,* can survive and multiply inside normal macrophages. Antibodies are ineffective against these organisms, so protection against this type of infection requires additional macrophage activation (Figure 18-12). Activated macrophages are functionally polarized. Classically activated or M1 macrophages are proinflammatory effector cells. Alternatively activated or M2 macrophages have anti-inflammatory effects and play a role in tolerance induction and in resolving inflammation.

Classical Macrophage Activation

Classically activated macrophages (M1 cells) become fully activated in two stages. Initial activation is triggered by exposure to invading bacteria as described previously. Complete activation, however, requires exposure to IFN-γ (Figure 18-13). This IFN-γ comes from two sources: NK cells and Th1 cells.

When macrophages encounter bacteria or viruses that activate their toll-like receptors (TLRs), signals are generated to produce cytokines. Two of these, TNF-α and IL-12, act on NK cells, causing them to produce large amounts of IFN-γ. Some TLR ligands can also activate pathways that result in IFN-β production. This endogenous IFN-β can also promote M1 cell polarization. Stimulation of Th1 cells by IL-12 will also trigger IFN-γ production. These Th1 cells also produce IL-2, which promotes M1 polarization and complete cell activation. It is likely that the NK cell–mediated pathway works in the early stages of an infection, whereas the Th1-mediated pathway comes into operation later (Figure 18-14).

M1 cells are activated by IFN-γ through the JAK/STAT pathway and IFN-γ exposure alters the expression of more than 1000 macrophage genes. Activated macrophages secrete proteases, which activate complement. They secrete interferons as well as thromboplastin, prostaglandins, fibronectins, plasminogen activator, and the complement components C2 and B. They increase expression of MHC class II, delay production of phagosomal proteases and promote antigen-loading onto MHC molecules, so enhancing antigen presentation. M1 macrophages are enlarged and show increased membrane activity (especially ruffling), increased formation of pseudopodia, and increased pinocytosis (uptake of fluid droplets) (Figure 18-15). They move more rapidly in response to chemotactic stimuli. They contain increased amounts of lysosomal enzymes and respiratory burst metabolites, and they are more avidly phagocytic than normal cells. They produce greatly increased amounts of nitric oxide synthase 2 (NOS2). As a result, they can kill intracellular organisms or tumor cells by generating high levels

of nitric oxide. The nitric oxide can destroy nearby tumor cells and intracellular bacteria such as *L. monocytogenes* (Figure 18-16). IFN-γ-activated macrophages can also inhibit the growth of intracellular bacteria such as *Legionella pneumophila* by limiting iron availability. They do this by downregulating their transferrin receptors (CD71) and by reducing the

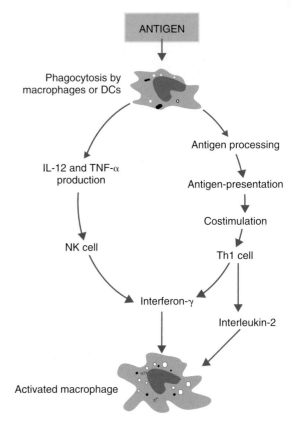

FIGURE 18-13 The two pathways by which macrophages can be activated. One involves IFN-γ production by natural killer cells and is thus an innate pathway. The other is mediated by IFN-γ from Th1 cells and is an adaptive response.

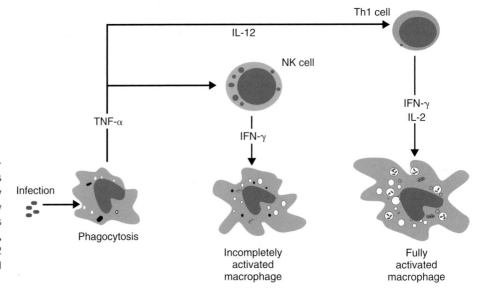

FIGURE 18-14 M1 macrophage activation probably develops in stages. Thus IFN-γ produced by NK cells probably activates macrophages in the early stages of an immune response. If this is insufficient, then Th1 cells are activated, and the combination of IFN-γ and IL-2 that they produce causes maximal M1 activation and polarization.

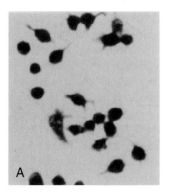
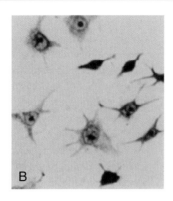

FIGURE 18-15 Stained cultures of mouse macrophages grown under identical conditions: *Left,* Normal unstimulated macrophages. *Right,* Macrophages activated by exposure to IFN-γ and acemannan. Note the cytoplasmic spreading of the activated cells. These cells secrete large quantities of cytokines and nitric oxide. Original magnification ×400.

(Courtesy Dr. Linna Zhang.)

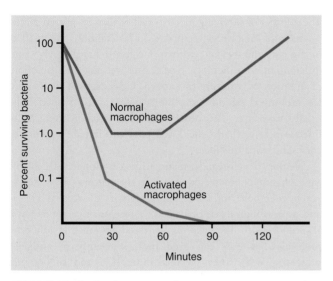

FIGURE 18-16 The destruction of *Listeria monocytogenes* when mixed in vitro with cultures of normal macrophages and "activated" macrophages from *Listeria*-infected mice.

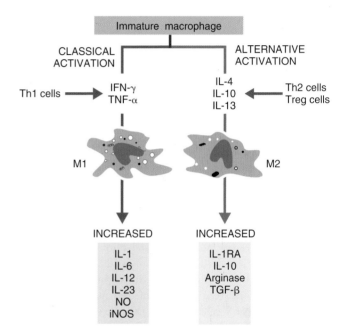

FIGURE 18-17 Depending on their cytokine exposure, macrophages may be classically activated (M1 cells) or become alternatively activated (M2 cells). M2 cells have a major regulatory role and are critical to granuloma formation and wound healing. They produce very different cytokine mixtures.

concentration of intracellular ferritin, the major iron storage protein in macrophages. All these changes reduce the ability of the cells to support microbial growth.

Alternative Macrophage Activation

Macrophages activated through their FcγR or under the influence of Th2 cytokines such as IL-4, IL-10, and IL-13 become M2 cells. These M2 cells differ in receptor expression, cytotoxic function, and cytokine production from M1 cells (Figure 18-17). M2 cells are regulatory and anti-inflammatory. They promote the resolution of inflammation and wound repair. They are protective in some parasitic diseases by walling off parasites such as schistosomes. Instead of producing nitric oxide, M2 cells use arginase to produce ornithine. They secrete low levels of the proinflammatory cytokines IL-1α, IL-12, IL-23, and caspase-1 but large quantities of IL-10 and IL-1RA. As a result, they tend to promote Th2 responses and tissue repair.

TGF-β secreted by M2 cells stimulates extracellular matrix (ECM) production by fibroblasts. M2 cells also secrete the matrix component fibronectin. They secrete transglutaminase, which promotes ECM cross-linking, and osteopontin, which promotes cell-binding to the ECM. Arginase is involved in proline and polyamine synthesis. Proline is required for ECM construction, whereas polyamines are required for cell proliferation. M2 cells secrete platelet-derived growth factor (PDGF), insulin-like growth factor (IGF), and TGF-β, all of which promote cell proliferation. They secrete fibroblast-like growth factor-β (FGF-β), TGF-α, and vascular endothelial growth factor (VEGF), which promote angiogenesis. Thus the molecules secreted by M2 cells promote resolution of inflammation and wound repair and have anti-inflammatory, fibrotic, proliferative, and angiogenic properties.

The importance of macrophage activation can be seen in tuberculosis. Thus mycobacteria that enter the lungs are readily phagocytosed by alveolar macrophages that mount a respiratory burst and secrete proinflammatory cytokines. These cytokines act on NK cells, triggering IFN-γ production and limited

□ Table 18-2 | Effects of Cytokines on Macrophage Function

CYTOKINE	MAJOR SOURCE	EFFECT
IL-2	Th1 cell	Activates
IFN-γ	Th1 cell, NK cell	Activates
IFN-α/β	Macrophages, T cells	Activates
TNF-α	Macrophages, Th1 cells	Activates
TNF-β	Th1 cells	Activates
GM-CSF	Many cell types	Activates
IL-4	Th2 cells	Suppresses
IL-10	Th2 cells, macrophages	Suppresses
IL-13	Th2 cells	Suppresses
TGF-β	T cells	Suppresses

macrophage activation. This rapid innate response can slow mycobacterial growth significantly. Nevertheless these macrophages cannot destroy the bacteria by these mechanisms alone. After several days, however, recruitment of T cells occurs. The T cells are stimulated by mycobacteria-infected dendritic cells secreting IL-12, TNF-α, and IFN-α. In response, Th1 cells are stimulated to secrete more IFN-γ and fully activate the M1 macrophages (Table 18-2). In most individuals, this level of activation is sufficient to control the infection.

Cytotoxic T cells can also kill infected macrophages. For example, cytotoxic T cells generated in cattle infected with *M. bovis* will kill infected macrophages. This cytotoxicity is mediated by both WC1+ γδ and CD8+ T cells. Presumably any *Mycobacteria* released are killed by granulysin.

Delayed Hypersensitivity Reactions

When certain antigens are injected into the skin of a sensitized animal, an inflammatory response, taking many hours to develop, may occur at the injection site. This is a T cell–mediated response called delayed hypersensitivity. Delayed hypersensitivity reactions are classified as type IV hypersensitivity reactions (Chapter 31). An important example of a delayed hypersensitivity reaction is the tuberculin response—the skin reaction that follows an intradermal injection of tuberculin.

Effector T Cell Memory

In contrast to the prolonged antibody response, the effector phase of T cell responses is relatively brief. Indeed, cytotoxicity is seen only in the presence of antigen. This is logical. Sustained cytotoxic activities or overproduction of cytokines could cause severe tissue damage.

Naïve CD8+T cells are long-lived resting cells that continuously recirculate between the bloodstream and lymphoid organs. Once they encounter antigen, they multiply rapidly in an effort to keep pace with the growth of invading pathogens. The number of responding cells may increase more than 1000-fold within a few days. They reach a peak 5 to 7 days after infection when pathogen-specific, cytotoxic T cells can make up 50% to 70% of the total CD8+ T cells. Once the infection has cleared, most of these cells are superfluous. Therefore the vast majority of them (90% to 95%) undergo apoptosis 1 to 2 weeks after infection. Elimination of excess cytotoxic T cells is a tightly controlled process involving the CD95 pathway. Cells surviving this stage differentiate into long-lived memory cells. The number of surviving memory cells is directly related to the intensity of the primary response. In general only 5% to 10% of the peak number of cytotoxic T cells produced survive and differentiate into memory T cells. Survival may be a function of duration of exposure to antigen. Cells exposed to antigen for prolonged periods may die, whereas cells exposed only briefly may live. The observation that overwhelming viral infections can exhaust the T cell pool and impair memory is consistent with this idea.

Memory T cells can be distinguished from naïve T cells by their phenotype, by secreting a different mixture of cytokines, and by their behavior. For example, memory T cells are CD44+ and express high levels of IL-2Rβ, a receptor that binds both IL-2 and IL-15. They express increased amounts of adhesion molecules, so they can bind more efficiently to antigen-presenting cells. They produce more IL-4 and IFN-γ and respond more strongly to stimulation of their TCR. They continue to divide very slowly, in the absence of antigen. This division requires cell-bound IL-15 and is inhibited by soluble IL-2. IL-15 is a unique cytokine that persists for very long periods attached to its receptor on T cells. It thus acts as a persistent stimulus for the memory cell microenvironment and stimulates nearby cells by cell-cell contact. The balance between IL-15 and IL-2 regulates the persistence of memory T cells. In the absence of IL-15, memory cells undergo apoptosis. In humans the CD8+ memory cell half-life is 8 to 15 years.

Over an animal's lifetime, immunological memories accumulate. Older animals have more memory cells than young animals and are thus much better prepared to respond to antigens than younger animals. It has been suggested that the number of memory T cells in an animal has a maximum limit so that new memory cells have to compete with older memory cells for limited space, and that vaccines that stimulate excessive memory T cells have an adverse effect on other immunological memories. That has been shown to be incorrect. Repeated vaccination does indeed generate new memory cells. However, the size of the memory cell compartment expands to accommodate them. Previously generated memory cells are not removed to make space for the newcomers.

For sources of additional information, please visit http:// evolve.elsevier.com/tizard/immunology/

19

The Third Lymphocyte Population: Natural Killer Cells

Key Points

- There exists a third major population of lymphocytes, distinct from B cells and T cells, that plays a key role in the innate immune responses to some infections and cancers. These lymphocytes are called natural killer (NK) cells.
- NK cells can kill virus-infected target cells, tumor cells, stressed cells, and some bacteria without prior activation.
- NK cells act as a first line of defense against pathogens such as viruses.
- In some species, NK cells are large granular lymphocytes.
- NK cells use several different types of receptors to recognize their targets.
- NK cells employ the "missing-self" recognition strategy. That is, they recognize and attack target cells that fail to express MHC class I molecules.
- NK cells also recognize and attack target cells that express certain stress-associated molecules.
- The most important mechanism of destruction of spontaneous tumors probably involves killing by NK cells.
- Natural killer T (NKT) cells are a population of cells that, as their name suggests, share properties with both NK and T cells.

Most lymphocytes participate in adaptive immune responses. These cells, the T and B cells, are responsible for cell-mediated and antibody-mediated immunity, respectively (Chapters 18 and 15). There is, however, a third major population of lymphocytes called natural killer (or NK) cells. NK cells constitute an important subsystem engaged in innate immunity. As such they serve as a first line of defense against pathogens such as viruses, some bacteria, and parasites. They eliminate stressed or damaged cells and play a major role in immunity to tumors.

Natural Killer Cells

Morphology

In most mammals, NK cells are large, granular, nonphagocytic lymphocytes (Figure 19-1). In cattle, NK cells are large cells, although they may not contain large intracytoplasmic granules. There is debate about NK cell morphology in the pig. Some investigators claim that they are large granular lymphocytes, whereas others believe that they are small lymphocytes without obvious cytoplasmic granules (Box 19-1).

Origins and Location

NK cells develop from bone marrow stem cells. NK cells are distributed widely throughout both lymphoid and nonlymphoid tissues. They are found in peripheral blood, lymph nodes, spleen, and bone marrow. NK cells are not found in the thymus. They range from 2% of the lymphocytes in mouse spleen to 15% in human blood.

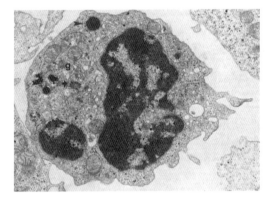

FIGURE 19-1 A transmission electron micrograph of a human NK cell. The nucleus is indented and rich in chromatin. The cytoplasm is abundant and contains many granules. Numerous mitochondria, centrioles, and a Golgi are visible. Original magnification ×17,000.

(From Carpen O, Virtanen I, Saksela E: Ultrastructure of human natural killer cells: nature of the cytolytic contacts in relation to cellular secretion, *J Immunol* 128:2691, 1982.)

□ **Box 19-1** | **Natural Killer Dendritic Cells**

A subset of dendritic cells in humans and mice is cytotoxic. They carry the NK cell marker NK1.1 as well as the dendritic cell marker CD11c. They are found in the spleen, liver, lymph nodes, and thymus of normal mice. Their activity is induced by interferons, LPS, and signals through TLR7, TLR8, and TLR9. They can kill apoptotic and tumor cells but also present antigens to naïve, antigen-specific T cells. They produce copious amounts of IFN-γ on stimulation with CpG nucleotides. These cells may play a key role in linking innate and adaptive immunity. They may be important in killing senescent cells in tissues.

Target Cell Recognition

NK cells recognize and kill abnormal cells using totally different mechanisms than do T or B cells. T and B cells use a strategy requiring the recognition of new and foreign antigens. NK cells, in contrast, employ two distinct strategies. One is a "missing-self" strategy. MHC class I molecules expressed on the surface of healthy normal cells can block NK cell killing by sending inhibitory signals. Thus normal cells are not killed. If, however, even a single MHC class I allele is missing, these inhibitory signals are no longer generated, and the target cells are killed. Viruses may suppress MHC class I expression in an attempt to hide from cytotoxic T cells, and tumor cells often fail to express MHC class I. Such cells are prime targets for NK cell attack. Their second strategy involves the use of activating receptors that can recognize that cells are in distress by the presence of stress-induced proteins on their surfaces. By binding to these proteins, NK cells receive signals that cause them to kill their targets (Figure 19-2).

There are three families of these NK cell receptors: the killer cell immunoglobulin (Ig)-like receptor (KIR or CD158) proteins classically expressed in primates, two families of C-type lectin receptors—Ly49 primarily expressed in rodents, and NKG2D receptors expressed in both rodents and primates. All three receptor families contain both inhibitory and activating receptors (Figure 19-3).

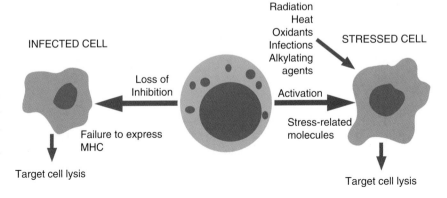

FIGURE 19-2 The activation of NK cells is triggered by two situations. Target cells may fail to express MHC class I molecules. As a result, NK cells lose their inhibitions about attacking such cells. Alternatively, NK cells may be activated by the expression of stress-related proteins on target cells.

NK cells also express CD2, CD16 (FcγRIII), CD178 (CD95L or Fas ligand), CD40L (CD154), toll-like receptors (TLR3 and TLR9), and leukocyte function-associated antigen-1 (LFA-1) (Figure 19-4). NK cells do not express conventional

rearranged V-region antigen receptors such as the B cell antigen receptors (BCRs) or T cell antigen receptors (TCRs), nor do they express a CD3 complex.

Receptors

KIR receptors In humans, the major NK cell MHC class I receptors belong to a multigene family of highly polymorphic proteins called killer cell Ig-like receptor (KIR or CD158) proteins. These are type I transmembrane proteins with two or three extracellular Ig-like domains encoded by a cluster of genes located within the leukocyte receptor gene complex. Through binding to inhibitory KIR receptors, certain MHC class I molecules can protect healthy cells from destruction by NK cells. Other KIR receptors have an opposite effect and stimulate the activity of NK cells. Thus, KIR molecules play a central role in controlling the NK cell response.

The *KIR* gene locus shows extreme structural diversity as a result of the use of multiple alleles. Allelic polymorphism is so extensive that unrelated individuals with identical *KIR* haplotypes are very rare. The variations in *KIR* gene sequences occur at positions that influence their interaction with their MHC class I ligands and as a result influence MHC allelic specificity. These variations tend to occur throughout the gene, unlike the pattern observed in MHC class I and II genes, in which nucleotide variation is restricted to one or two exons. *KIR* gene expression patterns also vary clonally, so NK cell subsets express

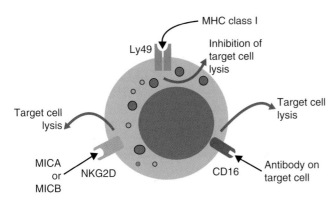

FIGURE 19-3 The three major receptor types found on mouse NK cells. Ly49 recognizes MHC class I molecules and suppresses NK cytotoxicity. NKG2D is a receptor for molecules such as MICA and MICB. These molecules are commonly expressed on stressed, virus-infected, or tumor cells. CD16 binds immunoglobulins and triggers target cell death by antibody-dependent cellular cytotoxicity. Remember that in other mammals, Ly49 may be replaced by KIR receptors.

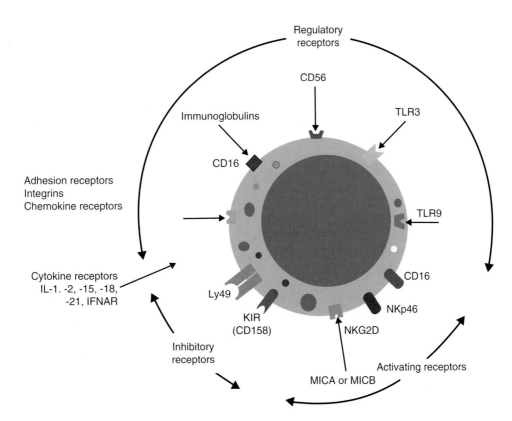

FIGURE 19-4 Some of the receptors on NK cells.

random combinations of KIR receptors. This extreme diversity at the KIR locus may be the result of selection pressure, in a manner analogous to that seen in MHC loci. Thus, disease resistance conferred by the KIR locus will vary depending on an animal's haplotype.

Although human KIR loci vary in their number and diversity, four are present in virtually all haplotypes and are called framework loci. The number of *KIR* genes expressed by a single individual ranges between 7 and 12, depending on the presence or absence of activating KIR loci. Other members of the KIR protein family include the leukocyte immunoglobulin-like receptors (LILRs) and NKp46 (CD335). NKp46 is only expressed on NK cells. The LILRs are expressed on other types of leukocytes. The KIR and LILR families include not only cellular activating receptors but also inhibitors and receptors with no known ligand.

The distinct binding affinities of activating compared with inhibitory KIR may also contribute to the dominance of inhibition. NK cells become activated when inhibition is removed, so activation must involve stimulatory receptors. Stimulatory KIR probably mediate NK cell activity through recognition of MHC ligands, but little direct binding of activating KIR molecules to these ligands has been detected.

Ly49 Receptors In rodents and horses, in contrast to humans and cattle, the predominant NK cell MHC class I receptors belong to the Ly49 family. There are at least 23 members (Ly49A to Ly49W) of this family. They are homomeric type II transmembrane proteins belonging to the C-type lectin family and are functionally equivalent to primate KIRs. The Ly49 molecules are encoded by genes located within the natural killer receptor gene complex. Ly49 haplotypes also contain variable numbers of inhibitory and stimulatory genes, some of which can recognize MHC class I molecules. Ly49 molecules also show specificity for specific MHC alleles. Genomes of humans and other primates contain a single Ly49-like gene. This is a pseudogene in humans, gorilla, and chimpanzee but may be functional in cow, baboon, and orangutan. NK1.1 is another member of the Ly49 family that serves as an activation receptor on mouse NK cells.

NKG2 receptors The third family of MHC-binding receptors on NK cells are activating molecules belong to the NKG2 receptor system. The NKG2 proteins are also C-type lectins. NKG2D, found on all NK cells, recognizes nonclassical MHC class I proteins produced by stressed cells. Two of the most important of these ligands are polymorphic MHC class I–like molecules called MICA (*m*ajor histocompatibility complex, class *I* chain-related *A*) and MICB coded for by MHC class Ic genes (Chapter 11). Unlike normal class I molecules, these are not associated with antigenic peptides. In addition, they have limited tissue distribution and are minimally expressed on normal, healthy cells but are expressed in large amounts on stressed cells. Stresses may include DNA damage due to ionizing radiation or alkylating agents, heat shock, and oxidative stress (see Figure 19-2). MICA and MICB are especially

overexpressed in tumor cells and virus-infected cells. When these ligands are engaged, NKG2D overrides the inhibitory effects of conventional MHC class I molecules and triggers NK cytotoxicity. NKG2D is also expressed on activated γ/δ and α/β T cells, suggesting that they too may have a role in innate immunity. It may be that on surfaces, the combination of γ/δ T cells and NK cells kills tumors, whereas within the body, a combination of α/β T cells and NK cells is most effective.

Fc Receptors NK cells can also recognize and kill target cells by an antibody-dependent pathway acting through CD16 (FcγRIII). CD16 is expressed on NK cells, granulocytes, and macrophages. On macrophages and NK cells, CD16 is a 38-kDa transmembrane protein linked to either the γ chain of FcγRI (in macrophages) or to the zeta chain of CD3 (in NK cells). When target cell surface antigens are bound by specific antibodies, these antigen-antibody complexes bind to NK cell CD16. This triggers NK cytotoxicity and kills the target cells. NK cells can spontaneously release their CD16 so that the NK cell may detach from an antibody-coated target cell after it has delivered its lethal hit.

Effector Mechanisms

NK cell functions are regulated by many different cytokines as well as some pathogen-associated molecular patterns (PAMPs). For example, IL-2 and IL-4 enhance their cytotoxicity, whereas IL-3 enhances their survival. Although NK cells are active in the nonimmunized animal, virus infections or interferon inducers can promote their activity (see Figure 19-5). These activated NK cells are called lymphokine-activated killer (LAK) cells (Figure 33-6). When macrophages phagocytose invading organisms and produce tumor necrosis factor-α (TNF-α) and

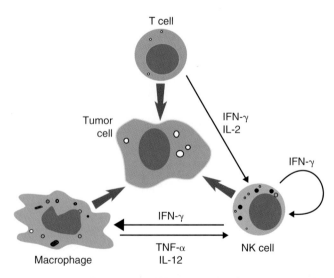

FIGURE 19-5 The interactions between NK cells, macrophages, T cells, and abnormal cells. IFN-γ is a potent stimulant of both NK cells and macrophages.

IL-12, these cytokines induce interferon-γ (IFN-γ) production by NK cells. The IFN-γ then enhances NK activity further by promoting the rapid differentiation of pre-NK cells. It also activates macrophages so that production of TNF-α is augmented by IFN-γ. This NK cell–IFN-γ system probably plays a role in resistance to some tumors since neutralization of interferon by specific antisera enhances tumor growth in mice. IL-21 from activated CD4+ T cells also regulates NK cell function. The IL-21 terminates NK cell responses by triggering their apoptosis, and initiating T cell– and B cell–mediated adaptive immunity.

Once triggered, NK cell killing is mediated, like T cells, through two pathways. One involving perforins, granulysin and NK-lysin, and the other involving CD95L. NK cell granules are specialized secretory lysosomes. They are preformed and stored in resting NK cells (in contrast to cytotoxic T cells, which only produce theirs on demand). Once contact is made with target cells, a synapse forms at the contact site. The KIRs induces MHC molecules to form a ring around a cluster of adhesion molecules. At the center of the synapse, there is a cSMAC through which NK cell granule contents can pass. Receptors and signaling molecules also segregate to the cSMAC, whereas integrins and cytoskeletal components such as talin accumulate in the pSMAC. Inhibitory KIR in contrast prevent the localization of lipid rafts to the immune synapse.

Perforins, granulysin, and NK-lysin are constitutively expressed in NK cell granules, and their expression is increased by exposure to IL-2 and IL-12. The NK cell perforin is a molecule of 70 to 72 kDa (slightly larger than that produced by T cells). It produces characteristic small (5 to 7 nm) channels in target cell surfaces. Presumably granzymes are injected into the target cells in association with the perforin channels.

Function

Unlike T and B cells that circulate as resting cells and so require several days to become fully activated, NK cells are "on call" and can be rapidly activated by IFNs released from virus-infected cells or by IL-12 from stimulated macrophages. As a result, NK cells promptly attack tumors and virus-infected cells. They participate in innate defenses long before antigen-specific primary adaptive responses can be generated (Box 19-2).

NK cells are active against some tumor cells, xenografts, and some virus-infected cells (Figure 19-6). Thus they are active against herpesviruses, influenza, and pox viruses. Some Ly49 molecules on mouse NK cells can recognize viruses directly so that, for example, they can kill cytomegalovirus-infected cells. NK cells can also kill bacteria such as *Staphylococcus aureus* and *Salmonella typhimurium*, protozoa such as *Neospora caninum*, and some fungi.

Most of the evidence that supports a role for NK cells in immunity to tumors is derived from studies on tumor cell lines grown in vitro. NK cells can destroy some cultured tumor cells, and there is a positive correlation between this NK activity measured in vitro and resistance to tumor cells in vivo.

□ **Box 19-2** | **NK-22 Cells**

A subset of NK cells is found in mucosa of the gastrointestinal tract (tonsils, Peyer's patches, and appendix) that produce IL-22 in response to IL-23. These have been designated NK-22 cells. They proliferate in response to IL-1β, IL-2, and IL-7 and secrete B cell–activating factor, suggesting that they may promote B cell–mediated immunity in the mucosa. Their IL-22 plays a role in the defense of mucosal barriers since stimulation of the IL-22 receptor induces the production of antimicrobial defensins and stimulates epithelial cells to secrete the anti-inflammatory cytokine, IL-10. As a result, IL-22 can protect the intestine against bacterial infections.

Experimentally, it is possible to increase resistance to tumor growth in vivo by passive transfer of NK cells from a resistant animal. NK cells destroy human leukemia, myeloma, and some sarcoma and carcinoma cells in vitro, and this activity is enhanced by IFN-γ. NK cells can also invade small primary mouse tumors. Some carcinogenic agents, such as urethane, dimethylbenzanthracene, and low doses of radiation, inhibit NK activity. Stressors such as surgery may also depress NK activity and thus promote tumor growth.

Memory NK cells A typical acquired immune response mediated by cytotoxic T cells can be divided into four phases. First, antigen-stimulated T cells increase greatly in number in response to antigen. This is followed, after antigen elimination, by a phase during which 90% to 95% of these activated T cells undergo apoptosis. This is followed by a memory maintenance phase during which long-lived stable populations of memory cells persist in lymphoid tissues. Finally, a secondary response occurs when the memory T cells re-encounter their cognate antigen. NK cells have long been known to increase in numbers in response to stimulation and are removed once invaders have been eliminated. It is now clear that they can also develop a

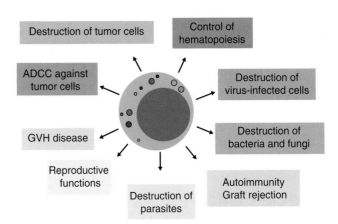

FIGURE 19-6 A schematic diagram showing the many functions of NK cells. ADCC, antibody-dependent cellular cytotoxicity; GVH, graft-versus-host.

memory and mount a form of secondary response to some antigens. For example, NK cells bearing a KIR specific for cytomegalovirus can expand and contract their numbers in response to viral antigen. Thereafter NK memory cells reside in both lymphoid and nonlymphoid tissues for several months. These self-renewing memory cells degranulate and produce cytokines on re-exposure to the antigen. Adoptive transfer of these reactivated NK cells leads to a rapid expansion of numbers and protective immunity to cytomegalovirus. T and B cells, of course express a single antigen receptor, whereas NK cells, in contrast, employ multiple receptors with distinct specificities. An NK cell activated through one receptor may well be reactivated through a different receptor. For example, NK cells initially activated through Ly49 may be reactivated through NKG2D. This NK "memory" response could be more accurately described as training the cells rather than the cells developing specific memory.

Regulation

NK cells interact with dendritic cells. For example, IL-12 and IL-15 from antigen-stimulated dendritic cells activate some NK cells. Thus dendritic cells turn on NK cells, activating them and stimulating them to divide. The activated NK cells in turn secrete cytokines such as IFN-γ that promote maturation of dendritic cells, activate M1 cells, and enhance T cell priming.

NK cell subsets have been identified in many species. Some of these subsets may simply represent cells at different stages of development, and differences in phenotype may simply represent maturation markers. Some NK cell diversity probably reflects site-specific subpopulations such as those found in the liver or the thymus. NK phenotypes may also change with increasing age. In mice some NK cells express Ly49 molecules on their surface, whereas others do not. In humans some subsets differentially express CD56 and CD16. Cells that express both are primarily cytotoxic, whereas those that express CD56 in the absence of CD16 are mainly cytokine producers. This second population predominates in secondary lymphoid organs. In humans, there is also evidence of two NK subsets based on cytokine secretion. NK1 cells produce IFN-γ but almost no IL-4, IL-10, or IL-13. NK2 cells do not secrete IFN-γ but produce IL-13. Another subset of NK cells has a regulatory function, secretes IL-10, and dampens immune responses. It has been suggested that NK cells exposed to moderate levels of IL-12 secrete IFN-γ, but if exposed to very high levels of IL-12, they produce IL-10. In effect, overstimulation turns on a suppressive function. These regulatory NK cells may reduce the severity of virus-induced immunopathology.

Species Differences

NK cell expression of KIR and Ly49 receptors is species specific and mutually exclusive. In mammals it appears that a species may have either a diverse *Ly49* or a diverse *KIR* gene family,

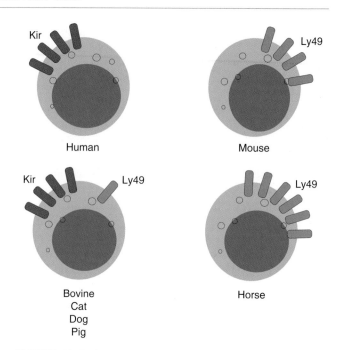

FIGURE 19-7 The species difference between the MHC class I receptors on NK cells. Humans possess a single, nonfunctional *Ly49* gene. Thus they rely totally on KIR molecules, whereas mice rely totally on Ly49 molecules for recognition of their MHC ligands.

but not both. For example, rodents do not express KIR, whereas humans have only a single, nonfunctional *Ly49* gene. Cattle, dogs, cats, and pigs also possess multiple *KIR* genes but only a single functional *Ly49* gene. This suggests that the use of Ly49 receptors by rodents and horses is not typical of mammals in general (Figure 19-7). Marine mammals such as seals and sea lions possess only a single *Ly49* gene and a single *KIR* gene. This is presumably the ancestral arrangement and suggests that some mammals may not require diverse Ly49 or KIR receptors to survive.

Horses

Equine NK cells are activated by recombinant human IL-2 and are active against human tumor cell targets. Horses have six transcribed *Ly49* genes but no transcribed *KIR* genes. Thus horse NK cell receptors resemble those of rodents rather than those of the other domestic mammals.

Cattle

NK cells constitute about 3.5% of blood lymphocytes in young calves and about 2% in older cattle. They are found in highest concentrations in the spleen, lymph nodes, and peripheral blood. Bovine NK cells can kill human cancer cell targets as well as bovine cells infected with parainfluenza-3, bovine leukemia virus (BLV), or bovine herpesvirus type 1 (BHV-1). They generate resistance to mycobacteria by preventing the replication of this organism within macrophages in a contact-dependent manner. They play a role in resistance to the protozoan parasite *Neospora caninum* by producing IFN-γ that kills infected cells. Three subpopulations have been described. Most bovine NK cells express both CD2 and NKp46, but subpopulations may be CD2 or NKp46 negative. Other NK cell surface molecules include CD16, perforin, CD5, CD94, WC1, MHC class II, and asialo-GM₁. (GM₁ is a ganglioside, which is a glycolipid molecule composed of a fatty ceramide residue buried in the lipid bilayer of a cell with at least three sugar groups projecting into the extracellular fluid. One of these is normally a sialic acid group. This is lacking in asialo-GM₁).

Cattle NK use KIR proteins as their MHC class I receptors. Cattle have at least six *KIR* genes, some of whose products are inhibitory, whereas others are activating. They have variable haplotype composition. Cattle NK cells express NKG2D. Cattle *MIC* genes are located close to three nonclassical BoLA MHC class I genes on chromosome 23. There are probably four MIC genes in total. One gene is consistently present, whereas the presence of the other three is variable. They possess one *Ly49* gene with three alleles, so cattle are the only species known to have both polymorphic *Ly49* genes in addition to a large polymorphic *KIR* gene family.

Cattle NK cells are activated by IL-2, IL-12, IL-15, IFN-α, and IFN-γ. Activation by IL-2 enables them to express CD25 and CD8 and lyse tumor cell lines. If activated by IL-12 and IL-15, their expression of granulysin, IFN-γ, and perforin increases, and they can kill both human tumor cells and bacille Calmette-Guérin (BCG)-infected macrophages.

Sheep

There is a population of CD16+, CD14− lymphocytes in sheep blood. More than 80% of these cells expressed perforin. They express NKp46 and are cytotoxic against mouse and sheep cell targets. They secrete IFN-γ in response to IL-12 stimulation. All features typical of NK cells.

Pigs

Pigs appear to have only a single *KIR* gene and a single *Ly49* gene. The latter may be inactive. Thus pigs appear to be unique in this respect, and it raises the question as to how pig NK cells recognize their targets. Porcine NK cells are found in spleen and peripheral blood, but very few are found in lymph nodes or thymus (Figure 19-8). They can lyse human cancer cells as well as cells infected with transmissible gastroenteritis virus or pseudorabies virus. Pigs have two *MIC* genes, one of which is a pseudogene.

Dogs

Canine NK cells can lyse distemper-infected target cells as well as cancer cells from melanomas, osteosarcomas, and mammary carcinomas. Canine NK cells stain weakly with anti-CD5, but their expression of other surface antigens is variable. In dogs, a subset of CD8+ TCR α/β cells also shows NK cell activity.

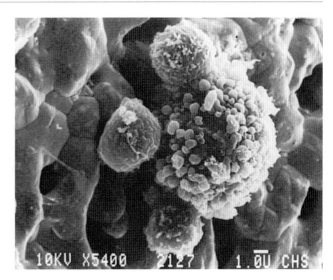

FIGURE 19-8 A scanning electron micrograph of NK cells from a pig (small round cells) attached to a target cell (a human tumor cell). Original magnification ×5400.

(From Yang WC, Schultz RD, Spano JS: Isolation and characterization of porcine natural killer [NK] cells, *Vet Immunol Immunopathol* 14:345–356, 1987.)

The presence of the T cell markers on these cells suggests that they may be of T cell lineage and, indeed, may be more closely related to NKT cells than to conventional NK cells.

Cats

Feline NK cells are large granular lymphocytes found in the blood and spleen. They are active against feline target cells infected with feline leukemia virus, herpesvirus, or vaccinia.

Natural Killer T Cells

NKT cells share properties with both NK and T cells and as such serve as a bridge between innate and adaptive immune responses. They appear to be typical lymphocytes without any unique structural features. NKT cells express NK cell markers such as NK1.1 and members of the Ly49 family, but they also express an invariant α/β TCR. NKT cells are produced in the thymus. Most are found in the sinusoids of the liver, where they make up about 30% of the population. They circulate in the bloodstream, where they make up 0.5% to 1% of mononuclear cells in humans.

NKT cells are activated by glycolipid antigens bound to the nonpolymorphic MHC class I molecule, CD1d (Figure 19-9). CD1d specifically binds and presents glycosphingolipid and diacylglycerol antigens. Cells that express CD1d include dendritic cells, Kupffer cells, endothelial cells, and hepatocytes. Binding of their invariant TCR to these glycolipid antigens stimulates NKT cells. NKT cells also require co-stimulation by IL-15. In the absence of prior antigenic stimulation, NKT cells respond more rapidly than conventional T cells and produce both IFN-γ and IL-4.

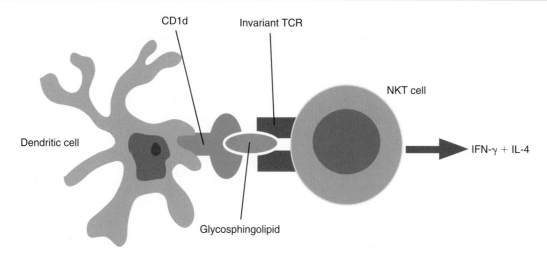

FIGURE 19-9 The mode of action of NKT cells using CD1d as an antigen-presenting molecule.

There are at least two subpopulations of NKT cells. Type 1 cells are classical NKT cells that use an invariant TCR. Type II NKT cells have a more diverse TCR repertoire, and their physiological functions are unclear. However, stimulation of type II cells reduced immunosurveillance, whereas stimulation of type I cells reduced tumor growth. The type II cells appear to suppress the type I cells, suggesting that they have an immunoregulatory role. NKT cells trigger chemokine and cytokine release, enhance NK function, and promote dendritic cell maturation and B cell responses. NKT cells inhibit the development of Th17 cells and regulate these IL-17 responses. NKT cells secrete IL-12 that acts on neutrophils to decrease their production of IL-10. They play a role in allergies, antitumor immunity, autoimmunity, and antimicrobial immunity, especially to mycobacteria. Thus they link the T-cell system with the innate NK cell system.

NKT cells have been well described in humans and mice. Pigs and horses possess functional *CD1d* genes that form receptors that are similar to those found in humans. The *CD1b* genes in cattle and other ruminants are pseudogenes. Therefore, functional NKT cells may not be present in all mammals.

For sources of additional information, please visit http:// evolve.elsevier.com/tizard/immunology/

Regulation of Adaptive Immunity

Key Points

- T cells must be made tolerant to self-antigens. This may be accomplished through central tolerance whereby self-reactive T cells are killed. Alternatively, it may be achieved through peripheral tolerance whereby these T cells are "turned off" by inappropriate signaling.
- B cells are much harder to tolerize than T cells. They are generally regulated by peripheral mechanisms and by the absence of T cell help.
- Antigens stimulate immune responses, although very low or very high doses of antigen may cause tolerance.
- Antibodies tend to regulate antibody production through negative feedback mechanisms. This can prevent the successful vaccination of newborn animals as a result of maternal immunity.
- Immune responses may also be controlled by the activities of regulatory T cells (Treg cells). These Treg cells secrete cytokines such as IL-10 and TGF-β.
- Another T cell subset, Th17 cells, regulates inflammation by secreting a cytokine called interleukin-17 (IL-17).
- The immune system and the central nervous system are closely interconnected and influence each other.

The adaptive immune system is a sophisticated defense system. It can recognize and respond to foreign invaders and can learn from the experience so that the body responds faster and more effectively when exposed to the invader a second time. There is, however, a risk associated with this—the risk of collateral damage. One of the reasons why the adaptive immune system is so complex is that much effort must be put into ensuring that it will only attack foreign or abnormal tissues and will ignore normal healthy tissues. As might be anticipated, many different mechanisms minimize the chances of developing autoimmunity. In addition, immune responses are regulated to ensure that they are appropriate with respect to both quality and quantity (Figure 20-1).

Since both T and B cells generate antigen-binding receptors at random, it is clear that the initial production of self-reactive cells cannot be prevented. An animal cannot control the amino acid sequences and hence the binding specificity of these receptors. As a result, when first generated, as many as 50% of the T cell antigen receptors (TCRs) and B cell antigen receptors (BCRs) may bind self-antigens. If autoimmunity is to be avoided, lymphocytes with these inappropriate receptors must either be destroyed or turned off.

Tolerance

Tolerance is the name given to the situation in which the immune system will not respond to a specific antigen. Tolerance is primarily directed against self-antigens from normal tissues. In 1948 two Australian immunologists, Burnet and Fenner, recognized this need for self-tolerance and suggested that immature lymphocytes would become tolerant to an antigen if they first met it early in fetal life.

Support for this suggestion came from observations on chimeric calves. In 1945 Owen noted that when cows are carrying twin calves, blood vessels in the two placentas commonly fuse. As a result, the blood of the twins intermingles freely, and bone marrow stem cells from one animal colonize the other. Each calf is born with a mixture of blood cells, some of its own and some originating from its twin. In dizygotic (nonidentical) twins, this is called a chimera. These "foreign" blood cells persist indefinitely because each chimeric calf is fully tolerant to the presence of its twin's cells (Figure 20-2). Burnet and

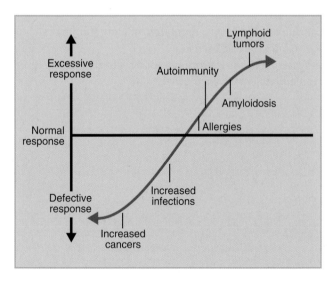

FIGURE 20-1 Some of the bad things that can happen if the immune system is not carefully regulated.

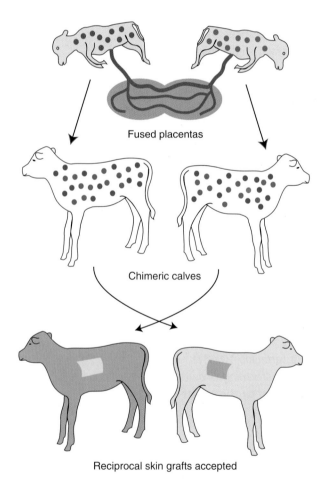

FIGURE 20-2 Fusion of the placentas of dizygotic twin calves results in the development of calf chimeras. Hematopoietic stem cells from each animal colonize the bone marrow of the other. Each chimera is tolerant to its twin's cells and will accept a skin graft from its twin despite the genetic differences.

Fenner suggested that this could only happen because each calf was exposed to the foreign cells early in fetal life during a period when lymphocytes become tolerant upon encountering antigens. Cells from an unrelated calf would be rejected normally if administered after birth.

Subsequent studies have shown that self-tolerance is of two types, central and peripheral. In central tolerance, immature self-reactive lymphocytes within the thymus, bursa, or bone marrow either die or alter their receptor specificity. In peripheral tolerance, mature lymphocytes that encounter self-antigens either die, are turned off, or are suppressed by Treg cells. By reconstituting lethally irradiated mice with T or B cells derived from normal or tolerant donors, tolerance can be shown to occur in both cell populations. However, their susceptibility to peripheral tolerance differs. T cells can be made tolerant rapidly and easily within 24 hours and remain in that state for more than 100 days (Figure 20-3). In contrast, B cells develop tolerance in about 10 days and return to normal within 50 days.

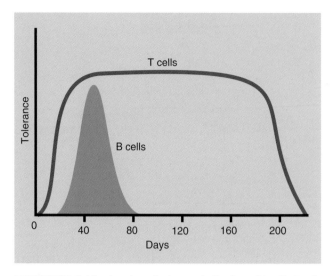

FIGURE 20-3 The duration of tolerance in T cells and B cells. T cells are much more easily rendered tolerant than B cells. Once tolerant, they remain that way for much longer.

T Cell Tolerance

Central T Cell Tolerance

Negative Selection. Tolerance will result if there are no functional T cells with receptors that can bind self-antigens (Figure 20-4). Although the body generates an enormous diversity of TCRs, far fewer receptors are actually used by mature T cells than might be anticipated. Several processes serve to limit receptor diversity. First, the mechanisms used to generate diverse TCRs inevitably result in the production of nonfunctional receptors. For example, two thirds of possible gene arrangements will be out of frame. Cells with these nonfunctional TCRs undergo apoptosis. As T cells mature within the thymus, positive selection ensures that the cells that

recognize self-MHC molecules survive. At this point, however, the cells whose receptors bind too strongly to self-antigens die by apoptosis (Figure 20-5). The timing and extent of this apoptosis depend on the affinity of the TCR for a self-antigen. T cells that bind self-antigens strongly die earlier and more completely than weakly binding cells. Thus the T cells that eventually leave the thymus have been purged of dangerous, self-reactive cells.

The negative selection process is assisted by the presence of many different self-antigens in the thymus. Normally each tissue possesses its own tissue-specific antigens. Thus "skin antigens" are usually restricted to the skin, whereas "liver antigens" are restricted to the liver, and so forth. However, the epithelial cells in the thymic medulla show uniquely

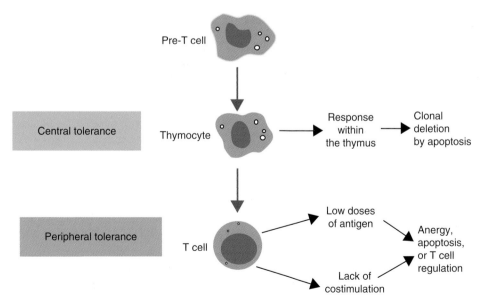

FIGURE 20-4 The principal ways by which T cells are made tolerant.

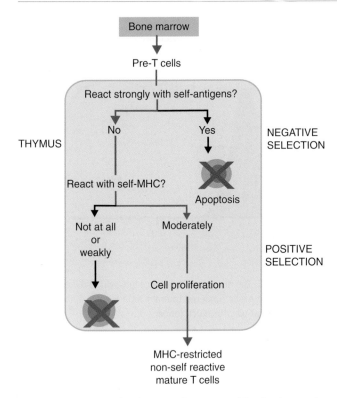

FIGURE 20-5 How the thymus induces central T cell tolerance by negative selection. Surviving T cells are unreactive to autoantigens yet can still respond to foreign antigenic peptides in association with MHC molecules as a result of positive selection.

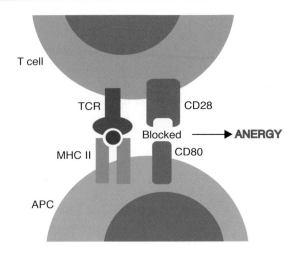

FIGURE 20-6 Peripheral tolerance through clonal anergy will develop if a TCR is stimulated by antigen in the absence of simultaneous co-stimulation through the CD28/CD80 or CD28/CD86 pathway.

"promiscuous" gene expression. Thymic epithelial cells use a transcription regulator, called the autoimmune regulator (AIRE), that promotes the expression of many different proteins once thought to be restricted to other tissues. Examples include insulin, thyroglobulin, and myelin basic protein. In this way, the thymic epithelial cells ensure that self-reactive T cells encounter many normal tissue antigens and are therefore eliminated. In addition, some normal tissue antigens may be taken up by macrophages and carried to the thymus. Self-reactive T cells that respond to these antigens are also eliminated. However, this raises another question: What about self-antigens that are not expressed in, or do not enter, the thymus? For example, antigens in the eye, testis, or brain are not processed in this way, and as a result central tolerance to these antigens does not develop.

Positive and negative selection acting together ensure that cells that can bind self-MHC molecules are positively selected and those that bind the MHC molecules with very low or very high affinity are subsequently deleted. As a result, the moderate-affinity clones survive and can recognize foreign antigens. An additional factor that probably determines thymocyte survival is the dose of antigen presented to the cells. If the amount of a specific antigen is high (as one might anticipate for a self-antigen), multiple TCRs will be occupied on each thymocyte and trigger apoptosis. In contrast, if the amount of an antigen is low, this will occupy only a few TCRs, and the weak signal may cause positive selection and thymocyte proliferation.

Receptor Editing. When the antigen receptors of a developing T cell bind to self-antigens, another strategy employed to prevent autoimmunity is receptor editing (Chapter 34). Although cell maturation stops when it leaves the thymus, the *RAG* genes remain active and as a result, V(D)J recombination continues. Consequently, the *TCR* genes continue to diversify, and changed receptors are expressed on the cell surface. This process is called receptor editing. If a cell successfully edits its receptors, its maturation can proceed. Failure to do so will result in its apoptosis. This is a potentially hazardous process since it permits the development of self-reactive T cells that have not undergone careful selection within the thymus.

Peripheral T Cell Tolerance

Clonal Anergy. Low-affinity self-reactive T cells may survive the selection process and leave the thymus and must then be suppressed by peripheral tolerance mechanisms. One form of peripheral tolerance is clonal anergy, the prolonged, antigen-specific suppression of T cell function. Clonal anergy can be triggered by the signals received by the T cell. T cells normally require multiple signals from several sources in order to respond to antigen. If these signals are insufficient or inappropriate, T cell responses to antigen will be suppressed.

As pointed out in Chapter 14, binding of an antigen to a TCR is by itself insufficient to trigger T cell responses. Indeed, occupation of the TCR in the absence of co-stimulation causes tolerance. For example, protein solutions normally contain some aggregated molecules. These aggregated molecules are readily taken up and processed by dendritic cells and thus are highly immunogenic. If a solution of such a protein, such as bovine γ-globulin, is ultracentrifuged so that all the aggregates are removed, then the aggregate-free solution will induce anergy. This is due to the lack of co-stimulation from antigen-presenting cells (APCs) (Figure 20-6).

Binding to the TCR by an antigen alone activates the tyrosine kinases and phospholipase C of the T cell and raises its

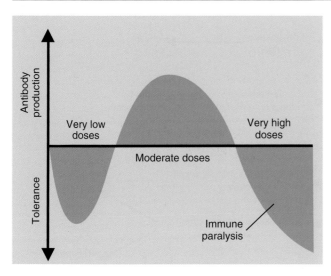

FIGURE 20-7 The ability of different doses of antigen to induce peripheral tolerance. Both very low and very high doses can induce tolerance. Moderate doses, in contrast, induce an immune response.

intracellular Ca²⁺. This results in enhanced production of IκB that inhibits NF-κB and effectively prevents the cell from making cytokines, especially IL-2. Tolerant Th1 cells produce about 1% to 3% of normal IL-2 levels and much less IFN-γ and TNF-α. Once induced, their anergy can last for several weeks. Induction of the transcription factor FoxP3 also silences anti-inflammatory cytokine genes and leads to the production of Treg cells.

Triggering of T cell responses normally requires prolonged interactions with antigen-presenting cells. Tolerance induction, on the other hand, is characterized by relatively short interactive episodes. Thus a key difference between T cell activation and anergy may simply be the duration of their encounter with APCs.

Very high doses of an antigen can induce a form of clonal anergy called immune paralysis (Figure 20-7). The high doses of the antigen probably bypass APCs, reach the Th cell receptors directly, and in the absence of co-stimulation trigger anergy.

B Cell Tolerance

Unlike the TCR repertoire, B cell antibody diversity is generated in two phases. The first phase involves VDJ rearrangement or gene conversion in the primary lymphoid organs; the second phase involves random somatic mutation in secondary lymphoid organs. B cells therefore have several opportunities to generate receptors that can bind self-antigens. It has been estimated that 55% to 75% of early immature B cells have self-reactive receptors, so suppression of these self-reactive B cells must begin at an early stage in an animal's development.

Immature B cells within the bone marrow can be made tolerant once they have arranged their V-region genes and are committed to express complete immunoglobulin M (IgM) molecules. When these immature cells encounter and bind antigen, the BCR transmits a signal that arrests cell development, blocks synapse formation, and triggers apoptosis. An immature B cell population can be rendered tolerant by one millionth of the dose of an antigen required to make mature B cells tolerant. Immature B cells may also undergo receptor editing as described previously. If receptor editing fails to generate a non-self-reactive B cell, it will die.

Peripheral B Cell Tolerance

Peripheral B cell tolerance is induced by multiple mechanisms, including apoptosis, clonal anergy, clonal exhaustion, and blockage of BCRs.

Because BCRs undergo random somatic mutation within germinal centers, self-reactive B cells can still develop in secondary lymphoid organs. These cells will not, however, make autoantibodies if APCs and helper T cells are absent or if Treg cells are active (Figure 20-8). This is not, however, a foolproof method of preventing self-reactivity. In the absence of T cell help, B cells may be activated by pathogen-associated molecular patterns (PAMPs) such as bacterial lipopolysaccharide (LPS), flagellins, or unmethylated CpG DNA acting through their toll-like receptors (TLRs). B cells may also be activated by either cross-reacting epitopes or a foreign carrier molecule stimulating nontolerant helper T cells (Figure 34-2).

As with T cells, B cell anergy occurs when the B cells encounter antigens in the absence of co-stimulation. B cells are difficult to maintain in a tolerant state, however, and will reactivate rapidly unless steps are taken to maintain tolerance. Self-reactive B cells must also bind to a critical threshold of self-antigen to be made tolerant. This results in selective silencing of high-affinity B cells. Presumably the failure of low-affinity anti-self B cells to become tolerant poses little threat of autoimmune disease because the low-affinity antibodies will not cause tissue destruction.

B cells subjected to repeated exhaustive antigenic stimulation may differentiate into short-lived plasma cells. If all B cells develop into such plasma cells, no memory B cells will remain to respond to antigen, and tolerance will result. Some polymeric antigens such as pneumococcal polysaccharide can bind irreversibly to BCRs, freezing the B cell membrane and blocking any further responses by these cells. The B cells recover once the antigen is removed.

Orally administered proteins may also induce tolerance. The mechanisms depend on the amount of an antigen fed. High doses induce clonal deletion and anergy, whereas lower doses induce the development of Treg cells.

Duration of Tolerance

The duration of tolerance depends on the persistence of an antigen and on the ability of the bone marrow to generate fresh T or B cells. When an antigen is completely eliminated,

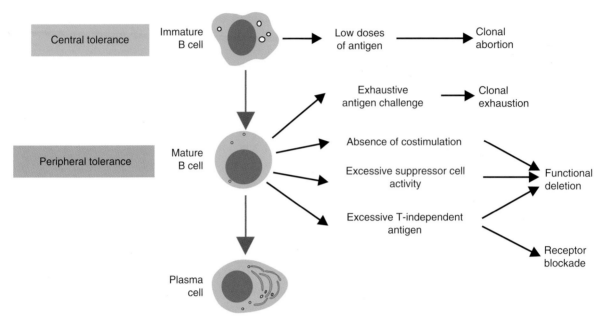

FIGURE 20-8 Central and peripheral tolerance mechanisms in B cells.

tolerance fades. If, however, an antigen is persistent, such as occurs in calf chimeras or with an animal's own self-antigens, tolerance persists. In the continued presence of an antigen, newly formed antigen-sensitive cells will undergo apoptosis as soon as their receptors bind self-antigen. Treatment that promotes bone marrow activity, such as low-dose X-irradiation, hastens the fading of tolerance, whereas immunosuppressive drug treatment has the opposite effect.

Control of Immune Responses

Tolerance is not the only mechanism of immune regulation employed by the body. The magnitude of immune responses must also be regulated. An inadequate immune response may lead to immunodeficiency and increased susceptibility to infection. An excessive immune response may result in the development of allergies or autoimmunity (Chapters 28 and 34). Failure to control the lymphocyte proliferation that occurs during immune responses may permit development of lymphoid cell tumors. Failure to control the immune response to the fetus may lead to abortion (Chapter 32). The immune responses must therefore be carefully regulated to ensure that they are appropriate in both quality and quantity. As might be anticipated, many different control mechanisms exist.

Antigen Regulation of Immune Responses

Adaptive immune responses are antigen driven. They commence only on exposure to an antigen, and once its concentration drops below a critical threshold, they stop. If an antigen

persists, the stimulus persists and the immune response is prolonged. Prolonged responses occur after immunization with slowly degraded antigens such as the bacterial polysaccharides, or with antigens incorporated in oil or insoluble adjuvants. Antigens that do not reach organized lymphoid tissues, irrespective of their origin, fail to induce either immunity or tolerance. Thus self-antigens restricted to sites such as the brain, or infectious agents such as papillomaviruses that never enter lymphoid organs, are usually ignored by the immune system.

Antibody responses are also regulated by antigen. Rigid polymeric antigens such as those on a bacterial surface or antigens linked to TCR activators such as LPS can induce B-cell responses in the absence of T cell help. On the other hand, nonpolymeric, flexible antigens such as soluble proteins induce B cell responses only in the presence of CD4+ T cells. Antigen concentration also affects this because the lower the antigen concentration, the greater is the need for T cell help.

Antigen Processing and Immune Regulation

The nature of the immune response may vary in different parts of the body as a result of processing by different dendritic cell populations. Langerhans cells seem especially suited for promoting T cell responses, whereas follicular dendritic cells prime B cells. DC1 cells are optimized to present antigens to Th1 cells, whereas DC2 cells present antigens to Th2 cells. Adjuvants also influence the type of immune response through their effects on APCs (Chapter 23). Thus, lipids conjugated to protein antigens commonly induce cell-mediated responses rather than antibody production and localize in T cell rather than B cell areas of lymphoid tissues.

Antibody Regulation of Immune Responses

Antibodies generally suppress B cell responses. IgG antibodies tend to suppress the production of both IgM and IgG, whereas IgM antibodies tend to suppress only the synthesis of IgM. Specific antibodies tend to suppress a specific immune response better than nonspecific immunoglobulins. An excellent example of this is seen in the method employed to prevent hemolytic disease of the newborn in humans (Chapter 29). In this disease, a mother who lacks the Rhesus (Rh) antigen makes antibodies against the Rh antigens expressed on the red blood cells of her fetus. If the mother is given antibodies against this antigen at the time of her exposure to fetal red blood cells at birth, she will be completely prevented from making responding to this antigen.

This negative effect of antibodies on B cell functions is mediated through the inhibitory B cell receptor CD32b (FcγRIIb). In diseases in which serum immunoglobulin levels are abnormally high, as in patients with myelomas (Chapter 15), this feedback depresses normal antibody synthesis, and patients become susceptible to infections. A similar phenomenon occurs in newborn animals that acquire antibodies from their mother. The presence of maternal antibodies, while conferring protection, inhibits immunoglobulin synthesis and so prevents the successful vaccination of newborn animals (Figure 20-9).

Serum IgG levels are also regulated through the FcRn immunoglobulin receptor. FcRn is widely distributed on endothelial cells in muscle, vasculature, and hepatic sinusoids. Immunoglobulins that bind to FcRn are protected from degradation. If FcRn expression remains constant, IgG levels remain stable. If IgG levels rise, the surplus will fail to bind FcRn and be degraded. Conversely, if IgG levels drop, a greater proportion will bind to FcRn and be protected.

The class, as well as the quantity, of immunoglobulins produced during an immune response is also regulated. Most unstimulated B cells express both IgM and IgD BCRs. During an immune response, these cells switch to the production of IgM, IgG, IgA, or IgE. This class switch is controlled by helper T cells. In animals given T-independent antigens, there is no class switch, and a persistent low-level IgM response ensues (Figure 15-11).

Inhibitory Receptors

A key feature of the adaptive immune system is that, while poised to launch a potent array of destructive mechanisms against invaders, the body maintains control of the process. It is critically important to limit and eventually terminate a response by inactivating or eliminating pathways that are no longer required. This regulation involves the extensive use of inhibitory receptors. These are especially important in diminishing the activity of lymphocytes once they have completed their task and provide a crucial safeguard against inappropriate immune responses. Thus activation and inhibition must be paired to initiate and terminate immune responses. In some cases activating and inhibitory receptors recognize similar ligands, so the net outcome is a product of the relative strength of these signals. Loss of inhibitory signals is often associated with autoimmunity or hypersensitivity.

An excellent example of an inhibitory receptor is CD32b (FcγRIIb) expressed on B cells. Any antibodies present will occupy these receptors. If these receptor-bound antibodies are linked to a BCR through an antigen, the BCR and CD32 come together (Figure 20-10). As a result, their signal transduction pathways interact, and BCR signal transduction is blocked. This prevents B cell activation and triggers its apoptosis. The CD32 pathway serves as a feedback mechanism whereby B-cell activation is suppressed by antibody and so prevents

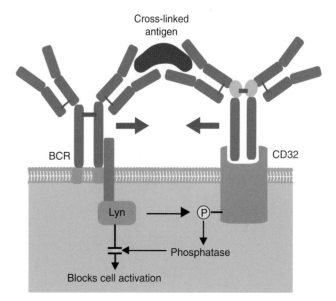

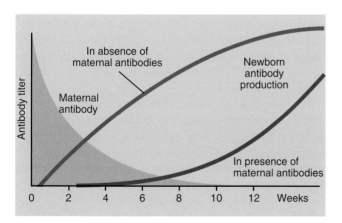

FIGURE 20-9 The presence of maternal antibody in a newborn animal effectively delays the onset of immunoglobulin synthesis through a negative feedback process.

FIGURE 20-10 Cross-linkage between a BCR and CD32, an Fc receptor, by antibody and antigen can turn off a B cell by activating a phosphatase that in turn blocks signaling by tyrosine kinase.

uncontrolled B-cell responses. Since another receptor, FcγRIII, stimulates B cells, B cell responses can be regulated by altering the ratio of FcγRIIb to FcγRIII. Macrophage activation is regulated in a similar manner, and activated macrophages have a high FcγRIII-to-II ratio.

CD28 and CTLA4 on T cells both bind the same ligand (CD80) but deliver antagonistic signals. CD28 is an activator, whereas CTLA4 is an inhibitor. A deficiency of CTLA4 leads to uncontrolled T cell proliferation and autoimmunity.

Regulatory Cells

Although much immune regulation is "passive" in that self-reactive lymphocytes are eliminated by central tolerance, cells in peripheral tissues also "actively" regulate the immune system. Cells with regulatory functions include T cells, macrophages, dendritic cells, and natural suppressor cells.

Regulatory T Cells

Regulatory T cells play a master role in regulating the immune system and maintaining the balance between peripheral tolerance and immunity (Figure 20-11). In their absence, multiorgan autoimmune disease results. Some of these Treg cells develop naturally, whereas others must be induced by cytokine exposure.

Treg cells are typical lymphocytes that characteristically express CD4 and CD25 (the α chain of the IL-2 receptor). (All activated T cells express CD25, but Treg cells are the only

ones that express it when naïve.) Their most characteristic feature, however, is their use of a specialized transcription factor FoxP3. This is yet another example of a situation in which cattle are different from mice and humans. Foxp3+, CD4+, and CD25+ cells are found in cattle but do not appear to function as Tregs. The Treg cells in cattle are WC1.1+, WC1.2+, and γ/δ T cells.

Natural Treg cells (nTreg) originate in the thymus, whereas induced Treg cells (iTreg) are produced in secondary lymphoid organs, especially the intestine. The intestine is a major site of iTreg development, and specialized intestinal dendritic cells promote this through pathways that use a combination of transforming growth factor-β (TGF-β) and retinoic acid, a metabolite of vitamin A. The retinoic acid is generated by the normal bacterial flora in the gut. Changes in the gut flora may therefore reduce the Treg population while increasing the Th17 cell population. It is possible that Treg and Th17 cells are alternative fates of a single cell lineage. Intestinal Treg cells develop in response to antigen and co-stimulation by IL-2 and TGF-β. These signals induce the transcription of FoxP3. FoxP3 in turn induces transcription of the genes for CTLA-4, TGF-β, and IL-10. Tregs are scattered throughout the body. They account for roughly 5% of circulating T cells and 10% of lymph node T cells in the dog.

The mechanisms of Treg action appear to be of two major types. Inhibition through direct cell-cell contact is used predominantly by nTreg cells. This may be mediated by delivery of suppressive molecules through gap junctions, by membrane-bound suppressive cytokines such as TGF-β, by production of cytotoxic granzymes and perforins, or by CTLA-4 reverse signaling through CD80. Inhibition through the production of soluble suppressive cytokines is used predominantly by iTreg cells. These cytokines include TGF-β, IL-10, or IL-35 as well as soluble competitors for cytokine receptors. They may also induce APCs to produce these molecules. As a result of all these mechanisms, Treg cells suppress the response of helper T cells to antigens and prevent inappropriate T cell activation in the absence of an antigen. Treg cells can also suppress CD4 and CD8 T cell responses by pathways independent of IL-10 and TGF-β. For example, they appear to shorten the interaction time between T cells and APCs and thus prevent activation.

Oral administration of an antigen may induce iTreg cells. Treg cells from the mesenteric lymph nodes of orally tolerant animals secrete TGF-β, with various amounts of IL-4 and IL-10. Since it is now recognized that the gut flora influences iTreg activity, this may support the hygiene hypothesis (Chapter 28). This hypothesis suggests that reduced microbial exposure in the gut depresses Treg production, accounting for the increased prevalence of allergies and autoimmunity.

Treg cells are not the only ways in which cellular control of immune responses is exercised. Many of the regulatory activities of T cells reflect the antagonistic functions of Th1 and Th2 cells. For example, IFN-γ from Th1 cells can suppress IgE production, whereas IL-10 from Th2 cells is suppressive for dendritic cell IL-12 production and thus for the production of Th1 cytokines.

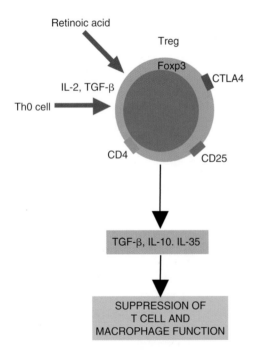

FIGURE 20-11 The production and functions of regulatory T cells. They are generated by the combined actions of IL-2 and TGF-β as well as the presence of retinoic acid. They characteristically produce the suppressive cytokines, TGF-β, IL-10, and IL-35.

Interleukin-10. IL-10 is an immunoregulatory cytokine that inhibits both innate and adaptive immune responses (Figure 20-12). It is a protein of about 178 amino acids produced by macrophages (especially M2 macrophages) and myeloid dendritic cells in response to microbial products. It is also produced by multiple T cell subsets, including all three populations of helper T cells in response to high antigen doses and IL-12. It is produced in especially large amounts by Treg cells in response to TGF-β stimulation. Small amounts of IL-10 can also be produced by B cells, mast cells, neutrophils, and natural killer (NK) cells.

IL-10 suppresses the production of IL-1, IL-6, tumor necrosis factor-α (TNF-α), and oxidants by macrophages. It stimulates production of IL-1RA, an anti-inflammatory cytokine. It also induces apoptosis in developing macrophages and mast cells. It downregulates MHC class II and co-stimulatory molecule expression on dendritic cells and macrophages and hence impairs antigen presentation. IL-10 or IL-10-treated dendritic cells can induce a long-lasting, antigen-specific, anergic state when both CD4 and CD8 T cells are activated in its presence. IL-10 inhibits the synthesis of the Th1 cytokines, IL-1, IFN-γ, and TNF-α and the Th2 cytokines IL-4 and Il-5. Thus it can regulate both Th1 and Th2 responses. IL-10 also inhibits the production of IL-5, CXCL8, IL-12, granulocyte-macrophage colony-stimulating factor (GM-CSF), and granulocyte colony-stimulating factor (G-CSF). IL-10 downregulates the production of IFN-γ and TNF-α by NK cells.

Other members of the IL-10 family include IL-19, IL-20, IL-22, IL-24, Il-26, IL-28, and IL-29. They share a common three-dimensional structure but have limited sequence similarity, and their biological activities may be quite different.

Transforming Growth Factor-β. TGF-β comprises a family of five glycoproteins; three (TGF-β1, TGF-β2, and

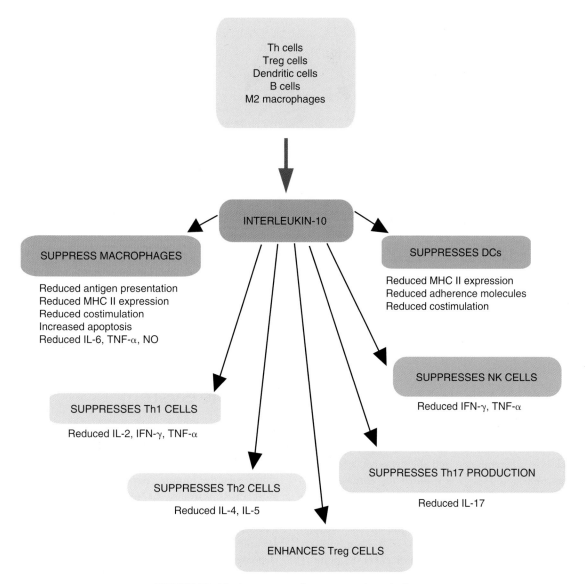

FIGURE 20-12 The origins and properties of interleukin-10.

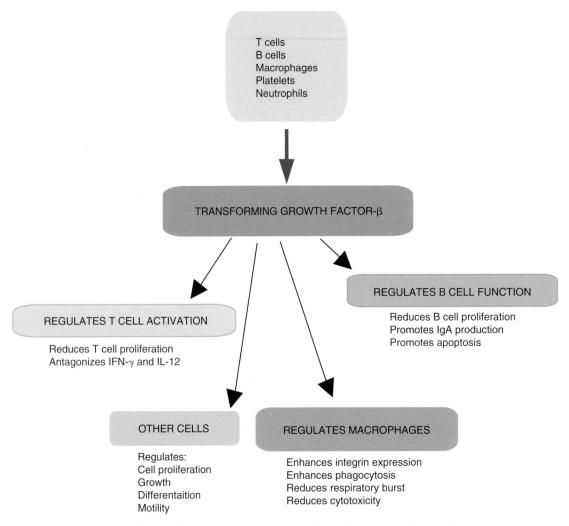

FIGURE 20-13 The origins and properties if transforming growth factor-β.

TGF-β3) are found in mammals, and two others (TGF-β4 and TGF-β5) have been described in chickens and *Xenopus* toads. They are secreted as inactive complexes that are activated on the cell surface by proteases after binding to integrins. TGFs are produced by platelets, activated macrophages, neutrophils, B cells, and T cells and act on T and B cells, dendritic cells, macrophages, neutrophils, and fibroblasts (Figure 20-13).

TGF-β regulates macrophage activities. It may be either inhibitory or stimulatory, depending on the presence of other cytokines. Thus it can enhance integrin expression as well as phagocytosis by blood monocytes. On the other hand, it suppresses the respiratory burst and nitric oxide production and blocks monocyte differentiation and the cytotoxic effects of activated macrophages. TGF-β is required for optimal dendritic cell development and regulates the interaction between follicular dendritic cells and B cells.

TGF-β inhibits T and B cell proliferation and stimulates their apoptosis. Apoptotic T cells release TGF-β, contributing to the suppressive environment. TGF-β influences the differentiation of Th subsets. It tends to promote Th1 responses and the production of IL-2 in naïve T cells, but it also antagonizes

the effects of IFN-γ and IL-12 on memory cells. It also controls the development and differentiation of B cells, inhibiting their proliferation, inducing apoptosis, and regulating IgA production.

Regulation by the Innate Immune System

The triggering of innate immune responses through pattern recognition receptors (PRRs) activates many intracellular pathways. These pathways may influence an animal's ability to mount adaptive immune responses. For example, signaling by most PRRs activates the transcription factors NF-κB and NFAT. These can activate both T and B cells. Stimulation of TLR4 can also induce Th1, Th2, and Th17 responses. The cytosolic PRRs such as the RLRs and NLRs can activate Th1 responses and trigger CD8+ cytotoxicity (Chapter 2). Thus if a virus infects dendritic cells and is recognized by cytosolic PRRs, not only will it trigger a type I interferon response but it also may trigger the production of cytokines and other co-stimulators needed to activate T cells. The cell surface TLRs can also activate B cells.

Th17 Cells

Naïve CD4+ T cells differentiate into Th17 cells when exposed to IL-6 plus TGF-β. Th17 cells play an important role in host defense and are potent inducers of acute inflammation (Figure 20-14). Th17 cells are conventional small lymphocytes that are abundant in mucosal surfaces. Their presence in these surface tissues is regulated by the gut microflora.

Dendritic cells and macrophages activated by microbial PAMPs through TLR2 secrete IL-23 (Box 20-1). IL-23 promotes the survival and activation of Th17 cells. Th17 cells secrete IL-17 and IL-22 (Figure 20-15; Box 20-2). IFN-γ suppresses the development of Th17 cells and inhibits IL-17-mediated inflammation.

Interleukin-17 There are six members of the IL-17 family (IL-17A through IL-17F), but the two most important members of the family are IL-17A and IL-17F. IL-17A is involved in the development of autoimmunity, inflammation, and some tumors. IL-17F is mainly involved in mucosal defense. IL-17E (also known as IL-25) promotes Th2 responses. The functions of the others are unclear. IL-17A is a homodimer of 35 kDa produced by Th17 cells. Endothelial cells and macrophages appear to be the main targets of these cytokines since IL-17A or IL-17F plus TNF-α can stimulate them to produce proinflammatory molecules (Figure 20-16). These include the CXC chemokines, G-CSF, GM-CSF, IL-1, and IL-6, inflammatory mediators such as acute-phase and complement proteins, and antibacterial defensins. IL-17A, IL17-B, and IL17-C are especially potent in triggering inflammation in autoimmune diseases such as rheumatoid arthritis.

□ Box 20-1 | Interleukin-23

IL-23 is closely related to IL-12. Both are heterodimers consisting of an identical p40 subunit and a second smaller subunit, IL-23p19 or IL-12p35, respectively. Both cytokines are produced by macrophages and dendritic cells in response to LPS, and both enhance T cell proliferation and the production of IFN-γ. Whereas IL-12 drives a pathway leading to Th1 cell production, IL-23 drives a pathway leading to the stabilization of IL-17-producing CD4+ T cells. IL-23 recruits diverse inflammatory cells in addition to Th17 cells and is thus involved in the pathogenesis of several immune-mediated diseases. The production of IL-23 is increased in some tumors, where it promotes inflammation and enhances angiogenesis (Chapter 33).

□ Box 20-2 | Interleukin-22

IL-22 is a member of the IL-10 family produced by Th17 cells, activated T cells, and NK cells. It acts on many different leukocytes and on many different tissues. It stimulates acute-phase protein production by hepatocytes. IL-22 acts on cells of the skin and the digestive and respiratory systems to increase expression of several β-defensins, and it presumably promotes innate immunity in these tissues.

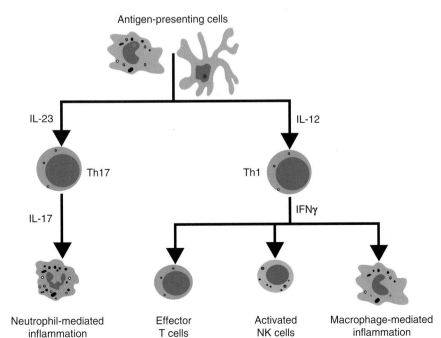

FIGURE 20-14 The generation of Th1 and Th17 cells depends upon the production of IL-12 or IL-23 by antigen-presenting cells. Th1 cells promote cell-mediated responses, Th17 cells promote innate responses.

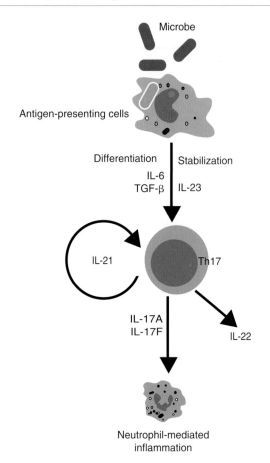

FIGURE 20-15 The production of Th17 cells. The original differentiation signal comes from TGF-β and IL-6. This signal is amplified by IL-21 and then the cell phenotype is stabilized by IL-23.

IL-17 regulates neutrophil accumulation in acute inflammation and is crucial for coordinating host defenses against many bacteria and fungi. For example, Th17 cells play a key role in defense against pathogens such as *Klebsiella pneumoniae, Citrobacter rodentium, Salmonella enterica, Mycobacterium tuberculosis,* and *Candida albicans.* It is believed that it does so by triggering inflammation and recruitment of inflammatory cells early in infection, leading to rapid pathogen eradication. Engagement of dectin-1 and -2 drives Th17 responses in fungal infections.

Regulatory Macrophages

Activation of macrophages by IFN-γ leads to the development of proinflammatory classically activated M1 cells. Exposure of macrophages to IL-4 or IL-13, in contrast, leads to the development of M2 cells (Chapter 5). M2 cells participate in tolerance induction, suppress inflammation, and participate in tissue repair. M2 cells increase expression of the macrophage mannose receptor, the β-glucan receptor, and CD163; enhance endocytosis and antigen processing; and increase MHC class II expression. M2 macrophages produce large amounts of anti-inflammatory cytokines such as IL-10, TGF-β,

and IL-1RA. They are not killer cells because they produce arginase, which generates ornithine rather than nitric oxide (Figure 5-7).

In healthy animals, M2 cells may be found in the placenta and lung, where they inhibit unwanted inflammatory reactions. Thus placental and alveolar macrophages inhibit dendritic cell antigen presentation and can inhibit mitogen responses in lymphocytes. M2 macrophages are responsible for control of granuloma formation as well as for skin tolerance induced by ultraviolet B radiation. They can also be found in healing tissues, where they are associated with angiogenesis.

Indoleamine 2,3-Dioxygenase and Tolerance Many regulatory cells, including Tregs, dendritic cells, some macrophages, fibroblasts, trophoblast giant cells, endothelial cells, and some tumor cell lines produce indoleamine 2,3-dioxygenase (IDO). This enzyme catalyzes the oxidative degradation of the amino acid tryptophan, leading to its local depletion. Tryptophan is an essential amino acid, and T cells undergo cell cycle arrest and apoptosis when deprived of tryptophan. IDO is therefore an inhibitor of T cell activation, proliferation, and survival within tissues and a promoter of peripheral tolerance. Th1 cells appear to be more sensitive to tryptophan depletion than are Th2 cells. Treg cells may induce IDO expression in trophoblast cells and some dendritic cell subsets. IDO activity has also been documented in T cell tolerance to tumors, as a negative regulator in autoimmune diseases, and in some experimental allergies. IDO plays a key role in preventing immunological rejection of the fetus and of liver and corneal allografts (Chapter 32). IDO can also act as a defensive enzyme since by removing tryptophan it prevents the growth of *Toxoplasma gondii, Chlamydia pneumoniae,* streptococci, and mycobacteria.

Tolerogenic Dendritic Cells

The normal function of dendritic cells is to capture and process foreign antigens for presentation to T cells. However, the precise signals generated by dendritic cells depend on their state of maturity, on their display of co-stimulating molecules, and on the presence or absence of inflammatory cytokines. Thus proteins from dead and dying cells that are captured by immature dendritic cells in the absence of inflammation may cause dendritic cells to trigger apoptosis in responding T cells or cause the T cells to differentiate into IL-10-producing Treg cells. Treatment of dendritic cells with IL-10 can block their ability to activate Th1 cells while preserving their ability to promote Th2 responses.

Natural Suppressor Cells

Natural suppressor (NS) cells are large granular lymphocytes that produce cytokines with Treg-inducing activity. They suppress B and T cell proliferation as well as immunoglobulin production. NS cells occur normally in the adult bone marrow

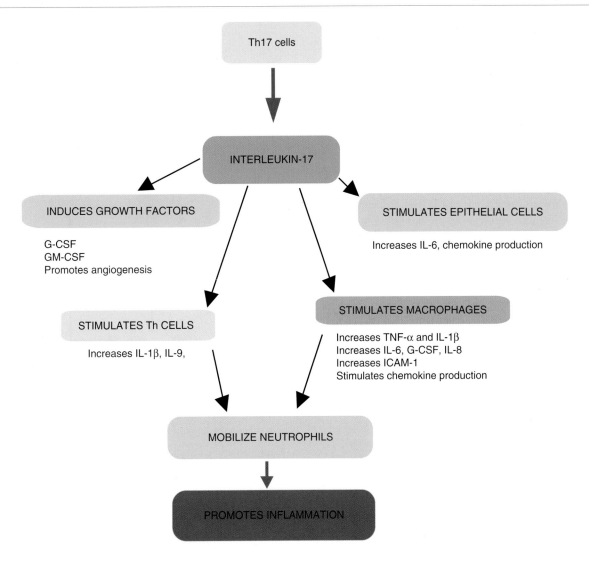

FIGURE 20-16 The origins and properties of interleukin 17.

and neonatal spleen and possibly regulate innate immune responses.

When Do Regulatory Cells Work?

Regulatory cell activities have been described as regulating almost all aspects of immune reactivity. Treg cells, for example, work constantly throughout an animal's life to prevent self-reactivity. They are responsible for lack of immune responses in the newborn; immunosuppression following trauma, burns, or surgery; prevention of autoimmunity; some cases of hypo-gammaglobulinemia; and blocking of responses to mitogens. Regulatory cells are found in some tumor-bearing animals, in which they block tumor rejection, and in pregnant animals, in which they block rejection of the fetus.

Regulation of Apoptosis

The thymus of the mouse releases about 1 million new T cells into the circulation every day. (Presumably a cow would produce many more.) To keep the number of mouse lymphocytes relatively constant, a million must also die. Likewise, the mouse bone marrow releases about 10^7 B cells daily, and a similar number must die. In addition, lymphocytes divide in response to antigens. All this proliferation must be balanced by the removal of cells by apoptosis. Apoptosis also removes autoreactive lymphocytes and limits the clonal expansion of lymphocytes during an immune response. This homeostatic system is carefully regulated because if it fails, excess lymphocytes may cause lymphoid tumors or autoimmunity. The regulatory process depends on providing cells with survival signals. If these are inadequate, cells will die. These regulatory signals are provided by cytokines such as IL-2, IL-4, IL-9, and IL-21.

Apoptosis is mediated by intracellular caspases. Caspases are expressed as inactive precursors in lymphocytes. Proteins of the bcl-2 family modulate their activity. Thus, in a quiescent cell, survival depends on the ongoing presence of bcl-2. Animals lacking bcl-2 lose their lymphocytes and become immunodeficient. External signals also regulate apoptosis. Survival is signaled through IL-2, IL-4, IL-7, and IL-15, whereas cell death is signaled through Fas (CD95) and TGF-β. Adherence receptors such as integrins also regulate the survival of quiescent B and T cells. Thus if a lymphocyte does not traffic to a lymphoid organ, it may be destroyed by apoptosis. Secondary lymphoid organs contain adhesion receptor ligands that allow long-term lymphocyte survival. Together these cytokine and adhesion receptors ensure the survival of quiescent lymphocytes.

Once a lymphocyte has been activated, it becomes less likely to undergo apoptosis unless it gets inappropriate or conflicting signals. The stronger the antigenic signals, the greater is its resistance to apoptosis. Activated lymphocytes also become more susceptible to killing through the TNF receptors and CD95. Thus, activation of T cells by antigen causes expression of CD95L, and they become sensitive to CD95-mediated killing. However, the CD95 pathway is normally blocked by stimulatory signals such as those transmitted through CD28 on T cells and CD40 on B cells. Once an antigen or co-stimulatory signal is lost, the activated cell will undergo CD95-induced apoptosis. This is why lymphocytes are eliminated at the end of the immune response. Lymphocyte activation, while temporarily protecting lymphocytes against apoptosis, will also ensure that these cells can eventually be removed.

Neural Regulation of Immunity

The central nervous and immune systems communicate extensively. The central nervous system communicates with the immune system through parasympathetic and sympathetic nerves and by soluble neurotransmitters. Neuroendocrine hormones such as corticotrophin-releasing factor and α-melanocyte-stimulating hormones, as well as some neurotransmitters, act on cells of the immune system to regulate cytokine balances. Conversely, cytokines and chemokines modulate central nervous system activities such as appetite, body temperature, and sleep behaviors.

Stress

Mental attitudes, especially stress, influence resistance to infectious diseases (Figure 20-17). Small bouts of stress are believed to enhance immune responses, but prolonged stress is detrimental. One obvious example occurs in shipping fever. This is a complex pneumonia of cattle primarily caused by several viral

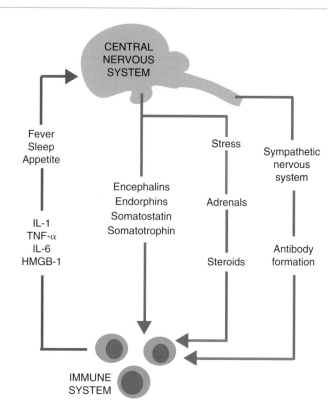

FIGURE 20-17 Some of the ways in which the central nervous system and the immune system interact.

respiratory pathogens with secondary infection by *Mannheimia hemolytica*. It develops in cattle that have been transported in confined spaces for long distances (and hence, many hours) with minimal feed and water and usually after rapid weaning and castration. The stress involved in the shipping process is sufficient to make these cattle highly susceptible to pneumonia. Stress can depress T cell responses, NK cell activity, IL-2 production, and expression of IL-2R on lymphocytes. Reduction in stress can have a reverse effect.

Stress can be due to something as simple as early weaning, which reduces IL-2 production in piglets. Stress in pregnant sows results in immunosuppression of their offspring. Thus confinement stress late in pregnancy results in the birth of piglets whose T and B cells have a reduced ability to respond to mitogens. Both morbidity and mortality are increased in piglets from stressed sows. A different form of stress may result from mammalian social structures. A dominance hierarchy regulates many mammalian populations. The rank of an individual animal within such a hierarchy influences its quality of life. Depending on the way the hierarchy is established, some members may be very highly stressed. Animals of high rank will be stressed if it requires constant fighting to maintain dominance. This occurs, for example, in wild dogs, lemurs, and mongooses. In hierarchies in which dominant members intimidate through psychological intimidation, such as in mice, rats, and many monkeys, low-ranking individuals may be stressed and immunosuppressed. If new individuals are introduced into a group, or a dominant animal loses its position, stresses occur as a result of the reorganization. In pigs, it has been shown that there is a relationship between social status and disease susceptibility. Thus morbidity and mortality among pigs challenged with pseudorabies virus were highest among subordinate animals. Dominant pigs had lymphocytes that were more responsive to virus antigens. This of course makes sense from an evolutionary point of view in that the least reproductively fit animals were more likely to die of disease, but it is difficult to separate cause and effect in this phenomenon. Were subordinate animals immunosuppressed because they were under stress as a result of their lowly status? Alternatively, could it be that those animals with a highly effective immune system were healthier and thus better able to reach high social status within the population? Were dominant animals better fed than subordinates? Certainly high levels of social stress are found in confined, crowded animal populations.

When the behavior of pigs is examined, they can be divided into two groups: aggressive animals that tend to fight other animals and then may flee rapidly, and passive animals that tend to cope with stress by withdrawing gradually from stressful situations. These differences are associated with different behavioral, physiological, and endocrine responses to stress. Aggressive pigs had higher in vitro and in vivo cell-mediated immune responses but lower humoral responses than passive animals. This suggests that there were differences in their relative Th1 and Th2 responses. However, when these animals were stressed, the aggressive ones showed a much greater drop in these responses than the passive animals. Differences in the way animals cope with stress are reflected in differences in immune reactivity.

This stress effect is mediated by two major pathways. One involves the autonomic nervous system producing its neurotransmitters, epinephrine, norepinephrine, and acetylcholine, and the other is the hypothalamic-pituitary-adrenal cortical axis producing glucocorticoids. Stress signals the brain to activate these pathways.

Autonomic Nervous System

Almost all primary and secondary lymphoid organs are supplied by nerves through the autonomic nervous system, and many cells of the immune system express receptors for the neurotransmitters released by both arms of the autonomic nervous system. This may occur either through adrenergic signals from the sympathetic nervous system or cholinergic signals from the parasympathetic nervous system.

The sympathetic nerves act through the neurotransmitter norepinephrine. They innervate the thymus, the splenic white pulp, and the lymph nodes. They influence blood flow, vascular permeability, and lymphocyte migration and differentiation. Surgical or chemical sympathectomy of the spleen enhances antibody production and can induce changes in the distribution of lymphocyte subpopulations. NK cell activity appears to be modulated directly by the hypothalamus through the splenic nerve. Autonomic nerves innervate Langerhans cells in

the skin. By releasing neuropeptides, these nerves can depress the antigen-presenting ability of these Langerhans cells. This might explain why "hot spots" in dogs worsen with anxiety. Denervated skin shows reduced inflammation after tissue damage and heals more slowly. Most important, sympathetic nerves innervate the adrenal medulla.

Immune cells have a complete set of cholinergic receptors. Efferent activity in the vagus nerve activates a cholinergic anti-inflammatory pathway. Vagal stimulation suppresses the systemic shock response to endotoxin by downregulating hepatic TNF-α synthesis. Activation of acetylcholine receptors on macrophages inhibits production of IL-1 and TNF-α.

The production of antimicrobial proteins such as the defensins is regulated by the autonomic nervous system, and stress reduces cutaneous epithelial antimicrobial activity. This appears to result from increased glucocorticoid and acetylcholine production.

Both adrenergic and cholinergic stimulation increase epinephrine signaling, leading to NF-κB activation in mononuclear cells. The sympathetic nervous system can alter the Th1/Th2 balance through the β-adrenergic receptor. Propranolol, a β-adrenergic antagonist, prevents the macrophage-mediated release of IL-10. Stimulation of sympathetic nerves enhances production of Th2 cytokines while inhibiting production of Th1 cytokines. Norepinephrine suppresses production of IL-6 and TNF-α.

CD4+, FoxP3 Treg cells play a central role in the regulation of immunity as described earlier in this chapter. If the sympathetic nervous system is experimentally destroyed by a selective neurotoxin, the numbers of spleen and lymph node Treg cells increase significantly. This effect is due to increased TGF-β production. Events such as stress that influence sympathetic nervous system function may well affect the number of cells available to regulate the immune system.

Hypothalamic-Pituitary-Adrenal Cortical Axis

The adrenal cortex is stimulated by adrenocorticotropic hormone (ACTH) from the pituitary under the influence of corticotrophin-releasing hormone from the hypothalamus. As a result, glucocorticoids are secreted and suppress T cell function by blocking the NF-κB pathway. IL-1 and IL-6 act on both the hypothalamus and the pituitary to increase ACTH production and subsequent cortisol release.

Neuropeptides and Lymphocytes

Cells of the immune system have receptors for neuropeptides such as the enkephalins and endorphins. These influence lymphocyte activity. The generation of cytotoxic T cells is enhanced by metenkephalin and β-endorphin, whereas α-endorphin suppresses antibody formation and β-endorphin reverses this suppressive effect. Other neuropeptides that influence the immune system include ACTH, oxytocin, vasoactive intestinal peptide, somatostatin, prolactin, and substance P. The brain may influence immune function by controlling neurotransmitter function or the autonomic nervous system.

Many neuropeptides such as vasoactive intestinal peptide and neurokinin-1 (NK-1) have a similar structure to the antimicrobial peptides so that they also have antimicrobial properties and may be involved in host defense. For example NK-1 (also known as substance P), not only mediates pain and inflammation but also has significant antibacterial activity. Other neuropeptides have similar effects. As a result, appropriate nervous stimulation can promote neuropeptide release that enhances local antibacterial activity. The pain associated with acute inflammation may well reflect local resistance to infection. Some neuropeptides can promote Th17 activity by triggering monocyte production of IL-23.

Immune responses are also modulated by environmental factors. Changes in day length (photoperiod) influence immune responses. These effects can be complex, but in general reduced day length appears to promote immune reactivity. The effect appears to be mediated through the hormone melatonin.

Finally, the innate immune system can influence nervous function. For example, cytokines such as IL-1, IL-6, and TNF-α induce "sickness behavior," including fever, fatigue, depressed activity, and excessive sleep. All these are closely associated with the systemic response to infectious agents and chronic inflammation (Chapter 6).

For sources of additional information, please visit http:// evolve.elsevier.com/tizard/immunology/

Immunity in the Fetus and Newborn

Key Points

- The immune system is fully formed at birth but has never been used. Hence all adaptive immune responses in the newborn are slow primary responses.
- Newborn mammals are temporarily protected against infection by transfer of immunoglobulins from their mother.
- Immunoglobulins are derived from the mother either by direct transfer across the placenta as in primates, or by ingestion of immunoglobulin-rich colostrum immediately after birth.
- Failure of this passive transfer may result in the newborn animal suffering from overwhelming infections.
- Milk provides a constant supply of immunoglobulin (immunoglobulin A [IgA] in most species) that helps protect the newborn against intestinal infections.
- Vaccination protocols in newborn mammals must take into account their inability to generate antibody responses in the presence of persistent maternal immunity.

When a mammal is born, it emerges from the sterile uterus into an environment where it is immediately exposed to a host of microorganisms. Its surfaces, such as the gastrointestinal tract, acquire a complex microbial flora within hours. If it is to survive, the newborn animal must be able to control this microbial invasion. In practice, the adaptive immune system takes some time to become fully functional, and innate mechanisms are responsible for the initial resistance to infection. In some species with a short gestation period, such as mice, the adaptive immune system may not even be fully developed at birth. In animals with a long gestation period, such as the domestic mammals, the adaptive immune system is fully developed at birth but cannot function at adult levels for several weeks. The complete development of adaptive immunity depends on antigenic stimulation. The proper development of B cells and B cell receptor (BCR) diversity requires clonal selection and antigen-driven cell multiplication (Chapter 15). Thus, newborn mammals are vulnerable to infection for the first few weeks of life. They need assistance in defending themselves at this time. This temporary help is provided by the mother in the form of antibodies and possibly T cells. The passive transfer of immunity from mother to newborn is essential for survival.

Development of the Immune System

The development of the immune system in the mammalian fetus follows a consistent pattern. The thymus is the first lymphoid organ to develop, followed closely by the secondary lymphoid organs. B cells appear soon after the development of the spleen and lymph nodes, but antibodies are not usually found until late in fetal life, if at all (Box 21-1). The ability of

the fetus to respond to antigens develops very rapidly after the lymphoid organs appear, but all antigens are not equally capable of stimulating fetal lymphoid tissue. The immune system develops in a series of steps, each step permitting the fetus to respond to more antigens. These steps are driven by a gradual increase in the use of gene conversion or somatic mutation to increase antibody diversity. The ability to mount cell-mediated immune responses develops at the same time as antibody production. T cell receptor (TCR) diversity is also limited in the fetus and neonate, and their cytokine production may be low. This may simply be due to their lack of exposure to foreign antigens.

Specific Animal Immune Systems

Foal The gestation period of the mare is about 340 days. Lymphocytes are seen first in the thymus at about 60 to 80 days postconception. They are found in the mesenteric lymph node and intestinal lamina propria at 90 days and in the spleen at 175 days. Blood lymphocytes appear at about 120 days. A few plasma cells may be seen at 240 days. Graft-versus-host disease, a cell-mediated response, has developed in immunodeficient foals transplanted with tissues from a 79-day-old fetus. The equine fetus can respond to coliphage T2 at 200 days postconception and to Venezuelan equine encephalitis virus at 230 days. Newborn foals have detectable quantities of IgM and IgG and occasionally IgG3 in their serum, but IgE production in the horse does not begin until foals are 9 to 11 months of age. Like other large herbivores, the foal has a well-developed ileal Peyer's patch that serves as a primary lymphoid organ and eventually involutes. Major B cell markers are expressed by 90 to 120 days gestation. *IGHM* and *IGLC* transcripts are expressed in liver, bone marrow, and spleen at all ages. The expression of essential B cell genes demonstrates that gene recombination and immunoglobulin class switching occur during equine fetal life. As a result, small amounts of IgM and IgG are detectable at birth. Despite this competence, B cell functions may be actively suppressed by regulatory T (Treg) cells during the first few months of a foal's life.

Calf Although the gestation period of the cow is 280 days, the fetal thymus is recognizable by 40 days postconception. The bone marrow and spleen appear at 55 days. Lymph nodes are found at 60 days, but Peyer's patches do not appear until 175 days (Figure 21-1). Blood lymphocytes are seen in fetal calves by day 45, IgM+ B cells by day 59, and IgG+ B cells by day 135. The time of appearance of serum antibodies depends on the sensitivity of the techniques used. It is therefore no accident that the earliest detectable immune responses are

☐ Box 21-1 | Immunity in Marsupials

Although the immune responses of marsupials are usually slower to develop than those of placental mammals, their immune system may develop remarkably early. The opossum, *Monodelphis domestica*, is born after only 15 days of gestation, and newborn opossums have neither immunological tissues nor organs. Nevertheless, young opossums can make antibodies by 7 days postpartum. During their first 7 days of life, they rely totally on passive immunity from their mother's milk and suckle permanently until 16 days. They suckle intermittently after that and are weaned at 60 days when absorption of antibodies across the intestinal epithelium ceases.

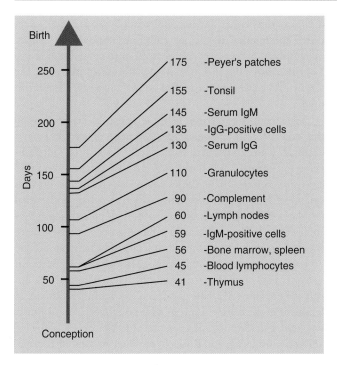

FIGURE 21-1 Progressive development of the immune system in the fetal calf.

The proportions of α/β and γ/δ T cells change as lambs mature. Thus, 1 month before birth, 18% of blood T cells are γ/δ positive. By 1 month after birth, they constitute 60% of blood T cells.

Piglet The gestation period of the sow is about 115 days. B cells appear in the yolk sac at day 20, progress to the fetal liver by day 30, and progress to the bone marrow by day 45. The first SWC3+ leukocytes can be found in the yolk sac and liver on day 17. The thymus develops by 40 days postconception and is colonized by two waves of T cell progenitors beginning on day 38. γ/δ T cells appear first in the thymus and in peripheral blood about 10 days later. α/β T cells develop by day 55, but their numbers grow rapidly so that they predominate late in gestation. The intestinal lymphoid tissues are devoid of T cells at birth. CD4+ T cells appear in the intestine at 2 weeks of age, and CD8+ T cells appear at 4 weeks. Their proliferation appears to be driven by the intestinal microflora. IgM+ B cells can be found in liver at 40 days, spleen by day 50, and bone marrow by day 60. Fetal piglets can produce antibodies to parvoviruses at 58 days and can reject allografts at about the same time. Blood lymphocytes can respond to mitogens between 48 and 54 days. Natural killer (NK) cell activity does not develop until several weeks after birth, although cells with an NK phenotype can be identified at 45 days' gestation in spleen and umbilical blood.

B cells are the first lymphocytes to appear in peripheral blood. The number of circulating B cells rises significantly between 70 and 80 days' gestation. The response to antigens in the fetus is of the IgM type, but newborn and fetal piglets also produce a small immunoglobulin that may not have light chains. It is interesting to note that B cells can be found in the thymus of newborn pigs.

The molecular development of the antibody repertoire has been followed in the developing pig. Thus, VDJ rearrangement is first seen in the fetal liver at day 30. However, the fetal piglet does not initially use all its *IGHV* or *IGHD* genes. Likewise, N-region addition does not occur before day 40, suggesting that the onset of terminal deoxynucleotidyltransferase activity occurs after that time. IgM, IgA, and IgG transcripts are present from 50 days in all major lymphoid organs. Piglets are thus born with relatively limited B cell diversity. B cell numbers increase for the first 4 weeks after birth, but their antigen-binding repertoire does not begin to expand until 4 to 6 weeks of age. Similar studies on rabbits have shown that the fetal immunoglobulin repertoire does not diversify until after birth, and this appears to be triggered by bacterial colonization of the gastrointestinal tract.

Puppy The gestation period of the bitch is about 60 days. The thymus differentiates between days 23 and 33, and fetal puppies can respond to phage φX174 by day 40. Blood lymphocytes can respond to phytohemagglutinin by 45 days postconception, and these cells can be detected in lymph nodes by 45 days and in the spleen by 55 days. The ability to reject allografts also develops at about day 45, although rejection is

those directed against viruses, using highly sensitive virus neutralization tests. Fetal calves have been reported to respond to rotavirus at 73 days, to parvovirus at 93 days, and to parainfluenza 3 virus at 120 days. Fetal blood lymphocytes can respond to mitogens between 75 and 80 days, but this ability is temporarily lost near the time of birth as a result of high serum steroid levels. T cell subpopulations are present in calves at levels comparable to adults, but B cell numbers increase significantly during the first 6 months after birth.

Lamb The gestation period of the ewe is about 145 days. Major histocompatibility complex (MHC) class I–positive cells can be detected by day 19, and MHC class II positive cells can be found by day 25. The thymus and lymph nodes are recognizable by 35 and 50 days postconception, respectively. Gut-associated follicles appear in the colon at 60 days, jejunal Peyer's patches at about days 75 to 80, and ileal Peyer's patches at days 110 to 115. Blood lymphocytes are seen in fetal lambs by day 32, and CD4+ and CD8+ cells appear in the thymus by 35 to 38 days. B cells are detectable at 48 days in the spleen and by that time have already begun to rearrange their *IGLV* genes. C3 receptors appear by day 120, but Fc receptors do not appear until the animal is born. Fetal liver lymphocytes can respond to phytohemagglutinin by 38 days. Lambs can produce antibodies to phage φX174 at day 41 and reject skin allografts by day 77. Some fetal lambs can produce antibodies to Akabane virus by as early as 50 days postconception. Antibodies to Cache Valley virus can be provoked by day 76, to SV40 virus by day 90, to T4 phage by day 105, to bluetongue virus by day 122, and to lymphocytic choriomeningitis virus by day 140.

slow at this stage, and fetal puppies may be made tolerant by intrauterine injection of an antigen before day 42. Thymic seeding of T cells to the secondary lymphoid organs and the development of humoral immune responses are therefore relatively late phenomena in the dog compared with the situation in the other domestic mammals.

Kitten Data on the ontogeny of the kitten are limited. Lymphocytes are seen in the blood at 25 days postconception. B cells are seen in the fetal liver at 42 days. Fetal kittens do make some IgG that can be detected in their serum before suckling, although this may be due to antibodies crossing the placenta.

Chick Stem cells arise in the yolk sac membrane and migrate to the thymus and bursa at 5 to 7 days' incubation. These cells differentiate within the bursa, and follicles develop by day 12. Lymphocytes with surface IgM may be detected in the bursa by day 14, and antibodies to keyhole limpet hemocyanin and to sheep erythrocytes may be produced by 16 and 18 days' incubation, respectively. Lymphocytes with surface IgY develop on day 21 around the time of hatching, whereas IgA-positive cells first appear in the intestine 3 to 7 days after hatching. Vaccination of 18-day embryonated eggs is commonly employed in the modern poultry industry. The major in ovo vaccine is against the Marek's disease herpesvirus, but others against Newcastle disease and coccidiosis are available, and those against infectious bronchitis and infectious bursal disease are under development.

The Immune System and Intrauterine Infection

Although a fetus is not totally defenseless, it is less capable than an adult of combating infection. Its adaptive immune system is not fully functional; as a result, some infections may be mild or unapparent in the mother but severe or lethal in the fetus. Examples include bluetongue, infectious bovine rhinotracheitis [bovine herpesvirus 1 (BHV-1)], bovine viral

diarrhea, rubella in humans, and toxoplasmosis. Fetal infections commonly trigger an immune response as shown by lymphoid hyperplasia and elevated immunoglobulin levels. For this reason the presence of any immunoglobulins in the serum of a newborn, unsuckled animal suggests infection in utero.

In general, the response to these viruses is determined by the state of immunological development of the fetus. For example, if live bluetongue virus vaccine, which is nonpathogenic for normal adult sheep, is given to pregnant ewes at 50 days postconception, it causes severe lesions in the nervous system of fetal lambs, including hydranencephaly and retinal dysplasia, whereas if it is given at 100 days postconception or to newborn lambs, only a mild inflammatory response is seen. Bluetongue vaccine virus given to fetal lambs between 50 and 70 days postconception may be isolated from lamb tissues for several weeks, but if given after 100 days, reisolation is not usually possible. Akabane virus acts in a similar fashion in lambs. If given before 30 to 36 days postconception, it causes congenital deformities. If given to older fetuses, it provokes antibody formation and is much less likely to cause malformations. Piglets that receive parvovirus before 55 days postconception will usually be aborted or stillborn. After 72 days, however, piglets will normally develop high levels of antibodies to the parvovirus and survive. Prenatal infection of calves with BHV-1 results in a fatal disease, in contrast to postnatal infections, which are relatively mild. The transition between these two types of infection occurs during the last month of pregnancy.

The effects of the timing of viral infection are well seen with bovine viral diarrhea virus (BVDV). If a cow is infected early in pregnancy (up to 50 days), she may abort. On the other hand, infections occurring between 50 and 120 days, before the fetus develops immune competence, lead to asymptomatic persistent infection because the calves develop tolerance to the virus (Figure 21-2). These calves are viremic yet, because of their tolerance, fail to make antibodies or T cells against the virus. Some of these calves may show minor neurologic problems and failure

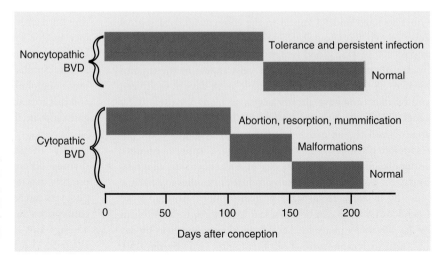

FIGURE 21-2 The effects of bovine viral diarrhea virus infection on development of the fetal calf depend on the timing of infection. As with adult animals, there is considerable individual variation in resistance to infection. Persistently infected calves may show minor neurological problems or failure to thrive.

to thrive, but many are clinically normal. If the cow is infected with BVDV between 100 and 180 days postconception, calves may be born with severe malformations involving the central nervous system and eye, as well as jaw defects, atrophy, and growth retardation. Vaccines containing modified live BVDV may have a similar effect if administered at the same time. Calves infected after 150 to 180 days' gestation are usually clinically normal.

Since they are specifically tolerant to BVDV, persistently infected calves shed large quantities of virus in body secretions and excretions and so act as a major source of infectious virus. The persistently infected calves may also produce neutralizing antibodies if immunized with a live BVDV vaccine of a serotype different from that of the persistent virus. Despite this, the original virus will persist in these animals. These persistently infected calves grow slowly and often die of opportunistic infections such as pneumonia before reaching adulthood. (BVDV has a tropism for lymphocytes and is immunosuppressive.) Their neutrophil phagocytic and bactericidal functions are also depressed.

BVD viruses occur in two distinct biotypes: cytopathic and noncytopathic. (The name derives from their behavior in cell culture, not their pathogenicity in animals.) Noncytopathic strains do not trigger type I interferon (IFN) production and therefore can survive in calves and cause persistent infections. Cytopathic strains induce IFN production and cannot cause persistent infection. These cytopathic strains, however, do cause mucosal disease (MD), a severe enteric disease leading to profuse diarrhea and death (Figure 21-3). Mucosal disease develops as a result of a mutation in a nonstructural viral gene that changes the BVDV biotype from noncytopathic to cytopathic while the animal fails to produce neutralizing antibodies or T cells. The cytopathic strain can spread between tolerant animals and lead to a severe mucosal disease outbreak. Both cytopathic and noncytopathic viruses can be isolated from these animals. Recombination may also occur between persistent noncytopathic strains and cytopathic strains in vaccines and lead to MD outbreaks. Although some of the lesions in MD are attributable to the direct pathogenic effects of BVDV, glomerulonephritis and other immune complex–mediated lesions also develop. The reasons for this are unclear but may reflect superinfection or the production of non-neutralizing antibodies. Because persistently infected calves can reach adulthood and breed, it is possible for BVD infection to persist indefinitely within carrier animals and their progeny. Epidemiological studies suggest that between 0.4% and 1.7% of cattle in the United States are persistently infected in this way.

Immune Response of Newborn Mammals

After developing in the sterile environment of the uterus, newborn mammals first encounter a diverse population of microbes at the time of birth. They must be able to combat

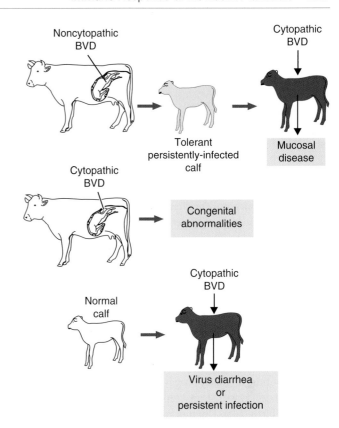

FIGURE 21-3 The relationship of mucosal disease to persistent infection with bovine viral diarrhea virus (BVDV) in tolerant cattle. Calves persistently infected with noncytopathic BVDV and then superinfected with cytopathic BVDV develop mucosal disease.

any attempted invasion immediately. The young mammals are capable of mounting both innate and adaptive immune responses at birth. However, any adaptive immune response mounted by a newborn must be a primary response with a prolonged lag period and low concentrations of antibodies. Innate immune responses are therefore critical for survival in the first weeks of life.

Role of the Intestinal Microflora

The development of the newborn immune system is largely driven by the intestinal microflora (Chapter 22). In its absence, "germ-free" mammals fail to fully develop their mucosal lymphoid tissues. The commensal flora generates a complex mixture of pathogen-associated molecular patterns (PAMPs) that act through epithelial cell toll-like receptors (TLRs). Likewise, microbial antigens are taken up by dendritic cells and presented to CD4+ T cells. These signals collectively promote the functional development of the immune system. The intestinal microflora also plays a key role in determining any Th1 or Th2 bias in immune function. This is the basis of the "hygiene hypothesis," the idea that the development of allergies is influenced by microbial exposure early in life (Chapter 28).

Innate Immunity

Newborns can produce a diverse array of antimicrobial molecules, including lectins such as the pentraxins and collectins, peptides such as the defensins, and lactoferrin and lysozyme. Surfactant proteins A and D as well as β-defensin 1 and TLR4 are produced in the preterm lamb lung. As a result, invaders can be killed relatively efficiently. TLRs are present and functional in the newborn. In the fetal pig, neutrophils at 90 days postconception are fully capable of phagocytosing bacteria such as *Staphylococcus aureus*. However, they are deficient in bactericidal activity, which only reaches adult levels 10 days later. Near birth, the phagocytic and bactericidal capacity of these neutrophils declines as a result of increased steroid levels. The neutrophils of newborn foals move relatively slowly compared with their dams. The serum of newborn mammals, however, is deficient in some complement components, resulting in a poor opsonic activity. Serum C3 increases rapidly after birth in newborn piglets and reaches adult levels by 14 days of age.

After birth, macrophages are able to support the growth of some viruses that macrophages from adult animals do not. Virucidal activity is gradually acquired. Changes also occur in the distribution of macrophages. Newborn piglets have few pulmonary intravascular macrophages. During the first few days after birth, blood monocytes adhere to the pulmonary capillary endothelium and differentiate into macrophages. In the newborn piglet, 75% of particles are removed from the blood by the liver and spleen, but by 2 months of age, 75% are removed by the lungs. The alveolar macrophages of newborn pigs have poor phagocytic activity, but this is effectively acquired by 7 days.

Newborn calves have fewer NK cells than adults, but these respond more strongly to simulation with interleukin-2 (IL-2) or IL-15 and are more cytotoxic! Age-dependent changes occur in the level of acute-phase proteins in newborn calves. Serum amyloid A (SAA), lipopolysaccharide-binding protein, haptoglobin and α_1-acid glycoprotein are present in high concentrations immediately after birth but gradually decline by 21 days. In developing piglets, IL-8 and tumor necrosis factor-α (TNF-α) production by blood monocytes increased significantly during the postnatal period, whereas monocyte production of IL-1β was unchanged.

Adaptive Immunity

The early development of the adaptive immune system has been especially well analyzed in newborn foals since some are highly susceptible to lethal *Rhodococcus equi* infection (Box 21-2). Newborn mammals, including foals, mount adaptive responses skewed toward Th2 rather than Th1 cells. Thus they favor antibody responses over cell-mediated immunity. This imbalance is a result of the delayed development of IL-12-producing DC1 cells and the activities of IL-4 and IL-13 from DC2 cells. Mononuclear cells from newborn foals are unable to express IFN-γ. Their Th2 cells rapidly differentiate, whereas neonatal Th1 cells are slow to develop. IFN-γ may cause

□ **Box 21-2** | *Rhodococcus equi*

Rhodococcus equi is a ubiquitous bacterium found in soil and bedding. Newborn foals are exposed to this bacterium soon after birth. Most foals then mount a protective immune response, but a minority are susceptible to this infection. They develop severe pneumonia at a time when maternal antibodies are waning. Multiple defects have been identified in both the innate and adaptive immune systems of neonatal foals. Foal neutrophils have a phagocytic ability similar to that in adult horses, but the opsonic activity of their serum is low. The killing activity of these cells is also reduced since they mount a weak respiratory burst. Dendritic cell function is also defective, possibly owing to decreased expression of MHC class II molecules. Bacterial glycolipid antigens are normally presented to antigen-sensitive T cells through CD1b, but reduced CD1b expression in foals may also increase their susceptibility

Because this disease is associated with declining maternal antibody levels, it is possible that antibodies are critical in determining resistance or susceptibility to *R. equi*. Foals generally lack IgA on their mucosal surfaces for the first 28 days of life. Likewise their synthesis of IgG4 tends to be reduced at the time of disease onset. While production of IL-8, IL-10, IL-12, and IL-23 in newborns is comparable to that in older foals, IFN-γ and IL-6 production is impaired. On stimulation with *R. equi*, foal mononuclear cells increase their production of IFN-γ, IL-6, and IL-23, but the size of this increase is much less in cells from neonates than in those from older foals. In prospective studies, foals destined to develop *R. equi* pneumonia were born with fewer leukocytes, fewer segmented neutrophils, a lower proportion of CD4+ T cells, and a lower CD4/CD8 ratio than normal foals. It has long been accepted that a Th1 response is essential for protection against *R. equi*. Since it is an intracellular organism, activation of phagocytic cells by IFN-γ is required for its elimination. Unfortunately, foals younger than 3 to 4 months have reduced IFN-γ expression compared with adults. It is likely that in susceptible foals, a combination of multiple immune defects permits this otherwise innocuous organism to cause disease.

placental damage, so this skewing is not accidental. IFN-γ production gradually increases through the first 6 months of life to reach adult levels within a year when the acquired responses revert to the balanced adult pattern.

During the first 3 months of life, puppies have a higher lymphocyte count than adult dogs. Much of the difference is due to CD21+ B cells. The proportion of puppy CD8+ T cells is low at birth but gradually climbs to reach adult proportions. A similar gradual increase in lymphocyte numbers is seen in newborn kittens. Thymic involution begins at around 6 months of age in both dogs and cats.

Unless additional immunological assistance is provided, however, organisms that present little threat to an adult may kill newborn mammals. This immunological assistance is provided by antibodies transferred from the mother to her offspring through colostrum. Maternal lymphocytes may also be transferred to the fetus through the placenta or to newborn mammals through colostrum.

Transfer of Immunity from Mother to Offspring

The route by which maternal antibodies reach the fetus is determined by the structure of the placenta. In humans and other primates, the placenta is hemochorial; that is, the maternal blood is in direct contact with the trophoblast. This type of placenta allows maternal IgG but not IgM, IgA, or IgE to transfer directly to the fetus. Maternal IgG can enter the fetal bloodstream, and the newborn human infant has circulating IgG levels comparable to those of its mother.

Dogs and cats have an endotheliochorial placenta in which the chorionic epithelium is in contact with the endothelium of the maternal capillaries. In these species, 5% to 10% of IgG is directly transferred from the mother to the puppy or kitten, but most must be obtained through colostrum.

The placenta of ruminants is syndesmochorial; that is, the chorionic epithelium is in direct contact with uterine tissues, whereas the placenta of horses and pigs is epitheliochorial and the fetal chorionic epithelium is in contact with intact uterine epithelium. In mammals with both these types of placenta, the transplacental passage of immunoglobulin molecules is totally prevented. Thus their newborns are entirely dependent on antibodies received through the colostrum.

Secretion and Composition of Colostrum and Milk

Colostrum contains the accumulated secretions of the mammary gland over the last few weeks of pregnancy together with proteins actively transferred from the bloodstream under the influence of estrogens and progesterone. Therefore, it is rich in IgG and IgA and contains some IgM and IgE (Table 21-1). The predominant immunoglobulin in the colostrum of most of the major domestic mammals is IgG, which may account for 65% to 90% of its total antibody content; IgA and the other immunoglobulins are usually minor but significant components. As lactation progresses and colostrum changes to milk, differences among species emerge. In primates, IgA predominates in both colostrum and milk. In pigs and horses, IgG predominates in colostrum, but its concentration drops rapidly as lactation proceeds so that IgA predominates in milk. In ruminants, IgG1 is the predominant immunoglobulin in both milk and colostrum (Figure 21-4).

All of the IgG, most of the IgM, and about half of the IgA in bovine colostrum are derived by transfer from the bloodstream. In milk, in contrast, only 30% of the IgG and 10% of the IgA are so derived; the rest is produced locally by lymphoid tissue within the udder. Colostrum also contains secretory component both in the free form and bound to IgA. Colostrum is rich in cytokines. For example, bovine colostrum contains significant amounts of IL-1β, IL-6, TNF-α, and IFN-γ. These cytokines may promote the development of the immune system in the young animal.

Absorption of Colostrum

Young mammals that suckle soon after birth ingest colostrum. Thus naturally suckled calves ingest an average of 2 L of colostrum, although individual calves may ingest as much as 6 L. In these young mammals, protease activity in the digestive tract is low and is further reduced by trypsin inhibitors in colostrum. Therefore, colostral proteins are not degraded but can reach the small intestine intact. Colostral immunoglobulins also bind to FcRn receptors on intestinal epithelial cells. FcRn receptors are also expressed on mammary gland ductal and acinar cells and are probably involved in the active secretion of IgG into

◻ Table 21-1 | Colostral and Milk Immunoglobulin Levels in Domestic Animals

SPECIES	FLUID	IMMUNOGLOBULIN (mg/dL)				
		IGA	IGM	IGG	IGG3	IGG6
Horse	Colostrum	500-1500	100-350	1500-5000	500-2500	50-150
	Milk	50-100	5-10	20-50	5-20	0
Cow	Colostrum	100-700	300-1300	2400-8000		
	Milk	10-50	10-20	50-750		
Ewe	Colostrum	100-700	400-1200	4000-6000		
	Milk	5-12	0-7	60-100		
Sow	Colostrum	950-1050	250-320	3000-7000		
Bitch	Colostrum	500-2200	14-57	120-300		
	Milk	110-620	10-54	1-3		
Queen	Colostrum	150-340	47-58	4400-3250		
	Milk	240-620	0	100-440		

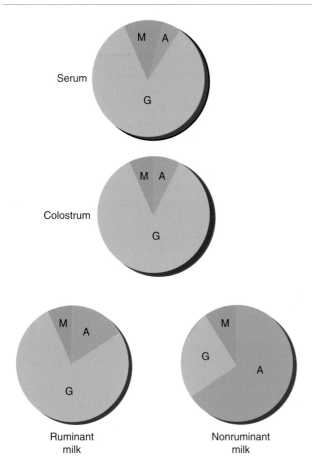

FIGURE 21-4 Relative concentrations of the major immunoglobulin classes in serum, colostrum, and the milk of ruminants and nonruminants.

colostrum. Once bound to FcRn, immunoglobulin molecules are taken up by intestinal epithelial cells and transferred to the lacteals and possibly the intestinal capillaries. Eventually the absorbed immunoglobulin reaches the bloodstream, and newborn mammals obtain a massive transfusion of maternal immunoglobulins.

Newborn mammals differ in the selectivity and duration of intestinal permeability. In the horse and pig, protein absorption is selective. IgG and IgM are preferentially absorbed, whereas IgA mainly remains in the intestine. In ruminants, immunoglobulin absorption is unselective, and all classes are absorbed, although IgA is gradually excreted. Young pigs and probably other young mammals have large amounts of free secretory component in their intestine. Colostral IgA and, to a lesser extent, IgM can bind this secretory component, which may then inhibit their absorption. The duration of intestinal permeability varies among species and immunoglobulin classes. In general, permeability is highest immediately after birth and declines after about 6 hours, perhaps because of the replacement of FcRn-bearing intestinal epithelial cells by cells that do not express this receptor. As a rule, absorption of all immunoglobulin classes drop to a very low level after about 24 hours. Feeding colostrum tends to hasten this closure, whereas a delay

in feeding results in a slight delay in closure (up to 33 hours). In piglets, the ability to absorb immunoglobulins may be retained for up to 4 days if milk products are withheld. The presence of the mother may be associated with increased immunoglobulin absorption. Thus calves fed measured amounts of colostrum in the presence of the mother will absorb more immunoglobulins than calves fed the same amount in her absence. In laboratory studies in which measured amounts of colostrum are fed, there is a great variation (25% to 35%) in the quantity of immunoglobulins absorbed. Management should ensure that foals or calves ingest at least 1 L of colostrum within 6 hours of birth.

Unsuckled mammals normally have very low levels of immunoglobulins in their serum. The successful absorption of colostral immunoglobulins immediately supplies them with serum IgG at a level approaching that found in adults (Figure 21-5). Peak serum immunoglobulin levels are normally reached between 12 and 24 hours after birth. After absorption ceases, these passively acquired antibodies decline through normal metabolic processes. The rate of decline differs among immunoglobulin classes, and the time taken to decline to nonprotective levels depends on their initial concentration.

As intestinal absorption is taking place, a simultaneous proteinuria may occur. This is due to intestinal absorption of very small proteins such as β-lactoglobulin that can be excreted in the urine. In addition, the glomeruli of newborn mammals are permeable to macromolecules. Thus the urine of neonatal ruminants contains intact immunoglobulin molecules. This proteinuria ceases spontaneously with the termination of intestinal absorption. In another example, urine from puppies collected 24 hours after birth contains relatively large amounts of IgG, IgM, and IgA. The amount excreted declines over time so that IgM is undetectable by 14 days, although there may still be significant amounts of IgG and IgA present. It is believed that the immunoglobulins enter the urine because glomerular filtration is insufficient. Over the first 2 weeks of life, the puppy's glomeruli mature and acquire the ability to filter macromolecules.

The secretions of the mammary gland gradually change from colostrum to milk. Ruminant milk is rich in IgG1 and IgA. Nonruminant milk is rich in IgA. For the first few weeks in life, while protease activity is low, these immunoglobulins can be found throughout the intestine and in the feces of young mammals. As the digestive ability of the intestine increases, eventually only secretory IgA molecules remain intact. The amount of IgA provided by milk can be large; for instance, a 3-week-old piglet may receive 1.6 g daily from sow's milk.

Although IgE is present in mare's milk and transmitted to the suckling foal, its level in foal serum drops to a very low level by 6 weeks of age. IgE synthesis by foals begins at about 9 to 11 months of age, and at that time a pattern of relatively high or low IgE levels is established. These levels are not correlated with the levels resulting from suckling. Thus maternal IgE levels have waned long before the onset of IgE synthesis in the foal, and there is no evidence of maternal priming. Total

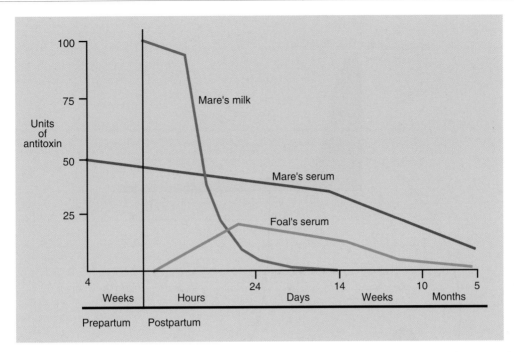

FIGURE 21-5 *Clostridium perfringens* antitoxin levels in serum, colostrum, and milk of six pony mares and in the serum of their foals from birth to 5 months.

(After Jeffcott LB. Studies on passive immunity in the foal. 1. γ-globulin and antibody variations associated with the maternal transfer of immunity and the onset of active immunity. *J Comp Pathol* 84:93–101, 1974.)

levels of IgE in young horses (and their susceptibility to allergies) are most likely mainly determined by genetic factors. IgE is also transferred in sheep colostrum. Colostral IgE levels are significantly higher than in ewe's serum. IgE is absent from presuckling lamb serum but can rise to adult levels by 2 days after birth. It then declines steadily over several weeks.

The IgG transferred through a mother's colostrum represents the results of her history of antigen exposure, B cell responses, and somatic mutation. This maternal IgG in effect represents the immunological experiences of the mother. Maternal antibodies act on the immune system of the newborn during a critical imprinting period and appear to exert a lifelong influence on the newborn's immune development. This influence may be stronger than some genetic predispositions! Thus maternal antibodies can enhance the newborn immune responses to some antigens and suppress their responses to others. They may also influence Th1/Th2 polarization and the subsequent development of allergies.

Failure of Passive Transfer

The absorption of IgG from colostrum is required for the protection of a newborn against septicemic disease. The continuous intake of IgA or IgG1 from milk is required for protection against enteric disease (Figure 21-6). Failure of these processes predisposes a young animal to infection.

There are three major reasons for failure of passive transfer through colostrum. First, the mother may produce insufficient or poor-quality colostrum (production failure). Second, there may be sufficient colostrum produced but inadequate intake by the newborn animal (ingestion failure). Third, there may be a failure of absorption from the intestine despite an adequate intake of colostrum (absorption failure).

Production Failure

Since colostrum represents the accumulated secretions of the udder in late pregnancy, premature births may mean that insufficient colostrum has accumulated. Valuable colostrum may also be lost from mammals as a result of premature lactation or excessive dripping before birth. Colostral IgG levels also vary among individuals, with up to 28% of mares producing low-quality colostrum. It is not possible to assess colostral quality simply by looking at it. Its IgG content should be assessed using a colostrometer (a modified hydrometer) to measure its specific gravity. This is normally in the range of 1.060 to 1.085, equivalent to an IgG concentration of 3000 to 8500 mg/dL. Colostrum with an IgG level of less than 3000 mg/dL may be inadequate to protect a foal, and feeding supplemental, high-quality colostrum may become necessary.

Ingestion Failure

In sheep or pigs, an inadequate intake may result from multiple births simply because the amount of colostrum produced does not rise in proportion to the number of newborn. It may be due to poor mothering, an important problem among young,

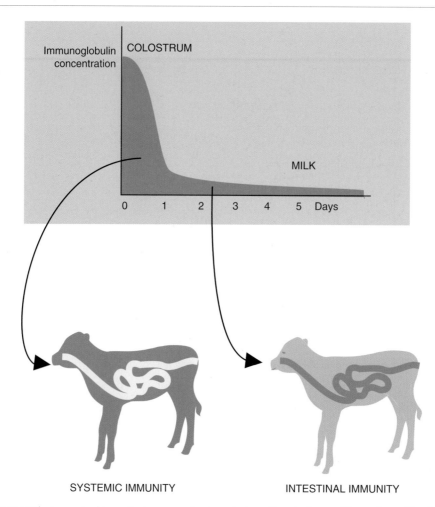

SYSTEMIC IMMUNITY   INTESTINAL IMMUNITY

FIGURE 21-6 Colostrum intake is required to protect young animals against septicemic disease. The prolonged intake of milk is necessary to ensure protection of the gastrointestinal tract against enteric infection.

inexperienced mothers. It also may be due to weakness in the newborn, to a poor suckling drive, or to physical problems such as damaged teats or jaw defects.

Absorption Failure

Failure of intestinal absorption is a major cause for concern in any species. It is especially important in horses not only because of the value of many foals but also because even with good husbandry, about 25% of newborn foals fail to absorb sufficient quantities of immunoglobulins. Alpacas also appear to experience a disproportionate number of cases of failure of passive transfer. Foals require serum IgG concentrations of at least 800 mg/dL 18 to 24 hours after receiving colostrum to ensure protection. Foals that have less IgG than this are at increased risk for infection. If their IgG level fails to reach 400 mg/dL, severe infections are assured (Figure 21-7).

Diagnosis of Failure of Passive Transfer

The success of passive transfer cannot be evaluated in a foal until 18 to 24 hours after birth, when antibody

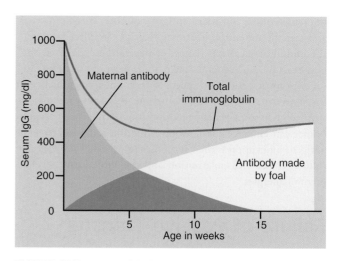

FIGURE 21-7 Immunoglobulin levels in newborn serum during the first 15 weeks of life indicating the relative contributions of maternal antibody and antibody synthesized by the newborn animal.

□ Table 21-2 | Tests for Failure of Passive Transfer in Horses

TEST EMPLOYED	RELATIVE SENSITIVITY (FALSE NEGATIVES)	RELATIVE SPECIFICITY (FALSE POSITIVES)
Glutaraldehyde coagulation	100	59
Latex agglutination	72	79
Snap test	90	79
Turbidimetric immunoassay	81	86
Infrared spectroscopy	93	97

From Crisman MV and Scarratt WK, Immunodeficiency disorders in horses. Vet Clin North Am Equine Pract. 2008, 24:299–310.

absorption is essentially complete. Several assays for serum immunoglobulins are available (Table 21-2). The most rapid and economic procedure is the zinc sulfate turbidity test, which involves mixing a zinc sulfate solution with foal serum. Zinc sulfate makes globulins insoluble. In total failure of transfer, the reaction mixture remains clear. In sera with an IgG level of more than 400 mg/dL, the mixture becomes cloudy. As an alternative to visual inspection, the optical density of the mixtures can be read in a spectrophotometer and the IgG concentration read off a standard curve. Other similar techniques include precipitation by glutaraldehyde or by sodium sulfite.

Single radial immunodiffusion is a more accurate method in that it is both quantitative and specific for IgG. As described in Chapter 41, known standards are compared with the test serum by measuring the diameter of precipitation produced in agar gel containing an antiserum to equine IgG. A diagnosis of failure of passive transfer is made in foals if IgG levels are less than 400 mg/dL and partial failure of passive transfer if IgG levels are between 400 and 800 mg/dL. Unfortunately radial immunodiffusion is slow. It takes 18 to 24 hours to give a result and is thus impractical when a rapid diagnosis is required.

A third method of measuring IgG levels is by use of a latex agglutination test. The latex particles are coated with anti-equine IgG. In the presence of IgG, they agglutinate. This test can be performed in about 10 minutes using either whole foal blood or serum. It appears to be reliable and rapid but is somewhat insensitive.

It is also possible to use a semiquantitative membrane-filter enzyme-linked immunosorbent assay (ELISA) test to measure IgG in a foal's serum. The color intensity of the reaction on the test filter is compared with color calibration spots. A variant technique uses a dipstick ELISA. Less satisfactory techniques include serum protein electrophoresis and refractometry. (Refractometry is an effective and practical test in calves but is less reliable in foals, in which the wide range of values leads to inaccuracy.)

Management of Failure of Passive Transfer

In foals, an IgG concentration higher than 800 mg/dL is preferred, but foals with immunoglobulin levels higher than 400 mg/dL will generally remain healthy and do not require treatment. About 75% of foals with IgG levels between 200 and 400 mg/dL will also remain healthy. However, they should be watched and treated with antibiotics at the first signs of bacterial infection. Any foals with total failure of passive transfer or foals younger than 3 weeks with partial failure of passive transfer should be treated. Foals with plasma IgG concentrations less than 200 mg/dL, foals that have not nursed within 6 hours of birth, and foals that have received colostrum with IgG of less than 1000 mg/dL (specific gravity less than 1.050) should receive additional colostrum. Two to 3 L of good-quality colostrum (IgG of more than 7000 mg/dL) should be given by bottle or nasogastric tube in three or four doses at hourly intervals. The colostrum must be free of antibodies to the foal's erythrocytes (Chapter 29). Colostrum may be obtained from mares that have more than is needed for their own young. It can be stored frozen at −15° to −20° C for up to 1 year. If stored colostrum is unavailable, fresh colostrum from primiparous mares can be used. If colostrum is not available, serum or plasma may be administered orally. A large volume (up to 9 L) may be required since serum IgG is not well absorbed and its concentration is much less than that found in colostrum.

In foals that are older than 15 hours, oral absorption ceases, and an intravenous plasma infusion must be given. Ideally the dose to be used can be calculated to attain an IgG level of at least 400 mg/dL. Frozen horse plasma is available commercially, although this may not contain antibodies against local pathogens. Alternatively, the plasma may be obtained from local donors. Blood should be collected aseptically with heparin or sodium citrate. The plasma is collected after the erythrocytes settle and is stored frozen until used. The plasma must be prechecked for antierythrocyte antibody and must be free of bacterial contamination. The transfusion should be given slowly while the foal is monitored for untoward reactions. All foals receiving supplemental colostrum or plasma should have their IgG levels rechecked 12 to 24 hours later.

Considerations similar to those described previously apply to failure of passive transfer in the calf. Calves with serum IgG of less than 1000 mg/dL at 24 to 48 hours of age have mortality rates more than twice those of calves with higher IgG levels. A minimum of 150 to 200 g of colostral IgG is required for optimal passive transfer. Three liters of colostrum should be administered by oropharyngeal tube to calves within 2 hours of birth. Substantially larger quantities of IgG must be administered after 2 hours to achieve optimal protection. Commercially available colostrum may be enriched in specific antibodies to protect the calf against potential pathogens such as K99 *Escherichia coli*, rotaviruses, and coronaviruses, the major causes of calf diarrhea.

Colostral transfer of immunity is essential for the survival of young mammals, but it may also cause disease. If a mother becomes immunized against the red cells of her fetus, colostral antibodies may cause erythrocyte destruction in the newborn, a condition called hemolytic disease (Chapter 29).

Cell-Mediated Immunity and Colostrum

Colostrum is full of lymphocytes, but milk is not. For example, sow colostrum contains between 1×10^5 and 1×10^6 lymphocytes/mL. Of these lymphocytes, 70% to 80% are T cells. The CD4/CD8 ratio is approximately 0.57, which is lower than the ratio in blood (~2.5). Bovine colostrum also contains up to 10^6 lymphocytes/mL, about half of which are T cells. Colostral lymphocytes may survive up to 36 hours in the intestine of newborn calves, and some may penetrate the epithelium of Peyer's patches and reach the lacteal ducts or the mesenteric lymph nodes. Within 2 hours after receiving colostrum that contained labeled cells, maternal lymphocytes appeared in the bloodstream of piglets. It is possible that cell-mediated immunity is transferred to newborn mammals in this way. Piglets that had received these colostral cells showed enhanced responses to mitogens compared with control mammals. Cell-containing and cell-free colostrum have been compared for their ability to protect calves against enteropathic *E. coli*. The calves receiving colostral cells excreted significantly fewer bacteria than the mammals receiving cell-free colostrum. The concentration of IgA- and IgM-specific antibodies against *E. coli* in the serum of neonatal calves was higher in those that received colostral cells than in those that did not. The calves that received colostral cells had better responses to the mitogen concanavalin A and to foreign antigens such as sheep erythrocytes. The mechanisms of this protective effect are unclear.

The CD8+ T cells in bovine colostrum can produce large quantities of IFN-γ, which may influence the early development of Th1 responses in neonatal calves. Thus ingestion of maternal colostral cells appears to accelerate the development of activated calf lymphocytes. The monocytes of calves that received colostral cells were more capable of processing and presenting antigens.

Transfer of cell-mediated immunity by bovine milk lymphocytes has been demonstrated. Pregnant cows were vaccinated against BVDV. Blood lymphocytes from calves that received cell-free colostrum from these cows were unresponsive to BVDV antigen. In contrast, lymphocytes from calves that received colostrum containing live cells showed enhanced responses to BVDV antigen at 1 and 2 days after colostral ingestion. The lymphocytes of calves that received whole colostrum showed enhanced mitogenic responses to maternal and unrelated leukocytes after 24 hours. They also responded to the nonspecific stimulant staphylococcal enterotoxin B. In contrast, the lymphocytes of calves that received acellular colostrum did not. Clearly, ingestion of maternal colostral leukocytes immediately after birth stimulates the development of the neonatal immune system.

Development of Adaptive Immunity in Neonatal Mammals

Local Immunity

The intestinal lymphoid tissues of neonatal mammals respond rapidly to ingested antigens. For example, calves vaccinated orally with coronavirus vaccines at birth are resistant to virulent coronavirus within 3 to 9 days. Likewise, piglets vaccinated orally 3 days after birth with transmissible gastroenteritis virus (TGE) vaccines develop neutralizing antibodies in the intestine 5 to 14 days later. Much of this early resistance is attributable to innate production of IFN-α/β, but there is an early intestinal IgM response that switches to IgA by 2 weeks. In the young animal, the IgA response appears earlier and reaches adult levels well before the other immunoglobulins. This rapid response of the unprimed intestinal tract is also seen in germ-free pigs. In these mammals, antibody synthesis in the intestine can be detected by 4 days after infection with *E. coli*.

Systemic Immunity

The antibodies acquired by a young animal as a result of ingesting its mother's colostrum, maternal antibodies, will inhibit the ability of the newborn to mount its own immune response (Figure 21-8). As a result, very young animals

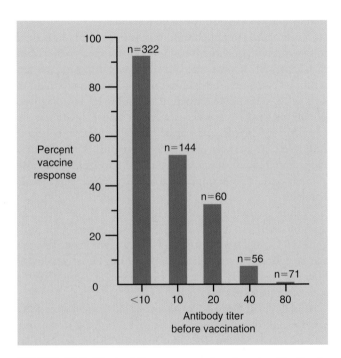

FIGURE 21-8 Effect of the presence of maternal antibodies to canine parvovirus in 653 puppies on their response to a modified live parvovirus vaccine. The prevaccination antibody titer profoundly inhibits the response of the puppies to the vaccine.

(From Carmichael LE: Immunization strategies in puppies—why failures? *Compend Contin Educ Pract Vet* 5:1043–1054, 1983.)

are unable to respond to active immunization using vaccines. This inhibition is B cell specific, and T cell responses are largely unaffected. It depends on the relative concentrations of maternal antibody and the dose of vaccine administered.

Several different mechanisms have been suggested as mediating this suppression. One of the simplest is the rapid neutralization of live viral vaccines by the maternal antibody. This would prevent viral replication and provide insufficient antigen to prime B cells. However, data from human infants and domestic mammals indicate that sufficient antigen is present to prime T cells. Likewise, this mechanism could not account for inhibition of the immune response to nonliving vaccines.

A second proposed mechanism suggests that the inhibition results from antibodies binding to B cell Fc receptors (CD32) and blocking BCR signaling (Figure 20-10). However, studies of mice whose Fc receptors have been deleted (FcR knockout mice) have shown that the ability of maternal antibodies to inhibit antibody responses is unaffected. This clearly cannot be the mechanism involved. Likewise, the suggestion that maternal antibodies bind antigen, which is then removed by Fc-dependent phagocytosis, cannot be correct.

A third suggested mechanism is that maternal antibodies simply mask the epitopes on vaccine antigens, preventing their recognition by the animal's B cells. This suggestion is compatible with the selective inhibition of B cell responses, the lack of inhibition of T cell responses, and the evidence that, at least in humans and mice, high doses of antigen can overcome maternal immunity. Thus for a given vaccine dose, an immune response can be elicited only when maternal antibody titers fall below a critical threshold.

In the absence of maternal antibodies, the newborn animal is able to make antibodies soon after birth. For example, if calves fail to suckle and are therefore hypogammaglobulinemic, they begin to make their own antibodies by about 1 week of age. In calves that have suckled and thus possess maternal antibodies, antibody synthesis does not commence until about 4 weeks of age. Likewise, colostrum-deprived piglets respond well to pseudorabies virus by 2 days after birth, but if they have suckled, antibody production does not begin until 5 to 6 weeks after birth. Colostrum-deprived lambs synthesize IgG1 at 1 week and IgG2 by 3 to 4 weeks. In colostrum-fed lambs, however, IgG2 synthesis does not occur until 5 to 6 weeks.

Passively acquired maternal antibodies not only protect newborns before their immune system becomes fully functional but also may shape the B cell repertoire of the offspring. Mice pups nursed by mothers producing antibodies to vesicular stomatitis virus developed higher endogenous antibody titers of this specificity as they matured. As a result, these pups developed higher titers of protective antibody when infected as adults. Passively acquired maternal antibodies have a very significant influence on the way in which a newborn's immune system develops.

Vaccination of Young Animals

Because maternal antibodies inhibit neonatal immunoglobulin synthesis, they prevent the successful vaccination of young animals. This inhibition may persist for many months, its length depending on the amount of antibodies transferred and the half-life of the immunoglobulins involved. This problem can be illustrated using the example of vaccination of puppies against canine distemper.

Maternal antibodies, absorbed from the puppy's intestine, reach maximal levels in serum by 12 to 24 hours after birth. Their levels then decline slowly through normal protein catabolism. The catabolic rate of proteins is exponential and is expressed as a half-life. The half-life of antibodies to distemper and canine infectious hepatitis is 8.4 days, and the half-life of antibodies to feline panleukopenia is 9.5 days. Experience has shown that, *on average*, the level of maternal antibodies to distemper in puppies declines to insignificant levels by about 10 to 12 weeks, although this may range from 6 to 16 weeks. In a population of puppies, the proportion of nonimmune animals therefore increases gradually from a very few or none at birth to almost all at 10 to 12 weeks. Consequently, very few newborn puppies can be successfully vaccinated, but most can be protected by 10 to 12 weeks. Rarely, a puppy may be 15 or 16 weeks old before it can be successfully vaccinated. If virus diseases were not so common, it would be sufficient to delay vaccination until all puppies were about 12 weeks old, when success could be almost guaranteed. In practice, a delay of this type means that an increasing proportion of puppies, fully susceptible to disease, would be without immune protection—an unacceptable situation. Nor is it feasible to vaccinate all puppies repeatedly at short intervals from birth to 12 weeks, a procedure that would ensure almost complete protection; therefore, a compromise must be reached.

The earliest recommended age to vaccinate a puppy or kitten with a reasonable expectation of success is at 8 weeks. Colostrum-deprived orphan pups may be vaccinated at 2 weeks of age. Essential vaccines for normal puppies should include distemper, two adenovirus, and parvovirus vaccines. In puppies a second dose should be given 3 to 4 weeks after the first and a third at 14 to 16 weeks of age. Rabies is an essential vaccine that should be given at 14 to 16 weeks. In kittens an appropriate protocol would be to use three doses of the essential vaccines (viral rhinotracheitis [herpesvirus 1], calicivirus, and panleukopenia) at 8 to 9 weeks, 3 to 4 weeks later, and at 14 to 16 weeks; feline leukemia vaccine can be given at 8 weeks and 3 to 4 weeks later; and rabies vaccine can be given at 8 to 12 weeks depending on the type of vaccine used (Figure 21-9).

Similar considerations apply when vaccinating large farm animals. The prime factor influencing the duration of maternal immunity is the level of antibodies in the mother's colostrum. Thus in foals, maternal antibodies to tetanus toxin can persist for 6 months and antibodies to equine arteritis virus for as long as 8 months. Antibodies to BVDV may persist for up to 9 months in calves. The half-lives of maternal antibodies against equine influenza and equine arteritis virus antigens in the foal are 32 to

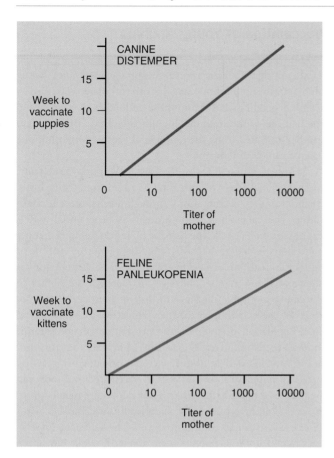

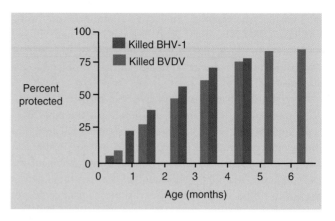

FIGURE 21-10 Effectiveness to two inactivated viral vaccines in calves between birth and 6 months of age.

(Data courtesy Dr. R.J. Schultz.)

FIGURE 21-9 Nomographs showing the relationship between the antibody titer of the mother and the age at which to vaccinate her offspring with modified live virus vaccine.

(Data from Scott FW, Csiza CK, Gillespie JH: Maternally derived immunity to feline panleukopenia. *J Am Vet Med Assoc* 156:439–453, 1970 [FPL]; and Baker JA, Robson DS, Gillespie JH, et al: A nomograph that depicts the age to vaccinate puppies for distemper. *Cornell Vet* 49:158–167, 1959 [CD].)

39 days. As in puppies, a young foal may have nonprotective levels of maternal antibodies long before it can be vaccinated. Maternal antibodies, even at low levels, effectively block immune responses in young foals and calves, so premature vaccination may be ineffective. The effectiveness of vaccines increases progressively after the first 6 months of life (Figure 21-10). A safe rule is that calves and foals should be vaccinated no earlier than 3 to 4 months of age followed by one or two revaccinations at 4-week intervals. The precise schedule will depend on the vaccine used and the species to be vaccinated. Animals vaccinated before 6 months of age should always be revaccinated at 6 months or after weaning to ensure protection.

Some live recombinant vaccines such as canarypox-vectored distemper in dogs or influenza in horses appear to be able to effectively prime young animals in the face of significant maternal immunity. DNA vaccines against pseudorabies also appear to be effective in priming cell-mediated responses in the face of maternal immunity, whereas a DNA vaccine against bovine respiratory syncytial virus vaccine is not. Thus the ability of DNA vaccines to overcome maternal immunity varies among species and infections.

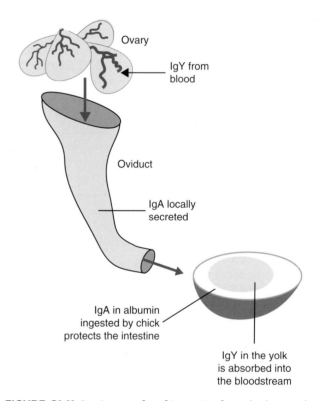

FIGURE 21-11 Passive transfer of immunity from the hen to the chick.

Passive Immunity in the Chick

Newly hatched birds emerge from the sterile environment of the egg and, like mammals, require temporary immunological assistance. Serum immunoglobulins are actively transported from the hen's serum to the yolk while the egg is still in the ovary. IgY in the fluid phase of egg yolk is therefore found at levels equal to or greater than those in hen serum. In addition, as the fertilized ovum passes down the oviduct, IgM and IgA from oviduct secretions are acquired with the albumin (Figure 21-11). As the chick embryo develops in ovo, it absorbs the yolk

IgY, which then appears in its circulation. At the same time, the IgM and IgA from the albumin diffuse into the amniotic fluid and are swallowed by the embryo. Thus when a chick hatches, it possesses IgY in its serum and IgM and IgA in its intestine. The newly hatched chick does not absorb all its yolk sac antibodies until about 24 hours after hatching.

These maternal antibodies effectively prevent successful vaccination until they disappear between 10 and 20 days after hatching.

For sources of additional information, please visit http:// evolve.elsevier.com/tizard/immunology/

Immunity at Body Surfaces

Key Points

- Because it is essential to prevent microbial invasion of the body, many of its immune defenses are located on surfaces such as those in the respiratory and digestive tracts.
- Surface defenses exclude invaders by preventing them from penetrating surface epithelia.
- γ/δ T cells are T cells that are specialized for epithelial defense.
- Immunoglobulin A (IgA), the major immunoglobulin produced on surfaces, prevents microbial invasion by blocking pathogen adherence.
- IgE is a backup surface defense. It triggers local acute inflammation in response to parasites that have succeeded in evading IgA.
- The normal intestine does not mount an inflammatory response to the intestinal microflora unless these organisms succeed in penetrating the intestinal wall.
- The body responds in a limited fashion to antigens in food. However, unless allergies develop, this is rarely noticed.

Although mammals possess an extensive array of innate and adaptive defense mechanisms within tissues, it is at their surfaces that invading microorganisms are first encountered and largely repelled or destroyed (Figure 22-1). Although the skin is the most obvious of these surfaces, it in fact represents only a small fraction of the area of the body exposed to the exterior. The areas of the mucous membranes of the intestine and respiratory tracts are at least 200 times larger. While the immune systems ensure that the interior of the body remains free of microbial invaders, it is not possible to keep the surfaces of the body sterile. Indeed a vast number of microorganisms live in a symbiotic relationship on body surfaces. These organisms are not a major threat to healthy individuals. Many are commensals whose presence is beneficial. This complex microflora is present in large numbers on all the body's surfaces, including the skin, gastrointestinal tract, respiratory tract, and urogenital tract.

The Body's Microflora

The immune system functions on the basis that microorganisms that invade the body must be eliminated. Organisms that penetrate the epithelial barriers are promptly detected, attacked, and destroyed by innate and adaptive mechanisms. The situation is different outside the body. Almost every surface is teeming with a large stable population of microorganisms collectively called the microflora or microbiota. This is an example of symbiosis—the living together in close union of very dissimilar organisms. Animal surfaces are a stable, nutrient-rich ecosystem where microbes can thrive. Because animals also benefit from the presence of these symbiotic microbes, as, for example, in the bovine rumen, these organisms can be considered commensals.

The Superorganism

Of the microbes that live on the skin and mucosal surfaces, the largest such community is found in the intestine. The intestinal microflora consists of more than 1000 bacterial species in humans, with each individual housing about 160 species and about a hundred trillion (10^{14}) bacterial cells. (Thus nine out of ten cells in the human body are bacterial. The figure for domestic mammals is unlikely to be very different!) Given the large number of bacterial species involved, they contain about 100 times more genes than the human genome. Because of the enormous number of microorganisms involved, the concept has emerged that animals together with their microflora form "superorganisms" in which enormous numbers of genes act together to promote survival and the whole is regulated by the immune system. In addition to considering the bacteria as part of the animal microbiome, it is also apparent that many viruses live within the body, collectively constituting a virome of unknown significance.

The presence of large stable populations of symbiotic bacteria implies that their elimination is neither feasible nor desirable. The immune system must therefore adapt to the presence of this microflora while at the same time retaining its ability to fight pathogens. The first bacteria to colonize body surfaces are acquired by a newborn animal from its mother at the time of birth. Within days, these are followed by many different environmentally acquired bacteria, generally as a result of chance microbial encounters. These organisms compete and adapt to their environment so that over the first months of life, their composition gradually changes to the stable adult-like microflora. The size and complexity of this microflora is greatest in the gastrointestinal tract. Most intestinal microbes are bacteria (Gram-positive and Gram-negative, facultative aerobic and anaerobic), but there are some archaea, a few eukaryotes,

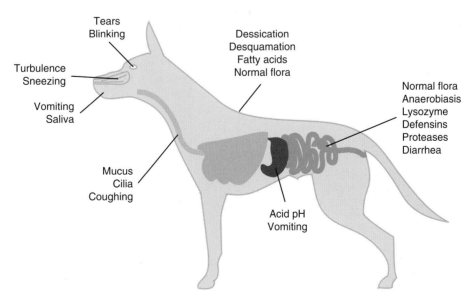

FIGURE 22-1 The wide diversity of innate surface protection mechanisms.

and many viruses and bacteriophages. The composition of the microflora varies among surfaces and even among locations on those surfaces. Additionally, the composition of the intestinal microflora differs among individuals and depends on their diet. The bacterial density is relatively low in the stomach but rises in the rumen, the distal small intestine, and especially the colon (Figure 22-2). The rumen mainly contains anaerobic bacteria, with some protozoa and fungi. In the large intestine, the microflora mainly consists of strict anaerobes. It has been estimated that this microbial population can eventually reach a density of 10^{12} organisms per gram of intestinal contents.

As commensals, the intestinal microflora helps to break down plant cell walls and digest complex carbohydrates such as cellulose and other plant polysaccharides. These commensals synthesize some essential vitamins and, by maintaining an appropriate balance within the microbial population, restrict the growth of potential pathogens. In addition, they play a

central role in the development and regulation of the immune system.

Although essential for the health and proper functioning of the animal body, it must not be assumed that the normal microflora does not present a threat to an animal. Microbes can only be excluded by continual vigilance. Many members of the microflora can be considered pathobionts, which retain the potential to cause disease. Remember too that the decomposition of a dead animal is initiated by its own microflora around the time of death immediately after the failure of its immune defenses.

Controlling the Microflora

Animals and their microflora have coevolved as a result of the benefits gained by each partner, but the huge mass of commensal bacteria within the intestine is a potential threat to host integrity and must be closely watched by the immune system. There are two obvious threats facing any animal. The first is the critical importance of ensuring that the normal microflora is kept in its place and prevented from any attempt at invasion. The second is that the microflora and the molecules it releases might trigger innate responses such as inflammation. If these organisms can invade, and especially if they cause inappropriate inflammation, bad things will happen.

Exclusion of Commensals The first cellular barrier to microbial invasion consists of intestinal epithelial cells (enterocytes). These cells maintain barrier integrity by having tight junctions between cells and a coating of attached mucins that form a glycocalyx, and they produce multiple antimicrobial peptides. Specialized intestinal epithelial cells called Paneth cells express toll-like receptors (TLRs) (Figure 22-3). When triggered by the microflora, they secrete multiple antimicrobial peptides. These enteric defensins, known as cryptdins, accumulate within intestinal crypts and achieve very

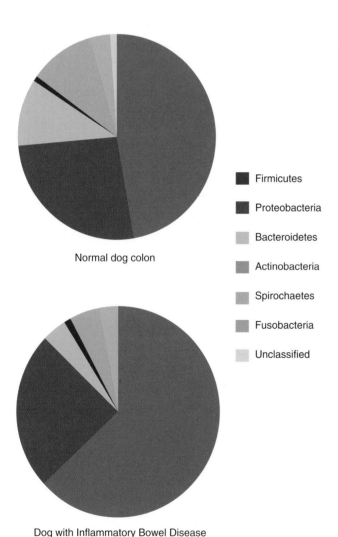

Firmicutes

Proteobacteria

Bacteroidetes

Actinobacteria

Spirochaetes

Fusobacteria

Unclassified

Normal dog colon

Dog with Inflammatory Bowel Disease

FIGURE 22-2 The enormous diversity of the gut flora in the dog is well seen in this comparison of the composition of the colon microflora in normal dogs and dogs with inflammatory bowel disease.

(Courtesy Dr. Panagiotis Xenoulis.)

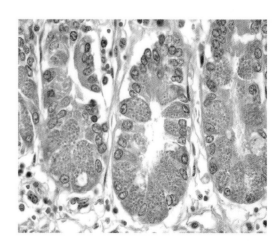

FIGURE 22-3 Paneth cells from the intestine of a horse. The cells are filled with large eosinophilic granules and are the major source of intestinal defensins. Original magnification ×60.

(Courtesy Dr. Brian Porter.)

high local concentrations. They prevent commensals from entering the crypt space and so protect enterocytes from invasion. In cattle, expression of cryptdin genes occurs throughout the small intestine and colon. These cryptdins are secreted as active molecules, as opposed to the human and mouse molecules that are secreted as inactive precursors and subsequently activated by trypsin within the intestine. Parasitic or other intestinal infections may increase production of α- and β-defensins. Cryptdins serve a barrier function since they are found in highest concentrations in the fluid layer closest to the epithelium and therefore reduce microbial contact with enterocytes. The cryptdin mixture selectively kills some bacterial species and as a result regulates the precise composition of the microflora.

The gastrointestinal mucus layer is also critical to the exclusion of both commensals and pathogens. The mucus layer consists of a gel made of mucins, glycoproteins, and lipids that prevents bacteria from contacting the epithelium. This mucus acts as a lubricant, blocks chemical insults, and can capture and then expel pathogens. The mucus forms an inner and outer layer. The inner layer next to the enterocytes consists of firm mucus rich in defensins and lysozyme and contains few bacteria. The looser mucus in the intestinal lumen is composed primarily of mucins produced by intestinal goblet cells. Many bacteria are embedded in this mucus, where it prevents their washout. Its thickness and composition vary, but it tends to be thickest where the microflora is abundant.

The epithelial cell brush border is also covered by a glycocalyx—a layer of acidic polysaccharides and glycoproteins that binds to the apical surface of the cells and serves as a protective barrier while still permitting the absorption of nutrients.

Suppression of Inflammation   As pointed out, constant inflammation is undesirable and must somehow be suppressed. The huge mass of bacteria in the intestine would be expected to produce plentiful amounts of bacteria-associated molecular patterns, and these would be expected to bind pattern-recognition receptors. Intestinal epithelial cells express pattern-recognition receptors (PRRs) such as the TLRs and NLRs. These can bind microbial-associated molecular patterns and in response trigger the production of antimicrobial peptides and cytokines but not inflammation. This is because the PRRs are not expressed on the luminal side of the epithelia, where they would normally come into contact with commensals. They are located at the base of the cells and at intracellular locations. Thus they are only triggered after bacteria penetrate the epithelial barrier. By preventing microbial invasion, they also prevent the development of inflammation within the intestinal epithelium.

Some commensal bacteria actively suppress inflammation in the intestinal wall. For example, commensal bacteria such as *Lactobacillus* and *Bacteroides* species inhibit the innate signaling pathways triggered by TLRs and NLRs. A common commensal, *Bacteroides thetaiotamicron* inhibits NF-κB signaling by blocking the migration of one of its subunits out of the nucleus, and intestinal lactobacilli prevent degradation of the inhibitor I-κB.

Other mechanisms such as desensitization of TLRs to bacterial PAMPs and bacterial stimulation of IL-10 and IL-2 production by regulatory Treg cells also help minimize inflammation. IL-10 inhibits the TLR-MyD88 pathway, whereas IL-2 inhibits TLR-independent pathways. Mice deficient in either IL-10 or IL-2 develop severe colitis.

Despite its defenses, however, the epithelial barrier is somewhat porous to microbial products. As a result, there is a constant interplay between the intestinal microflora and the mucosal immune system. In effect, the mass of the intestinal microflora provide a constant source of microbial products that keeps both the innate and acquired immune responses in a state of constant readiness. The intestinal microflora is especially necessary for the differentiation and recruitment of T cells since it acts as a massive source of antigenic stimulation. As a result, intestinal lymphoid tissues must be relatively unresponsive to the microflora while still being responsive to potential pathogens. Under steady-state conditions, the intestinal immune system must recognize commensal bacteria but respond in a highly regulated manner somewhat short of full activation. It is likely that the development of some forms of inflammatory bowel disease in humans and other animals is due to dysfunction in these regulatory pathways.

Although most intestinal bacteria probably suppress inflammation, others may have an opposite effect. Thus some unculturable segmented filamentous bacteria (SFBs) trigger Th17 responses in mice and promote innate responses in the intestine. In the absence of these SFBs, mice mount weaker immunoglobulin A (IgA) responses and poorer intestinal T cell responses. Unlike most intestinal bacteria that are excluded by the mucus layer and have minimal contact with the enterocytes, the SFBs attach directly to the epithelium of the ileum and Peyer's patches and can be readily sampled by dendritic cells. SFBs have been detected in humans, rodents, chickens, and fish, so they may play an important role in shaping the development of the intestinal immune system.

Benefits of the Microflora

Exclusion of Pathogens   The intestinal microflora acts competitively against potential invaders and supplements the physical defenses of this system (Figure 22-4). By occupying and exploiting the intestinal microenvironment, commensals block subsequent colonization by pathogenic bacteria. (It is, for example, possible to block *Salmonella* species colonization of the chicken intestine by administering an appropriate mixture of commensal bacteria to birds.) The microflora determines local environmental conditions by, for example, keeping the pH and oxygen tension low. The microflora is also influenced by the diet; as a result, the intestine of milk-fed animals is colonized largely by lactobacilli, which produce bacteriostatic lactic and butyric acids. These acids inhibit colonization by potential pathogens such as *Escherichia coli*, so young animals suckled naturally tend to have fewer digestive

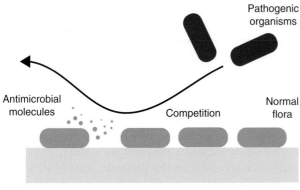

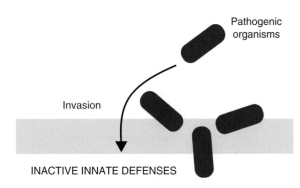

FIGURE 22-4 The role of the normal bacterial flora in excluding pathogens from body surfaces by competition. In the absence of a normal flora, the invading organisms face no competition and can readily colonize and invade surfaces.

disturbances than animals weaned early in life. Genetically identical pigs housed in an outdoor environment, an indoor environment, or experimental isolators have had their intestinal flora studied. It has been found that 90% of the bacteria within the intestine of the outdoor group were Firmicutes, especially lactobacilli. In contrast, Firmicutes constituted less than 70% of the intestinal flora in the indoor group and about 50% in the isolated pigs. Pigs from cleaner environments had smaller proportions of lactobacilli. There is a strong negative correlation between the level of lactobacilli and the level of pathogens in the intestine. These differences also influence the expression of immune system genes. For example, animals raised in isolation express more genes involved in inflammatory immune responses such as type I interferons. In contrast, genes associated with T cell function are expressed more highly in the pigs housed outdoors.

Development of Lymphoid Organs The immune system fails to develop properly in some germ-free animals. Thus pigs or mice that are microbiologically sterile have fewer and smaller Peyer's patches, smaller mesenteric lymph nodes, and fewer cells in their lamina propria than animals with a complete microflora. The natural development of the Peyer's patches in

the pig, and the appendix in rabbits depends upon the stimulation provided by the intestinal microflora. In the absence of this microflora, their enterocytes express fewer TLRs and MHC class II molecules. Intestinal lymphocyte numbers are reduced, and they are less cytotoxic. Systemic defects are also apparent. There are fewer CD4+ T cells in the spleen, they have fewer and smaller germinal centers as a result of reduced B cell numbers, and their immunoglobulin levels are only about 2% of normal.

Although the initial development of the mucosal lymphoid organs occurs before birth, the complete maturation of the mucosal immune system and the recruitment of IgA-producing B cells and activated T cells occurs after birth in response to signals from the intestinal microflora. These signals modulate the crosstalk between enterocytes and dendritic cells. In general the intestinal microflora stimulate the production of secretory IgA and the production of all three helper T cell subsets as well as Treg cells.

Regulation of B Cell Function Although the microflora are separated by the glycocalyx from direct contact with enterocytes, intestinal dendritic cells can extend their processes into the intestinal lumen and capture commensal bacteria. These bacteria can persist within the dendritic cells for several days while the cells carry them into the mucosa and the mesenteric lymph nodes and present them to B cells. This induces a local IgA response that also serves to block mucosal penetration by these commensals. In addition, some commensal bacteria are taken up by specialized antigen capturing M cells, penetrate the Peyer's patches, and become resident within the tissues. Although most of these invading bacteria are killed by macrophages, some are also presented to B cells. The repertoire of these B cells is regulated by the interaction between the intestinal microflora and the intestinal-associated lymphoid tissues. The B cells produce IgA, which may modify the composition of the intestinal microflora. The commensals are prevented from breaching the mucosal barrier by the ongoing IgA response, and the mesenteric lymph nodes form an additional barrier that prevents the commensals from reaching the systemic immune system. It is likely that a similar type of local IgA response occurs against food antigens. As a result, there is more immune activity in the intestine than in all other lymphoid tissues combined. It has been estimated, for example, that more than 80% of the body's activated B cells are found in the intestine.

Many dendritic cells in the intestinal lymphoid tissues produce retinoic acid, a metabolite of dietary vitamin A. The ability to synthesize retinoic acid is a property of many mucosal immune cells, and this appears to be a central regulator of mucosal immunity and homeostasis. Retinoic acid induces the expression of the intestinal homing receptors α4β7 and CCR9 on T cells and B cells. In association with transforming growth factor-β (TGF-β), it enhances T cell proliferation and cytotoxicity and is especially important in promoting Th2 and Treg differentiation in the intestine and in the homing of IgA+ B cells to mucosal surfaces (Chapter 38). Retinoic acid, therefore, normally suppresses Th1 and Th17 responses and favors tolerance to food antigens.

Regulation of T Cell Function Molecules produced by commensal bacteria can influence the functions of all the major T cell subsets. For example, Treg cells producing IL-10 are present in the intestine. Several commensal bacteria such as *Bacteroides fragilis* and some clostridia seem especially effective in inducing these FoxP3+, IL-10-producing T cells. The bacterial molecule polysaccharide A (PSA) is key to this process. PSA suppresses proinflammatory cytokine responses in the intestine and inhibits lymphocyte infiltration. Treg populations are reduced in germ-free mice.

Th17 cell development in the intestine is also affected by the microflora (Figure 22-5). Germ-free mice are deficient in IL-17. Segmented filamentous bacteria drive T cell development and stimulate Th17 production. SFBs also promote germinal center development, IgA production, and recruitment of intraepithelial lymphocytes. Because it is believed that Th17 cells may originate from T reg precursors, it is suggested that the microflora regulates the Th17-Treg switch.

Dysbiosis and the Hygiene Hypothesis

Changes in the composition of the intestinal microflora have been implicated in the development of allergies. The hygiene hypothesis suggests that a lack of exposure to certain commensal bacteria early in life affects the development of the immune system and increases an individual's chances of developing allergic diseases. In support of this, it has been shown that children who develop allergic disease have different intestinal microflora than children who do not. Studies on piglets exposed to differing levels of intestinal colonization have shown that the complexity of the intestinal flora influences gene expression in the immune system. Animals with a limited intestinal flora expressed more genes involved in inflammation. Conversely, piglets with a more diverse intestinal flora expressed more genes related to T cell function. Alterations in the intestinal microflora also influence the development of autoimmune diseases such as rheumatoid arthritis, some mouse models of autoimmune arthritis, ankylosing spondylitis, insulin-dependent diabetes mellitus, and experimental autoimmune encephalitis (Chapter 35).

Mucosal Lymphoid Tissues

Because of the importance of preventing invasion through the mucosa, these surfaces contain large amounts of lymphoid tissue. Mucosal lymphoid tissues fall into two groups: sites where antigens are processed and immune responses are initiated (inductive sites), and sites where antibodies and cell-mediated responses are generated (effector sites).

Inductive Sites

The mucosa-associated lymphoid tissues (MALTs) possess the three cell types required to initiate immune responses: T cells, B cells, and dendritic cells. These tissues include lymphoid tissues in the eyelids, nasal mucosa, tonsils, pharynx, tongue, and palate (collectively called Waldeyer's ring); Peyer's patches; solitary lymphoid nodules; the appendix in the intestine; and numerous lymphoid nodules in the lung. These lymphoid tissues are known by their acronyms. Thus GALT (gut-associated lymphoid tissue) is the collective term for all the lymphoid nodules, Peyer's patches, and individual lymphocytes found in the intestinal walls. Similarly, BALT is the acronym used for the bronchus-associated lymphoid tissue in the lungs. These organized lymphoid tissues, unlike lymph nodes, do not react to foreign antigens delivered through afferent lymph but rather sample them directly from the surface.

The tonsils are especially important in inducing immunity on mucosal surfaces. Some organisms, however, can overcome the defenses of the tonsils and use them as a portal of entry into the body. For example, pathogens such as bovine herpesvirus-1, *Mannheimia hemolytica*, *Streptococcus suis,* and *Mycobacterium tuberculosis* can persist indefinitely within the tonsils.

The surface of the intestine is covered by a layer of enterocytes that form intercellular tight junctions and which thus form an effective barrier to both microbes and macromolecules (Figure 22-6). (Molecules larger than about 2 kDa are excluded.) Obviously, some aggressive invasive bacteria may damage this barrier and trigger local inflammatory and immune responses. There are two alternative routes by which organisms

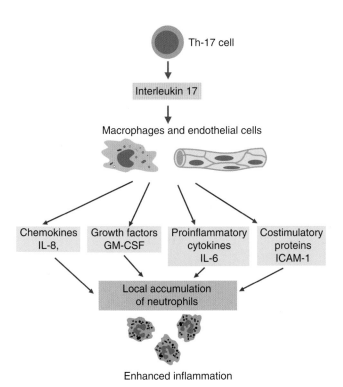

FIGURE 22-5 The role of Th17 cells in attracting neutrophils and promoting inflammation.

and macromolecules can penetrate the intact intestinal wall and be directed toward the intestinal lymphoid tissues. One route involves penetrating specialized epithelial cells (M cells) found in the epithelium directly over aggregates of lymphoid tissue or Peyer's patches; the other involves dendritic cells that reside in the submucosa but extend their cytoplasmic processes between the enterocytes into the intestinal lumen. The tight junctions remain intact, but antigen samples can enter within the dendritic cell cytosol. This route provides a mechanism whereby noninvasive bacteria and macromolecules can be sampled and presented to nearby T cells.

Peyer's patches are the largest of the mucosal lymphoid tissues. A newborn calf normally has about 100 Peyer's patches, and these may cover as much as half of the ileal surface. Collectively, therefore, the intestine contains more lymphocytes than the spleen. In ruminants and pigs, there are two types of Peyer's patch that differ in location, structure, and functions. The ileocecal Peyer's patches of ruminants are primary lymphoid organs, whereas the jejunal Peyer's patches are secondary lymphoid organs (Figure 12-8). In lambs, the ileocecal patches increase in size from birth to 6 months of age and then regress, leaving only a small scar. In contrast, the jejunal patches persist throughout adult life and continue to play a major role in intestinal defense. Both types of Peyer's patch consist of masses of lymphocytes arranged in follicles and covered with an epithelium that contains M cells. M cells are specialized epithelial cells involved in antigen transportation. They have microfolds (M) rather than microvilli on their surface (Figure 22-7). The mucus layer tends to thin out over Peyer's patches so that the M cells protrude into the lumen. M cells phagocytose the macromolecules and microbes they encounter, but rather than destroy them, they transport the antigens to their underlying lymphoid tissue. M cells may transport soluble macromolecules such as IgA, small particles, and even whole organisms. (Some pathogens, such as salmonellae, *Yersinia* and *Listeria*

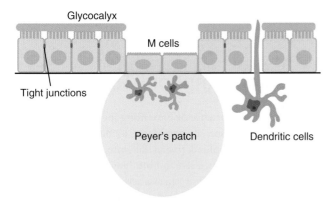

FIGURE 22-6 The epithelial defenses of the gut and the ways by which microbial antigens can enter the body.

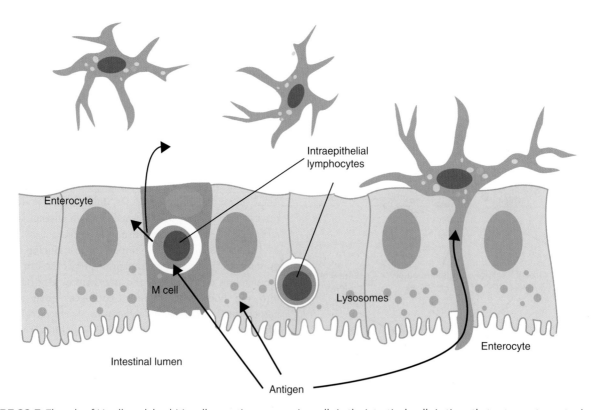

FIGURE 22-7 The role of M cells and dendritic cells as antigen-processing cells in the intestinal wall. Antigen that enters enterocytes is usually rapidly degraded in lysosomes. Antigen that enters M cells is not degraded. It may be presented directly to intraepithelial lymphocytes within the M cell or, alternatively, permitted to pass along the intercellular space to the tissue fluid. From here, it will be carried to the draining lymph nodes.

species, *M. tuberculosis,* and the reoviruses may take advantage of the M cells and use them to gain access to the body.) The proportion of M cells in the follicle-associated epithelium varies from 10% in humans and mice to 50% in rabbits and to 100% in the terminal ileum of pigs and calves.

Effector Sites

Although Peyer's patches are full of lymphocytes, most IgA is produced in diffuse lymphoid nodules and in isolated plasma cells scattered throughout the walls of the intestine, in bronchi, in salivary glands, and in the gallbladder. These cells constitute at least 80% of all plasma cells in the body, and more IgA is produced than all other immunoglobulin classes combined.

B Cells The intestinal wall contains B cells that divide repeatedly in response to antigen. Some of these responding B cells migrate to regional lymph nodes and into intestinal lymphatics, from which they reach the thoracic duct and enter the bloodstream. These circulating IgA-positive B cells have an affinity for all body surfaces. As a result, they colonize not only in the intestinal tract but also the respiratory tract, urogenital tract, and mammary gland. Thus antigen priming at one location will permit antibodies to be synthesized and secondary responses to occur at locations remote from the priming site (Figure 22-8). The movement of IgA-positive B cells from the intestine to the mammary gland is especially important since it provides a route by which antibodies directed against intestinal pathogens can be transferred to the newborn through milk. Oral administration of antigen to a pregnant animal will thus result in the appearance of IgA antibodies in its milk. In this way, antibodies directed against intestinal pathogens will flood the intestine of the newborn animal. T cells originating within the Peyer's patches also home specifically to

the intestinal mucosa by using specialized vascular adhesive molecules. For example, mucosal addressin cell-adhesion molecule-1 (MAdCAM-1) is an adhesion molecule expressed on the high endothelial venules of Peyer's patches and on venules in intestinal lamina propria and the mammary gland. Its ligand is the lymphocyte integrin $\alpha 4/\beta 7$. B and T cells that express this integrin migrate preferentially to the intestine and the mammary gland.

T Cells Both α/β and γ/δ T cells are found in the intestinal wall but in two very different locations. Thus α/β T cells are scattered throughout the lamina propria and in Peyer's patches. γ/δ T cells, in contrast, are situated between enterocytes immediately below the mucosal surface, where they are known as intraepithelial lymphocytes (IELs) (Figure 22-9). Their location suggests that they play an early, critical role in the defense of the mucosa. IELs regulate host-microbial interactions at the intestinal mucosal surface and are critical components in preventing invasion by the commensal microbiota.

γ/δ IELs originate in the bone marrow and mature within cryptopatches, clusters of cells located just under the enterocytes. Cryptopatches each contain several hundred immature T cells. Located between epithelial cells, IELs can recognize antigens directly, possibly through the TLR-MyD88 pathway as well as their T cell receptors (TCRs), and secrete cytokines such as interferon-γ (IFN-γ) in response. The interferon in turn, stimulates macrophages and nearby enterocytes to secrete protective nitric oxide.

There are major differences in the properties of IELs between species. Five percent of IELs in humans, 50% in mice, and up to 90% in ruminants carry γ/δ TCR. A high proportion of the IELs are CD8+ (85% in humans, 77% in pigs, 24% in sheep). These CD8 molecules are α/α homodimers, in contrast to the CD8 α/β heterodimers found on conventional α/β T

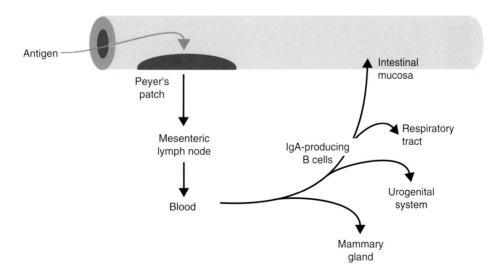

FIGURE 22-8 When stimulated by antigen, IgA-producing B cells are produced in inductive sites, such as the Peyer's patches. They then leave the intestine and circulate in the bloodstream. They all eventually settle on other surfaces, such as the lung, the mammary gland, and other regions of the gastrointestinal tract effector sites. This transfer of antibody-producing cells in the mammary gland ensures that milk contains IgA antibodies directed against intestinal pathogens.

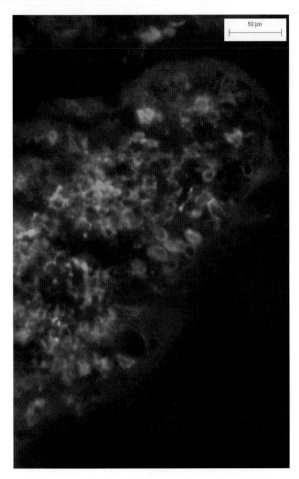

FIGURE 22-9 Double-color immunofluorescence showing a canine duodenal villous tip stained with monoclonal antibodies to αβ TCR and γδ TCR. The αβ T cells are stained green and are located in the interior of the villus. The γδ T cells are stained red and are clearly located within the intestinal epithelium.

(From German AJ, Hall EJ, Moore PF, et al: The distribution of lymphocytes expressing alpha/beta and gamma/delta T-cell receptors, and the expression of mucosal addressin cell adhesion molecule-1 in the canine intestine, *J Comp Pathol* 121:249–263, 1999.)

cells. IELs tend to use unusual *TRGV* and *TRDV* genes to form the TCR antigen-binding site. These genes are not expressed in other lymphoid organs, suggesting that the intraepithelial T cells are specialized for epithelial surveillance. IELs are MHC class II positive and may act as antigen-presenting cells. They regulate B cell IgA responses. Some have natural killer (NK) cell activity, whereas others are cytotoxic T cells that may attack parasites within the intestinal lumen. They also play a role in the repair of damaged epithelia.

Globule leukocytes are a subset of γ/δ T cells found in the cat and goat. They contain large eosinophilic cytoplasmic granules, but their nucleus resembles that in lymphocytes. Their function is unknown.

Ruminant γ/δ T cells recirculate continuously between epithelial surfaces such as the skin or intestinal epithelium and the bloodstream. In sheep, they are located in skin near the basal layer of the epidermis and in the dermis close to hair

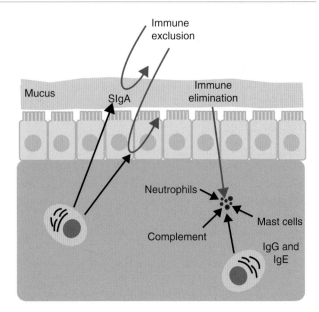

FIGURE 22-10 Two key defensive mechanisms are employed on mucosal surfaces. The most important is immune exclusion, an effect primarily mediated by IgA. If antigens gain access to the mucosa, they are destroyed through IgG- and IgE-mediated processes by immune elimination.

follicles and sebaceous glands. They are uncommon in wool-covered skin but are present in large numbers in bare and hairy skin. They are also found in the epithelium of the tongue, esophagus, trachea, and bladder.

Adaptive Protective Mechanisms

Both antibody- and cell-mediated immune processes protect body surfaces. The antibodies produced on mucosal surfaces include IgA, IgM, IgE, and IgG. Some of these, most notably IgA and possibly IgM, act by immune exclusion (Figure 22-10). The others, especially IgE and IgG, destroy antigen within the surface tissues by immune elimination.

Immune Exclusion

Immunoglobulin A IgA predominates in surface secretions; it is found in enormous amounts in saliva, intestinal fluid, nasal and tracheal secretions, tears, milk, colostrum, urine, and the secretions of the urogenital tract (Figure 22-11; Table 22-1). Thus, in swine, 90% of immunoglobulin-containing cells in the intestinal lamina propria contain IgA.

To undergo a class switch and thus produce IgA, mucosal B cells must receive signals from other cells. Some IgA production is T cell independent and requires signals from antigen-presenting dendritic cells and epithelial cells. Other B cells require help from Th2 cells to make the switch to IgA production. Dendritic cells secrete soluble B cell–stimulating cytokines including BAFF and APRIL (Chapter 15). The dendritic cells themselves are activated by some intestinal neuropeptides, such as vasoactive intestinal peptide (VIP). These signals, together with CD40-CD154 interactions, can trigger B cell IgA production in the absence of antigen. Enterocytes and intraepithelial lymphocytes also produce APRIL in response to exposure to commensal bacteria and promote B cell differentiation. B cells that require both antigen and Th2 cell to make the switch to IgA are stimulated by TGF-β (Figure 22-12). Other Th2 cytokines that promote this switch include IL-4, IL-5, IL-6, and even IL-10. The IgA response is relatively slow to develop and has a very high threshold for induction (10^9 bacteria). When boosted, the IgA response does not increase exponentially but rather in an additive manner.

IgA monomers are about 160 kDa in size and are typical four-chain, Y-shaped molecules (see Figure 16-6). They are usually secreted as dimers or larger polymers linked by a J-chain. IgA has several extra cysteine residues in its heavy chains. As a result, the short interchain disulfide bonds compact the chains and shield vulnerable bonds from proteases.

IgA is synthesized and secreted by plasma cells in the intestinal submucosa, especially in the crypt region. This dimeric IgA binds to a glycoprotein receptor for polymeric immunoglobulins (pIgR) on the basal surface of enterocytes (Figure 22-13). The receptor binds covalently to the Cα2 domain of one of the IgA monomers. The membrane-bound IgA-pIgR complex is then endocytosed and actively transported across the enterocyte. When it reaches the exterior surface, the endocytic vesicle fuses with the plasma membrane and exposes the complex to the intestinal lumen. The extracellular domains of the pIgR are then cleaved by proteases so that the IgA, with the receptor peptide still attached (secretory IgA), is released into the lumen. The receptor peptide is called secretory component. The production, transport, and secretion of secretory component occur even in the absence of IgA so that free secretory component is found in high concentrations in intestinal contents.

IgA is not bactericidal and does not activate complement. It can neutralize viruses as well as some viral and bacterial enzymes. IgA-antigen complexes can bind to monocytes and macrophages, neutrophils, and eosinophils through a low-affinity receptor, FcγR1 (CD89). When IgA-opsonized particles bind to this receptor, they trigger superoxide production, opsonization, antibody-dependent cell-mediated cytotoxicity, and the release of inflammatory mediators. Its most important function is to prevent the adherence of bacteria and viruses to epithelial surfaces—immune exclusion. If bacteria or viruses cannot adhere to enterocytes, they simply pass along with the intestinal contents and are expelled without doing any harm.

Because IgA is transported through enterocytes, it can also act inside these cells (Figure 22-14). Thus IgA can bind to newly synthesized viral proteins inside these cells and interrupt viral replication. In this way, the IgA can prevent viral growth before the integrity of the epithelium is damaged. This is a

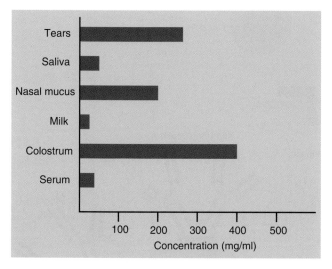

FIGURE 22-11 Typical IgA levels in bovine body fluids. In other species, milk and colostral IgA concentrations may be considerably higher.

☐ Table 22-1 | Approximate IgA Levels in the Serum and Various Secretions of the Domestic Animals

ANIMAL	SERUM	COLOSTRUM	MILK	NASAL MUCUS	SALIVA	TEARS
		SECRETION (mg/dL)				
Horse	170	1000	130	160	140	150
Cow	30	400	10	200	56	260
Sheep	30	400	10	50	90	160
Pig	200	1000	500	—	—	—
Dog	100	250	400	—	—	—
Cat	200	100	24	—	54	—
Chicken	50	—	—	—	20	15

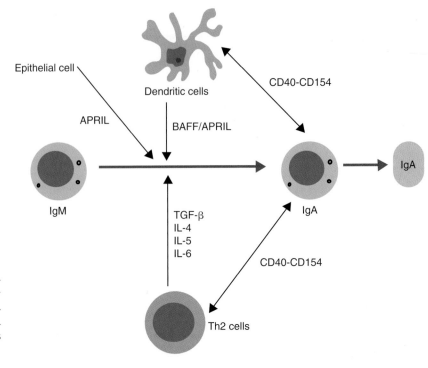

FIGURE 22-12 The control of IgA production. Multiple Th2 cytokines, especially TGF-β, are primarily responsible for the IgM-to-IgA switch. Co-stimulation is provided by BAFF and APRIL from epithelial cells and dendritic cells as well as CD40-CD154 interactions.

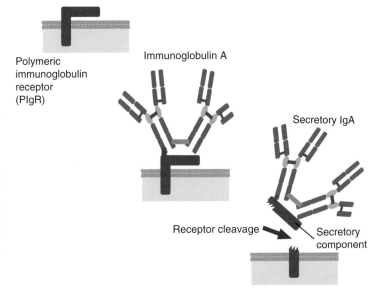

FIGURE 22-13 IgA is secreted by mucosal plasma cells and binds to receptors (pIgR) on the interior surface of intestinal enterocytes. The bound IgA is taken into the enterocytes and passed in vesicles to the cell surface. Once in the intestinal lumen, the pIgR is cleaved from the cell and remains bound to the IgA. In this state it is called secretory component and serves to protect the IgA from degradation.

unique example of an antibody acting in an intracellular location. The second unique function of intracellular IgA is to excrete foreign antigens. Thus IgA can bind to antigens that have penetrated to the submucosa. Once bound, the IgA-antigen complexes will bind to pIgR and be actively transported back across the enterocytes into the intestinal lumen. IgA can therefore act at three different levels to exclude foreign antigens: within the submucosa, within enterocytes, and within the intestinal lumen.

In some species, such as rats, rabbits, and chickens, up to 75% of the IgA produced within the intestinal wall may diffuse into the portal blood circulation and be carried to the liver (Figure 22-15). In these species, hepatocytes express pIgR. The

blood-borne IgA can bind to these hepatocytes and is carried across their cytosol to be released into the bile canaliculi. Bile is therefore the major route by which IgA reaches the intestine in these species. It is also a route by which antigens bound to circulating IgA can be removed from the body. However, in the major domestic mammals (dogs, ruminants, and swine), less than 5% of IgA enters the bile.

Immunoglobulin M The earliest immunoglobulins found in the intestine of the newborn are of the IgM class. IgM will also bind to pIgR and is carried through the enterocyte to the lumen. Because of its structure, however, secretory IgM is much more susceptible to proteases than secretory IgA.

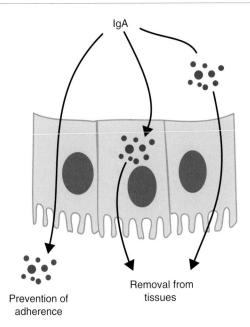

FIGURE 22-14 IgA is unique in that it can act in three locations. It can bind antigen in tissue fluid or in enterocytes as well as in the intestinal lumen. The bound antigen in tissues or enterocytes is carried to the intestinal lumen.

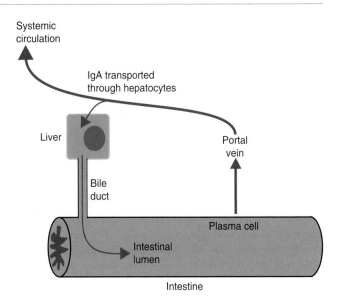

FIGURE 22-15 Some IgA, instead of being secreted directly into the intestine, as shown in Figure 22-14, may be carried to the liver, where it is passed through the hepatocytes into the bile duct. In some species, such as the rat, this is a very important pathway. In others, it is much less significant. For example, only about 5% of IgA reaches the intestine by this route in humans.

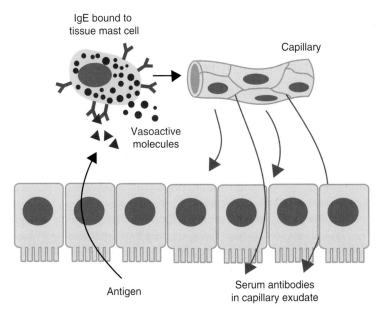

FIGURE 22-16 The IgE response in the intestinal wall. Antigen reaches IgE-sensitized mast cells to cause their degranulation. As a result of this, vasoactive factors are released. These cause increased vascular permeability and exudation of serum IgG antibodies.

Immune Elimination

Immunoglobulin E Because IgA does not activate complement, it functions by immune exclusion. There is a second line of defense, however, that destroys antigen that penetrates the mucosal barrier (immune elimination). This is mediated by IgE. Cells producing IgE are mainly found on body surfaces rather than in the lymph nodes or spleen. IgE binds to mast cell Fc receptors in the mucosa of the intestine, respiratory tract, and skin. If invading organisms evade the IgA and gain

access to the tissues, IgE-mediated responses will be triggered (Figure 22-16). These responses involve rapid degranulation of mast cells and the release of their vasoactive molecules into the surrounding tissues. As described in Chapter 3, these vasoactive molecules cause acute inflammation, increase the permeability of small blood vessels, and promote fluid leakage between enterocytes, leading to the outflow of mucus containing large quantities of IgG.

This process occurs, for example, when parasitic worms invade the intestinal mucosa. IgA has little effect on these invaders, so they have no difficulty in burrowing into the superficial layers of the mucosa. When parasite antigens encounter sensitized mast cells, however, the release of vasoactive molecules, together with the intense local inflammation, changes in blood flow, and intestinal motility, may be sufficient to force the parasite to disengage—a phenomenon called self-cure (Chapter 27).

Thus IgA and IgE work in concert. IgA normally is the first line of defense, and IgE serves as a backup system. If IgA production is defective, the IgE response may be triggered to excess. As a result, low levels of IgA result in increased IgE production and the development of allergic responses to food and inhaled antigens.

Immunoglobulin G In ruminants (especially cattle), IgG1, not IgA, is the major secretory immunoglobulin in colostrum and milk. This is due to selective transfer from the bloodstream into the mammary gland. On other body surfaces in ruminants, however, IgA remains the predominant immunoglobulin, although IgG1 is also present. IgG2 is also transferred into the intestine and saliva in ruminants. IgG may be of greater protective significance in the respiratory tract than in the intestine because there it is less likely to be degraded by proteases.

Immunity on Specific Surfaces

Immunity in the Gastrointestinal Tract

Saliva is rich in IgA and hence protects the mouth against infections. Small amounts of IgG are secreted into the crevicular groove between the gums and the base of the teeth. As a result it has proved possible to make a vaccine against caries-causing bacteria. Immunization of dogs with these organisms reduces microbial colonization of this area and prevents plaque formation and periodontitis. The flushing activity of saliva may be complemented by the generation of peroxidases from streptococci. The tonsils also produce much IgA, but because of the thin epithelium over the tonsillar clefts, they are very vulnerable to microbial invasion (Figure 22-17).

In single-stomach animals, the gastric pH may be sufficiently low to have a bactericidal or virucidal effect, although this varies among species and among meals. The dog, for instance, has a low gastric pH relative to that of the pig. Similarly, the pH in the center of a mass of ingested food may not necessarily drop to low levels, and some foods such as milk are potent buffers. In addition to antimicrobial peptides, lysozyme is synthesized in the gastric mucosa and in macrophages within the intestinal mucosa. As a result, it is found in large quantities in intestinal fluid.

Immunity to Food Although it is now fairly clear how the immune response to commensal bacteria is regulated, it remains unclear how this applies to food. Secretory IgA responses are not usually generated against food antigens.

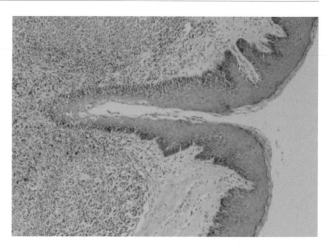

FIGURE 22-17 A section of pig tonsil showing a tonsillar crypt. Note how thin the epithelium is at the base of the crypt. This is an easy invasion route for many organisms. Original magnification ×150. (Courtesy Dr. S. Yamashiro.)

Likewise, soluble food proteins are unlikely to trigger intense TLR responses. (Although TLR4-deficient mice readily develop food allergies.) It may be that Treg cells play a major role in tolerance to food antigens.

It has been estimated that about 2% of ingested food protein is absorbed as peptide fragments large enough to be recognized by the immune system, although a very much smaller fraction of these molecules (<0.002%) is absorbed intact. This protein readily reaches the portal circulation, but little passes the liver and enters the systemic circulation. Presumably the Kupffer cells of the liver effectively capture blood-borne food antigens. Antibodies produced locally may bind to this adsorbed antigen and generate immune complexes that are removed as the blood passes through the liver. If a calf is fed a defined dietary antigen such as soy protein, although it is initially well absorbed, the animal soon begins to make IgA antibodies to soy. Once antibodies are produced, immune exclusion occurs, and the amount of protein absorbed drops significantly. If another novel protein is introduced into the feed, it too will be initially absorbed until IgA is produced against it. Thus IgA may serve to exclude intact food antigens from the body. The extent to which normal animals make antibodies against proteins in their food has been unclear. Cats fed soy and casein produced high levels of IgG and IgA antibodies in their serum against both these proteins. For unknown reasons, however, proteins from canned food appear to be more immunogenic than unprocessed proteins.

If a small amount of dietary antigen gains access to the general circulation in adults, a systemic immune response may be prevented by the activities of Treg cells, and oral tolerance may develop. Oral tolerance may involve either cellular suppression or clonal anergy and is generally directed against Th1 cells. The determining factor in deciding which mechanism is involved in this tolerance is probably the dose of antigen. Low doses invoke active suppression; high doses provoke clonal anergy.

Intestinal Inflammatory Disease Inflammatory bowel diseases probably result from a combination of genetic and environmental factors that result in dysregulation of the immune responses to the intestinal microflora and subsequent development of intestinal inflammation. Other changes, such as increased bacterial adherence to the mucosa, reduced bacterial diversity, changes in the bacterial mixture, and overgrowth of other bacteria, may all contribute to the process. As pointed out, commensal bacteria within the intestine are prevented from invading the intestinal wall by a glycocalyx, by high concentrations of defensins, and by an ongoing IgA response. They also suppress inflammation by blocking NF-κB activation and generating IL-10–secreting Treg cells. If these control mechanisms fail and the animal responds aggressively to its commensals, severe inflammation may result, making the intestine much more susceptible to bacteria-induced injury.

Canine inflammatory bowel diseases are a group of diseases characterized by persistent or recurrent gastrointestinal inflammation of undetermined cause. The most common form is a lymphocytic-plasmacytic enteritis. The disease presents with a history of chronic vomiting, diarrhea, and weight loss. This is characteristically associated with an increase in T cell and IgA+ plasma cells in the small intestine. The T cells are primarily α/β CD4+ cells. There is also an increased in the numbers of intestinal mast cells. Affected small intestine shows increased messenger RNA for IL-12, IFN-γ, tumor necrosis factor-α (TNF-α), and TGF-β. A hypoallergenic diet may result in clinical improvement and strongly suggests that the disease results from a food hypersensitivity. It may also respond well to glucocorticoids and the immunosuppressive drug azathioprine. A monoclonal gammopathy has been associated with this condition. Lymphocytic-plasmacytic enteritis has also been described in cats, horses, and a cow.

Histiocytic ulcerative colitis in Boxers is a severe form of inflammatory bowel disease. The lesions are characterized by the presence of large macrophages that stain intensely with periodic acid–Schiff stain. It is possible that this disease is triggered by an unidentified infectious agent since it somewhat resembles Johne's disease. The lesions also show accumulations of IgG+ plasma cells, MHC class II–positive cells, macrophages, and granulocytes.

Immunoproliferative enteropathy of Basenji dogs is an inherited autosomal disease that presents as gastric mucosal hypertrophy with lymphoid cell infiltration and ulceration. The whole small intestine may show villous blunting, crypt elongation, and infiltration of the mucosa with lymphocytes, plasma cells, and some neutrophils. Dogs show a polyclonal increase in serum IgA. The disease may be controlled by high doses of corticosteroids.

Protein-losing enteropathy of soft-coated Wheaten Terriers is also an inherited disease. Histological examination shows an inflammatory bowel disease. The cellular infiltrates are mainly lymphocytes and plasma cells, but neutrophils and eosinophils are often present. This disease may result from food hypersensitivity, possibly to wheat gluten.

Gluten-sensitive enteropathy of Irish Setters is an autosomal recessive small intestinal disease also caused by exposure to wheat gluten. As with the diseases described previously, affected small intestine is infiltrated with lymphocytes and other inflammatory cells. The mucosa shows increased numbers of CD4+ cells and decreased CD8+ T cell numbers. Affected dogs may also have elevated serum IgA levels.

Immunity in the Respiratory Tract

The respiratory tract differs from other body surfaces in that it is in intimate connection with the interior of the body yet is required by its very nature to allow unhindered access of air to the alveoli. The system obviously requires a filter. Particles suspended in the air entering the respiratory tract are largely removed by turbulence that directs them onto its mucus-covered walls, where they adhere. The turbulence is caused by the conformation of the turbinate bones, the trachea, and the bronchi. This turbulence filter serves to remove particles as small as 5 μm before they reach the alveoli (Figure 22-18).

A blanket of mucus produced by goblet cells covers the walls of the upper respiratory tract. The mucus gel serves as a matrix for soluble host defense molecules such as lysozyme, lactoferrin, surfactant proteins, and cationic peptides such as the defensins and cathelicidins. Most microorganisms that encounter this fluid layer are likely to be killed rapidly. There are four major surfactant proteins in lung fluid (SP-A, -B, -C, -D) produced by alveolar type II cells. SP-B and -C are extremely hydrophobic. Their function is to reduce surface tension at the alveolar surface so that a thin film of fluid forms on the surface and prevents lung collapse. The functions of SP-A and -D, in contrast, are to defend the lungs against microbial invasion. They are hydrophilic collectins that bind to microbial surface carbohydrates and act as opsonins. SP-A and -D also activate macrophages, promote chemotaxis, enhance the respiratory burst, and promote the production of inflammatory cytokines. SP-A thus regulates the production of TNF-α, the respiratory burst, and nitric oxide. These surfactant proteins enhance the clearance of apoptotic cells from the lung. This is especially important in the resolution of inflammation, in which apoptotic neutrophils should be removed by macrophages as promptly as possible. Surfactant proteins can also modulate the functions of dendritic cells and T cells. SP-A inhibits the maturation of dendritic cells, whereas SP-D enhances their uptake and presentation of antigen. Both SP-A and SP-D inhibit T cell proliferation.

The mucus layer is in continuous flow, being carried from the bronchioles up the bronchi and trachea by ciliary action or backward through the nasal cavity to the pharynx. Here the dirty mucus is swallowed and presumably digested in the intestinal tract. Particles that bypass this mucociliary escalator and reach the alveoli are phagocytosed by alveolar macrophages. Once these cells have successfully ingested particles, they migrate to the mucus escalator and are also carried to the pharynx.

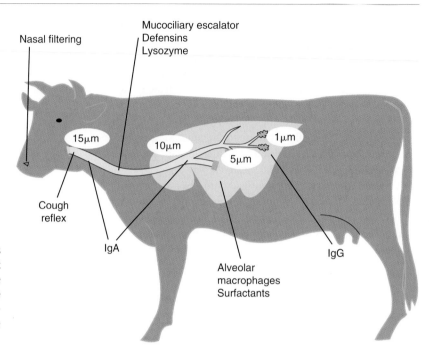

FIGURE 22-18 Some of the innate mechanisms involved in the protection of the respiratory tract against infection and the influence of particle size on the site of deposition of particles within the respiratory tract. Note that only the smallest particles can penetrate deeply and gain access to the alveoli.

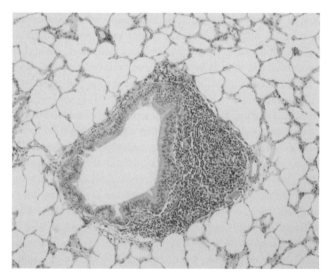

FIGURE 22-19 Lymphoid follicle found in the bifurcation of an airway in a section of calf lung. This type of bronchus-associated lymphoid tissue is a key component of the defenses of the respiratory tract.

(From a specimen kindly provided by Drs. N.H. McArthur and L.C. Abbott.)

The respiratory tract contains lymphoid nodules in the walls of the bronchi as well as lymphocytes distributed diffusely throughout the lung and the walls of the airways (Figure 22-19). The mucosa of the larynx contains many immunologically active cells, including large numbers of T cells. M cells may be associated with these lymphoid nodules as well as with nasal mucosal lymphoid tissues. The immunoglobulin synthesized in these tissues is mainly secretory IgA, especially in the upper regions of the respiratory tract. This IgA is bound to the

mucus layer through secretory component and enhances the clearance of adherent bacteria. pIgR is expressed at low levels on bronchial epithelial cells. In the bronchioles and alveoli, however, the secretions contain a large proportion of IgG, the concentration of which is intermediate between the levels in the trachea and in serum. IgE is also synthesized in significant amounts in the lymphoid tissues of the upper respiratory tract. As on other body surfaces, IgA in the respiratory tract probably protects by immune exclusion, whereas IgG and IgE act by immune elimination (see Figure 22-10).

Many cells may be washed out of the airways of the lung with saline. In dogs, about 80% of bronchoalveolar cells obtained in this way are macrophages, and 13% are lymphocytes, of which about half are T cells (Table 22-2). In healthy horses, about 50% of the cells in bronchoalveolar washes are macrophages, 40% are lymphocytes, and 2% are neutrophils. In sheep, B cells are less than 10% of the lung lymphocyte population. Lung T cells can produce cytokines, and alveolar macrophages are activated following infection with *Listeria monocytogenes*. Cell-mediated immune reactions are therefore readily provoked among the cells within the lower respiratory tract.

The lungs of most domestic species (pigs, horses, sheep, goats, cattle, cats) differ from rodent, human, or dog lungs in that they contain large numbers of intravascular macrophages (Chapter 5). It has been estimated that these macrophages cover 16% of the lung capillary surface in young pigs. As a result, the lungs of these species can remove more bacteria from the blood than can the liver and spleen. In pigs, pulmonary intravascular macrophages are damaged by porcine reproductive and respiratory syndrome virus. As a result, infected animals are more likely to develop *Streptococcus suis* pneumonia. There is debate as to whether lung macrophages are

□ Table 22-2 | Composition of Cells in Canine Bronchoalveolar Lavage Fluid

CELL	PERCENTAGE (RANGE)
Macrophages	79.4 (71-87)
Lymphocytes	13.5 (7-20)
Eosinophils	3.6 (0-14)
Mast cells	2.1 (0-5)
Epithelial cells	0.8 (0-6)
Neutrophils	0.6 (0-2)
Lymphocyte Percentages	
T cells	52.0 (34-69)
CD4+	21.9 (10-32)
CD8+	17.8 (6-25)
CD4/CD8 ratio	1.3 (0.8-2.4)

From Vail DM, Mahler PA, Soergel SA: Differential cell analysis and phenotypic subtyping of lymphocytes in bronchoalveolar lavage fluid from clinically normal dogs, *Am J Vet Res* 56:282–285, 1995.

□ Box 22-1 | **Skin Microbiome**

The skin is an inhospitable environment—it is very dry, with an acidic pH, continuous shedding of skin cells, and the presence of multiple antimicrobial molecules. The skin microenvironment, however, is very diverse. Some skin is hairless, and some in the groin and axilla or within the ears is moist, whereas that on an animal's back may be very dry. As a result, many diverse microbial communities live on the skin of animals. The development of new methodologies has permitted investigators to examine these microbial communities by means of large-scale genomic analysis. Much of the flora consists of permanent residents that can protect against pathogens, but there are also many different transient residents. Anatomically distinct sites can harbor very different bacterial communities. This skin microbiome may fluctuate over time and change with the age of the individual. Although most are innocuous, some of the pathobionts in the skin microflora may contribute to skin disease or delayed wound healing.

Data from Hong HH: Skin microbiome: genomics-based insights into the diversity and role of skin microbes, *Trends Mol Med* 17:320–328, 2011.

effective antigen-presenting cells. A dense network of dendritic cells is found within airway epithelium and alveoli.

Although it has long been believed that the respiratory tract is sterile, growing evidence suggests that it too has a normal bacterial flora. The composition of this flora appears to have a direct influence on the development of allergic respiratory disease (Chapter 28).

Immunity in the Urogenital Tract

In the urinary system, the flushing action and low pH of urine generally provide adequate protection; however, when urinary stasis occurs, urethritis resulting from the unhindered ascent of pathogenic bacteria is not uncommon. In adult animals, the vagina is populated almost exclusively by commensal lactobacilli. The vagina is lined by a squamous epithelium composed of cells rich in glycogen. When these cells desquamate, they provide a substrate for the lactobacilli that, in turn, generate large quantities of lactic acid, and reduce the pH to a level that protects the vagina against invasion by pathogenic bacteria and yeasts. Glycogen storage in the vaginal epithelial cells is stimulated by estrogens and thus occurs only in sexually mature animals.

The predominant immunoglobulin in cervicovaginal mucus is IgA, whereas within the uterus, it is IgG. If bacteria such as *Campylobacter fetus* infect the genital tract, vaginal IgA antibodies immobilize and agglutinate the organisms. If the mucous membrane becomes inflamed, IgG antibodies from serum will also assist in protection. Surfactant protein A is also important in protecting the vagina from infection. *C. fetus*

infections are associated with the presence of many mononuclear cells as well with delayed skin reactions (type IV hypersensitivity) so that cell-mediated immunity is also involved in resistance to this local infection. Similar local immune responses may also be directed against other organisms that infect the cervix and vagina, and the presence of agglutinating antibodies in vaginal mucus may be used as a diagnostic test for brucellosis, campylobacteriosis, and trichomoniasis. (The local immune response to trichomoniasis is largely mediated by IgE; see Chapter 27.) IgG also reaches the uterine lumen and the vagina by active transport mediated by FcRn. This receptor is pH dependent. It picks up IgG in the tissues where the pH is relatively high and releases it in the vagina where the pH is very low.

Preputial washings of bulls infected with *C. fetus* may contain IgG1 antibodies with some IgM and IgA. IgA is present in small amounts in normal urine, produced presumably by lymphoid tissues in the walls of the urinary tract. IgG may be present in large amounts in the urine of animals with nephritis because of the breakdown in the glomerular barrier.

Immunity on the Skin

The skin is the first line of defense against many microbial invaders. It carries out this function effectively, and few bacteria can penetrate intact skin unaided. It serves as a strong physical barrier supplemented by continuous desquamation, desiccation, and a low pH because of fatty acids in sebum (Box 22-1). In addition, the skin carries a resident bacterial flora that excludes pathogenic bacteria and fungi. If this skin flora is disturbed, its protective properties are reduced, and microbial invasion may result. Thus skin infections tend to occur in areas such as the axilla or groin, where both pH and humidity are high. Similarly, animals forced to stand in water or mud show an increased frequency of foot infections as the skin becomes sodden, its structure breaks down, and its resident flora changes in response to alterations in the local environment.

The skin has a multitude of innate defenses ranging from its own microbial flora to the production of potent antimicrobial peptides by keratinocytes. Large numbers of genes for antimicrobial peptides have been identified in normal skin, and these are expressed at multiple locations on the surface of the body.

The skin also participates in the adaptive immune system through antigen-trapping by a network of several populations of dermal dendritic cells. The best known of these are Langerhans cells. Langerhans cells can bind exogenous antigen and may present it to nearby helper T cells. They account for 50% to 70% of the dendritic cells in pig skin.

Healthy skin contains a population of T cells mainly located in the basal layer associated with the Langerhans cells. CD4+ and CD8+ cells are present in equal numbers. In humans and mice they are predominantly α/β T cells. In the domestic mammals many are γ/δ T cells. In cattle, for example, 44% of dermal T cells are γ/δ positive. The three major Th cell subsets are present. Th1 and Th2 play a key role in defense. Th17 cells are of importance in inflammatory skin disease such as atopic dermatitis. A subset of circulating T cells that home to the skin and produce IL-22 (Th22 cells) have also been identified. IL-22 appears to play an important role in maintaining barrier function on exposed body surfaces. It promotes antimicrobial immunity, inflammation, and tissue repair.

If an antigen is injected intradermally, such as occurs when a tick bites an animal, the antigen is captured by Langerhans cells and is presented to skin T cells, thus stimulating a rapid and effective immune response. A similar reaction occurs when reactive chemicals are painted on the skin. Skin washings contain immunoglobulins. For example, in cattle, serum IgM, IgG1, and IgG2 cross the skin by transudation, but the IgA appears to be locally synthesized.

The major epidermal skin cells, the keratinocytes, serve as immune sentinels and are active participants in the defense of the skin. Under normal conditions keratinocyte precursor cells divide and continually renew the epidermis in a coordinated manner. If the skin is wounded or inflamed, alterations in adhesion molecules, surface receptors, and the cytokine environment change the behavior of the keratinocytes. If inflammation is prolonged, severe skin lesions may develop. Damage-associated molecular patterns (DAMPs) generated by trauma or ultraviolet light will trigger inflammasome formation. Keratinocytes express multiple PRRs such as the TLRs and C-type lectin receptors, so they are well able to recognize PAMPs associated with microbial invasion. Upon appropriate stimulation, they can produce a complex mixture of interleukins, interferons, and other cytokines, growth factors, chemokines, cathelicidins, and multiple defensins, all of which assist

in excluding microbes seeking to penetrate the skin. Keratinocytes express MHC class II and can serve as antigen-presenting cells.

Immunity in the Mammary Gland

The protective mechanisms of the udder are presumably not at their most effective in that biological anomaly, the modern dairy cow. In a nonlactating animal, a keratin plug blocks the teat orifice and excludes bacteria. In a lactating animal, the flushing action of the milk helps to prevent invasion by some potential pathogens, whereas milk itself contains many innate antibacterial molecules. These antibacterial agents include complement, lysozyme, lactoferrin, and lactoperoxidase. Lactoferrin competes with bacteria for iron and makes it unavailable for the animal's growth. It also enhances the neutrophil respiratory burst. Milk contains lactoperoxidase and thiocyanate (SCN^-) ions. In the presence of exogenous hydrogen peroxide, lactoperoxidase can oxidize the SCN^- to bacteriostatic products such as $OSCN^-$.

$$H_2O_2 + SCN^- \rightarrow OSCN^- + H_2O$$

The hydrogen peroxide may be produced by bacteria such as streptococci or by the oxidation of ascorbic acid. Phagocytic cells released into milk in response to inflammation also contribute to antimicrobial resistance not only through their phagocytic efforts but also by providing additional lactoferrin, hydrogen peroxide, and lysosomal peroxidases. The binding of bovine lactoferrin to *Streptococcus agalactiae* can activate C1q of the classical complement pathway.

Milk also contains IgA, secretory component, and IgG1. The IgA and secretory component are closely associated with the milk fat globules. In simple-stomach animals, IgA predominates, whereas in ruminants, IgG1 does. IgA is synthesized in the mammary tissue, although many of the IgA-producing cells in the gland are derived from precursors originating in the intestine. These cells are a source of antibodies against intestinal pathogens. Colostral IgG1, in contrast, is selectively transferred by active transport from serum using FcRn on mammary gland epithelial cells.

If antigen is infused into a lactating mammary gland, it tends to be promptly flushed out again in the milk. If it is infused into a nonlactating gland, a local antibody response develops. Unfortunately, because of the continuous removal of milk, antibody concentrations in this fluid remain low (<100 mg/dL) even though, over a period of time, the amount of immunoglobulin produced in the udder may be considerable. In acute mastitis, the inflammatory response leads to the influx of actively phagocytic cells, especially neutrophils, and to the exudation of serum proteins. As a result immunoglobulin levels in mastitic milk may rise to levels at which they can exert a protective influence (~8000 mg/dL).

Because the local immune response in the udder is relatively ineffective in preventing infection, attempts to vaccinate against mastitis-causing organisms have been generally unsuccessful. Nevertheless, recent advances have produced encouraging results. Thus a *Staphylococcus aureus* vaccine that stimulates the production of antibodies against the pseudocapsule appears to be effective. This pseudocapsule interferes with the ability of milk leukocytes to phagocytose *S. aureus*. Antibodies induced by the vaccine promote opsonization and destruction of the bacteria. A vaccine designed to stimulate antibody production against staphylococcal α toxin, as well as the pseudocapsule, has reduced the incidence of mastitis following challenge by 50%. Encouraging results have also been obtained by the use of a J5 mutant vaccine against coliform bacteria (Chapter 25). The vaccine is given to cattle at drying off, 30 days later, and at calving.

Colostrum is rich in macrophages and lymphocytes. These macrophages can process antigen, and when cultured, their supernatant fluids can enhance IgA production from blood lymphocytes. Milk lymphocytes may survive for a short time in the intestine and may transfer some immunity to the newborn animal (Chapter 21).

Vaccination on Body Surfaces

When animals are vaccinated against organisms that infect body surfaces, such as the intestinal or respiratory tracts, it makes sense to stimulate a mucosal IgA response. To do this, the vaccine antigen can simply be ingested or inhaled. Unfortunately, such vaccines are not always effective. Inactivated antigens commonly fail to trigger an IgA response because they are immediately washed or sneezed off when applied to mucous membranes. (A notable exception occurs when high levels of vaccine antigens are incorporated in feed.) The only way a significant IgA response can be triggered is to use live vaccines, in which the vaccine organism can invade mucous membranes. The vaccine must persist for a sufficient time to trigger an immune response yet not cause significant damage. Because of the abundant intestinal microflora, intestinal IgA responses also have a high threshold, tend to lack memory, and tend to fade rapidly. The body tightly regulates antigen input across epithelial cells. Regulatory effects on IgA production constantly adapt the IgA response to the intestinal microflora. Good examples of such vaccines are the respiratory tract vaccines against bovine or feline rhinotracheitis. Even some of these vaccines may cause a transient conjunctivitis or tracheitis. Other examples of effective live oral vaccines include polio vaccine in humans and transmissible gastroenteritis vaccine in piglets. Oral tolerance also remains a challenge for mucosal vaccines. Thus administration of some antigens to the respiratory or intestinal tracts may promote mucosal and T cell systemic unresponsiveness.

Systemic vaccination against these surface infections may provide adequate immunity (as in human influenza and polio vaccines) since some IgG may be transferred from serum to the mucosal surface. Indeed, many available vaccines simply work by stimulating high levels of IgG antibodies in blood. These are effective because once an invading organism causes tissue damage and triggers inflammation, the site of invasion is flooded by IgG. Nevertheless, this is not the most efficient way of providing immunity.

Once a protective IgA response has been stimulated, other difficulties may arise. For example, secondary immune responses are sometimes difficult to induce on surfaces, and multiple doses of vaccine may not increase the intensity or duration of the local immune response. This is not caused by any intrinsic defect but occurs because high levels of IgA can block antigen absorption and prevent it from reaching antigen-presenting cells.

For sources of additional information, please visit http://evolve.elsevier.com/tizard/immunology/

Vaccines and Their Production

Key Points

- An animal can be made immune to infection in two general ways—passive immunization and active immunization.
- Passive immunization by administering preformed antibodies made in a normal animal provides immediate protection, but the resulting immunity is short lived.
- Active immunization using vaccines containing live or dead organisms produces slowly developing but long-lasting immunity.
- Live vaccines tend, in general, to stimulate a more effective immune response than vaccines containing killed organisms. However, vaccines containing killed organisms have tended to be somewhat safer.
- Innovative molecular techniques, such as the use of DNA vaccines or reverse vaccinology, may permit the development of vaccines against diseases for which current vaccines are ineffective or not available.
- Adjuvants are substances added to vaccines to enhance their effectiveness.

Vaccination is by far the most efficient and cost-effective method of controlling infectious diseases in humans and animals. The eradication of smallpox and rinderpest from the globe, the elimination of hog cholera and brucellosis from many countries, and the control of diseases such as foot-and-mouth disease, canine distemper, rabies, influenza, and pseudorabies would not have been possible without the use of effective vaccines. Vaccine technology continues to advance rapidly, especially through the use of modern molecular techniques and through our increased understanding of immune mechanisms and ways to optimize immune responses to achieve maximal protection.

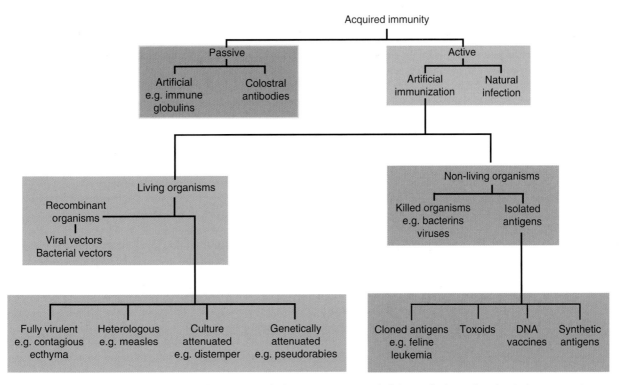

FIGURE 23-1 A classification of the different types of adaptive immunity and of the methods employed to induce protection.

Types of Immunization Procedures

There are two basic methods by which any animal may be made immune to an infectious disease (Figure 23-1): passive and active immunization. Passive immunization produces temporary immunity by transferring antibodies from a resistant to a susceptible animal. These passively transferred antibodies give immediate protection, but since they are gradually catabolized, this protection wanes, and the recipient eventually becomes susceptible again.

Active immunization, in contrast, involves administering antigen to an animal so that it responds by mounting an immune response. Reimmunization or exposure to infection in the same animal will result in a secondary immune response and greatly enhanced immunity. The disadvantage of active immunization is that, as with all adaptive immune responses, protection is not conferred immediately. However, once established, immunity is long-lasting and capable of restimulation (Figure 23-2).

Passive Immunization

Passive immunization requires that antibodies be produced in donor animals by active immunization and that these antibodies be given to susceptible animals to confer immediate protection. Serum containing these antibodies (antisera) may be produced against a wide variety of pathogens. For instance,

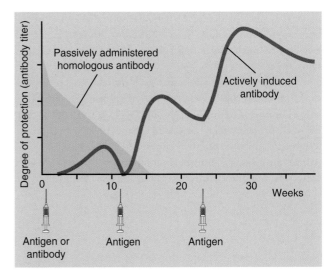

FIGURE 23-2 The levels of serum antibody (and hence the degree of protection) conferred by active and passive methods of immunization.

they can be produced in cattle against anthrax, in dogs against distemper, in cats against panleukopenia, and in humans against measles. They are most effective protecting animals against toxigenic organisms such as *Clostridium tetani* or *Clostridium perfringens*, using antisera raised in horses. Antisera made in this way are called immune globulins and are commonly produced in young horses by a series of immunizing injections. The clostridial toxins are proteins that can be denatured and made nontoxic by treatment with formaldehyde.

Formaldehyde-treated toxins are called toxoids. Donor horses are initially injected with toxoids, but once antibodies are produced, subsequent injections may contain purified toxin. The responses of the horses are monitored, and once their antibody levels are sufficiently high, they are bled. Bleeding is undertaken at intervals until the antibody level drops, when the animals are again boosted with antigen. Plasma is separated from the horse blood, and the globulin fraction that contains the antibodies is concentrated, titrated, and dispensed.

To standardize the potency of different immune globulins, comparison must be made with an international biological standard. In the case of tetanus immune globulin, this is done by comparing the dose necessary to protect guinea pigs against a fixed amount of tetanus toxin with the dose of the standard preparation of immune globulin required to do the same. The international standard immune globulin for tetanus toxin is a quantity held at the State Serum Institute in Copenhagen. An international unit (IU) of tetanus immune globulin is the specific neutralizing activity contained in 0.03384 mg of the international standard. The U.S. standard unit (AU) is twice the international unit.

Tetanus immune globulin is given to animals to confer immediate protection against tetanus. At least 1500 IU of immune globulin should be given to horses and cattle; at least 500 IU to calves, sheep, goats, and swine; and at least 250 IU to dogs. The exact amount should vary with the amount of tissue damage, the degree of wound contamination, and the time elapsed since injury. Tetanus immune globulin is of little use once the toxin has bound to its target receptor and clinical signs appear.

Although immune globulins give immediate protection, some problems are associated with their use. For instance, when horse tetanus immune globulin is given to a cow or dog, the horse proteins will be perceived as foreign, elicit an immune response, and be rapidly eliminated (Figure 23-3). To reduce antigenicity, immune globulins are usually treated with pepsin to destroy their Fc region and leave intact only the portion of the immunoglobulin molecule required for toxin neutralization—the $F(ab)'_2$ fragment.

If circulating horse antibody is still present by the time the recipient animal mounts an immune response, the immune complexes formed may cause a type III hypersensitivity reaction called serum sickness (Chapter 30). If repeated doses of horse immune globulin are given to an animal of another species, this may provoke immunoglobulin E (IgE) production and anaphylaxis (Chapter 28). Finally, the presence of high levels of circulating horse antibody may interfere with active immunization against the same antigen. This is a phenomenon similar to that seen in newborn animals passively protected by maternal antibodies. Sometimes passive immunization may have unexpected side effects (Box 23-1).

Monoclonal antibodies are another source of passive protection for animals. These are, however, mainly made by mouse-mouse hybridomas and thus are mouse immunoglobulins. They will therefore be antigenic when given to other species. Nevertheless, mouse monoclonal antibodies against the K99 pilus antigens of *Escherichia coli* may be given orally to calves to protect them against diarrhea caused by this organism. A mouse monoclonal antibody to lymphoma cells has been successfully used in the treatment of dogs with this tumor.

Active Immunization

Active immunization has several major advantages over passive immunization. These include the prolonged period of protection and the recall and boosting of this protective response by repeated injections of antigen or by exposure to infection. An ideal vaccine for active immunization should therefore give prolonged strong immunity. This immunity should be

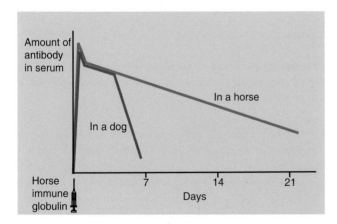

FIGURE 23-3 The fate of passively administered immune globulin when given to a homologous species (horse) or to a heterologous species (dog).

> ▫ **Box 23-1 | Serum Hepatitis of Horses**
>
> On rare occasions, horses may develop acute hepatic necrosis 30 to 70 days after vaccination. It has followed administration of horse plasma, equine immune globulin against tetanus, anthrax, strangles, influenza, and equine encephalitis. It has also occurred after active immunization against equine encephalitis and rhinopneumonitis when the vaccines were prepared using fetal equine cells. Certain serum mixtures or a single vaccine batch may be associated with a high incidence of the disease. Its etiology, mechanism of transmission, and pathogenesis are unknown. Occasional cases have been described in untreated horses living with affected animals, suggesting that a virus may transmit the disease. Nevertheless, experimental transmission and serological testing have failed to reveal a causal agent. The disease is severe, with 53% to 88% mortality. Clinical signs include anorexia, icterus, excessive sweating, and neurological abnormalities. Clinical chemistry confirms severe liver damage with high liver enzyme levels, ammonia, and bilirubin.

conferred on both the animal immunized and any fetus carried by it. In obtaining this strong immunity, the vaccine should be free of adverse side effects. (In effect it should stimulate adaptive immunity without triggering the inflammation associated with innate immunity.) The ideal vaccine should be cheap, stable, and adaptable to mass vaccination; ideally, it should stimulate an immune response distinguishable from that due to natural infection so that immunization and eradication may proceed simultaneously.

In addition to the requirements listed previously, effective vaccines must have other critical properties. First, antigen must be delivered efficiently so that antigen-presenting cells can process antigen and release appropriate cytokines. Second, both T and B cells must be stimulated so that they generate large numbers of memory cells. Third, helper and effector T cells must be generated to several epitopes in the vaccine so that individual variations in MHC class II polymorphism and epitope properties are minimized. Finally, the antigen must be able to stimulate memory cells in such a way that protection will last as long as possible.

Living and Killed Vaccines

Unfortunately, two of the prerequisites of an ideal vaccine—high antigenicity and absence of adverse side effects—are often incompatible. Modified live vaccines infect host cells and undergo viral replication. The infected cells then process endogenous antigen. In this way live viruses trigger a response dominated by CD8+ cytotoxic T cells, a Th1 response. This may be hazardous because the vaccine viruses may themselves cause disease or persistent infection (called residual virulence). Killed organisms, in contrast, act as exogenous antigens. They commonly stimulate responses dominated by CD4+ Th2 cells. This may not be the most appropriate response to some organisms, but it may be safer. It also appears that dendritic cells respond in a different fashion to live and killed bacteria. For example, live organisms such as salmonella upregulate more CD40, CD86, IL-6, IL-12, and GM-CSF than do killed organisms.

The practical advantages and disadvantages of vaccines containing living or killed organisms are well demonstrated in the vaccines available against *Brucella abortus* in cattle. *B. abortus* is a cause of abortion in cattle, and vaccination has been used historically to control the disease. Brucella infections are best controlled by a T cell–mediated immune response, and a vaccine containing a living avirulent strain of *B. abortus* is required for the control of this infection. Older live *Brucella* vaccines, especially strain 19, caused a lifelong immunity in cows and successfully prevented abortion. Unfortunately, strain 19 vaccine also caused systemic reactions: swelling at the injection site, high fever, anorexia, listlessness, and a drop in milk yield. Strain 19 could cause abortion in pregnant cows, orchitis in bulls, and undulant fever in humans. To eradicate brucellosis, serological tests are used to identify infected animals, and strain 19 causes an antibody response that is difficult to distinguish from a natural infection.

Because of the disadvantages associated with the use of strain 19, considerable efforts have been made to find a better alternative. Unfortunately, killed vaccines (strain 45/20) protected cattle for less than 1 year. A live attenuated strain of *B. abortus* called RB-51 has been used in cattle in the United States. This is a rough mutant that fails to produce the lipopolysaccharide O antigen. As a result, it produces a strong Th1 response, but unlike strain 19, it does not induce false-positive results in the standard diagnostic tests such as card agglutination, complement fixation, or tube agglutination. It is therefore possible to distinguish between vaccinated and infected cattle. RB-51 is less pathogenic for cattle than strain 19, and it is not shed in nasal secretions, saliva, or urine. RB-51 will not cause abortion in pregnant cattle. It will, however, cause disease in accidentally exposed humans, and because of its failure to stimulate antibody production, this may be difficult to diagnose.

The advantages of vaccines such as brucella strain 45/20 that contain killed organisms are that they are safe with respect to residual virulence and are relatively easy to store since the organisms are already dead (Box 23-2). These advantages of killed vaccines correspond to the disadvantages of live vaccines, such as strain 19 or RB-51. That is, some live vaccines may possess residual virulence, not only for the animal for which the vaccine is made but also for other animals. They may revert to a fully virulent type or spread to unvaccinated animals. Thus some vaccine strains of porcine reproductive and respiratory syndrome virus (PRRSV) vaccine may be transmitted to unvaccinated pigs, causing persistent infection and disease. Live vaccines always run the risk of contamination with unwanted organisms; for instance, outbreaks of reticuloendotheliosis in chickens in Japan and Australia have been traced to contaminated Marek's disease vaccines. A major outbreak of bovine leukosis in Australia resulted from contamination of a batch of babesiosis vaccine containing whole calf blood.

□ Box 23-2 | **Relative Merits of Living and Inactivated Vaccines**

Living Vaccines	Inactivated Vaccines
Fewer doses required	Stable on storage
Adjuvants unnecessary	Unlikely to cause disease through residual virulence
Less chance of hypersensitivity	
Induction of interferon	Do not replicate in recipient
Relatively cheap	Unlikely to contain live contaminating organisms
Smaller dose needed	
Can be given by natural route	Will not spread to other animals
Stimulate both humoral and cell-mediated response	Safe in immunodeficient patients
Longer-lasting protection	Easier to store
	Lower development costs
	No risk of reversion

Abortion and death have occurred in pregnant bitches that received a parvovirus vaccine contaminated with bluetongue virus. Contaminating mycoplasma may also be present in some vaccines. Scrapie has been spread in mycoplasma vaccines. Finally, vaccines containing living attenuated organisms require care in their preparation, storage, and handling to avoid killing the organisms. Maintaining the cold chain can account for 20% to 80% of the cost of a vaccine in the tropics.

The disadvantages of killed vaccines parallel the advantages of living vaccines. The use of adjuvants to increase effective antigenicity can cause severe inflammation or systemic toxicity, whereas multiple doses or high individual doses of antigen increase the risk of producing hypersensitivity reactions, as well as increasing costs.

Inactivation

Organisms killed for use in vaccines must remain as antigenically similar to the living organisms as possible. Therefore crude methods of killing that cause extensive changes in antigen structure as a result of protein denaturation are usually unsatisfactory. If chemicals are used, they must not alter the antigens responsible for stimulating protective immunity. One such chemical is formaldehyde, which cross-links proteins and nucleic acids and confers structural rigidity. Proteins can also be mildly denatured by acetone or alcohol treatment. Alkylating agents that cross-link nucleic acid chains are also suitable for killing organisms since by leaving the surface proteins of organisms unchanged, they do not interfere with antigenicity. Examples of alkylating agents include ethylene oxide, ethyleneimine, acetyl ethyleneimine, and β-propiolactone, all of which have been used in veterinary vaccines. Many successful vaccines containing killed bacteria (bacterins) or inactivated toxins (toxoids) can be made relatively simply by the use of these agents. Some vaccines may contain mixtures of these components. For example, some vaccines against *Mannheimia hemolytica* contain both killed bacteria and inactivated bacterial leukotoxin.

Attenuation

Virulent living organisms cannot normally be used in vaccines. Their virulence must be reduced so that, although still living, they can no longer cause disease. This process of reduction of virulence is called attenuation. The level of attenuation is critical to vaccine success. Underattenuation will result in residual virulence and disease; overattenuation may result in an ineffective vaccine. The traditional methods of attenuation were empirical, and there was little understanding of the changes induced by the attenuation process. They usually involved adapting organisms to growth in unusual conditions so that they lost their adaptation to their usual host. For example, the bacille Calmette-Guérin (BCG) strain of *Mycobacterium bovis* was rendered avirulent by being grown for 13 years on bile-saturated medium. The vaccine strain of anthrax was rendered avirulent by growth in 50% serum agar under an atmosphere

rich in CO_2 so that it lost its ability to form a capsule. *B. abortus* strain 19 vaccine was grown under conditions in which there was a shortage of nutrients. Unfortunately, genetic stability cannot always be guaranteed in these attenuated strains. Back-mutation may occur, and attenuated organisms may redevelop virulence.

A more reliable method of making bacteria avirulent is by genetic manipulation. For example, a modified live vaccine is available that contains streptomycin-dependent *M. hemolytica* and *Pasteurella multocida*. These mutants depend on the presence of streptomycin for growth. When they are administered to an animal, the absence of streptomycin will eventually result in the death of the bacteria, but not before they have stimulated a protective immune response.

Viruses have traditionally been attenuated by growth in cells or species to which they are not naturally adapted. For example, rinderpest virus, which is normally a pathogen of cattle, was first attenuated by growth in rabbits. Eventually, a successful tissue culture–adapted rinderpest vaccine devoid of residual virulence was developed. Widespread and systematic use of this vaccine eventually permitted the global eradication of rinderpest. Similar examples include the adaptation of African horse sickness virus to mice and of canine distemper virus to ferrets. Alternatively, mammalian viruses may be attenuated by growth in eggs. For example, the Flury strain of rabies was attenuated by prolonged passage in eggs and lost its virulence for normal dogs and cats.

The traditional method of virus attenuation has been prolonged tissue culture. In these cases virus attenuation is accomplished by culturing the organism in cells to which they are not adapted. For example, virulent canine distemper virus preferentially attacks lymphoid cells. For vaccine purposes, therefore, this virus was cultured repeatedly in canine kidney cells. In adapting to these culture conditions, it lost its ability to cause severe disease.

Under some circumstances it is possible to use fully virulent organisms for immunization just as the Chinese once did with smallpox. Vaccination against contagious ecthyma of sheep is of this type. Contagious ecthyma (orf) is a viral disease of lambs that causes massive scab formation around the mouth, prevents feeding, and results in a failure to thrive. The disease has little systemic effect. Lambs recover completely within a few weeks and are immune from then on. It is usual to vaccinate lambs by rubbing dried, infected scab material into scratches made in the inner aspect of the thigh. The local infection at this site has no untoward effect on the lambs, and they become solidly immune. Because the vaccinated animals may spread the disease, however, they must be separated from unvaccinated animals for a few weeks.

Modern Vaccine Technology

Although both killed and modified live vaccines have been successful in controlling many infectious diseases, there is always a need to make them more effective, cheaper, and safer

(Figure 23-4). The use of modern molecular techniques can produce new and improved vaccines. These vaccines can be divided into several categories (Table 23-1).

Antigens Generated by Gene Cloning (Category I)

Gene cloning can be used to produce large quantities of purified antigen in culture. In this process, DNA coding for an antigen of interest is first isolated from the pathogen. This DNA is then inserted into a bacterium or yeast in such a way that it is functional and the recombinant antigen is expressed in large amounts. The first successful use of gene cloning to prepare an antigen in this way involved foot-and-mouth disease virus (Figure 23-5). This virus is extremely simple. The protective antigen (VP1) is well recognized, and the genes that code for this protein have been mapped. The RNA genome of the foot-and-mouth disease virus was isolated and transcribed into DNA by the enzyme reverse transcriptase. The DNA was then carefully cut by restriction endonucleases so that it only contained the gene for VP1. This DNA was then inserted into a plasmid, the plasmid inserted into *E. coli*, and the bacteria grown. The bacteria synthesized large quantities of VP1, which was harvested, purified, and incorporated into a vaccine. The process is highly efficient since 4×10^7 doses of foot-and-mouth vaccine can be obtained from 10 L of *E. coli* grown to 10^{12} organisms per milliliter. Unfortunately, the immunity produced is inferior to that produced by killed virus and requires a 1000-fold higher dose to induce comparable protection.

The first commercially available category I recombinant veterinary vaccine was made against feline leukemia virus. The major envelope protein of FeLV, gp70, is the antigen largely responsible for inducing a protective immune response in cats. Thus the gene for gp70 (a *glyco*protein of 70 kDa) plus a small portion of a linked protein called p15e (a *p*rotein of 15 kDa from the *e*nvelope) was isolated and inserted into *E. coli,* which then synthesized large amounts of p70. This recombinant p70 is not glycosylated and has a molecular weight of just over 50 kDa. Once cloned, the recombinant protein is harvested, purified, mixed with a saponin adjuvant, and used as a vaccine.

Another example of a recombinant vaccine is that directed against the Lyme disease agent, *Borrelia burgdorferi.* Thus the

□ Table 23-1 | **USDA Classification of Genetically Engineered Veterinary Biologics**

CATEGORY	DESCRIPTION
I	Vaccines that contain inactivated recombinant organisms or purified antigens derived from recombinant organisms
II	Vaccines containing live organisms that contain gene deletions or heterologous marker genes
III	Vaccines that contain live expression vectors expressing heterologous genes for immunizing antigens or other stimulants
IV	Other genetically engineered vaccines such as polynucleotide vaccines.

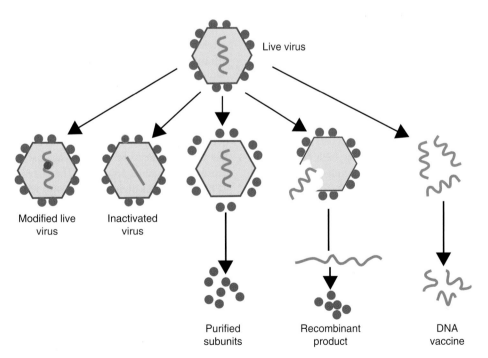

FIGURE 23-4 A schematic diagram showing some of the different ways in which a virus and its antigens may be treated in order to produce a vaccine.

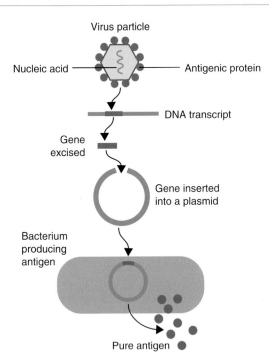

FIGURE 23-5 The production of a recombinant viral protein for use in a vaccine. The gene coding for the viral antigen of interest is cloned into another organism, in this case a bacterium, and expressed and produced in very large quantities.

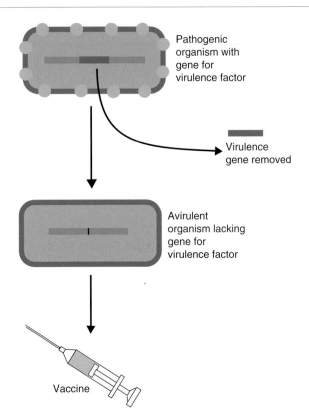

FIGURE 23-6 The production of an attenuated virus by removal of a gene required for virulence. Genes coding for major antigens detected by serological techniques can also be removed, ensuring that vaccinated animals can be distinguished from naturally infected ones.

gene for OspA, the immunodominant outer surface lipoprotein of *B. burgdorferi*, has been cloned into *E. coli*. The recombinant protein expressed by the *E. coli* is purified and used as a vaccine when combined with adjuvant. This vaccine is unique since ticks feeding on immunized animals ingest the antibody. The antibodies then kill the bacteria within the tick midgut and prevent their dissemination to the salivary glands. They thus prevent transmission by the vector.

Rather than cloning the gene of interest in another microorganism, it is possible to clone vaccine antigen genes in plants. This has been successfully achieved for viruses such as transmissible gastroenteritis, Norwalk virus, and Newcastle disease. The plants employed include tobacco, potato, soybean, rice, and corn. In some cases these plants contain very high concentrations of antigen and so can simply be fed to recipients. Although results have been mixed, a tobacco plant–based Newcastle disease vaccine has been licensed in the United States. It is unclear just how these vaccines will be best employed in animals.

Gene cloning techniques are useful in any situation in which pure protein antigens need to be synthesized in large quantities. Unfortunately, pure proteins are often poor antigens because they are not effectively delivered to antigen-sensitive cells and may not be correctly folded. In addition, they may be inefficient antigens because of MHC restriction. An alternative method of delivering a recombinant antigen is to clone the gene of interest into an attenuated living carrier organism.

Genetically Attenuated Organisms (Category II)

Attenuation by prolonged tissue culture can be considered a primitive form of genetic engineering. The desired result is the development of a strain of organism that cannot cause disease. This may be difficult to achieve, and reversion to virulence is an ever-present risk. Molecular genetic techniques, however, make it possible to modify the genes of an organism so that it becomes irreversibly attenuated. These are classified as category II vaccines. They are available against the herpesvirus that causes pseudorabies in swine. The enzyme, thymidine kinase (TK), is required by herpesviruses to replicate in nondividing cells such as neurons. Viruses from which the *TK* gene has been removed can infect nerve cells but cannot replicate and cannot therefore cause disease (Figure 23-6). As a result, these vaccines not only confer effective protection but also block cell invasion by virulent pseudorabies viruses, preventing the development of a persistent carrier state.

Genetic manipulation can also be used to make "marker vaccines." For example, pseudorabies virus synthesizes two glycoprotein antigens called gX and gI. These are potent antigens, yet neither is essential for viral growth or virulence. They are expressed by all field isolates of this virus. Animals infected with the field virus will make antibodies to both gX and gI.

An attenuated pseudorabies vaccine has been produced that lacks these proteins. Vaccinated pigs will not make antibodies to gX or gI, but naturally infected pigs will. The vaccine will not cause positive serological reactions in enzyme-linked immunosorbent assay tests for gX or gI, and the presence of antibodies to gX and gI in a pig is evidence that the animal has been exposed to field strains of pseudorabies virus. This type of vaccine, called a DIVA vaccine (*d*ifferentiate *i*nfected from *v*accinated *a*nimals), should assist in eradicating specific infectious diseases much more economically and rapidly than conventional methods.

Live Recombinant Organisms (Category III)

Genes coding for protein antigens can be cloned directly into a variety of organisms. Instead of being purified, the recombinant organism itself may then be used as a vaccine. These are classified as category III vaccines (Figure 23-7). Experimental recombinant vaccines have used adenoviruses, herpesviruses, and bacteria such as BCG or salmonella as vectors, but the organisms that have been most widely employed for this purpose are poxviruses such as vaccinia, fowlpox, and canarypox. These viruses are easy to administer by dermal scratching or by ingestion. They have a large stable genome that makes it relatively easy to insert a new gene (up to 10% of its genome can be replaced by foreign DNA), and they can express high levels of the new antigen. Moreover, these

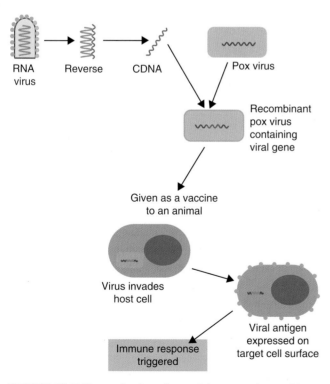

FIGURE 23-7 The production of a vaccinia-vectored recombinant vaccine. Vaccinia is selected because it has room to spare in its genome, and it is easy to administer to an animal. Thus rabies-vaccinia recombinants can be given orally.

recombinant proteins undergo appropriate processing steps, including glycosylation and membrane transport within the poxvirus. The avian poxviruses such as canarypox are especially effective vectors in mammals. They do not replicate, and antigen expression only lasts about 6 hours. As a result, these vaccines are very safe, they cannot be transmitted by arthropods, and they are not excreted in body fluids. It is of interest to note that they do not stimulate immunity to the vector virus, a feature that occurs with the use of other vectors and hence can prevent subsequent immunizations. Canarypox-vectored vaccines appear in many cases to be able to overcome blocking by maternal antibodies and thus prime young animals. They cannot revert to virulence. As a result, canarypox-vectored vaccines are widely employed for such diseases as feline leukemia, West Nile virus, canine parvovirus, canine distemper, equine influenza, and rabies. Another example of a live recombinant vaccine is vaccinia-vectored rabies. The gene for the rabies envelope glycoprotein, or G-protein, is inserted into vaccinia. This glycoprotein is the only rabies antigen capable of inducing virus-neutralizing antibody and conferring protection against rabies. Infection with this rabies-vaccinia recombinant results in the production of antibodies to the G-protein and the development of immunity. This vaccine has been successfully used as an oral vaccine administered to wild carnivores in bait. This form of the vaccine can be distributed by dropping from aircraft. Thus in Belgium, oral rabies vaccine dropped from the air effectively terminated fox rabies, spreading through the Ardennes (Figure 23-8). It has been used in Ontario to prevent the spread of fox rabies, in New Jersey to prevent the spread of raccoon rabies, and in Texas to block the spread of coyote rabies. For example, since 1995, 17.5 million doses of vaccinia-vectored rabies vaccine have been air-dropped over 255,500 square miles (661,745 sq km) of Texas with great success (Box 23-3).

Highly effective category III vaccines have also been developed for rinderpest; these consist of a vaccinia or capripox vector containing the hemagglutinin *(H)* or fusion *(F)* genes of rinderpest virus. These vaccines have been so effective that their systematic use has led to the global eradication of rinderpest. The recombinant capripox vaccine has also had the benefit of protecting cattle against lumpy skin disease. Vaccinia virus can be further attenuated by inactivation of its thymidine kinase and hemagglutinin genes. This has the advantage that it does not cause skin lesions in vaccinated animals. Another example of a category III vaccine involves the use of a yellow fever viral chimera to protect against West Nile virus. This technology uses the capsid and nonstructural genes of the attenuated yellow fever vaccine strain 17D to deliver the envelope genes of other flaviviruses such as West Nile virus. The resulting virus is a yellow fever–West Nile virus chimera that is much less neuroinvasive and hence much safer than either of the parent viruses. The margin of safety can be increased even further by introducing targeted point mutations into the envelope genes.

The first category III vaccine approved by the U.S. Department of Agriculture (USDA) was against the Newcastle disease

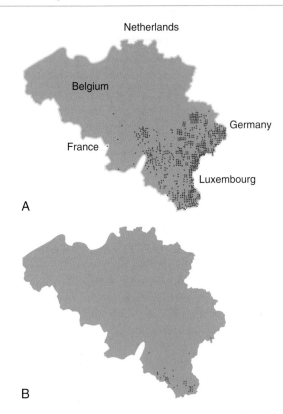

A

B

FIGURE 23-8 The geographical distribution of cases of wild animal rabies in Belgium. **A,** In 1989. **B,** In 1992 and 1993, following the introduction of an oral rabies-vaccinia recombinant vaccine. This is a remarkable example of the effectiveness of a recombinant vaccine.

(From Brochier B, Boulanger D, Costy F, Pastoret PP: Towards rabies elimination in Belgium by fox vaccination using a vaccinia-rabies glycoprotein recombinant virus, *Vaccine* 12:1368–1371, 1994.)

☐ Box 23-3 | **Cost Benefits of Vaccination**

Rabies is an expensive disease. If an unvaccinated animal bites a human, costs include those of postexposure vaccination of the victim as well as quarantine or euthanasia of the biting animal. The brain of the animal must be examined for the presence of the virus. These costs, of course, do not account for the stress and worry associated with this disease. In Texas, aerial vaccination by dropping vaccinia-vectored rabies vaccine enclosed in food bait has been employed to vaccinate coyotes against rabies. The costs of this were the total expenditures on the program—vaccine, food, planes, fuel, and so forth. The benefits were the savings associated with prevented human postexposure prophylaxis and animal rabies tests within the affected area. It was calculated that the rabies vaccination program cost about $26 million. The benefits were estimated at between $89 million and $346 million! Depending on the frequency of postexposure prophylaxis and animal testing, the benefit-to-cost ratio therefore ranged from 3.38 to 33.13.

Shwiff SA, Kirkpatrick KN, Sterner RT: Economic evaluation of an oral rabies vaccination program for control of a domestic dog-coyote rabies epizootic: 1995-2006, *J Am Vet Med Assoc* 233: 1736–1741, 2008.

virus. The vector is a fowlpox virus, into which Newcastle disease *HA* and *F* genes have been incorporated. It has the benefit of conferring immunity against fowlpox as well.

Polynucleotide Vaccines (Category IV)

Another method of vaccination involves injection, not of a protein antigen, but of DNA that encodes foreign antigens. For example, the DNA coding for a vaccine antigen can be inserted into a bacterial plasmid, a piece of circular DNA that acts as a vector (Figure 23-9). The vaccine antigen gene is placed under the control of a strong mammalian promoter sequence. When the genetically engineered plasmid is injected intramuscularly into an animal, it will be taken up by host cells. The DNA is then transcribed into messenger RNA and translated into endogenous vaccine protein (Figure 23-10). The plasmid, unlike viral vectors, cannot replicate in mammalian cells. Experience has shown that plasmid incorporation is enhanced by the use of some "adjuvants." These may include lipid complexes, microcapsules, and nonionic copolymers. Aluminum phosphate seems especially effective in improving vaccine efficiency. Transfected host cells process the vaccine

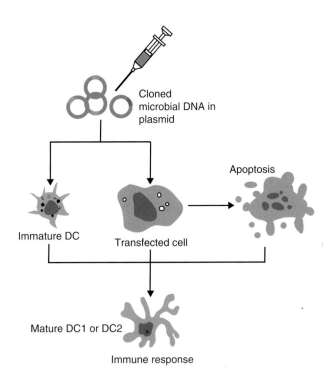

FIGURE 23-9 The mechanism by which polynucleotide vaccines can work. The DNA that enters a cell is functional and can code for endogenous antigens.

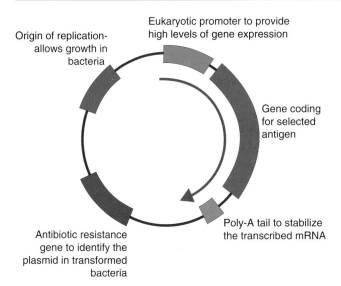

Origin of replication- allows growth in bacteria

Eukaryotic promoter to provide high levels of gene expression

Gene coding for selected antigen

Poly-A tail to stabilize the transcribed mRNA

Antibiotic resistance gene to identify the plasmid in transformed bacteria

FIGURE 23-10 The structure of a typical DNA plasmid used for vaccination purposes. In this case the plasmid codes for protective antigens of West Nile virus. In addition to coding for the antigen in question, the plasmid carries an antibiotic resistance marker so that its fate may be traced.

protein and present it, as an endogenous antigen, in association with MHC class I molecules. This leads to the development not only of neutralizing antibodies but also, since the antigen is endogenous, of cytotoxic T cells. Expressed antigens have an authentic tertiary structure and posttranslational modifications such as glycosylation. The immune response is also enhanced since the bacterial DNA contains unmethylated CpG motifs that are recognized by toll-like receptor 9 (TLR9) and activate dendritic cells. These in turn promote a strong Th1 response. This type of vaccine is used to protect horses against West Nile virus infection. The commercial vaccine consists of a plasmid vector engineered to express high levels of the virus envelope (E) and premembrane (prM) proteins. In addition the plasmid contains gene promoters and marker genes. Upon injection together with a biodegradable oil adjuvant, this plasmid enters cells and causes them to express the viral protein. A second DNA vaccine has been approved to prevent infectious hematopoietic necrosis in Atlantic salmon. Another approved DNA vaccine is designed to treat dogs with the lethal cancer, melanoma. It significantly extends the life of vaccinated animals (Chapter 33). This approach has also been applied experimentally to produce vaccines against avian influenza, lymphocytic choriomeningitis, canine and feline rabies, canine parvovirus, bovine viral diarrhea, feline immunodeficiency virus, feline leukemia virus, pseudorabies, foot-and-mouth disease virus, bovine herpesvirus-1, and Newcastle disease. Although theoretically producing a response similar to that induced by attenuated live vaccines, these nucleic acid vaccines are ideally suited to protect against organisms that are difficult or dangerous to grow in the laboratory. DNA vaccines cannot, of course, be used to induce immunity to polysaccharide antigens. Some

DNA vaccines can induce immunity even in the presence of very high titers of maternal antibody. Although the maternal antibodies block serological responses, the development of strong memory responses is not impaired.

Polynucleotide vaccines must be delivered inside target cells. This can be done by intramuscular injection or by "shooting" the DNA plasmids directly through the skin adsorbed onto microscopic gold beads fired by a "gene gun." Although intramuscular injection is very inefficient because the transfection rate is low (about 1% to 5% of myofibrils in the vicinity of an intramuscular injection site), the expression can persist for at least 2 months. The gene products are either treated as endogenous antigens and displayed on the cell surface or secreted and presented to antigen-processing cells. This processed antigen thus preferentially stimulates a Th1 response associated with IFN-γ production. The use of a gene gun is more efficient than injection since some of this DNA is taken up by the animal's dendritic cells directly, and it minimizes degradation. By bypassing TLR9, the DNA preferentially stimulates a Th2 response. Viral DNA in eye drops can induce an IgA response in the tears and bile of recipients.

Immunization with purified DNA allows presentation of viral antigens in their native form. They are synthesized in the same way as antigens during a viral infection. This is more effective than the use of recombinant proteins since it has proved difficult to create the proteins in the correct conformation. Another advantage is that it is possible to select only the genes for the antigen of interest rather than using a complex carrier organism with its own large gene pool and antigenic mass.

As far as safety is concerned, one theoretical problem is the potential for the vaccine DNA to integrate into the host genome and possibly activate oncogenes or inhibit tumor suppressor genes. Experience suggests that this is a low risk. The presence of an antibiotic-resistant gene in these plasmids also risks transferring this resistance to bacteria. This may be avoided by the use of other markers. Adding cytokines or cytokine genes such as those for IL-3 may also result in improved responses. The risks of DNA vaccination appear to be minimal at this time.

Prime-Boost Strategies It has long been normal practice to use exactly the same vaccine for boosting an immune response as was employed when first priming an animal. This approach has many advantages, not the least of which is simplicity in manufacturing and regulating vaccine production. There is, however, no reason why different forms of a vaccine should not be used for priming and for boosting. This approach is known as a prime-boost strategy. Under some circumstances this may result in significantly improved vaccine effectiveness. The prime-boost approach is somewhat empirical, and researchers may simply test numerous vaccine combinations to determine which combination yields the best results. Prime-boosting has been most widely investigated in attempts to improve the effectiveness of DNA vaccines. Combinations usually involve priming with a DNA vaccine but boosting with either another DNA vaccine, perhaps in another vector, or with recombinant protein antigens.

Reverse Vaccinology

Now that many complete microbial genomes are available, it is possible to identify all the proteins of a pathogen by computer analysis. This analysis can then be used to select potential protective epitopes from this repertoire. This can lead to the identification of unique or unsuspected antigens that may then be experimentally tested—a process called reverse vaccinology (Figure 23-11). The procedures involved include complete sequencing of the antigens of interest, followed by identification of their important epitopes, especially those that bind to common MHC molecules and are likely recognized by CD4+ and CD8+ T cells. These epitopes may be predicted by the use of computer models of the protein or by the use of monoclonal antibodies to identify critical protective components. Once identified, the protective epitopes may be chemically synthesized and tested in animals. Experimental T cell vaccines have been developed in this way against foot-and-mouth disease virus, canine parvovirus, and influenza A.

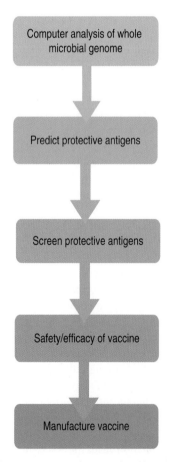

FIGURE 23-11 Reverse vaccinology involves the use of our detailed knowledge of an organism's genome to predict the structure of protective epitopes. These can be synthesized and then tested.

Adjuvants

To maximize the effectiveness of vaccines, especially those containing poorly antigenic killed organisms or highly purified antigens, it has been common practice to add substances called adjuvants to the vaccine (*adjuvare* is the Latin verb for "to help"). Adjuvants can increase the speed or the magnitude of the body's response to vaccines, they may permit reductions in the amount of antigen injected or the numbers of doses administered, and they are essential if long-term memory is to be established to soluble antigens. The mechanisms of adjuvant action are only poorly understood, a problem that has hampered rational development and that has made adjuvant selection somewhat empirical. In general, however, adjuvants belong to one of three groups depending on their mode of action (Table 23-2). The first group, depot adjuvants, simply protect antigens from rapid degradation and thus prolong immune responses. A second group consists of particles that effectively deliver antigen to antigen-presenting cells such as dendritic cells. A third group, immunostimulatory adjuvants, consists of molecules that enhance cytokine production and that selectively stimulate Th1 or Th2 proliferation by providing improved co-stimulation. Some adjuvants may act directly on T or B cells, improving their proliferation or their conversion into memory cells. Adjuvants may be employed to selectively bias Th1 or Th2 responses and optimize the immune response to a specific antigen. Thus the choice of adjuvant can affect the nature of antibodies and the T cells produced and significantly enhance the effectiveness of a vaccine.

Depot Adjuvants

Some adjuvants simply delay the elimination of antigens and thus permit an immune response to last longer. The immune system, being antigen driven, responds to the presence of antigen and terminates once the antigen is eliminated. The rate of antigen elimination can be slowed by mixing it with an insoluble, slowly degraded adjuvant. Examples of depot-forming adjuvants include aluminum salts, such as aluminum hydroxide, aluminum phosphate, and aluminum potassium sulfate (alum) as well as calcium phosphate (Figure 23-12). When antigen is mixed with one of these salts and injected into an animal, a macrophage-rich granuloma forms in the tissues. The antigen within this granuloma slowly leaks into the body and provides a prolonged antigenic stimulus. Antigens that normally persist for only a few days may be retained in the body for several weeks by this technique. These depot adjuvants influence only the primary immune response and have little effect on secondary immune responses. Aluminum-based adjuvants also have the disadvantage that while promoting antibody responses, they have little stimulatory effect on cell-mediated responses. Alum adjuvant clearly enhances Th2 responses to protein antigens. Recruitment of mature myeloid dendritic cells to the sites of injection is greatly increased. Likewise activated macrophages are attracted to sites of alum

Table 23-2 | Some Common Adjuvants

TYPE	ADJUVANT	MODE OF ACTION
Depot adjuvants	Aluminum phosphate	Slow-release antigen depot
	Aluminum hydroxide	Slow-release antigen depot
	Alum	Activate DAMPs
	Freund's incomplete adjuvant	Slow antigen release depot
Microbial adjuvants	Anaerobic corynebacteria	Macrophage stimulator
	BCG	Macrophage stimulator
	Muramyl dipeptide	Macrophage stimulator
	Bordetella pertussis	Lymphocyte stimulator
	Lipopolysaccharide	Macrophage stimulator
Immune stimulators	Saponin	Stimulates antigen processing
	Lysolecithin	Stimulates antigen processing
	Pluronic detergents	Stimulates antigen processing
	Acemannan	Macrophage stimulator
	Glucans	Macrophage stimulator
	Dextran sulfate	Macrophage stimulator
Delivery systems	Liposomes	Stimulates antigen processing
	ISCOMS	Stimulates antigen processing
	Microparticles	Stimulates antigen processing
Mixed adjuvants	Freund's complete adjuvant	Depot plus immune stimulant

injection, and these macrophages may develop into dendritic cells. Studies on the peritoneal fluid of immunized mice showed that alum strongly induced the production of uric acid, a very potent damage-associated molecular pattern (DAMP) and activator of macrophages and dendritic cells.

An alternative method of forming a depot is to incorporate the antigen in a water-in-oil emulsion (called Freund's incomplete adjuvant). The light mineral oil stimulates a local, chronic inflammatory response, and as a result, a granuloma or abscess forms around the site of the inoculum. The antigen is slowly leached from the aqueous phase of the emulsion. These depot adjuvants may cause significant tissue irritation

and destruction. Mineral oils are especially irritating. Nonmineral oils, although less irritating, are also less effective. Tissue damage induced by adjuvants may also promote immune responses since the DAMPs generated by inflammation and cellular necrosis stimulate both dendritic cells and macrophages. Significant irritant activity of adjuvants is not, however, acceptable in modern vaccines, and it is essential to reduce this irritation while retaining adjuvant effectiveness.

Particulate Adjuvants

The immune system can trap and process particles such as bacteria or other microorganisms much more efficiently than soluble antigens. As a result, successful adjuvants may incorporate antigens into readily phagocytosable particles. These adjuvants include emulsions, microparticles, immunostimulating complexes (ISCOMs), and liposomes, and all are designed to deliver antigen efficiently to antigen-presenting cells. The particles are usually of similar size to bacteria and are readily endocytosed. Liposomes are lipid-based synthetic microparticles containing encapsulated antigens that are effectively trapped and processed yet are also protected from rapid degradation. ISCOMS, described later, are complex lipid-based microparticles. All of these particulate adjuvants may be made more potent by incorporating microbial immunostimulants. They are not yet widely employed in veterinary vaccines.

Immunostimulatory Adjuvants

Immunostimulatory adjuvants exert their effects by promoting cytokine production. Many of them are complex microbial products that often present PAMPS, and they are designed to target specific PRRs. As a result, they activate dendritic cells and macrophages through TLR and other PRRs and stimulate the production of key cytokines such as IL-1 and IL-12. These cytokines in turn promote helper T cell responses and drive and focus the adaptive immune responses. Depending on the specific microbial product, they may enhance either Th1 or Th2 responses. TLR ligands alone are not usually effective adjuvants since they induce excessive inflammation. Indeed, much of the difficulty encountered in developing adjuvants is to stimulate adaptive immunity without provoking excessive innate immunity.

Double-stranded RNA (dsRNA) is the ligand for TLR3, and synthetic dsRNA (e.g., polyIC) is an effective adjuvant. TLR4 ligands such as bacterial lipopolysaccharides (or their derivatives) have long been recognized as having adjuvant activity. Their toxicity, however, has limited their use. Lipopolysaccharides enhance antibody formation if given at about the same time as the antigen. They have no effect on cell-mediated responses, but they can break T cell tolerance, and they have a general immunostimulatory activity. Killed anaerobic corynebacteria, especially *Propionibacterium acnes,* have a similar effect. When used as adjuvants, these bacteria enhance antibacterial and antitumor activity. The TLR5 ligand bacterial flagellin is an adjuvant that promotes mixed Th1 and Th2

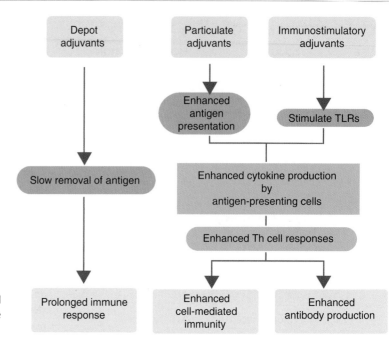

FIGURE 23-12 The three major groups of adjuvants and the ways in which these may act to enhance immune responses triggered by vaccine antigens.

responses. The ligand for TLR7 and TLR8 is single-stranded RNA. Unfortunately it is rapidly degraded and therefore impractical. Some synthetic ligands, such as the imidazoquinolines, and some guanosine and adenosine analogs may be effective adjuvants. Microbial CpG oligodinucleotides that bind TLR9 are potent immunostimulatory adjuvants for Th1 responses. There are multiple classes of CpG-oligodinucleotides, each of which has slightly different immunostimulatory effects. In practice it has been found that multiple innate stimuli may be more effective than a single stimulus and that combination adjuvants that have multiple mechanisms of action appear to be most effective.

Another group of immunostimulatory adjuvants are the saponins (triterpene glycosides), derived from the bark of the soapbark tree (*Quillaja saponaria*). Crude saponins have both toxic and adjuvant activities, although it is possible to purify those with potent adjuvant activity and minimal toxicity. Saponin-based adjuvants selectively stimulate Th1 responses since they direct antigens into endogenous processing pathways and enhance co-stimulatory activity. A purified saponin is used as an adjuvant in a recombinant feline leukemia vaccine. Saponin is also employed as an adjuvant for foot-and-mouth disease vaccines. Toxic saponin mixtures are used in anthrax vaccines, where they destroy tissue at the site of injection so that the anthrax spores may germinate. Modified dextran may be an effective substitute for saponins in some vaccines. Micelles may be constructed using protein antigens and a complex saponin mixture called Quil A. ISCOMs are stable complexes containing cholesterol, phospholipid, saponin, and antigen. ISCOMs are effective adjuvants with few adverse side effects. They are highly effective in targeting antigens to the professional antigen-processing cells, whereas the saponin activates these cells and promotes cytokine production and the expression of co-stimulatory molecules. Depending on the antigen employed, ISCOMs can stimulate either Th1 or Th2 responses.

Combined Adjuvants

Very powerful adjuvants can be constructed by combining a particulate or depot adjuvant with an immunostimulatory agent. For example, an oil-based depot adjuvant can be mixed with killed *Mycobacterium tuberculosis* incorporated into the water-in-oil emulsion. The mixture is called Freund's complete adjuvant (FCA). Not only does FCA form a depot, but the tubercle bacilli also contain muramyl dipeptide (*N*-acetylmuramyl-L-alanyl-D-isoglutamine), a molecule that activates macrophages and dendritic cells through NOD2. FCA works best when given subcutaneously or intradermally and when the antigen dose is relatively low. FCA promotes IgG production over IgM. It inhibits tolerance induction, favors delayed hypersensitivity reactions, accelerates graft rejection, and promotes resistance to tumors. FCA can be used to induce experimental autoimmune diseases, such as experimental allergic encephalitis and thyroiditis (Chapter 35). It also stimulates macrophage activation to M1 cells, promoting their phagocytic and cytotoxic activities.

Use of oil-based adjuvants in animals intended for human consumption is problematic since the oil may spoil the meat. Use of FCA is unacceptable in cattle, not only because of the mineral oil but also because its mycobacteria may induce a positive tuberculin skin test, a critical drawback in any area in which tuberculosis is controlled by skin testing. FCA is highly toxic in dogs and cats.

Given that many adjuvants act by stimulating cytokine production, it is logical that some cytokines may also be effective adjuvants. Most cytokines tested in this way have unacceptable toxicity. IL-12 appears to be especially effective since as a Th1 cell stimulator, it enhances IFN-γ production. IL-3 potentiates some DNA vaccines.

The most widely employed adjuvants in commercial veterinary vaccines remain the depot adjuvants, including aluminum hydroxide, aluminum phosphate, and aluminum potassium sulfate (alum). These adjuvants are produced in the form of a colloidal suspension to which the antigenic material is adsorbed. They are stable on storage, and although they produce a small local granuloma on inoculation, they do not track between muscles or make large parts of the carcass unsuitable for consumption.

For sources of additional information, please visit http:// evolve.elsevier.com/tizard/immunology/

The Use of Vaccines

Key Points

- Vaccine use should be determined by a careful assessment of the relative risks and benefits to an animal.
- Vaccines should only be administered in the doses and by the routes recommended by the manufacturer.
- Vaccines should not be given more often than necessary to provide effective protection.
- On occasion vaccines may cause adverse effects in animals. These are often mild but may be life-threatening.

Although the principles of vaccination have been known for many years, vaccines and vaccination procedures are continuously evolving as we seek to improve both efficacy and safety. The earliest veterinary vaccines were often of limited efficacy and induced severe adverse effects, although these effects were considered acceptable when measured against the risks of acquiring disease. The vaccination protocols developed at that time reflected the inadequacies of these vaccines. Ongoing developments in vaccine design and production have resulted in great improvements in both vaccine safety and effectiveness. These improvements have permitted a reassessment of the relative risks and benefits of vaccination and have resulted in changes in vaccination protocols. Vaccination is not always an innocuous procedure. For this reason, the use of any vaccine should be accompanied by a risk-to-benefit analysis conducted by the veterinarian in consultation with the animal's owner. Vaccination protocols should be customized to each animal, giving due consideration to the seriousness of the disease, the zoonotic potential of the agent, the animal's exposure risk, and any legal requirements relating to vaccination.

The two major factors that determine vaccine use are safety and efficacy. We must always be sure that the risks of vaccination do not exceed those associated with the chance of contracting the disease. Thus it may be inappropriate to use a vaccine against a disease that is rare, is readily treated by other means, or is of little clinical significance. In addition, because the detection of antibodies is a common diagnostic procedure, unnecessary use of vaccines may complicate diagnosis based on serology and perhaps make eradication of a disease impossible. The decision to use vaccines for the control of any disease must be based not only on the degree of risk associated with the disease but also on the availability of superior control or treatment procedures.

The second major consideration is vaccine efficacy. Vaccines may not always be effective. In some diseases, such as equine infectious anemia, Aleutian disease in mink, and African swine fever, poor or no protective immunity can be induced even with the best vaccines. In other diseases, such as foot-and-mouth disease in pigs, the immune response is transient and relatively ineffective, and successful vaccination is difficult to achieve.

As a result of these considerations, some investigators have recommended that animal vaccines be divided into categories based on their importance. The first category consists of essential (or core) vaccines—those that are required because they protect against common, dangerous diseases and because a failure to use them would place an animal at significant risk of disease or death. Which vaccines are considered essential may vary based on local conditions and disease threats. The second category consists of optional (or noncore) vaccines. These are directed against diseases for which the risks associated with not vaccinating may be low. In many cases, risks from these diseases are determined by the location or lifestyle of an animal. The use of these optional vaccines would be determined by a veterinarian on the basis of exposure risk. A third category consists of vaccines that may have no application in routine vaccination but may be used under very special circumstances. These are vaccines directed against diseases of little clinical significance or vaccines whose risks do not significantly outweigh their benefits. Of course, all vaccine use should be conducted on the basis of informed consent. An animal's owner should be made aware of the risks and benefits involved before seeking approval to vaccinate.

When vaccines are used to control disease in a population of animals rather than in individuals, the concept of herd immunity should also be considered. This herd immunity is the resistance of an entire group of animals to a disease as a result of the presence, in that group, of a proportion of immune animals. Herd immunity reduces the probability of a susceptible animal meeting an infected one so that the spread of disease is slowed or terminated. If it is acceptable to lose individual animals from disease while preventing epizootics, it may be possible to do this by vaccinating only a proportion of the population.

Administration of Vaccines

Most vaccines are administered by injection. All such vaccines should be injected carefully and with due regard to the anatomy of the animal. Care must be taken not to injure or introduce infection into any animal. All needles used must be clean and sharp. Dirty or dull needles can cause tissue damage and infection at the injection site. The skin at the injection site must be clean and dry, although excessive use of alcohol swabbing should be avoided. Vaccines are provided in a standard dose, and this dose should not be divided to account for an animal's size. Doses are not formulated to account for body weight or age. There must be a sufficient amount of an antigen to trigger the cells of the immune system and provoke an immune response. This amount is not related to body size. (Unfortunately, the risk of an adverse event occurring is increased in the smallest animals, so it may be necessary to make some adjustment in vaccine dose for safety reasons.) Vaccination by subcutaneous or intramuscular injection is the simplest and most common method of vaccine administration. This approach is obviously excellent for small numbers of animals and for diseases in which systemic immunity is important. In some diseases, however, systemic immunity is not as important as local immunity, and it is perhaps more appropriate to administer the vaccine at the site of potential invasions. Therefore, intranasal vaccines are available for infectious bovine rhinotracheitis of cattle; for *Streptococcus equi* infections in horses; for feline rhinotracheitis, *Bordetella bronchiseptica*, coronavirus, and calicivirus infections; for canine parainfluenza and *Bordetella* infection; and for infectious bronchitis and Newcastle disease in poultry. Unfortunately, these methods of administration require that each animal be dealt with on an individual basis. When animal numbers are large, other methods must be employed. For example, aerosolization of vaccines enables them to be inhaled by all the animals in a group. This technique is employed in vaccinating against canine distemper and mink enteritis on mink ranches and against Newcastle disease in poultry. Alternatively, the vaccine may be put in the feed or drinking water, as is done with *Erysipelothrix rhusiopathiae* vaccines in pigs and against Newcastle disease, infectious laryngotracheitis, and avian encephalomyelitis in poultry. Alternative routes of vaccine administration that are in development or employed in humans include liquid-jet injectors, microinjection, and topical skin application.

Vaccination is now the most important method of preventing infectious diseases in farmed fish. Most commercial fish vaccines consist of inactivated products that are administered either by intraperitoneal injection or, preferably, by immersing the fish in a dilute antigen solution. Immersion results in the antigen being deposited on mucosal surfaces such as the gills or oral cavity, and some may be swallowed.

Multiple-Antigen Vaccines

For convenience, it has become common to employ mixtures of organisms within single vaccines. For respiratory diseases of cattle, for example, vaccines are available that contain infectious bovine rhinotracheitis (BHV-1), bovine virus diarrhea (BVDV), parainfluenza 3 (P13), and even *Mannheimia hemolytica*. Dogs may be given vaccines containing all of the following organisms: canine distemper virus, canine adenovirus 1, canine adenovirus 2, canine parvovirus 2, canine parainfluenza virus, leptospira bacterin, and rabies vaccine. These mixtures may be used when exact diagnosis is not possible and may protect animals against several infectious agents with economy of effort. However, it can also be wasteful to use vaccines against organisms that may not be causing problems. When different antigens in a mixture are inoculated simultaneously, competition occurs between antigens. Manufacturers of multiple-antigen vaccines take this into account and modify their mixtures accordingly. Vaccines should never be mixed indiscriminately since one component may dominate the mixture or interfere with the response to the other components.

Some veterinarians have questioned whether the use of complex vaccine mixtures leads to less than satisfactory protection or increases the risk for adverse side effects. They are concerned that the use of 5- or 7-component vaccines in their pets will somehow overwhelm the immune system, forgetting that we and our animals encounter hundreds of different antigens in daily living. The suggestion that these multiple-antigen vaccines can overload the immune system is unfounded, nor is there any evidence to support the contention that the risk for adverse effects increases disproportionately when more components are added to vaccines. The success of a 23-component pneumococcal vaccine in AIDS patients should serve as a reassurance that multiple component vaccines are not overwhelming. Certainly such vaccines should be tested to ensure that all components induce a satisfactory response. Licensed vaccines provided by a reputable manufacturer will generally provide satisfactory protection against all components.

Vaccination Schedules

Although it is not possible to give exact schedules for all veterinary vaccines available, certain principles are common to all methods of active immunization. Most vaccines require an initial series in which protective immunity is initiated, followed by revaccination (booster shots) at intervals to ensure that this protective immunity remains at an adequate level.

Initial Series Because maternal antibodies passively protect newborn animals, it is not usually possible to successfully vaccinate animals very early in life. If stimulation of immunity is deemed necessary at this stage, the mother may be vaccinated during the later stages of pregnancy, the vaccinations being timed so that peak antibody levels are achieved at the time of colostrum formation. Once an animal is born, successful active immunization is effective only after passive immunity has waned. Since it is impossible to predict the exact time of loss of maternal immunity, the initial vaccination series will generally require administration of multiple doses. Current guidelines for essential canine and feline vaccines, for example, indicate that the first dose of vaccine should be administered at 8 weeks of age, followed by a second dose 3 to 4 weeks later, and concluding at about 15 weeks of age. (These are not, strictly speaking, booster doses. They are simply designed to trigger a primary response as soon as possible after maternal immunity has waned.) All animals should then receive a booster dose 12 months later. Administration of vaccines to young animals is discussed in Chapter 21.

The timing of initial vaccinations may also be determined by the disease. Some diseases are seasonal, and vaccines may be given before disease outbreaks are expected. Examples of these include the vaccine against the lungworm *Dictyocaulus viviparus* given in early summer just before the anticipated lungworm season, the vaccine against anthrax given in spring, and the vaccine against *Clostridium chauvoei* given to sheep before turning them out to pasture. Bluetongue of lambs is spread by midges (*Culicoides variipennis*) and is thus a disease of midsummer and early fall. Vaccination in spring will therefore protect lambs during the susceptible period.

Revaccination and Duration of Immunity As pointed out in Chapter 18, the phenomenon of immunological memory is not well understood; yet it is the persistence of memory cells, B cells, plasma cells, and T cells after vaccination that provides an animal with long-term protection. The presence of long-lived plasma cells is associated with persistent antibody production so that a vaccinated animal may have antibodies in its bloodstream for many years after exposure to a vaccine. It is believed that these long-lived plasma cells are stimulated to survive by activation with microbial PAMPs acting through TLRs and that it is the antibodies that are mainly responsible for long-term protection.

Revaccination schedules depend on the duration of effective protection (Table 24-1). This in turn depends on specific antigen content, whether the vaccine consists of living or dead organisms, and its route of administration. In the past, relatively poor vaccines may have required frequent administration, perhaps as often as every 6 months, to maintain an acceptable level of immunity. Newer, modern vaccines usually produce a long-lasting protection, especially in companion animals; many require revaccination only every 3 years, whereas for others, immunity may persist for an animal's lifetime. Even killed viral vaccines may protect individual animals against disease for many years. Unfortunately, the minimal duration of immunity has, until recently, rarely been measured, and reliable figures are not available for many vaccines. Likewise, although serum antibodies can be monitored in vaccinated animals, tests have not been standardized, and there is no

☐ Table 24-1 | Estimated Minimum Duration of Immunity (DOI) of Select Commercially Available Canine Vaccine Antigens

VACCINE	ESTIMATED MINIMUM DOI	ESTIMATED RELATIVE EFFICACY (%)
Essential		
Canine distemper (modified live virus [MLV])	>7 yr	>90
Canine distemper (recombinant [R])	>1 yr	>90
Canine parvovirus-2 (MLV)	>7 yr	>90
Canine adenovirus-2 (MLV)	>7 yr	>90
Rabies virus (killed [K])	>3 yr	>85
Optional		
Canine coronavirus (K or MLV)	N/A	N/A
Canine parainfluenza (MLV)	>3 yr	>80
Bordetella bronchiseptica (ML)	<1 yr	<70
Leptospira canicola (K)	<1 yr	<50
Leptospira grippotyphosa (K)	<1 yr	N/A
Leptospira icterohaemorrhagiae (K)	<1 yr	<75
Leptospira pomona (K)	<1 yr	N/A
Borrelia burgdorferi (K)	1 yr	<75
Borrelia burgdorferi OspA (R)	1 yr	<75
Giardia lamblia (K)	<1 yr	N/A

From Paul MA, Appel M, Barrett R, et al: Report of the American Animal Hospital Association (AAHA) Canine Vaccine Task Force: executive summary and 2003 canine vaccine guidelines and recommendations, *J Am Anim Hosp Assoc* 39:119–131, 2003.

consensus regarding the interpretation of these antibody titers. Even animals that lack detectable antibodies may well have significant resistance to disease. Nor is there much information available regarding long-term immunity on mucosal surfaces. In general, immunity against feline panleukopenia, canine distemper, canine parvovirus, and canine adenovirus is considered to be relatively long-lasting (>5 years). On the other hand, immunity to feline rhinotracheitis, feline calicivirus, and *Chlamydophila* is believed to be relatively short. One problem in making these statements is variability among individual animals and among different types of vaccine. Thus recombinant canine distemper vaccines may induce immunity of much

shorter duration than conventional, modified live vaccines. There may be a great difference between the shortest and longest duration of immunological memory within a group of animals. Duration of immunity studies are confounded by the fact that in many cases older animals show increased innate resistance. Different vaccines within a category may differ significantly in their composition, and although all vaccines may induce immunity in the short term, it cannot be assumed that all confer long-term immunity. Manufacturers use different master seeds and different methods of antigen preparation. The level of immunity required for most of these diseases is unknown. A significant difference exists between the minimal level of immunity required to protect most animals and the level of immunity required to ensure protection of all animals.

Annual revaccination has been the rule for most animal vaccines since this approach is administratively simple and has the advantage of ensuring that an animal is regularly seen by a veterinarian. It is clear, however, that vaccines such as those against canine distemper or feline herpesvirus induce protective immunity that can last for many years and that annual revaccination using these vaccines is unnecessary. A growing body of evidence now indicates that most modified live viral (MLV) vaccines induce lifelong sterile immunity in dogs and cats. In contrast, immunity to bacteria is of much shorter duration and often may prevent disease but not infection. Old dogs and cats rarely die from vaccine-preventable disease, especially if they have been vaccinated as adults. Young animals, in contrast, may die from such diseases, especially if not vaccinated or if vaccinated at an incorrect age. A veterinarian should always assess the relative risks and benefits to an animal in determining the use of any vaccine and its frequency of administration. It may therefore be good practice to use serum antibody assays such as ELISAs, if available, to provide guidance on revaccination intervals. Persistent antibody titers may indicate protection, but this is not guaranteed, especially if cell-mediated immune mechanisms are important for protection. Likewise, animals with low or undetectable serum antibody levels may still be protected as a result of persistence of memory B and T cells capable of responding rapidly to reinfection.

Notwithstanding the previous discussion, animal owners should be made aware that protection against an infectious disease can only be maintained reliably when vaccines are used in accordance with the protocol approved by the vaccine-licensing authorities. The duration of immunity claimed by a vaccine manufacturer is the minimum duration of immunity that is supported by the data available at the time the vaccine license is approved. This must always be taken into account when discussing revaccination protocols with an owner.

Vaccination Strategies

Although vaccination is a powerful tool for the control of infectious disease, its potential to prevent the spread of a disease or to eliminate a disease depends on selecting correct control strategies. If an infectious disease outbreak, such as one caused by foot-and-mouth virus, is to be rapidly controlled, it is vitally important to select the correct population to be vaccinated. The success of any mass vaccination program depends both on the proportion of animals vaccinated and on the efficacy of the vaccine. Neither of these factors will reach 100%, so it is essential to target the vaccine effectively. It is also the case that vaccines do not confer immediate protection, so the strategy employed will depend on the rate of spread of an infection. Vaccines may thus be given prophylactically, in advance of an outbreak, or reactively, in response to an existing outbreak. Both strategies have advantages and disadvantages. In general, prophylactic vaccination greatly reduces the potential for a major epidemic of a disease such as foot-and-mouth disease by reducing the size of a susceptible population. The effectiveness of this approach can be greatly enhanced by identifying high-risk individuals and ensuring that they are protected in advance of an outbreak.

It is generally not feasible to vaccinate an entire population of animals once a disease outbreak has occurred. However, two effective reactive vaccination strategies are *ring vaccination,* which seeks to contain an outbreak by establishing a barrier of immune animals around an infected area, and *predictive vaccination,* which seeks to vaccinate the animals on farms likely to contribute most to the future spread of disease. Reactive vaccination in this way can ensure that an epidemic is not unduly prolonged. A prolonged "tail" to an epidemic commonly results from the disease "jumping" to a new area. Well-considered, predictive vaccination may well prevent these jumps. Thus a combination of prophylactic and reactive vaccination will likely yield the most effective results.

Vaccine Assessment

To assess the efficacy of a vaccine, animals must first be vaccinated and then challenged. The percentage of vaccinated animals that survive this challenge can then be measured. It is important, however, to determine the percentage of nonvaccinated control animals that also survive the challenge. The true efficacy of a vaccine, called the preventable fraction (PF), is calculated as follows:

$$PF = \frac{(\% \text{ of controls dying} - \% \text{ of vaccinates dying})}{\% \text{ of controls dying}}$$

For example, a challenge that kills 80% of controls and 40% of vaccinates shows that the PF of the vaccine is as follows:

$$PF = \frac{80 - 40}{80} = 50\%$$

Good, effective vaccines should have a PF of at least 80%. Obviously, less effective vaccines are acceptable if safe and if nothing better is available. In determining vaccine efficacy.

however, large challenge doses may overwhelm any reasonable level of vaccine-induced immunity. It is also important to determine what degree of protection is desired. It may be much easier to prevent deaths rather than illness.

Failures in Vaccination

There are many reasons that a vaccine may fail to confer protective immunity on an animal (Figure 24-1).

Incorrect Administration

In many cases vaccine failure is due to unsatisfactory administration. For example, a live vaccine may have died as a result of poor storage, the use of antibiotics in conjunction with live bacterial vaccines, the use of chemicals to sterilize the syringe, or the excessive use of alcohol when swabbing the skin. Sometimes animals given vaccines by nonconventional routes may not be protected. When large flocks of poultry or mink are to be vaccinated, it is common to administer the vaccine either as an aerosol or in drinking water. If the aerosol is not evenly distributed throughout a building, or if some animals do not drink, they may receive insufficient vaccine. Animals that subsequently develop disease may be interpreted as cases of vaccine failure.

Failure to Respond

Occasionally, a vaccine may actually be ineffective. The method of production may have destroyed the protective epitopes, or there may simply be insufficient antigen in the vaccine. Problems of this type are uncommon and can generally be avoided by using only vaccines from reputable manufacturers.

More commonly, an animal may simply fail to mount an immune response. The immune response, being a biological process, never confers absolute protection and is never equal in all members of a vaccinated population. Since the immune response is influenced by a large number of genetic and environmental factors, the range of immune responses in a large random population of animals tends to follow a normal distribution. This means that most animals respond to antigens by mounting an average immune response, whereas a few will mount an excellent response, and a small proportion will mount a poor immune response (Figure 24-2). This group of poor responders may not be protected against infection despite having received an effective vaccine. Therefore, it is essentially impossible to protect 100% of a random population of animals by vaccination. The size of this unreactive portion of the population will vary between vaccines, and its significance will depend on the nature of the disease. Thus, for highly infectious diseases against which herd immunity is poor and in which infection is rapidly and efficiently transmitted, such as foot-and-mouth disease, the presence of unprotected animals could permit the spread of disease and would thus disrupt control programs. Likewise, problems can arise if the unprotected

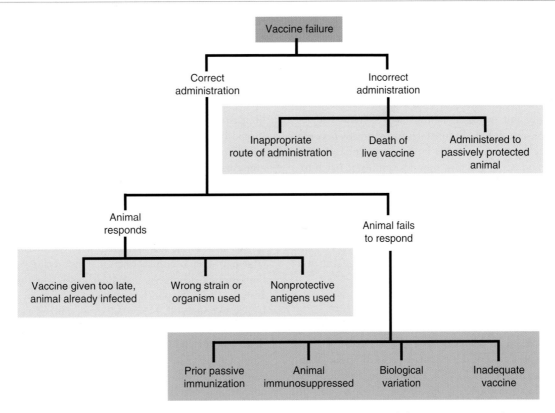

FIGURE 24-1 A simple classification of the ways in which a vaccine may fail to protect an animal.

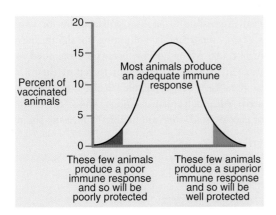

FIGURE 24-2 The normal distribution of protective immune responses in a population of vaccinated animals. No vaccine can be expected to protect 100% of a population.

animals are individually important, such as companion animals. In contrast, for diseases that are inefficiently spread, such as rabies, 70% protection may be sufficient to effectively block disease transmission within a population and may therefore be quite satisfactory from a community health viewpoint.

Another type of vaccine failure occurs when the normal immune response is suppressed. For example, heavily parasitized or malnourished animals may be immunosuppressed and should not be vaccinated. Some virus infections induce profound immunosuppression. Animals with a major illness or high fever should not normally be vaccinated unless for a compelling reason. Stress may reduce a normal immune response, probably because of increased steroid production; examples of such stress include pregnancy, fatigue, malnutrition, and extremes of cold and heat.

Other studies have shown that neutering at or near the time of first vaccination does not impair the antibody responses of kittens. This type of immunosuppression is discussed in detail in Chapter 38. The most important cause of vaccine failure of this type is passively derived maternal immunity in young animals, as described in Chapter 21.

Analysis of an outbreak of influenza in racehorses has shown some interesting and important factors that appeared to determine disease susceptibility. Thus when the effect of age was analyzed, it appears that 2-year-old horses were less susceptible than other animals. Further analysis suggested that this increased resistance resulted from recent vaccination of this age cohort despite other age groups possessing similar antibody levels. There was evidence of gender differences in resistance (62% of females and 71% of males were infected). There was also some evidence that vaccination at a young age (<6 months) in the presence of maternal antibody had detrimental long-term effects on protection when compared with foals first vaccinated between 6 and 18 months of age.

Recent studies have also analyzed data from 10,483 dogs of all ages and breeds vaccinated against rabies to determine the factors that influence seroconversion. It was found that a general relationship exists between a dog's size and its antibody level. Smaller dogs produced higher antibody titers than large dogs. Vaccine effectiveness also varied among breeds. Thus significant failure rates were seen in German Shepherds and Labradors. Young animals vaccinated before 1 year of age produced lower antibody levels than adults. The highest antibody titers were generated in dogs aged 3 to 4 years at time of vaccination. Primary vaccination of aged animals showed lower antibody levels and increased failure rates. Gender had no effect on failure rate or titer. Failure rates varied greatly between vaccines. They ranged from 0.2% in the worst case to 0.01% in the best, and some vaccines showed significant batch-to-batch variation in efficacy. Of the variation in antibody titers observed, 19% was due to vaccine differences, 8% was due to breed differences, 5% was attributed to size differences, and 3% to other differences. It is likely that similar variables influence the responses of dogs and cats to other vaccines. Perhaps vaccines should be reformulated to take these age, size, and breed differences into account.

Correct Administration and Response

Even animals given an adequate dose of an effective vaccine may fail to be protected. If the vaccinated animal was incubating the disease before inoculation, the vaccine may be given too late to affect the course of the disease. Alternatively, the vaccine may contain the wrong strain of organisms or the wrong (nonprotective) antigens.

Adverse Consequences of Vaccination

Vaccination continues to be the only safe, reliable, and effective way of protecting animals against the major infectious diseases. Vaccine-related toxicity is usually rare, mild, and transient, and

hypothetical side effects must not dominate our perceptions. Nevertheless, the use of vaccines is not free of risk. Residual virulence and toxicity, allergic responses, disease in immunodeficient hosts, neurological complications, and harmful effects on the fetus are the most significant risks associated with the use of vaccines (Figure 24-3). Veterinarians should use only licensed vaccines, and the manufacturer's recommendations should be carefully followed. Before using a vaccine, the veterinarian should consider the likelihood that an adverse event will happen, as well as the possible consequences or severity of this event. These factors must be weighed against the benefits to the animal. Thus a common but mild complication may require a different consideration than a rare, severe complication.

The issue of the risk associated with vaccination remains in large part a philosophical one since the advantages of vaccination are well documented and extensive, whereas the risk for adverse effects is poorly documented and, in many cases, largely hypothetical. Nevertheless, established facts should be recognized, unsubstantiated allegations rebutted by sound data, and uncertainties acknowledged. For example, there is absolutely no evidence that vaccination itself leads to ill health. Although difficult to prove a negative, competent statistical analysis has consistently failed to demonstrate any general adverse effect of vaccination.

Traditionally, adverse events resulting from vaccine administration have been reported voluntarily by veterinarians to manufacturers or government agencies. The resulting figures have been impossible to analyze satisfactorily for two major reasons. First, reporting is voluntary, so significant underreporting occurs. Many adverse events are regarded as insignificant, or it may be inconvenient to report them. Second, very few data have been available on the number of animals vaccinated. Although manufacturers know the number of doses of vaccine sold, they are unable to measure the number

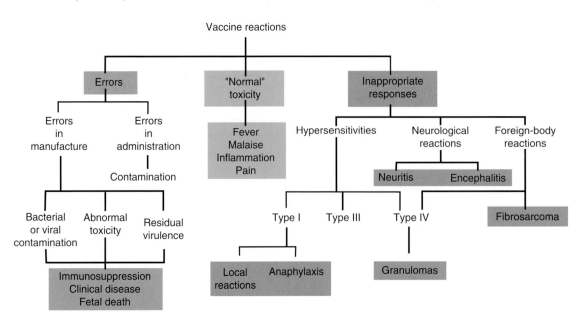

FIGURE 24-3 A simple classification of the major adverse effects of vaccination.

of animals vaccinated. Nevertheless, it has proved possible by examining the electronic records of a very large general practice to determine the prevalence of vaccine-associated adverse events in more than 1 million dogs. The use of a standardized reporting system within a very large population has permitted Dr. Larry Glickman and his colleagues to determine the prevalence of adverse events occurring within 3 days of vaccine administration. Out of 1,226,159 dogs vaccinated, there were 4,678 adverse events recorded (38.2/10,000 dogs); 72.8% of these events occurred on the same day the vaccine was administered, 31.7% were considered to be allergic reactions, and 65.8% were considered "vaccine reactions" and were likely due to toxicity. Additional analysis indicated that the risk of adverse events was significantly greater for small than for large dogs (Figure 24-4); for neutered than for sexually intact dogs; and for dogs that received multiple vaccines. Each additional vaccine dose administered increased the risk of an adverse event occurring by 27% in small dogs (<10 kg) and by 12% in dogs heavier than 12 kg. High-risk breeds included Dachshunds, Pugs, Boston Terriers, Miniature Pinschers, and Chihuahuas. Overall, the increased incidence of adverse events in small dogs and their relationship to multiple dosing suggests that veterinarians should look carefully at the practice of giving the same dose of vaccine to all dogs irrespective of their size.

A similar study examined the incidence of vaccine-associated adverse events following the administration of 1,258,712 doses

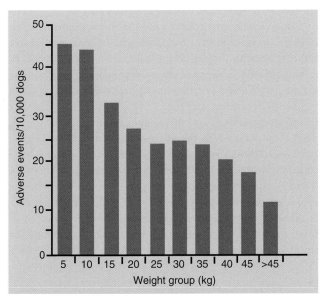

FIGURE 24-4 Vaccine-associated adverse events are much more likely to occur in small rather than in large dogs. Mean ± SEM vaccine-associated adverse event rates by 5-kg weight groups in 1,226,159 dogs vaccinated at 360 veterinary hospitals from January 1, 2002 to December 31, 2003. These adverse events were diagnosed within 3 days of vaccine administration.

(From Moore GE, Guptill LP, Ward MP, et al: Adverse events diagnosed within three days of vaccine administration in dogs, *J Am Vet Med Assoc* 227:1102–1108, 2005.)

of vaccine to 496,189 cats. The investigators reported 2560 adverse events (51.6/10,000 cats vaccinated). The risk was greatest for cats 1 year old. For unknown reasons, risk was greater in neutered than in sexually intact cats. Lethargy was the most commonly reported event (Figure 24-5). The number of adverse events increased significantly when multiple vaccines were given during a single visit.

Identification of an adverse event is based on the clinical judgment of the attending veterinarian and is subject to bias. Standard case definitions of a vaccine-associated adverse event are not yet available. On the other hand, the significance of such bias is reduced by the use of such a large database.

"Normal" Toxicity

Vaccines commonly elicit transient inflammatory reactions, and some degree of inflammation is required for the efficient induction of protective immune responses. This may cause pain. Thus the sting produced by some vaccines may present problems not only to the animal being vaccinated but also, if the animal reacts violently, to the vaccinator. More commonly, local swellings may develop at the reaction site. These may be firm or edematous and may be warm to the touch. They appear about 1 day after vaccination and can last for about a week. Unless an injection-site abscess develops, these swellings leave little trace. Vaccines containing killed Gram-negative organisms may be intrinsically toxic owing to the presence of endotoxins that can cause cytokine release, leading to shock, fever, and leukopenia. Although such a reaction is usually only a temporary inconvenience to male animals, it may be sufficient to provoke abortion in pregnant females. Thus it may be prudent to avoid vaccinating pregnant animals unless the risks of not giving the vaccine are considered to be too great.

Inappropriate Responses

Vaccines may cause rare but serious allergic reactions. For example, type I hypersensitivity can occur when an animal produces immunoglobulin E (IgE) in response not only to the immunizing antigen but also to other antigens found in vaccines, such as egg antigens or antigens from tissue culture cells. All forms of hypersensitivity are more commonly associated with multiple injections of antigens and therefore tend to be associated with the use of killed vaccines. It is important to emphasize that a type I hypersensitivity reaction is an immediate response to an antigen and occurs within a few minutes or hours after exposure to an antigen. Reactions occurring more than 2 or 3 hours after administration of a vaccine are likely not type I hypersensitivity reactions.

Type III hypersensitivity reactions are also potential hazards. These may cause intense local inflammation, or they may present as a generalized vascular disturbance such as purpura. A type III reaction can occur in the eyes of dogs vaccinated against infectious canine hepatitis (Chapter 26). Some rabies vaccines may induce a local complement-mediated vasculitis leading to ischemic dermatitis and local alopecia. This type of

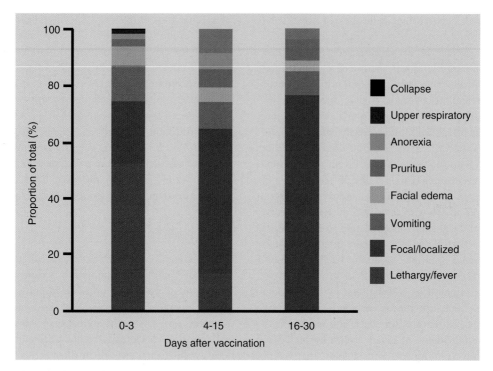

FIGURE 24-5 Distribution of types of vaccine-associated adverse events diagnosed during various periods after vaccination in 496,189 cats administered one or more vaccines from January 1, 2002 to December 31, 2004.

(From Moore GE, DeSantis-Kerr AC, Guptill LF, et al: Adverse events after vaccine administration in cats: 2,560 cases (2002-2005), *J Am Vet Med Assoc* 231: 94–100, 2007.)

reaction is most often seen in small dogs such as Dachshunds, Miniature Poodles, Bichon Frises, and Terriers.

Type IV hypersensitivity reactions may occur in response to vaccination, but a more common reaction is granuloma formation at the site of inoculation. This may be a response to depot adjuvants containing alum or oil. Vaccines containing a water-in-oil adjuvant produce larger and more persistent lesions at injection sites than vaccines containing alum and aluminum hydroxide. These lesions can be granulomas or sterile abscesses. If the skin is dirty at the injection site, these abscesses may become infected.

Postvaccinal canine distemper virus encephalitis is a rare complication that may develop after administration of a modified live canine distemper vaccine. The affected animal may show aggression, incoordination, and seizures or other neurological signs. The pathogenesis of this condition is unknown, but it may be due to residual virulence, increased susceptibility, or triggering of a latent paramyxovirus by the vaccine.

Errors in Manufacture or Administration

Some problems associated with vaccine use may be due to poor production or administration. Thus some modified live vaccines may retain the ability to cause disease. For example, some modified live herpes vaccines or calicivirus vaccines given intranasally may spread to the oropharynx and result in persistent infection. Indeed, such a virus vaccine may infect (and protect) other animals in contact. Even if these vaccines do not cause overt disease, they may reduce the rate of growth of farm animals with significant economic consequences.

Some vaccines may trigger a mild immunosuppression. For example, some modified live parvovirus vaccines may cause a transient decrease in lymphocyte responses to mitogens or even a lymphopenia in some puppies, although not all strains of canine parvovirus 2 are immunosuppressive. Some polyvalent canine viral vaccines can cause a transient drop in absolute lymphocyte numbers and their responses to mitogens (Figure 38-1). This occurs even though the individual components of these vaccines may not have this effect. Several vaccine combinations may result in transient immunosuppression between 5 and 11 days after vaccination. For example, a combination of canine adenovirus type 1 or type 2 with canine distemper virus is especially suppressive of canine lymphocyte responses to mitogens. This T cell suppression may be accompanied by simultaneous enhancement of B cell responses and raised immunoglobulin levels. Rather than being a pure immunosuppressive effect, it may simply reflect a transient change in the Th1/Th2 balance.

Vaccines such as bluetongue vaccine have been reported to cause congenital anomalies in the offspring of ewes vaccinated while pregnant. The stress from this type of vaccination may also be sufficient to reactivate latent infections; for example, activation of equine herpesvirus has been demonstrated following vaccination against African horse sickness. Mucosal disease may develop in calves vaccinated against bovine virus diarrhea (Chapter 21).

Vaccine-Associated Autoimmune Disease

It is widely believed that the prevalence of autoimmune disease in domestic pets, especially dogs, has risen in recent years. Some investigators have attributed this rise to excessive use of potent vaccines. This link is by no means proven; nevertheless, there is limited evidence that supports an association between vaccination and autoimmunity. A retrospective analysis of the history of dogs presenting with immune-mediated hemolytic anemia (IMHA) (Chapter 35) showed that 15 of 70 dogs with IMHA had been vaccinated within the previous month, compared with a randomly selected control group in which none had been vaccinated. Dogs with IMHA that developed within a month of vaccination differed in some clinical features from dogs with IMHA unassociated with prior vaccination. Epidemiological studies using very large databases tend to confirm this effect, in that they show an approximately three-fold increase in diagnoses of autoimmune thrombocytopenia, and a two-fold increase in diagnoses of IMHA, in dogs in the 30 days following vaccination, compared with other time periods. The overall incidence of these diseases, however, is low, and they can be diagnosed at times not temporally associated with vaccination. Vaccination may therefore serve as a stimulus for these diseases in some dogs, but other, undefined, stimuli must also exist.

Contaminating thyroglobulin found in some vaccines (usually from the presence of fetal bovine serum) can lead to the production of antithyroid antibodies in vaccinated dogs. Lymphocytic thyroiditis has been found in 40% of Beagles on necropsy, but there was no association detected between vaccination and the development of this thyroiditis.

It is well recognized that Guillain-Barré syndrome, an autoimmune neurological disease of humans, can be triggered by administration of some vaccines such as influenza vaccine. At least one case has been reported in a dog following vaccination with a polyvalent distemper-hepatitis-parvovirus vaccine (Chapter 35). In some animals, the administration of potent, adjuvanted vaccines may stimulate the transient production of autoantibodies to connective tissue components such as fibronectin and laminin.

Vaccine-Induced Osteodystrophy

Vaccination of some Weimaraner puppies with an MLV vaccine may lead to the development of a severe hypertrophic osteodystrophy. The disease appears within 10 days of administration of a vaccine containing MLV canine distemper vaccine. Systemic signs include anorexia, depression, fever, and gastrointestinal, nervous, and respiratory symptoms in addition to symmetrical metaphyseal lesions with painful swollen metaphyses. Radiological examination shows radiolucent zones in the metaphyses, flared diaphyses, and formation of new periosteal bone. Hind and fore limbs are equally affected. It is possible that the condition is triggered in genetically susceptible animals by MLV canine distemper vaccine. The disease responds well to corticosteroid therapy. In many cases, these dogs show a preexisting immune dysfunction with low concentrations of one or more immunoglobulin classes, recurrent infections, and inflammatory disease (Chapter 37). It has been suggested that Weimaraners are especially susceptible to this condition and that they receive only killed virus vaccines.

A mild transient polyarthritis has been reported to occur in other dogs following vaccination. Dogs show a sudden onset of lameness with swollen and painful joints within 2 weeks of vaccination. The dogs recover within 2 days. No specific breed or vaccine has been associated with this problem. Vaccination against calicivirus has been associated with polyarthritis and a postvaccination limping syndrome in cats.

Injection Site–Associated Sarcomas

Sarcomas associated with the site of vaccine injection are discussed in detail in Chapter 33.

Adverse Effect Principles

In determining whether a vaccine causes an adverse effect, the following three principles should apply. First, is the effect consistent? The clinical responses should be the same if the vaccine is given to a different group of animals, by different investigators, and irrespective of the method of investigation. Second, is the effect specific? The association should be distinctive and the adverse event linked specifically to the vaccine concerned. It is important to remember that an adverse event may be caused by vaccine adjuvants and additives other than the active component. Finally, there must be a temporal relationship. Administration of the vaccine should precede the earliest manifestations of the event or a clear exacerbation of a continuing condition.

Production, Presentation, and Control of Vaccines

The production of veterinary vaccines is controlled by the Animal and Plant Health Inspection Service of the USDA in the United States, by the Canadian Centre for Veterinary Biologics of the Canadian Food Inspection Agency, and by the Veterinary Medicines Directorate in the United Kingdom, as well as by appropriate government agencies in other countries. In general, regulatory authorities have the right to license establishments where vaccines are produced and to inspect these premises to ensure that the facilities are appropriate and that the methods employed are satisfactory. All vaccines must be checked for safety and potency. Safety tests include confirmation of the identity of the organism used and of the freedom of the vaccine from extraneous organisms (i.e., purity), as well as tests for toxicity and sterility. Because the living organisms or antigens found in vaccines normally die or degrade over a period of time, it is necessary to ensure that they will be effective even after storage. It is usual, therefore, to use an antigen in generous excess of the dose required to protect animals under laboratory conditions, and potency is tested both before and after accelerated aging. Vaccines that contain killed organisms, although much more stable than living ones, also contain an excess of antigens for the same reason. Vaccines approved for licensing on the basis of challenge exposure studies must usually show evidence of protection in 80% of vaccinated animals, whereas at least 80% of the unvaccinated controls must develop evidence of disease after challenge exposure (the 80:80 efficacy guideline). The route and dose of administration indicated on the vaccine label should be scrupulously heeded since these were probably the only route and dose tested for safety and efficacy during the licensing process. Vaccines usually have a designated shelf-life, and although properly stored vaccines may still be potent after the expiration of this shelf-life, this should never be assumed. Correct storage and handling are essential. All expired vaccines should be discarded. Adverse reactions should always be reported to the appropriate licensing authorities as well as to the vaccine manufacturer. Because MLV vaccines carry with them the risks for residual virulence and for contamination with other agents, certain countries will not approve their use.

Inactivated vaccines are commonly available in liquid form and usually contain suspended adjuvant. These should not be frozen, and they should be shaken well before use. The presence of preservatives such as phenol or merthiolate will not control massive bacterial contamination, and multidose containers should be discarded after partial use. Many vaccines containing MLV are susceptible to heat inactivation but are much more resistant if lyophilized. Remember, however, that intense sunlight and heat can destroy even lyophilized vaccines. They store well but should be kept cool and away from light and should only be reconstituted with the fluid provided by the manufacturer.

For sources of additional information, please visit http://evolve.elsevier.com/tizard/immunology/

Immunity to Bacteria and Fungi

Key Points

- Antibodies can neutralize bacterial toxins.
- Antibodies alone will opsonize bacteria. Antibodies and complement may opsonize bacteria or kill them directly through the terminal complement complex.
- T cell–mediated activation of macrophages is required to kill intracellular bacteria.
- Under some circumstances, especially in mycobacterial disease, an inappropriate Th2 response rather than the required Th1 response may lead to severe disease and death.
- Bacteria may resist destruction by multiple mechanisms.
- Cell-mediated immune responses are usually required to protect against fungal infections.

Although animals live in environments densely populated with bacteria, most of these organisms neither invade animal tissues nor cause disease. This is unsurprising for several reasons. First, the combined efforts of the innate and adaptive immune systems are sufficient to prevent invasion. Second, even organisms that successfully invade the animal body gain very little by harming their host. On the contrary, illness or death of the host animal may well reduce the survival of the bacteria and is therefore normally avoided. Indeed, many bacteria are essential for the animal's well-being since they maintain an environment on body surfaces that is hostile to other potential invaders. They also assist in the digestion of foods such as celluloses and promote the normal development of the immune system. Nevertheless, many commensal bacteria are also pathobionts. For example, *Clostridium tetani* and *Clostridium perfringens* are commonly found among the intestinal flora of horses, and *Bordetella bronchiseptica* is found in the nasopharynx of healthy swine. Bacterial disease is not, therefore, an inevitable consequence of the presence of pathogenic organisms on the body surface. The development of

LIVERPOOL JOHN MOORES UNIVERSITY
LEARNING SERVICES

disease is related to many other factors, including the response of the host, the presence of damaged tissues, the location of the bacteria within the body, and the disease-producing power (or virulence) of the bacteria. Only when the balance between host immunity and bacterial virulence is upset will disease or death result.

The adaptation of bacteria to a host depends on factors that enable the bacteria to survive and grow—virulence factors. Many of these virulence factors are encoded on mobile genetic elements that can be transmitted between species (e.g., plasmids). These virulence factors permit the bacteria to adapt to a specific environment and promote their transmission between hosts. Depending on their niche within the body, bacteria can use virulence factors to penetrate surface epithelia, to bind to cell surfaces, to acquire iron, to evade immune responses, to hide within cells, and to promote transmission to another host. Some of the strategies adopted by bacteria are associated with damage to host tissues and must be counteracted by the immune system.

Innate Immunity

Antimicrobial immunity consists of an early innate response followed by a sustained adaptive response. Recognition of invading bacteria through toll-like receptors (TLRs) and other receptors induces inflammation, cytokine release, and complement activation. If this is insufficient to eliminate the invaders, adaptive immune mechanisms take over. Thus dendritic cells and macrophages ingest invading bacteria and initiate adaptive immunity by secreting cytokines and triggering both T and B cell responses. The importance of these innate defenses is emphasized by the observation that the resistance of chickens to *Salmonella enterica* Typhimurium appears to be linked to allelic variations in TLR4, whereas the resistance of foals to *Rhodococcus equi* depends on TLR2.

TLRs are responsible in large part for the initial recognition of invading bacteria. Binding of microbial pathogen-associated molecular patterns (PAMPs) to TLRs triggers a signal cascade that activates genes that are critical in host defense.

The production of cytokines by horse neutrophils following exposure to *R. equi* provides an example of these responses. Thus after exposure to *R. equi*, neutrophils express increased amounts of interleukin-23 (IL-23). This IL-23 promotes Th17 cell differentiation. Driven by transforming growth factor-β (TGF-β) and IL-6, the Th17 cells then participate in inflammatory reactions. Th17 cells confer protection against extracellular bacteria and fungi, especially at epithelial surfaces. Not only do these Th17 cells produce IL-17 but also IL-6, GM-CSF, G-CSF, chemokines, and metalloproteases. They trigger inflammation and coordinate early neutrophil recruitment to infection sites. Type I interferons are also readily produced in response to bacterial PAMPS. IFN-α/β boosts macrophage responses enhancing their production of IFN-γ, nitric oxide, and TNF-α.

☐ **Box 25-1** | **Vitamin D and Immunity**

When an intracellular bacterium such as *Mycobacterium tuberculosis* interacts with TLR1 or TLR2 on the surface of macrophages, it upregulates many different genes and enhances their antimicrobial activity. In mice, this is mainly mediated by nitric oxide. In humans, however, nitric oxide is not elevated, and other mechanisms are involved (Figure 25-2). One gene activated by TLR1/2 signaling in humans is that coding for the vitamin D receptor. This receptor is therefore upregulated on activated macrophages. Binding of vitamin D to its receptor upregulates expression of the gene for the antibacterial peptide cathelicidin. The cathelicidin, in turn, can kill intracellular *M. tuberculosis*. It is no coincidence, therefore, that resistance to tuberculosis is directly related to serum vitamin D levels and that humans with a deficiency of vitamin D show significantly decreased resistance to this infection. It is of interest to recall that sanatorium treatment of tuberculosis classically involved exposure to fresh air and sunlight, a procedure that would be expected to increase vitamin D levels in human patients. Conversely, mice are nocturnal mammals that would not be expected to have high vitamin D levels and must rely on other pathways.

Natural killer (NK) cells play a protective role in some bacterial, protozoan, and fungal infections. For example, some bacteria may activate NK cells by upregulating expression of NKG2D ligands on cells. Activated NK cells produce a large amount of IFN-γ that in turn activates both macrophages and dendritic cells.

Although many bacteria are destroyed by phagocytosis, others are killed when free in the circulation. Bacteria can be destroyed by complement acting through the alternate or lectin pathways. Bacterial cell walls, lacking sialic acid, inactivate factor H and stabilize the alternate C3 convertase (C3bBbP). As a result, these bacteria are either opsonized or lysed. Activation of the terminal complement components leads to the development of terminal complement complexes (TCCs). These TCCs may be unable to insert themselves into the complex carbohydrates of the microbial cell wall. However, lysozyme in the blood may digest the cell wall and enable the TCCs to gain access to the lipid bilayer of the inner bacterial membrane.

Antimicrobial peptides are critical for the defense against some bacteria such as the mycobacteria (Box 25-1). Suppression of bacterial growth by withholding iron is discussed in Chapter 6.

Adaptive Immunity

There are five basic mechanisms by which the adaptive immune responses combat bacterial infections (Figure 25-1): (1) neutralization of toxins or enzymes by antibody; (2) killing of bacteria

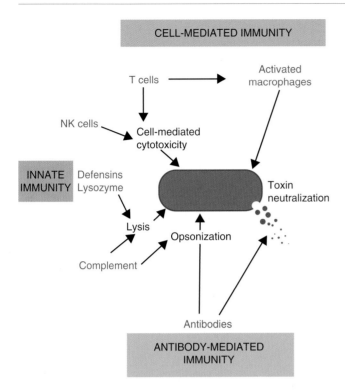

FIGURE 25-1 The mechanisms by which the immune responses can protect the body against bacterial invasion.

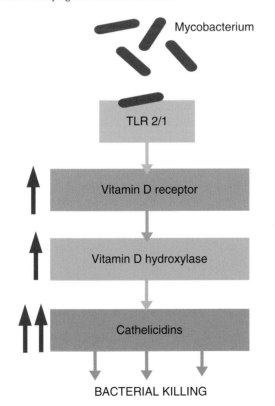

FIGURE 25-2 Immunity to tuberculosis is governed in many species by the availability of vitamin D. The vitamin D receptor is upregulated on activated macrophages. Binding of vitamin D to this receptor upregulates vitamin D hydroxylase, which in turn increases production of the antibacterial cathelicidins and enhances disease resistance.

by the classical complement pathway; (3) opsonization of bacteria by antibodies and complement, resulting in their phagocytosis and destruction; (4) destruction of intracellular bacteria by activated macrophages; and (5) direct killing of bacteria by cytotoxic T cells and NK cells. The relative importance of each of these processes depends on the species of bacteria involved and on the mechanisms by which they cause disease.

Immunity to Toxigenic Bacteria

In disease caused by toxigenic bacteria such as clostridia or *Bacillus anthracis*, the immune response must not only eliminate the invading bacteria but also neutralize their toxins. Destruction of the bacteria, however, may be difficult if they are embedded in a mass of necrotic tissue, and toxin neutralization is a priority. Neutralization occurs when antibody prevents the toxin from binding to its receptors on a target cell. The neutralization process therefore involves competition between receptors and antibodies for the toxin molecule. Once the toxin has bound to its receptors, antibodies are relatively ineffective in reversing this combination.

Immunity to Invasive Bacteria

Protection against invasive bacteria is usually mediated by antibodies directed against their surface antigens. Efficient phagocytosis requires that the bacteria be coated with opsonins that can be recognized by phagocytic cells. These opsonins include antibodies and C3b in addition to the innate opsonins such as MBL. Antibodies not only are effective opsonins in their own right but also increase the binding of C3b by activating the classical complement pathway. Antibodies directed against capsular (K) antigens may neutralize the antiphagocytic properties of bacterial capsules, thus permitting their destruction by phagocytic cells. In bacteria lacking capsules, antibodies directed against O antigens act as opsonins. Protection also results when antibodies are produced against the *Escherichia coli* pilus antigens F4 (K88) and F5 (K99). The antibodies may interfere with the expression of pili. Once the adherence pili are suppressed, these strains of *E. coli* cannot bind to the intestinal wall and thus are no longer pathogenic.

The importance of bacterial capsules in immunity is seen in anthrax. *B. anthracis* organisms possess both a capsule and an exotoxin. Antitoxic immunity is protective but slow to develop. In addition, toxin production tends to be prolonged since the organism is encapsulated and phagocytic cells have difficulty eliminating it. As a result, death is usually inevitable in unvaccinated animals. The vaccine commonly employed against animal anthrax contains an unencapsulated but toxigenic strain of *B. anthracis*. Given in the form of spores that can germinate, the unencapsulated bacteria are eliminated by phagocytic cells before dangerous amounts of toxin are synthesized but not before antitoxic immunity is established.

Molecule for molecule, immunoglobulin M (IgM) is about 500 to 1000 times more efficient than IgG in opsonization and about 100 times more potent than IgG in sensitizing bacteria for complement-mediated lysis. During a primary immune response, therefore, the quantitative deficiency of the IgM response is compensated for by its quality, ensuring early and efficient protection.

The traditional view of antibodies has been that they alone could not kill microorganisms, but simply could mark microorganisms for destruction. That view is now known to be incorrect. Many antibodies have direct antimicrobial activities. Antibodies against *E. coli* may be bacteriostatic since they interfere with production of the iron-binding protein enterochelin and thus prevent bacterial iron scavenging. IgM and IgG antibodies against *Borrelia burgdorferi* damage surface proteins on the bacteria and are bactericidal in the absence of complement. There is also evidence that antibodies are able to generate oxidants and may kill bacteria directly.

Heat-Shock Protein Response Many new proteins are induced in bacteria by stressors such as a heat, starvation, and exposure to oxidants; toxins such as heavy metals; protein synthesis inhibitors; and viral infections. The heat-shock proteins (HSPs) are the best understood of these new proteins. HSPs are present in all bacteria at very low levels at normal temperatures. Mild stress such as a low-grade fever will induce HSP production. For example, HSP levels climb from 1.5% to 15% of the total protein in stressed *E. coli*. There are three major bacterial HSPs: HSP 90, HSP 70, and HSP 60. (The number refers to their molecular weight.) When a bacterium is phagocytosed and exposed to the neutrophil respiratory burst, the resulting stress triggers the production of bacterial HSP. As a result, HSP 60 is the dominant antigen in infections caused by mycobacteria, *Coxiella burnetii*, legionella, treponema, and *Borrelia* species. These HSPs are highly antigenic for several reasons. First, they are produced in abundance within the infected host; second, they are readily processed by antigen-presenting cells; and third, the immune system may possess unusually large numbers of cells capable of responding to HSPs. In addition, some γ/δ T cells may preferentially recognize bacterial HSPs. Thus anti-HSP responses may induce significant protection against many bacterial pathogens.

Immunity to Intracellular Bacteria

As discussed in Chapter 18, some bacteria such as *Brucella abortus, Mycobacterium tuberculosis, Campylobacter jejuni, R. equi, Listeria monocytogenes, Corynebacterium pseudotuberculosis, C. burnetii,* and some serotypes of *S. enterica* can grow readily inside macrophages. In addition, *L. monocytogenes* can travel from cell to cell without exposure to the extracellular fluid through cytoskeletal membrane protrusions.

Autophagy, as described in Chapter 4, is also a key component of the destruction of intracellular bacteria. The same cellular machinery used to destroy unwanted organelles can be employed to eliminate intracellular organisms. Autophagy (or more correctly, xenophagy) may also play a key role in

delivering microbial antigens to the appropriate major histocompatibility complex (MHC) molecules.

Protection against intracellular bacteria is mediated by macrophages activated through the M1 pathway. Classically activated M1 macrophages are responsive to inflammatory cytokines and microbial products (Chapter 5). Although macrophages from unimmunized animals cannot usually destroy these bacteria, this ability is acquired about 10 days after onset of infection once the macrophages are activated (Chapter 18). IFN-γ, especially in association with TNF-α, greatly enhances the production of cytokines such as TNF-α, IL-6, IL-1β and IL-12, enzymes such as indoleamine 2,3-dioxygenase (IDO) and nitric oxide synthase 2 (NOS2), and the release of reactive oxygen and nitrogen intermediates. M1 polarization has been shown to be important in resistance to *L. monocytogenes, S. enterica* Typhi and Typhimurium, mycobacteria, and chlamydia. For example, IFN-γ and TNF-α produced by primed T cells generate M1 macrophages, acidify their phagosomes, and kill mycobacteria. Uncontrolled M1 activation by organisms such as streptococci and *E. coli,* however, can contribute to pathology by inducing, for example, sepsis, tissue damage, and organ failure. The response of these activated macrophages tends to be nonspecific, particularly in listerial infections, and M1 macrophages are able to destroy many normally resistant bacteria. Thus an animal recovering from an infection with *L. monocytogenes* develops increased resistance to infection by *M. tuberculosis*. The development of M1 macrophages often coincides with the appearance of delayed (type IV) hypersensitivity responses to intradermally administered antigen (Chapter 31).

Both CD4+ and CD8+ cells are also involved in immunity to Listeria. CD8+ cytotoxic T cells lyse listeria- or mycobacteria-infected cells and complement the Th1 cells that activate the macrophages. *R. equi*–infected macrophages are recognized and killed by CD8+ T cells in a MHC class I unrestricted manner.

It has been observed that protective immunity against intracellular bacteria cannot be induced by vaccines containing killed bacteria. Only vaccines containing living bacteria are protective. This is because of the differential stimulation of helper T cell populations by live and dead bacteria. Infection of mice with live *B. abortus* stimulates Th1 cells to secrete IFN-γ. Conversely, immunization of these mice with *Brucella* protein extracts induces Th2 cells to secrete IL-4. Likewise, live but not dead *L. monocytogenes* or *B. abortus* organisms induce macrophage secretion of TNF-α. Killed *Brucella* organisms stimulate IL-1 production to a greater extent than live bacteria. Resistance to these intracellular bacteria is generally short lived, persisting for only as long as viable bacteria remain in the body. (Tuberculosis is an exception, in which case memory is prolonged.)

If, in a bacterial disease, it is observed that dead vaccines do not give good protection, that serum cannot confer protection, that antibody levels do not relate to resistance, and that delayed hypersensitivity reactions can be elicited to the bacterial antigens, the possibility that cell-mediated immunity may play an important role in resistance to the causative organism should be considered, and the use of vaccines containing living bacteria should be contemplated.

Modification of Bacterial Disease by Immune Responses

The immune response clearly influences the course and severity of an infection. At best, it will result in a cure. In the absence of a cure, however, the infection may be profoundly modified. Much depends on whether a cell-mediated or antibody response is generated. Thus the type of helper T cells induced during infection may affect the course of disease. As described in Chapter 18, cell-mediated responses are required to control intracellular bacteria since only activated macrophages can prevent their growth. Macrophage activation requires that Th1 cells produce IFN-γ. Once activated, these M1 cells can localize or cure these infections. If an animal mounts an inappropriate Th2 response, cell-mediated immunity fails to develop, M2 macrophages are generated, and chronic progressive disease may result. This is readily seen in mycobacterial diseases. For example, in humans, leprosy occurs in two distinct forms called tuberculoid and lepromatous leprosy. Tuberculoid (or paucibacillary [PB]) leprosy is characterized by an intense cell-mediated immune response dominated by Th1 cells and M1 macrophages. Lesions of this form of the disease contain very few organisms. Lepromatous (or multibacillary [MB]) leprosy, in contrast, is characterized by very high antibody levels and poor cell-mediated responses. Humans with lepromatous leprosy employ Th2 cells secreting IL-4 and IL-10. The IL-10 reduces the production of IL-12, which in turn decreases IFN-γ secretion by Th1 cells and generates M2 macrophages. This reduces the patient's ability to control *Mycobacterium leprae,* and their lesions contain enormous numbers of bacteria. The prognosis of lepromatous leprosy is much poorer than for tuberculoid leprosy.

A similar diversity of lesions is seen in Johne's disease of sheep. Some animals develop MB disease, in which their intestinal lesions contain enormous numbers of bacteria (Figure 25-3) and little histological evidence of a cell-mediated response. Their granulomas tend to lack organization, with large numbers of bacteria-laden macrophages intermixed with lymphocytes. In contrast, other sheep may develop PB disease, in which the lesions contain very few bacteria but large numbers of lymphocytes. These are organized nodular lesions with epithelioid cells and multinucleated giant cells at the center surrounded by fibrous connective tissue. The two forms of the disease are associated with differential expression of cytokine and chemokine receptors. Thus animals with the PB disease have increased numbers of CD25+ T cells that produce more IL-2 and much more IFN-γ than sheep with the MB form of the disease (Figure 25-4). In contrast, sheep with the MB disease have higher antibody levels and a lack of cellular immune responses. It is likely, therefore, that sheep with PB lesions mount an immune response in which Th1 cells predominate, whereas those with MB disease use Th2 cells.

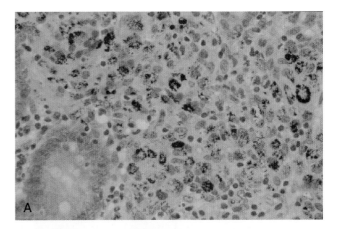

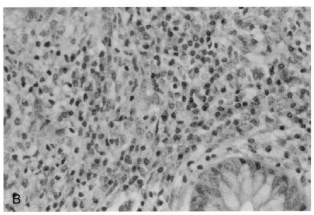

FIGURE 25-3 The two forms of Johne's disease in sheep. **A,** Section of terminal ileum from a case of multibacillary Johne's disease, showing abundant acid-fast organisms within large infiltrating macrophages. **B,** Section of terminal ileum from a case of paucibacillary Johne's disease, showing very few acid-fast bacteria and a significant lymphocyte infiltration. Ziehl-Nielsen stain.

(Courtesy Dr. C.J. Clarke.)

IL-4 is a key cytokine that regulates the balance between Th1 and Th2 responses. For example, conventional IL-4 triggers Th2 responses while suppressing Th1 responses. Some animals, however, produce structural variants of IL-4. For example, in addition to normal IL-4, cattle produce two variants, called IL-4δ2 and IL-4δ3, by alternative splicing of pre–messenger RNA. These splice variants may bind and block IL-4 receptors and regulate its activity. As a result, they can influence the resistance of cattle to bovine tuberculosis and may account for their different responses to this infection. Animals showing significant resistance to tuberculosis produced high levels of IL-4δ3 compared with susceptible cattle. Likewise transient increases in the ratio of IL-4δ3 to IL-4 have been observed after vaccination against bovine tuberculosis.

It must not be assumed from the previous discussion that the specific helper T cell subset involved in an immune response does not change once the response is established. Time-based studies have shown that immune responses to an organism can swing between Th1 and Th2 responses, perhaps several times, before a final response is established. This final response may

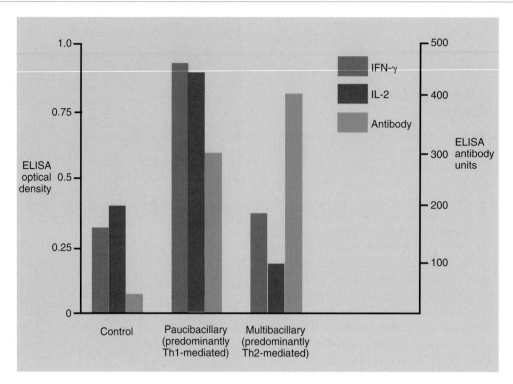

FIGURE 25-4 The differences in peripheral blood lymphocyte IL-2, IFN-γ, and antibody production between sheep with the paucibacillary (PB) form and sheep with the multibacillary (MB) form of Johne's disease. Note that there is a marked tendency for the T cells from animals with the PB form of the disease to produce more Th1 cytokines than those with the MB form. Despite this, animals with the latter form appear to produce more antibodies.

(From data kindly provided by Dr. Chris Clarke and Mr. Charles Burrells.)

well be a Th1 or Th2 response, or even some intermediate point in the Th1 to Th2 spectrum. This variation appears to be a common feature of chronic infections such as tuberculosis.

Evasion of the Immune Response

To survive within an animal, bacteria manipulate the immune system to their advantage. The complex interrelationships between bacteria and their animal hosts, described in Chapter 22, include the role of commensal bacteria on mucosal surfaces in regulating the growth and development of the immune system. These bacteria generally do not aggressively seek to invade the body, so equilibrium can be achieved. As pointed out previously, however, an invading microorganism becomes a pathogen because it can invade the body, evade the immune defenses, and survive at least for a time within its host. Pathogenic bacteria, like all organisms, try to avoid destruction. They have evolved a diverse array of mechanisms by which they overcome host innate and adaptive immune responses, especially inflammation and phagocytosis, and avoid elimination. Bacteria may employ several evasive mechanisms simultaneously or sequentially as infection progresses. For example, *Streptococcus pyogenes* can interfere with Fc-mediated opsoniza-

tion, block phagocytosis, and prevent the activities of the terminal complement complex—all at the same time.

Evasion of Innate Immunity

The key to successful microbial invasion, at least initially, is the evasion of innate immune responses. Bacteria employ a highly diverse set of mechanisms to prevent or at least delay an unpleasant fate.

Some pathogenic bacteria interfere with TLR signaling pathways (Figure 25-5). The methods used include the production of modified PAMPs that will not trigger TLRs, blockage of TLR signaling pathways, accelerated destruction of intermediate signaling molecules, destruction of NF-κB, and misdirection of signaling pathways toward anti-inflammatory pathways. Modified PAMPs are used by *Leptospira* and *Campylobacter* species. Leptospira have lipopolysaccharides that are recognized by TLR2, but not by TLR4. *C. jejuni* organisms make a form of flagellin that is not recognized by TLR5. Bacteria differ in the frequency of CpG dinucleotides in their DNA and, as a result, differ in their ability to trigger TLR9. Potent stimulators of TLR9 signaling include *M. tuberculosis* and *Pseudomonas aeruginosa*. Weak TLR9 stimulators include *C. jejuni* and *Staphylococcus epidermidis*.

Many bacteria interfere with intracellular signaling pathways. *Brucella* synthesize a protein called TcpB that closely

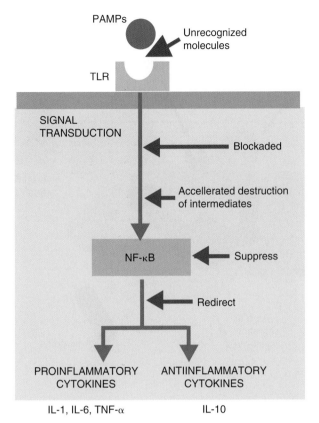

FIGURE 25-5 Bacteria can interfere with TLR signaling pathways in many different ways and at many different positions as described in the text. This can include redirecting the signaling pathways from proinflammatory to anti-inflammatory pathways.

resembles the mammalian Toll/IL-1 receptor. As a result, it causes accelerated degradation of an adaptor protein and blocks the TLR signaling pathway. *P. aeruginosa* secretes a molecule that impairs the regulation of NF-κB. The MAP kinase pathway can be weakened by proteolysis of MKK (anthrax), elimination of MAPK (*Shigella* species), or acetylation of MAPK (*Yersinia* species). Misdirection of signaling pathways occurs when products from candida, yersinia, or mycobacteria trigger signaling through TLR2, leading to production of IL-10.

Another useful skill for a bacterium to possess is the ability to resist antibacterial proteins. For example, staphylokinase from *Staphylococcus aureus* can bind and neutralize defensins. Another staphylococcal enzyme, aureolysin, destroys cathelicidins. Salmonella can bind defensins and respond by changing the negative charge and fluidity of the bacterial outer membrane resulting in decreased defensin binding. *Klebsiella pneumoniae* capsular polysaccharide blocks β-defensin expression by airway epithelial cells.

Many bacteria can block phagocytosis. Some prevent recognition by phagocytic receptors. For example, *S. aureus* inhibits phagocytosis by expressing protein A. Protein A attaches to the Fc region of IgG molecules and so prevents antibodies from binding to Fc receptors on phagocytic cells or activating the classical complement pathway. Encapsulated bacteria such as

pneumococci possess a thick hydrophilic capsule that cells find difficult to bind to. Many bacteria can evade opsonization by complement. Thus the M protein of streptococci binds fibrinogen and masks C3b-binding sites. It also binds factor H, thus inactivating bound C3b. *S. aureus* produces a protein that blocks C3 convertases. Other bacteria produce proteases that can destroy complement components. *S. enterica* Typhimurium has a gene called *Rck* that confers resistance to complement-mediated lysis by preventing insertion of the terminal complement complex into the bacterial outer membrane.

Bacteria can of course, avoid being eaten simply by killing phagocytic cells (Figure 25-6). Thus *Streptococcus canis* produces streptolysin O that lyses neutrophil cell membranes. Several Gram-negative bacteria of veterinary importance, such as *Mannheimia hemolytica* and *Fusobacterium necrophorum*, secrete leukotoxins that kill leukocytes, especially granulocytes. The most important leukotoxins are the RTX ("repeats in toxin") proteins. *M. hemolytica* secretes an RTX toxin that kills ruminant neutrophils, alveolar macrophages, and lymphocytes. This leukotoxin binds to CD18 as well as lipid rafts on leukocytes and induces their apoptosis. *Moraxella bovis* also secretes a leukotoxin for bovine neutrophils. *Actinobacillus pleuropneumoniae* secretes a toxin that kills porcine macrophages. *Mycoplasma mycoides* can kill bovine T cells. Other bacteria trigger lymphocyte death by activating apoptotic pathways. These include *B. anthracis*, streptococci, *Shigella* species, *L. monocytogenes*, *S. aureus*, and yersinia. Leukotoxins are a relatively crude method of assassination. Some bacteria use much more sophisticated methods. Thus some bacteria inject toxins into their targets. Gram-negative bacteria such as *Salmonella* and *Pseudomonas* species and *E. coli* have developed an elaborate needle complex—a type III secretion system, to convey effector molecules directly into the cytosol of effector cells. These injection systems are turned on when a bacterium is ingested by a cell and exposed to a low pH within the phagosome. Once the needle complex enters the cytosol and detects its neutral pH, injection of effector molecules occurs. These molecules activate guanosine triphosphatases and disrupt intracellular signaling pathways. At high concentrations, they produce transmembrane pores and cell necrosis.

Although killing leukocytes is an effective way to avoid being eaten, other bacteria are content to simply prevent intracellular destruction. Some bacteria generate a resistant cell wall to protect themselves against lysosomal enzymes (Table 25-1). For example, the cell wall waxes of *C. pseudotuberculosis* make that organism resistant to lysosomal enzymes. *S. aureus* uses a cell wall peptidoglycan that is completely resistant to lysozyme. Some bacteria produce antioxidants that neutralize the products of the respiratory burst. For example, the carotenoid pigments responsible for the yellow color of *S. aureus* can quench singlet oxygen. *S. enterica* Typhimurium can prevent assembly of the NOX complex and downregulate host NOS2 activity. *Pasteurella multocida* and *Histophilus somni* are also able to inhibit the respiratory burst. Anthrax toxins LF and EF can inhibit NAPDH oxidase activity. *S. aureus* produces catalase that inactivates hydrogen peroxide and the free radicals

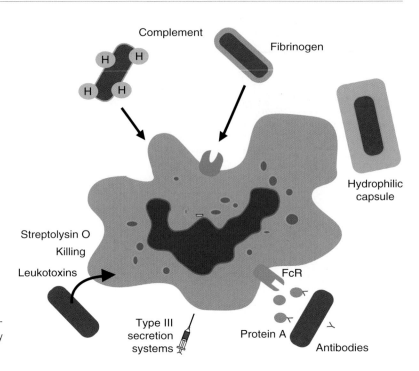

FIGURE 25-6 Some of the many different mechanisms by which bacteria can avoid being killed by phagocytic cells such as neutrophils.

◻ Table 25-1 | **Facultative Intracellular Bacteria and Their Mechanisms of Survival**

ORGANISM	METHOD OF INTRACELLULAR SURVIVAL
Brucella abortus	Resistant cell wall Prevents phagosome maturation
Corynebacterium pseudotuberculosis	Resistant cell wall
Listeria monocytogenes	Neutralizes respiratory burst Escapes into the cytosol
Mycobacterium tuberculosis	Lipid cell wall Prevents phagosome maturation Suppresses antigen presentation Detoxifies oxidants
Salmonella enterica	Prevents phagosome maturation Modifies endosomal trafficking Detoxifies oxidants Downregulates NOS2 and NOX
Rhodococcus equi	Survives in phagosomes

produced during the respiratory burst. It also produces lactate dehydrogenase that also helps it to resist NO^+-mediated oxidation. Some bacteria can defend themselves against hypochloride through the actions of a molecular chaperone called Hsp33. This protein unfolds on exposure to HOCl and then binds and protects essential proteins against bleach-induced aggregation.

Bacteria such as enteropathogenic *E. coli*, *Yersinia pestis*, *M. tuberculosis*, and *P. aeruginosa* secrete molecules that depress neutrophil killing. For example, *E. coli* produces lysozyme inhibitors. Other bacteria ensure that they are never exposed to these enzymes by interfering with phagosomal maturation (Figure 25-7). Mycobacteria, *Aspergillus flavus*, *B. abortus*, and *Chlamydophila psittaci* can establish themselves within vacuoles that exclude proteases and oxidants by blocking lysosome-phagosome fusion. In the case of *M. tuberculosis*, the bacterium enters the macrophage through cholesterol-enriched membrane microdomains that are coated on the cytosolic side with a protein (tryptophan-aspartate-containing coat protein, or TACO) that prevents phagosome maturation. Thus lysosomes cannot fuse with the phagosome. They remain distributed within the cytosol, and the bacteria continue to survive and grow. Mycobacteria also prevent acidification of phagosomes by preventing recruitment of the proton pump adenosine triphosphatase from the vacuolar membrane so that lysosomal cathepsins remain inactive. Another mechanism used by bacteria to avoid destruction is simply to escape from the phagosome by migrating into the cytosol surrounded by a coat of polymerized actin. This method is employed by some mycobacteria and by *L. monocytogenes*. Listeria secretes listeriolysin O that destroys cell membranes and so permits the organism to escape from the phagosome into the cytosol.

Even extracellular killing can be inhibited. Dying neutrophils release intranuclear DNA and associated proteins, leading to the formation of neutrophil extracellular traps (NETs) (see Figure 4-11). The extracellular DNA is studded with antimicrobial proteins, including granule components that can kill

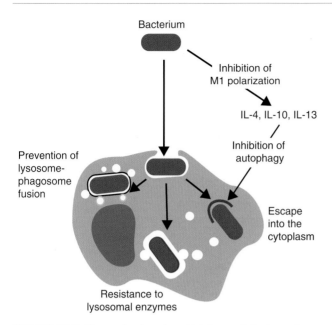

FIGURE 25-7 The mechanisms by which intracellular bacteria can evade intracellular destruction.

extracellular bacteria. However, bacteria such as the pneumococci can secrete an endonuclease, which degrades the DNA scaffold of the net.

Evasion of Adaptive Immunity

Bacteria also seek to avoid or modify adaptive immune responses—a more difficult task.

The body will not respond effectively to organisms it cannot detect or to organisms that it encounters for the first time. *C. fetus* subspecies *venerealis*, an organism that normally colonizes the genital tracts of cattle, prevents effective immune elimination by changing its surface coat. The destruction of most of these bacteria by a local immune response leaves a remnant population that possesses new and different antigens. This population multiplies but is largely eliminated in turn by a second immune response, leaving organisms of a third antigenic type. This process of cyclical antigenic variation may be repeated for a long time, resulting in a persistent infection. *Anaplasma marginale,* a bacterium that lives within bovine red cells, also shows sequential antigenic variation. As a result, the number of anaplasma in blood cycles at 6- to 8-week intervals. The number of bacteria gradually increases and then falls rapidly as a result of an antibody response. This is followed by development of a new antigenic variant that repeats the cycle. *A. marginale* is transmitted by ticks, so successful spread depends on maintenance of a high bacteremia. The persistence of a high bacteremia in bovine anaplasmosis is assisted by a dysfunctional memory CD4+ T cell response.

Some bacteria secrete proteases that can destroy immunoglobulins or cytokines. For example, proteases specific for IgA are produced by *Neisseria gonorrhoeae, Haemophilus influenzae,*

and *Streptococcus pneumoniae.* These organisms can thus prevent opsonization and Fc receptor–mediated phagocytosis. *M. haemolytica* secretes a protease specific for bovine IgG1. *P. aeruginosa* secretes a protease that destroys IL-2 *B. abortus* produces a B cell mitogen that stimulates the cells to secrete IL-10. This causes transient immunosuppression and permits the bacterium to successfully establish a chronic infection. Finally, it must be pointed out that bacteria growing on a surface in a biofilm are much more resistant to opsonization and phagocytosis than single bacteria growing in suspension. The biofilm matrix appears to be able to inhibit opsonic killing.

Pathogenic mycobacteria have evolved to survive within host macrophages, and *Mycobacterium avium paratuberculosis* (MAP) is highly adept at such survival. MAP interacts with receptors on macrophages to initiate cell signaling and phagocytosis. Mannosylated lipoarabinomannan (Man-lam) is a major component of the MAP cell wall. Man-lam binds to TLR2, triggering transcription of IL-10. The IL-10 suppresses production of proinflammatory cytokines and attenuates phagosome acidification and phagolysosome fusion. Thus Man-lam appears to be largely responsible for suppressing the inflammatory and antimicrobial responses against MAP.

Avirulent mycobacteria are taken up by macrophages and induce their apoptosis. This results in a "cellular corpse" with an impermeable envelope that prevents the bacteria from escaping. Thus the avirulent mycobacteria are killed only when the apoptotic cell is removed. Virulent mycobacteria, in contrast, when taken up by macrophages, cause necrosis. This produces a dead cell with a permeable cell membrane that enables the bacteria to escape and spread.

It has long been recognized that *M. tuberculosis* can survive within macrophages by blocking fusion of the phagosome with lysosomes. The Th1 cytokine IFN-γ can overcome this maturation block by triggering autophagy. Thus a new autophagosome forms around the blocked phagosome, and this then fuses with lysosomes, permitting the killing of the mycobacteria. Conversely Th2 cytokines such as IL-4 and IL-13 inhibit autophagy and permit mycobacterial survival. Several intracellular bacteria are eliminated by autophagy. These include *S. pyogenes* and *S. enterica* Typhimurium. Other organisms such as *Listeria* and *Shigella* species have evolved mechanisms to avoid autophagy. Likewise many bacteria have evolved mechanisms to survive within autophagosomes.

Bacteria may interfere with M1 polarization to promote their own survival. Some salmonella and mycobacteria can neutralize M1-related effectors, or inhibit M1 cytokine secretion or expression. *S. enterica* Dublin suppresses IL-18, and *B. suis* inhibits TNF-α production. Proteins from *M. tuberculosis* can inhibit activation of NF-κB. Responding mycobacteria may induce the synthesis of IL-6, IL-10, and TGF-β and hence prolong their own survival. IL-10 is especially effective in inhibiting macrophage activation, suppressing oxidant production, and reducing MHC class II expression. Some pathogens, such a *Yersinia enterocolitica* and *C. burnetii,* actually stimulate M2 polarization. The evolution of bacterial diseases into persistent chronic infections is associated with a tendency to M2 polarization mediated by IL-10. This occurs in chronic brucellosis, Q fever, and tuberculosis.

Some Antibacterial Vaccines

Toxoids

The immunoprophylaxis of tetanus is restricted to toxin neutralization. Tetanus toxoid in an aluminum hydroxide suspension is given for routine prophylaxis, and a single injection will induce protective immunity in 10 to 14 days. Conventional immunological wisdom would suggest that the previous use of tetanus immune globulin should interfere with the immune response to toxoid and must therefore be avoided. This is not a problem in practice, however, and both may be successfully administered simultaneously (at different sites) without problems. This may be because of the relatively small amount of immune globulin usually needed to protect animals.

Some veterinary vaccines combine both toxoid and killed bacteria in a single dose by the simple expedient of formolizing a whole culture. These products, sometimes called anacultures, are used to vaccinate against *Clostridium haemolyticum* and *C. perfringens*. Trypsinization of the anaculture may make it more immunogenic. Toxoids, usually incorporated with an alum adjuvant, are available for most clostridial diseases and for infections caused by toxigenic staphylococci.

Bacterins

Vaccines containing killed bacteria are called bacterins. It is usual to kill the bacteria with formaldehyde and to incorporate them with alum or aluminum hydroxide adjuvants. As with other dead vaccines, the immunity produced by bacterins is relatively short lived, usually lasting no longer than 1 year and sometimes considerably less. For instance, formolized swine erysipelas (*Erysipelothrix rhusiopathiae*) vaccine protects for only 4 to 5 months, and *Streptococcus equi* bacterins give immunity for less than 1 year, even though recovery from a natural case of strangles may confer a lifelong immunity in horses.

Bacterins may be improved by adding purified immunogenic antigens to the killed bacteria. *E. coli* bacterins against enteric colibacillosis may be enriched and made much more effective by the addition of K88 or K99 pilus antigens. Antibodies to these antigens block binding of *E. coli* to the intestinal wall and thus contribute significantly to protection. Similarly, *Mannheimia* species bacterins enriched with the leukotoxoid show improved efficacy over conventional bacterins. Purified bacterial components such as the surface antigens of *M. hemolytica* may also be effective vaccine components.

One problem encountered, especially when using coliform and *Campylobacter* species vaccines, is strain specificity. Several different antigenic types of each organism commonly occur, and successful vaccination requires immunization with appropriate bacterial strains. This is sometimes not possible if a commercial vaccine must be employed. One method of overcoming this difficulty is to use autogenous vaccines. These are vaccines that contain organisms obtained either from infected animals on the farm where the disease problem is occurring or from the infected animal itself. These can be very successful if carefully prepared since the vaccine will contain all the antigens required for protection in that particular location. As an alternative to the use of autogenous vaccines, some manufacturers produce polyvalent vaccines containing a mixture of antigenic types. For example, leptospirosis vaccines commonly contain up to five different serovars. This practice, although effective, is inefficient since only a few of the antigenic types employed may be appropriate in any given situation.

An alternative approach to the development of vaccines against Gram-negative bacteria is the use of common core antigens. As pointed out in Chapter 2, the outer layer of the Gram-negative bacterial cell wall consists of lipopolysaccharide. This lipopolysaccharide consists of a variable oligosaccharide (O antigen) bound to a highly conserved core polysaccharide and lipid A. The O antigen varies greatly among Gram-negative bacteria so that an immune response against one O antigen confers no immunity against bacteria expressing other O antigens. In contrast, the underlying core polysaccharide is similar between Gram-negative bacteria of different species and genera. Thus an immune response directed against this common core structure has the potential to protect against a wide variety of different gram-negative bacteria.

Mutant strains of *E. coli* (J5) and *S. enterica* Minnesota and Typhimurium (Re) have been used as sources of core antigen. J5 is a rough mutant that is deficient in uridine diphosphate galactose 4-epimerase. As a result, the organism makes an incomplete oligosaccharide side chain, having lost most of the outer lipopolysaccharide structure (see Figure 2-2). Immunization with J5 thus provides protection against *E. coli*, *K. pneumoniae*, *A. pleuropneumoniae*, and *H. influenzae* (type B). J5 has been reported to protect calves against organisms such as *S. enterica* Typhimurium and *E. coli* and pigs against *A. pleuropneumoniae*. The most encouraging results have been obtained in protection against coliform mastitis.

Living Bacterial Vaccines

Successful living bacterial vaccines include strains 19 and RB51 of *B. abortus*. Another successful living vaccine is that employed for the prevention of anthrax. Older anthrax vaccines used Pasteur's technique of culturing the bacteria at a relatively high temperature (42° to 43° C) to reduce their virulence. The anthrax vaccines currently available for animals contain capsuleless mutants that remain capable of forming spores. The vaccine is prepared as a spore suspension and is administered with saponin.

A rough strain of *S. enterica* Dublin (strain 51) is used in Europe to give good protection to calves when administered at 2 to 4 weeks of age. As discussed earlier, immunity to salmonellosis involves macrophage activation and is thus relatively nonspecific. For this reason, strain 51 may also give good protection against *S. enterica* Typhimurium.

Adverse Consequences of the Immune Responses

Although immune responses are beneficial in that they eliminate invading bacteria, this is not always the case. The immune responses can influence the course of a bacterial disease without producing a cure and in some situations may increase its severity. The adverse consequences of the immune responses correspond in their mechanisms to the hypersensitivity types described in Chapters 28 to 31. For example, a local type I hypersensitivity reaction is sometimes seen in sheep vaccinated against foot rot by means of *Dichelobacter nodosus* vaccine, but in this case it is believed that the hypersensitivity may assist in preventing reinfection.

Type II (cytotoxic) reactions may account for the anemia that occurs in animals with salmonellosis. In these infections, bacterial lipopolysaccharides from disrupted bacteria are adsorbed onto erythrocytes. The subsequent immune response against the bacterium and its products therefore results in red cell destruction.

Type III (immune complex) reactions may contribute to the development of arthritis in *E. rhusiopathiae* infections in pigs or to the development of intestinal lesions in Johne's disease due to *M. avium paratuberculosis*. In the former case, bacterial antigen tends to localize in joints, where local immune complex formation then results in inflammation and arthritis. Passively administered antiserum may therefore exacerbate the arthritis in these infected animals. In Johne's disease, type I or type III reactions occurring in the intestinal mucosa may increase the outflow of fluid and diarrhea. It is clear, however, that the intestinal lesions in this disease are etiologically complex since diarrhea can be transferred to normal calves by either plasma or leukocytes, and antihistamine drugs may reduce the diarrhea. Type III hypersensitivity reactions are involved in purpura hemorrhagica of horses, in which immune complex lesions result from *S. equi* infection.

Although cell-mediated (type IV) immune responses are manifestly beneficial, they do contribute to the development of granulomatous lesions in some chronic infections. The development of large granulomas, although serving to wall off invading bacteria and thus to prevent their spread, may also involve uninfected tissues. If these granulomas invade essential structures such as airways in the lungs or large blood vessels, damage may be severe.

Serology of Bacterial Infections

Bacterial infections are often diagnosed by detecting specific antibodies in serum. Thus the agglutination test is widely employed in the diagnosis of bacterial infections, particularly those involving Gram-negative bacteria such as *Brucella* and *Salmonella*. The usual procedure in bacterial agglutination tests is to titrate serum (antibody) against a standard suspension of antigen. Bacteria are not, of course, antigenically homogeneous but rather are covered by a mosaic of many different antigens. Thus, motile bacteria will have flagellar (H) antigens, and agglutination by antiflagellar antibodies will produce fluffy cotton-like floccules as the flagella stick together, leaving the bacterial bodies only loosely agglutinated. Agglutination of the somatic (O) antigens results in tight clumping of the bacterial bodies so that the agglutination is finely granular in character. Many bacteria possess several O and H antigens, as well as capsular (K) and pilus (F) antigens. By using a set of specific antisera, it is possible to characterize the antigenic structure of an organism and consequently to classify it. It is on this basis, for instance, that the 2400 or so different serovars of *S. enterica* are classified.

Flagella (H) antigens are destroyed by heating, whereas O antigens are heat resistant and therefore remain intact on heat-killed bacteria. K antigens vary in their heat stability: the L antigen of *E. coli*, which is a capsular antigen, is heat labile, whereas another K antigen, antigen A, is heat stable. *S. enterica* Typhi possesses an antigen called Vi that, although heat stable, is removed from the bacterial cells by heating. The presence of K or Vi antigens on an organism may render them O-inagglutinable and thus complicate agglutination tests. It should also be pointed out that rough forms of bacteria do not form stable suspensions and therefore cannot be typed by means of agglutination tests.

Bacterial agglutination tests may be performed by mixing drops of reagents on glass slides or by titrating the reagents in tubes or wells in plastic plates. Tube agglutination tests are commonly used for such diseases as salmonellosis, brucellosis, tularemia, and campylobacteriosis. Slide agglutination tests are commonly used as screening tests. These include the *Brucella*-buffered antigen tests, in which killed, stained *Brucella* organisms are suspended in an acid buffer (pH 3.6). The dye used, either the red dye rose-bengal or a mixture of crystal violet and brilliant green, enables the test to be easily read. At this low pH, nonspecific agglutination by IgM antibodies is eliminated. The *Brucella*-buffered plate agglutination test has a specificity of as high as 99% and a sensitivity of 95%. The efficient and widespread use of these tests has eliminated bovine brucellosis from so many countries.

S. enterica Pullorum infection in poultry can be diagnosed by a slide agglutination test, in which killed bacteria stained with gentian violet are mixed with whole chicken blood. Agglutination is readily seen if antibodies are present. Leptospirosis is diagnosed by a microscopic agglutination test, in which mixtures of living organisms and test serum are examined under the microscope for agglutination. This technique preferentially detects IgM antibodies and is thus an excellent test for detecting recent outbreaks as well as for distinguishing between infected and vaccinated animals.

It is not mandatory that serum be used as the source of antibody for diagnostic tests. The presence of antibodies in body fluids other than serum, such as milk whey, vaginal mucus, or nasal washings, may be of more significance, especially if the infection is of a local or superficial nature. One such example is the milk ring test used to detect the presence of antibodies to *B. abortus* in milk (Figure 25-8). Fresh milk is shaken with bacteria stained with hematoxylin or triphenyl tetrazolium and is allowed to stand. If antibodies, especially those of the IgM or IgA classes, are present, the bacteria will clump and adhere to the fat globules of the milk and rise to the surface with the cream. If antibodies are absent, the stained bacteria will remain dispersed in the milk, and the cream, on rising, will remain white.

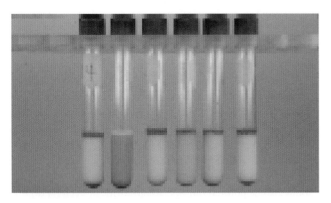

FIGURE 25-8 The milk ring test. Stained *Brucella* species remain suspended in the milk in a negative test but rise with the cream in a positive reaction (*second tube*).

(Courtesy Dr. John Huff.)

Immunity to Fungal Infections

Fungal infections are of three major types (Figure 25-9). The first are primary infections by fungi that affect the skin or other surfaces, such as *Microsporum* or *Candida* species, and cause diseases such as ringworm or thrush. The second type includes primary infections by dimorphic fungi that mainly cause respiratory infections, for example, *Histoplasma capsulatum, Blastomyces dermatitidis,* and *Coccidioides immitis.* The third type consists of secondary infections by opportunistic fungi in immunodeficient animals, such as the Mucorales (*Rhizopus, Mucor,* and *Absidia*) and *Pneumocystis.* The body uses both innate and adaptive immune mechanisms to defend itself against primary infections. Thus innate immune mechanisms against invasive fungi such as *Candida* or *Aspergillus* species include activation of the alternate complement pathway, resulting in attraction of neutrophils and attempts by these neutrophils to destroy the invading hyphae or pseudohyphae. Neutrophils are also activated by the IL-23/IL-17 axis during fungal infections. Fungal PAMPs acting either through TLR2 or through a cell-surface lectin called dectin-1 trigger IL-23 synthesis. IL-23 activates Th17 cells. The IL-17 produced by these cells then activates both neutrophils and endothelial cells and promotes acute inflammation. It is of interest to note that culturing T cells and monocytes in the presence of *Candida* hyphae promotes the generation of Th17 cells. In contrast,

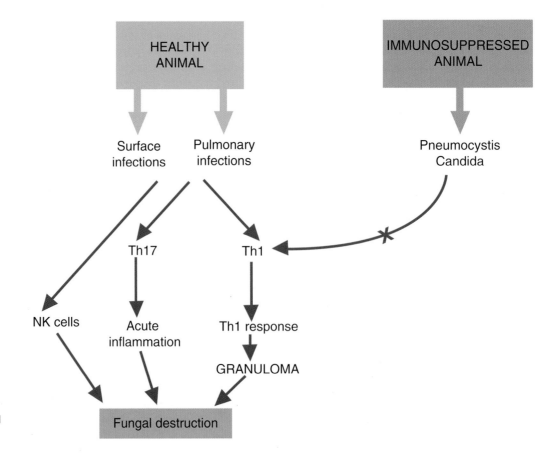

FIGURE 25-9 The mechanisms of antifungal immunity.

culture in the presence of the *Candida* yeast form promotes production of IL-12 and a Th1 response. Because of their size, neutrophils cannot totally ingest invading fungi. Nevertheless, by releasing enzymes and oxidants into the tissue fluid, neutrophils may severely damage fungal hyphae. Small fungal fragments or spores may be ingested and destroyed by macrophages or by NK cells.

Once established, fungal infections can be destroyed only by Th1-mediated mechanisms. Thus some species of *Aspergillus* are facultative intracellular parasites, and chronic or progressive fungal diseases are commonly associated with defects in the T cell system. Th1 cells function in fungal infections by activating macrophages and by promoting epidermal growth and keratinization. Some T and NK cells can exert a direct cytotoxic

effect on yeasts such as *Cryptococcus neoformans* and *Candida albicans*. It is not uncommon for recovered animals to develop a type IV hypersensitivity to fungal antigens. The critical importance of adaptive immunity to fungi is seen in the way that fungal infections, such as those caused by *P. jiroveci*, develop in immunosuppressed animals such as dogs with canine distemper. Although defense against *P. jiroveci* is critically dependent upon CD4+ T cell function, it is also dependent on Th17 cells. Depletion of IL-17 or IL-23 increases the severity of *P. jiroveci* pneumonia.

For sources of additional information, please visit http:// evolve.elsevier.com/tizard/immunology/

Immunity to Viruses

Key Points

- When sentinel cells detect foreign nucleic acids through their TLRs and other receptors, they are triggered to secrete the antiviral type I interferons.
- Antibodies are effective against extracellular viruses and can prevent them binding and infecting cells and thus neutralizing them.
- Cell-mediated responses are primarily responsible for antiviral immunity. The major mechanism involved is the killing of virus-infected cells by cytotoxic T cells.
- Because viruses are obligate intracellular parasites, they employ a wide variety of methods of evading the immune response.
- Some viruses may cause minimal disease themselves, but significant damage and disease may be caused by the immune response to these viruses.

Since viruses are obligate intracellular organisms, their very existence is threatened if they are destroyed by the immune system or by the death of their host. Because of this, both viruses and their hosts have been subjected to rigorous selection and adaptation. Viruses are selected for their ability to evade the host's immune responses, while at the same time animals are selected for resistance to virus-induced disease. Viruses that are eliminated before they replicate cannot spread. Hosts eliminated by viruses can no longer serve as hosts. An "oversuccessful" virus will reduce the availability of susceptible hosts, whereas a very successful host will be the largest target for the next generation of viruses. As a result, there can never be a "solution" to the problem of viruses. Virus diseases therefore tend to be lethal when the virus first encounters its host species or infects the wrong species. As time passes, however, virus infections tend to become less severe.

For example, in infections in which virus-host adaptation is poor, diseases tend to be lethal. Rabies is an excellent example of this. The virus is inevitably lethal in dogs, cats, horses, and cattle because they are unnatural hosts. On the other hand, in its natural hosts, especially bats and skunks, rabies virus persists and may be shed in saliva for a long period without causing disease. From the virus's "point of view," infection of dogs, cattle, or horses is unprofitable since those animals almost never transmit rabies to skunks. Other diseases of this type include feline panleukopenia, canine parvovirus-2, and the virulent forms of Newcastle disease. Vaccination is relatively successful in this type of infection since the virus has not adapted to the host's defenses.

When the virus and its host are more adapted, although disease may be severe, mortality may not be high, and the virus may be persistent. In this type of disease, further attacks may occur as a result of infection by variants of the same virus. Examples of this type of virus infection include foot-and-mouth disease and influenza. Vaccination against diseases of this type is complicated by the diversity of these viruses.

Even more adapted viruses can result in persistent infection, and the immune system is unable to eliminate the virus. Diseases of this type include the lentivirus infections, equine infectious anemia, maedi-visna of sheep, and AIDS in humans. The virus may constantly evade the immune system. Vaccination against these diseases is essentially unsuccessful. As their adaptation increases, viruses may cause latent infections and relatively mild, nonlethal disease. Some herpesvirus infections fall into this category. The most extreme examples of virus adaptation are those in which the viral genome becomes stably integrated into the host genome. These endogenous viruses are well recognized in domestic mammals such as the cat and pig.

In studying the nature of the host responses to viruses, it is well to recognize that this continuing selective pressure on both host and virus exists and profoundly influences the outcome of all viral infections (Box 26-1).

□ Box 26-1 | **The Virome**

The animal body plays host to enormous numbers of commensal bacteria. It also shelters very large numbers of diverse viruses. It has been estimated that the number of distinct viruses in human stool samples can range from 50 to almost 3000. This virome differs greatly between individuals and may be even more diverse than the bacterial microflora. It is possible that some of these viruses may be responsible for some of the unexplained fevers that occur in animals. In addition to mammalian viruses, the virome contains huge numbers of bacteriophages—perhaps as many as 100 phages for every bacterium. These phages prey on the bacteria and may play a role in transmitting genes between bacteria. When alterations in diet change the composition of the bacterial microflora, they also alter the composition of the phage population.

Pennisi E: Going viral: exploring the role of viruses in our bodies, *Science* 331:1513, 2011.

Virus Structure and Antigens

Virus particles, called virions, consist of a nucleic acid core surrounded by a layer of proteins (see Figures 9-2 and 38-2). This protein layer, called the capsid, is made up of subcomponents called capsomeres. An envelope containing lipoprotein may also surround virions. The complexity of viruses varies. Some, such as poxviruses, are complex, whereas others, such as foot-and-mouth disease virus, are relatively simple. Antibodies can be produced against epitopes on all the proteins situated inside and on the surface of the virion. Antibodies against the nucleoprotein components are not usually significant from a protective point of view, but they may be useful for serologic diagnosis.

Pathogenesis of Virus Infections

Adsorption, the first step in the invasion of a cell by a virus, occurs when a virus binds to receptors on the cell surface. These receptors have not evolved for the convenience of viruses but have some other physiological function. The rabies virus binds to the receptor for acetylcholine, a neurotransmitter. The Epstein-Barr virus (the cause of infectious mononucleosis) binds to a receptor for C3. Rhinoviruses that cause the common cold bind to cell-surface integrins. The chemokine receptor CCR5 has been identified as the receptor used by West Nile virus. The nature, number, and distribution of host cell receptors determine the host range and tissue tropism of a virus. The bound virion is taken into the cell through endocytosis or by fusion with the plasma membrane. Once inside a cell, the

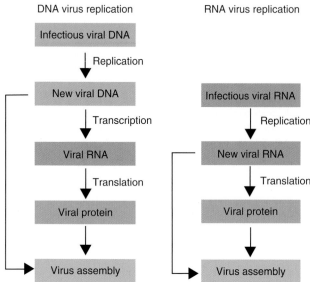

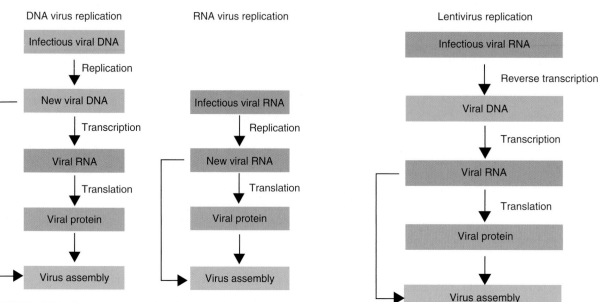

FIGURE 26-1 The mechanism of replication of DNA and RNA viruses.

FIGURE 26-2 The mechanism of replication of the retroviruses.

capsid is dismantled so that its nucleic acid is released into the cell cytoplasm, a process called uncoating. Once the virus genome is uncoated, replication begins (Figure 26-1). The host cell DNA, RNA, and protein synthesis are usually inhibited so that only viral genetic information is processed. If the virus, for example, a herpesvirus, contains DNA, this viral DNA is replicated. The new viral DNA is then transcribed into viral messenger RNA (mRNA), and this RNA is translated into new capsid proteins. These new proteins are then assembled into virions. The host cell also replicates the viral nucleic acid so that large quantities of viral DNA are produced. The viral DNA is packaged inside the new capsids so that complete virions are formed. If the virus is unenveloped, the infected cells rupture, and the virions are released into the environment. If the virions are enveloped, they leave the cell by budding through the cell surface. The cell membrane that encloses them serves as the new envelope. The released virions may then spread to nearby cells and invade them in turn.

If a virus contains RNA rather than DNA, its replication takes a slightly different course. For most RNA viruses, such as Newcastle disease or foot-and-mouth disease virus (FMDV), viral DNA is not used. Thus in FMDV infection, the viral single-stranded RNA (the "plus strand") is used as a template to synthesize a complementary "minus strand" of RNA. These minus strands are then used to generate new plus strands that can be translated into viral proteins. Some viruses contain double-stranded RNA (dsRNA) and use only one of the strands generated during replication. In other RNA viruses, the infecting virus RNA may be complementary to the newly synthesized viral RNA that will translate into viral proteins.

A different replication mechanism is employed in the case of some RNA tumor viruses and immunodeficiency viruses

(Figure 26-2). These are called retroviruses since their RNA is first reversely transcribed into DNA by an enzyme called a reverse transcriptase. The new viral DNA is then integrated into the host cell genome as a provirus. This proviral DNA can then be transcribed into RNA, as well as being able to copy itself. The proteins and RNA can then be packaged into a complete new virion.

Changes in virus-infected cells may be minimal, perhaps detectable only by the expression of new proteins on the cell surface. Sometimes, however, the changes may be extensive and result in either cell death or malignant transformation and the development of tumors.

Innate Immunity

Rapid, powerful innate immune responses limit many viral infections. Interferons are especially important in this process. Lysozyme can destroy several viruses, as can many intestinal enzymes and bile. Collectins bind to viral glycoproteins and block virus interaction with host cells. For example, conglutinin, MBL, SP-A, and SP-D can all inactivate influenza viruses. Defensins from leukocytes and mucosal epithelial cells play a dual role in antiviral defenses since they can act both on the virus and on the host cell. Thus defensins can inactivate enveloped virions by disrupting their envelopes or by interacting with their glycoproteins. Some defensins can act on virus-infected cells by blocking intracellular signaling pathways and interfering with transcription of viral RNA. Finally, cells invaded by viruses may undergo premature apoptosis, preventing successful viral invasion and replication.

Pattern-Recognition Receptors: Antiviral Sensors

Viruses, unlike bacteria and fungi, do not contain easily recognizable microbe-specific structures since they are constructed from host-derived components. For this reason, animal cells have evolved the ability to recognize their only virus-specific components, their nucleic acids. Two complementary receptor systems recognize viral nucleic acids. One system consists of nucleic acid sensor proteins found within the cytosol of all nucleated cells. These sensor proteins are called RIG-1 and MDA5. These molecules detect viral dsRNA produced by viral infection and then signal through several adaptor proteins to activate the interferon-β (IFN-β) gene. The second system is mediated by toll-like receptor (TLR)3, TLR7, TRL8, and TLR9. TLR3 recognizes dsRNA. TLR7 and TLR8 recognize single-stranded RNA viruses such as vesicular stomatitis and influenza viruses. TLR9 detects unmethylated CpG motifs in DNA. These motifs are common in both DNA viruses and bacteria. Mice deficient in either TLR7 or TLR9 or their adaptor protein MyD88 have a reduced ability to defend themselves against viruses. Plasmacytoid dendritic cells use a specialized signaling pathway that links TLR7 and TLR9 to the production of very large amounts of type I interferons.

Interferons

The interferons are cytokines that protect other cells against viral, bacterial, and protozoan invasion. They are all glycoproteins of 20 to 34 kDa. They are classified into three major types: I, II, and III. There are many type I interferons, each denoted by a greek letter. These include IFN-α, produced in large quantities by plasmacytoid dendritic cells and in much smaller amounts by lymphocytes, monocytes, and macrophages. Most mammals produce multiple isoforms of IFN-α. (There are 18 different isoforms in humans, 12 in pigs and cattle, 4 in horses, 2 in dogs). IFN-β is derived from virus-infected fibroblasts. (There are 5 isoforms in cattle and pigs and 1 in dogs and humans.) IFN-ω is produced by lymphocytes, monocytes, and human, horse, pig, rabbit, and dog trophoblast cells (6 to 7 in pigs, 5 in humans, 2 in horses, and none in dogs). A distinct form of type I interferon, IFN-τ, has been isolated from the ruminant trophoblast, and IFN-δ has been isolated from the pig trophoblast. IFN-δ is only distantly related to the other type I interferons. IFN-ε is a member of the type I family whose expression is limited to reproductive and brain tissues. It appears to play a role in mucosal and nervous system immunity. In most cases these molecules act on virus-infected cells to inhibit viral growth. The trophoblast interferons also regulate the maternal immune response to a fetus (see Figure 32-9).

There is only one type II interferon, IFN-γ, a produced by antigen-stimulated T cells. It is also produced in pig trophoblast cells (Box 26-2).

Three type III interferons have been identified, called IFN-λ1, IFN-λ2, and IFN-λ3 (also known as interleukin-29

◻ **Box 26-2** | **Measuring Interferons**

Interferons may be assayed by measuring their antiviral effects. For example, serum samples to be tested for interferon activity are added to fibroblast cultures at various dilutions and incubated for 18 to 24 hours. The fibroblast monolayers are then washed, and a standard quantity of bovine vesicular stomatitis virus is added to each culture. After 48 hours of incubation, the monolayers are stained, and virus plaques are seen as cleared areas in the monolayer. The presence of interferons in the test serum will reduce the number of plaques formed. This is called a plaque reduction assay.

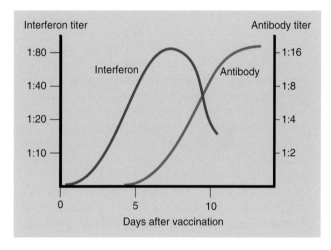

FIGURE 26-3 The sequential production of interferon and antibody following intranasal vaccination of calves with infectious bovine rhinotracheitis vaccine.

(From data kindly provided by Dr. M. Savan.)

[IL-29], IL-28A, and IL-28B). They are expressed in response to viral infections and TLR ligands. They signal through a unique receptor complex consisting of IL-10Rβ and IL-28Rα. While structurally unrelated to the type I interferons, they induce similar intracellular signals and a similar gene expression profile and can be produced by most appropriately stimulated cell types. Despite this, the type III interferons are probably more important as immune regulators. For example, IFN-λ1 inhibits Th2 responses, whereas IFN-λ2 enhances Th1 responses. Pigs lack IFN-λ2.

Antiviral Activities The two major type I interferons (IFN-α and IFN-β) are produced by virus-infected cells within a few hours after viral invasion, and high concentrations may be achieved in vivo within a few days, long before adaptive immunity develops. For example, in cattle infected intravenously with bovine herpesvirus-1 (BHV-1), peak interferon levels in serum are reached 2 days later and then decline, but they are still detectable by 7 days (Figure 26-3). In contrast, antibodies are not usually detectable in serum until 5 to 6 days after the onset of a virus infection.

Type I IFN-α and IFN-β are secreted by virus-infected cells, and both bind to a heterodimeric receptor (IFNAR) on nearby cells activating a JAK/STAT signaling pathway (see Figure 8-8) (Figure 26-4). Receptor binding results in the development of an "antiviral state" within a few minutes that peaks 5 to 8 hours later. This virus resistance is mediated through four major pathways.

- *The 2'5' A pathway:* Type I interferons upregulate transcription of the genes coding for 2'5'-oligoadenylate synthetases (2'5'-OAS). Expressed OAS enzymes are then activated by exposure to dsRNA. The activated enzymes act on adenosine triphosphate (ATP) to form 2'5' adenylate oligomers. These oligomers in turn activate a latent ribonuclease called RNAase L (Figure 26-5). RNAase L degrades viral RNA and inhibits viral growth.
- *The Mx guanosine triphosphatase (GTPase) pathway:* Mx proteins are interferon-induced GTPases that accumulate as oligomers on intracellular membranes such as the smooth endoplasmic reticulum. Following viral infection, Mx monomers are released. These bind and trap viral nucleocapsids and other essential viral components and so block the assembly of new viruses. Mx proteins are expressed in many different cell types such as hepatocytes, endothelial cells, and immune cells. They inhibit a wide range of RNA viruses, including the influenza viruses.
- *The protein kinase R (PKR) pathway:* PKR is induced by type I interferons. The inactive kinase accumulates in the cell nucleus and cytoplasm, where it is activated directly by viral RNAs. Activated PKR regulates several cell signaling pathways and phosphorylates an initiation factor called eIF2α, which then prevents translation initiation of viral mRNA.
- *The ISG15 pathway:* One of the most prominent of the interferon-stimulated genes is *ISG15*. This codes for a 17-kDa, ubiquitin-like protein that binds to many different proteins and enhances their destruction. It is not known how this results in increased antiviral resistance and reduced viral replication.

The ability of cells to produce interferons varies. Virus-infected leukocytes, especially plasmacytoid dendritic cells, produce large amounts of IFN-α; virus-infected fibroblasts produce IFN-β; and antigen-stimulated T cells are the major source of IFN-γ (Chapter 14). Kidney cells are poor interferon producers, and neutrophils produce no interferon.

Lymphocytes from normal, unsensitized donors can kill virus-infected cells. This innate cytotoxicity is due to natural killer (NK) cells (Chapter 19). NK cell cytotoxicity is stimulated by type I interferons and, as a result, is important early in a virus infection. Indeed NK cells provide a first line of defense against many viruses. NK cells also produce IFN-γ, and this too has a direct antiviral effect. NK cells may therefore reduce the severity of viral infections long before the development of adaptive immunity and the appearance of specific cytotoxic T cells.

IFN-α not only activates NK cells but it also stimulates the differentiation of monocytes into dendritic cells, as well as the

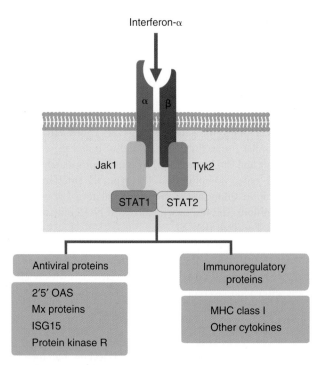

FIGURE 26-4 The receptor for the type I interferons. Ligand binding triggers the JAK-STAT transduction pathway and eventually activates both antiviral and immunoregulatory pathways.

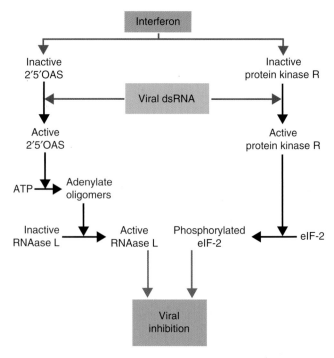

FIGURE 26-5 Some of the mechanisms by which the interferons can exert their antiviral activities.

maturation and activity of dendritic cells. IFN-α participates in the transition from innate to adaptive immunity and drives some γ/δ T cell responses. It stimulates memory T cell proliferation, activates naïve T cells, and enhances antigen-specific T cell priming.

Adaptive Immunity

Antibody-Mediated Immunity

Virus capsid and envelope proteins are antigenic, and it is against these that antiviral antibody responses are largely mounted (Figure 26-6). Antibodies can prevent cell invasion by blocking the adsorption of virions to target cells, by stimulating phagocytosis of viruses, by triggering complement-mediated virolysis, or by causing viral clumping and thus reducing the number of infectious units available for cell invasion. Binding of antibodies alone does not destroy viruses since the splitting of virus-antibody complexes may release infectious virions.

Antibodies are not only directed against proteins on free virions but are also directed against viral proteins expressed on infected cells. As a result, these infected cells may also be destroyed. Virus infections in which antibody-mediated destruction of infected cells occurs include Newcastle disease, rabies, bovine virus diarrhea, infectious bronchitis of birds, and feline leukemia. Antibodies may kill infected cells by complement-mediated cytolysis or by antibody-dependent cell-mediated cytotoxicity (ADCC). The cytotoxic cells include lymphocytes, macrophages, and neutrophils with Fc receptors through which they can bind to antibody-coated target cells.

Virus-neutralizing antibodies include immunoglobulin G (IgG) and IgM in serum and IgA in secretions. IgE may also be protective since IgE-deficient humans suffer from severe respiratory infections. As in antibacterial immunity, IgG is quantitatively the most significant immunoglobulin, whereas IgM is qualitatively superior.

Although most viruses infect cells by binding directly to receptors on target cells, some use an intermediate molecule. For instance, some antibody-coated viruses bind to cells through Fc receptors. This, of course, facilitates endocytosis of the virus and may thus enhance virus infection. Complement may enhance some virus infections in a similar fashion. Examples of viruses whose infections are enhanced by antibodies include feline infectious peritonitis, Aleutian disease of mink, African swine fever, and human immunodeficiency virus (HIV).

Cell-Mediated Immunity

Although antibodies and complement can neutralize free virions and destroy virus-infected cells, cell-mediated immune responses are much more important in controlling virus diseases. This is readily seen in immunodeficient humans (Chapter 37). Those who cannot mount an antibody-mediated response suffer from overwhelming bacterial infections but tend to recover from the common viral diseases. In contrast, humans with a T cell deficiency are commonly resistant to bacterial infection but highly susceptible to virus diseases.

Viral antigens may be expressed on the surface of infected cells long before progeny viruses are produced. When this endogenous antigen is presented by MHC class I molecules, virus-infected cells are recognized as foreign and killed. Viruses require host cells in which to replicate. Elimination of infected cells prevents viral spread. Although antibody and complement or ADCC can play a role in this process, T cell–mediated

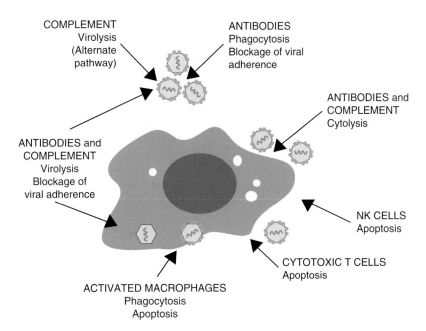

COMPLEMENT
Virolysis
(Alternate pathway)

ANTIBODIES
Phagocytosis
Blockage of viral adherence

ANTIBODIES and COMPLEMENT
Cytolysis

ANTIBODIES and COMPLEMENT
Virolysis
Blockage of viral adherence

NK CELLS
Apoptosis

CYTOTOXIC T CELLS
Apoptosis

ACTIVATED MACROPHAGES
Phagocytosis
Apoptosis

FIGURE 26-6 The ways in which the immune system can protect the body against viruses.

cytotoxicity is the major destructive mechanism. Cytotoxic T cells recognize peptide-MHC complexes and kill them. Type I interferons can sensitize virus-infected cells to this cytotoxic effect. Under some circumstances, cytotoxic T cells may kill intracellular viruses without killing the infected cells. This antiviral effect is mediated by T cell–derived IFN-γ and tumor necrosis factor-α (TNF-α). These cytokines activate two virucidal pathways. One pathway eliminates viral nucleocapsid particles, including their contained genomes. The second pathway destabilizes viral RNA.

Some viral antigens may act as superantigens by binding directly to TCR V_β chains. For example, rabies virus nucleocapsid binds to mouse $V_\beta 8$ T cells. By stimulating helper T cell activity, rabies viruses can switch on Th2 cells. This in turn can result in an enhanced immune response to rabies viruses, as well as a polyclonal B cell response sometimes seen in this disease.

Macrophages develop antiviral activity following activation. Viruses are readily endocytosed by macrophages and are usually destroyed. If the viruses are noncytopathic but can, however, grow inside macrophages, a persistent infection may result. Under these circumstances, the macrophages must be activated to eliminate the virus. Thus immunity mediated by IFN-γ is a feature of some virus diseases (Chapter 18). For example, macrophages from birds immunized against fowlpox show an enhanced antiviral effect against Newcastle disease virus and will prevent the intracellular growth of *Salmonella gallinarum*, a feature that is not a property of normal macrophages.

The duration of immunological memory to viruses is highly variable. Antibodies against viruses may persist for many years in the absence of the virus. On the other hand, because of the hazards of persistent cytotoxicity, cytotoxic T cells die soon after virus elimination. Memory T cells, however, can persist for many years.

Evasion of the Immune Response By Viruses

As discussed at the beginning of this chapter, during the millions of years they have coexisted with animals, viruses have evolved numerous ways by which to evade host immune responses (Figure 26-7). As a result, the relationship between host and virus must be established on the basis of mutual accommodation so that the long-term survival of both is ensured. Failure to reach this accommodation will result in the elimination of either host or virus; and death of the host automatically eliminates the virus.

Viruses in different families use different survival strategies. RNA viruses have a very small genome with little room to spare for genes dedicated to suppressing immunity. The proteins of RNA viruses therefore tend to be multifunctional. RNA viruses tend to rely on antigenic variation as their principal mechanism of immune evasion. On the other hand, DNA viruses have a larger genome and can afford to devote many different genes to immune evasion. In large DNA viruses such as the poxviruses and herpesviruses, as much as 50% of the total genome may be devoted to immunoregulatory genes.

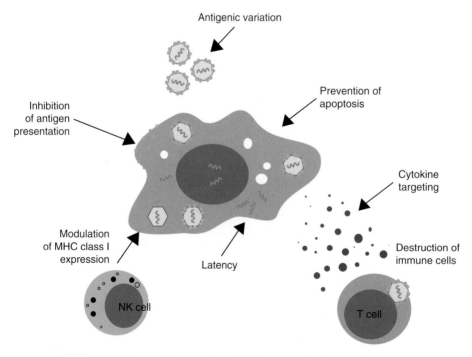

FIGURE 26-7 Some of the ways by which viruses evade immune destruction.

Negative Cytokine Regulation

Viruses use several methods to block the effectiveness of interferons. These range from blocking interferon receptor signal transduction to synthesizing soluble interferon receptors. Some viruses inhibit IFN-γ production by blocking the activities of IL-18 and IL-12, both of which are required for its production. Another example is the production of a protein related to the IFN-γR by myxoma and poxviruses. Presumably, by binding IFN-γ, the interferon is prevented from binding to cell receptors.

Some important viruses make viral versions of cytokines and chemokines and their receptors. These have been called virokines or immunoevasins. For example, equine herpesvirus makes CCR3, the receptor for CCL11. Marek's disease virus makes a protein related to CXCL8. Poxviruses make a version of the immunosuppressive cytokine IL-10. Cowpox virus also makes an IL-1β-binding protein that reduces the amount of IL-1β available to promote an immune response.

Alterations in Antigen Processing Pathways

Many viruses interfere with the expression of MHC class I molecules and inhibit antigen presentation. They use many different suppressive techniques, including reducing transcription of MHC genes; blocking TAP function and the transport of peptides into the endoplasmic reticulum; inhibiting proteasomal degradation of viral proteins; inhibiting the intracellular transport of MHC class I α chains; preventing delivery of the loaded MHC to the cell surface; and ubiquitinating and hence destroying MHC molecules. Thus BHV-1 downregulates the expression of MHC class I molecules by interfering with transporter protein functions and downregulating the expression of mRNA for MHC class I molecules. Other viruses may cause MHC class I molecules to be retained within a cell; they may prevent peptide binding to transporter proteins, prevent proteasomal degradation, redirect MHC molecules to lysosomes for degradation, or even encode inhibitors that block caspase activity. Influenza A viruses can block macrophage differentiation into dendritic cells. Other viruses may downregulate the expression of co-stimulating molecules such as ICAM-1, B7-2, CD4, and CD28.

Evasion of Natural Killer Cells

NK cells kill virus-infected cells at an early stage of infection before T and B cells are fully activated. Cytotoxic T cells kill targets that express foreign antigens on MHC class I molecules. NK cells kill targets that fail to express these MHC class I molecules. For a virus to survive, it must induce the selective downregulation of some MHC class I molecules, enabling the virus-infected cells to evade destruction by T cells while at the same time preventing NK cell activation. Some viruses may decrease the expression of the stress-related protein MICB and so inhibit NK cell mediated cytotoxicity.

Alterations in the B Cell System

One of the simplest mechanisms of viral immune evasion involves antigenic variation of RNA viruses. Rapidly occurring point mutations accompanied by poor editing functions of RNA polymerases permit the generation of large numbers of closely related but distinct viruses. The most significant examples of this occur among the influenza A viruses and the lentiviruses.

Influenza A viruses possess envelope proteins called hemagglutinins and neuraminidases. There are at least 16 different hemagglutinins and 9 neuraminidases found among the type A influenza viruses; they are identified according to a standard nomenclature system. The hemagglutinin of the swine influenza virus is called H1, and its neuraminidase is called N1. The two subtypes of the equine influenza viruses are typified by A/equine/Prague/56, which has H7 and N7, and A/equine/Hong Kong/92, which has H3 and N8 (Table 26-1).

As influenza viruses spread through a population, they undergo mutation and selection and gradually change the structure of their hemagglutinins and neuraminidases. These changes gradually lead to alterations in the antigenicity of the virus. This gradual change is called antigenic drift, and it permits the virus to persist in a population for many years. In addition, influenza viruses sporadically undergo a sudden, major genetic change in which a new strain develops whose hemagglutinins show no apparent relationship to the hemagglutinins of prior strains. Such a major change, called an antigenic shift, is not produced by mutation but results from

□ **Table 26-1 | Examples of Influenza A Virus Strains and Their Antigenic Structure**

SPECIES	VIRUS STRAIN	ANTIGENIC STRUCTURE
Human	A/New Caledonia/20/99*	H1N1
	A/California/7/2009 (swine flu)	H1N1
	A/Perth/16/2009	H3N2
Canine	A/Canine/Florida/04	H3N8
Equine	A/Equine/Prague/1/56	H7N7
	A/Equine/Miami/1/63	H3N8
	A/Equine/Suffolk/89	H3N8
	A/Equine/Hong Kong/1/92	H3N8
Swine	A/Swine/Iowa/15/30	H1N1
Avian	A/Fowl Plague/Dutch/27	H7N7
	A/Duck/England/56	H11N7
	A/Turkey/Ontario/6118/68	H8N4
	A/Chicken/Hong Kong/258/97	H5N1
	A/Chicken/Shantou/4231/2003	H5N1

*The first number is the isolate number; the second is the year of isolation.

recombination between two virus strains. This occurs readily since the influenza virus has a segmented genome. It is the development of these naturally recombinant influenza viruses with a completely new antigenic structure that accounts for the periodic major outbreaks of influenza in humans and poultry. In horses and pigs, in contrast, the rapid turnover of the population and the constant production of large numbers of susceptible young animals ensure the persistence of influenza viruses without the necessity for extensive antigenic drift. As a result, the antigenic structure of equine and swine influenza viruses has changed only slowly since they were first described. Nevertheless, the H3N8 equine influenza virus strains are evolving into two distinct lineages, one European and one American, based on the structure of the HA1 domain of their hemagglutinin. Viruses of both lineages can circulate in horse populations at the same time. Examples of the European strains include A/Suffolk/89 and A/Hong Kong/1/92. American strains include A/Kentucky/94 and A/Florida/93. All are distinctly different from the original strain A/Miami/1/63.

A second form of immune evasion by viruses is seen in caprine arthritis-encephalitis (CAE), Aleutian disease of mink, and African swine fever. Although infected animals respond to these viruses, the antibodies produced are incapable of virus neutralization. Thus virus-antibody complexes from Aleutian disease–infected mink are fully infectious. Goats with CAE make large amounts of antienvelope antibodies, but they develop negligible levels of neutralizing antibodies. In this case, goats fail to recognize and respond to the virus-neutralizing epitopes. If rabbits are immunized with CAE virus, they can readily produce virus-neutralizing antibodies; even goats will produce these antibodies if immunized with large amounts of an adjuvanted viral antigen. The antibodies produced in these hyperimmunized goats are very specific and will react only with the immunizing strain of the virus. Notwithstanding the absence of neutralizing antibodies, other antibodies can bind to CAE virions, and the opsonized virions are endocytosed by macrophages. Unfortunately, this virus grows within macrophages so that opsonizing antibodies merely speed up virus replication, an example of antibody-mediated enhancement. Attempts to vaccinate goats against CAE lead only to more severe disease.

A third mechanism by which viruses can evade destruction by antibodies is seen in yet another lentiviral infection, maedi-visna, a complex disease of sheep (maedi is a chronic pneumonia; visna is a chronic neurological disease caused by the same virus). In maedi-visna infections, neutralizing antibodies are produced slowly. These neutralizing antibodies are unable to reduce the viral burden in infected sheep, and cyclical relapses do not occur. The antibodies have a low affinity for viral epitopes and take at least 20 minutes to bind to the virus and 30 minutes to neutralize it. In contrast, it takes only 2 minutes for this virus to infect a cell. Thus the virus can spread between cells much faster than it can be neutralized. The maedi-visna virus also invades monocytes and macrophages. In most of these cells, the replication of the virus stops after its RNA has been reversely transcribed into proviral DNA. As a result, the cells are persistently infected by the virus without expressing viral antigens. The virus may therefore be disseminated without provoking immunological attack. Maedi-visna is associated with extensive infiltration of the lungs, mammary gland, and central nervous system with T cells and macrophages. Immunosuppression reduces the severity of the lesions, whereas immunization against the virus increases their severity. It is suggested that virus-infected macrophages stimulate the T cells to release cytokines. These cytokines delay the maturation of monocytes and restrict virus replication. They also enhance macrophage MHC class II expression and trigger T cell proliferation and chronic lymphoid hyperplasia.

Alterations in the T Cell System

Viruses may, of course, use the cells of the immune system as their hosts. Viruses like HIV, feline immunodeficiency virus (FIV), canine distemper (CDV) and feline leukemia virus (FeLV) infect lymphocytes and either kill them or otherwise impair their ability to function normally. Glucocorticoids are profoundly suppressive for T cells and T cell responses. Influenza virus triggers a generalized stress response leading to a sustained increase in serum glucocorticoid levels and resulting immunosuppression.

Viral Evasion Through Latency

Viruses causing a state of reversible nonproductive infection is called latency. It is a consistent feature of the herpesviruses. During latency, viruses express only the absolute minimum number of genes. Because they do not express viral antigens, they are not detected by the immune system and may remain in that state for many years.

In contrast to the short-lived immune response against bacteria, antiviral immunity is, in many cases, very long-lasting. The reasons for this are unclear, but they are often related to virus persistence within cells, perhaps in a slowly replicating or a nonreplicating form as typified by the herpesviruses. It is usually difficult to isolate viruses from an animal that has recovered from a herpesvirus infection. Some time later, however, especially when the individual is stressed, the herpesvirus may reappear and may even cause disease again. During the latent period, when it is present in the host but cannot be reisolated, the virus nucleic acid persists in host cells, but its transcription is blocked, and viral proteins are not made. The persistent virus may periodically boost the immune response of the infected animal and in this way generate long-lasting immunity to superinfection. The immune responses in these cases, although unable to eliminate viruses, may prevent the development of clinical disease and therefore serve a protective role. Immunosuppression or stress may permit disease to occur in persistently infected animals. The association between stress and the development of some virus diseases is well recognized. It is likely that the increased levels of steroid production in stressful situations may be sufficiently immunosuppressive to permit activation of latent viruses or infection by exogenous ones.

Sometimes viruses may interact with bacteria to overcome the immune system. For example, *Mannheimia hemolytica* and BHV-1, acting together, cause severe respiratory disease in cattle. BHV-1 infection increases expression of the β_2-integrin LFA-1 on lung neutrophils. The leukotoxin of *M. hemolytica* binds to this integrin and then kills the neutrophils, permitting growth of the invading bacteria.

Inhibition of Apoptosis

Apoptosis may be considered a protective response since viruses also die when a cell dies. This is especially significant if a cell dies before viruses are released. It is therefore to a virus's advantage to delay apoptosis until progeny viruses can be released. Thus poxviruses and some herpesviruses (including equine herpesvirus-2) produce caspase inhibitors that protect cells against death. Excessive lymphoid apoptosis is a feature of canine distemper, a disease characterized by severe immunosuppression.

Adverse Consequences of Immunity to Viruses

The immune response to viruses can, on occasion, be a disadvantage. Indeed, there are many virus diseases in which lesions develop as a result of inappropriate or excessive immune responses. For example, bovine respiratory syncytial virus (RSV) induces a Th2 response in infected cattle with production of IL-4 and specific IgE antibodies in the lungs. This may result in a local type I hypersensitivity reaction since there is a direct correlation between lung IgE levels and the severity of clinical disease.

The destruction of virus-infected cells by antibody is classified as a type II hypersensitivity reaction (Chapter 29) and, although normally beneficial, may exacerbate virus diseases. Thus viruses are removed at the cost of cellular destruction. The severity and significance of this destruction depend on how widespread the infection becomes. In some diseases in which the virus causes little cell destruction, most of the tissue damage may result from immunological attack. A good example of this is seen in distemper encephalitis, in which neurons are demyelinated as a result of an antiviral immune response. Thus macrophages, which are numerous in these brain lesions, ingest immune-complexes and infected cells. As a result they release oxidants and other toxic products. These toxic products damage nearby cells, especially oligodendroglia, causing demyelination. Old-dog encephalitis, a disease of middle-aged dogs, is perhaps a variant of this postdistemper lesion.

Type III (immune complex) lesions (Chapter 30) are associated with viral diseases, especially those in which viremia is prolonged. For example, a membranoproliferative glomerulonephritis resulting from the deposition of immune complexes is a common complication of equine infectious anemia, Aleutian disease of mink, feline leukemia, chronic hog cholera, bovine virus diarrhea-mucosal disease, canine adenovirus infections, and feline infectious peritonitis. A generalized vasculitis due to deposition of immune complexes throughout the vascular system is seen in equine infectious anemia, Aleutian disease of mink, malignant catarrhal fever, and possibly, equine viral arteritis.

In dogs infected with canine adenovirus-1 (infectious canine hepatitis), an immune complex–mediated uveitis and a focal glomerulonephritis both develop. The uveitis, commonly called blue-eye, is seen both in dogs with natural infections and in those vaccinated with live attenuated adenovirus vaccine (Figure 26-8). The uveitis results from the formation of virus-antibody complexes in the anterior chamber of the eye and in the cornea with complement activation and consequent neutrophil accumulation (Figure 26-9). The neutrophils release enzymes and oxidants that damage corneal epithelial cells, leading to edema and opacity. The condition resolves spontaneously in about 90% of affected dogs.

Finally, many virus diseases are associated with the occurrence of rashes. The pathology of these is complex but may reflect type II, III, or IV hypersensitivity reactions occurring as the host responds to the presence of viral antigens in the skin.

Antibody-Dependent Enhancement

There are many examples of virus infections in which the presence of antibodies results in increased susceptibility or severity of infection. Several mechanisms are involved in this, and many are poorly understood. One important mechanism observed in cats with feline coronavirus (FCV) or FIV is antibody-dependent enhancement. This can involve, as

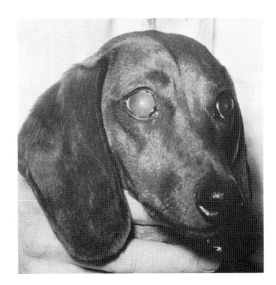

FIGURE 26-8 A case of blue-eye in a Dachshund. This is a type III hypersensitivity reaction to canine adenovirus 1 (ICH) occurring in the cornea.

(Courtesy Dr. H. Reed.)

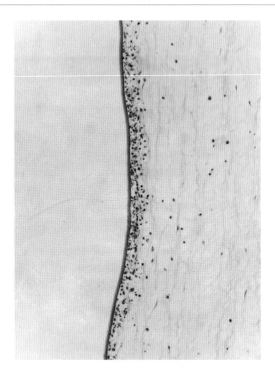

FIGURE 26-9 A section from the cornea of a dog with blue-eye. Note the neutrophil infiltration of the posterior surface of the cornea as a result of virus-antibody complex deposition in this region.

(From Carmichael LE: Pathogenesis of ocular lesions of infectious canine hepatitis: 1. Pathology and virological observations, *Pathol Vet* 1:73–95, 1964.)

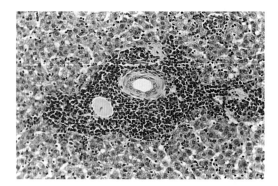

FIGURE 26-10 A section of liver from a mink infected with Aleutian disease. Note the marked plasma cell and mononuclear cell infiltration. Original magnification ×250.

(From a specimen kindly provided by Dr. S.H. An.)

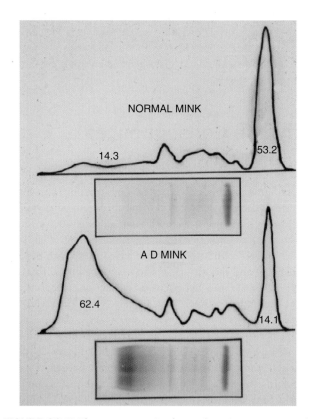

FIGURE 26-11 The serum protein electrophoretic patterns seen in normal and Aleutian disease–infected mink. The serum of the infected animal shows a polyclonal gammopathy, so the γ-globulins account for 62.4% of the serum proteins in contrast to the normal level of 14.3%.

(Courtesy Dr. S.H. An.)

described previously, antibody opsonizing virions such that their entry into cells through Fcγ receptors is enhanced. This FcR-mediated entry may be less potent than other routes in triggering antiviral responses such as interferon production. Some experimental FIV, simian immunodeficiency virus (SIV), and equine infectious anemia virus (EIAV) vaccines may increase disease susceptibility by a similar mechanism. FIV envelope-specific antibodies appear especially effective in enhancing infection.

Some Selected Viral Diseases

Aleutian Disease of Mink

Although immune complex–mediated lesions are usually only of passing interest in many infectious diseases, they generate the major pathological lesions in Aleutian disease of mink. Aleutian disease is a parvovirus infection that was first recognized in mink with the Aleutian coat color. Although all strains of mink are susceptible to this virus, Aleutian mink are genetically predisposed to the development of severe lesions since they are also affected by the Chédiak-Higashi syndrome (Chapter 37). Persistently infected mink develop a slowly progressive lymphoproliferative disease with a plasmacytosis that has been compared to a myeloma since it results in a polyclonal or monoclonal gammopathy (Figures 26-10 and 26-11). They also develop immune complex lesions (Chapter 30), including

glomerulonephritis and arteritis. They make autoantibodies to their own immunoglobulins (rheumatoid factors) and to DNA (antinuclear antibodies). Their serum IgG concentration increases, sometimes to very high levels. On occasion these elevated immunoglobulins are monoclonal in origin. They are directed against the Aleutian disease virus. The virus transforms B cells so that they proliferate and differentiate excessively.

The immune complex–mediated lesions of Aleutian disease include an arteritis, in which IgG, C3, and viral antigen are found within vessel walls, and a glomerulonephritis, in which deposits of immune complexes containing virus and antibody are found. In addition, infected mink are anemic. Their red cells are coated with antiviral antibodies. It is likely, therefore, that the red cells of infected animals adsorb virus-antibody complexes from plasma. These coated red cells are then removed from the circulation by macrophages. As might be predicted, the use of immunosuppressive agents such as cyclophosphamide or azathioprine in infected mink prevents the development of many of these lesions and prolongs survival, whereas experimental vaccination with inactivated Aleutian disease virus increases the severity of infections.

Feline Infectious Peritonitis

Feline coronavirus (FCV) is endemic in feral cat populations. Infection by this virus precedes outbreaks of feline infectious peritonitis (FIP). FIP is a fatal granulomatous disease of wild and domestic cats. There are two distinct genotypes of feline enteric coronavirus, avirulent and virulent. The avirulent genotype prefers to replicate within intestinal epithelial cells, whereas the virulent genotype prefers to replicate within macrophages. Macrophages also spread the virus throughout the body. FIP tends to infect relatively young cats between 6 months and 3 years of age. The disease presents in two major forms: (1) an effusive ("wet") form with peritonitis or pleuritis characterized by the presence of large amounts of proteinaceous fluid in the body cavities and associated with a vasculitis, and (2) a noneffusive ("dry") form characterized by multiple small granulomas on the surface of the major abdominal organs. Pleural lesions are uncommon in the noneffusive form of FIP. Some cats may show central nervous system involvement and ocular lesions. Both forms of the disease are uniformly lethal, with affected cats dying between 1 week and 6 months.

The pathogenesis of FIP differs between the two forms of the disease. After invading a cat, the virus first replicates in intestinal epithelial cells. The virus shed by epithelial cells is then spread by monocytes and taken up by phagocytic cells in the target tissues. These target tissues include the serosa of the peritoneum and the pleura, as well as the meninges and the uveal tract. The course of the infection then depends on the nature of the immune response to the virus—a phenomenon also seen in several bacterial diseases (Chapter 25). Immunity to FIP virus is entirely cell mediated, and a Th1 response is protective. A cat that mounts a good Th1 response will become immune, regardless of the amount of antibodies it makes. Some cats, however, mount a Th2 response to the viral spike proteins. In these animals, antibodies enhance virus uptake by macrophages, in which they then replicate. Virus-laden macrophages accumulate around the blood vessels of the omentum and serosa (Figure 26-12). These macrophages are activated in that they are strongly positive for CD18 and produce TNF-α and IL-1β. Endothelial cells upregulate MHC class II expression. These antibodies also

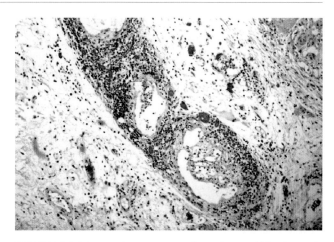

FIGURE 26-12 Granulomatous vasculitis of serosal blood vessels in a cat with feline infectious peritonitis. Note the marked cellular infiltration of the vessel adventitia and media. This reaction may be partially due to the deposition of virus-antibody complexes in the vessel walls.

(Courtesy Dr. R.C. Weiss.)

generate immune complexes that are deposited in the serosa, causing pleuritis or peritonitis, and in glomeruli, leading to glomerulonephritis. The serosal vasculitis is responsible for the effusion of fibrin-rich fluid into the serosal cavities. This massive production of immune complexes may also be responsible for the disseminated intravascular coagulation seen in these cats. IL-1 and IL-6 are found in unusually high concentrations in the peritoneal fluid from cats with effusive FIP. Cats with preexisting high levels of antibodies against FCV develop effusive FIP rapidly on challenge. Administering antiserum to FCV before FIP challenge may also enhance the peritonitis. Compared with cats with FIP, FCV-infected cats without FIP express higher levels of IL-10 and macrophage colony-stimulating factor (M-CSF) in their spleen, higher levels of IL-12 p40 in their lymphoid tissues, lower levels of IL-1β, IL-6, granulocyte colony-stimulating factor (G-CSF), and M-CSF, and higher levels of TNF-α in their mesenteric lymph nodes. It has been suggested that these FCV-infected cats do not develop FIP since they avoid excessive macrophage activation by upregulating IL-10.

A modified live intranasal vaccine is available against FIP. The vaccine contains a temperature-sensitive mutant virus that replicates in the upper respiratory tract and induces a local IgA response in the mucosa. This local mucosal response should prevent coronavirus invasion without inducing high levels of serum antibodies. This vaccine, however, will only be effective if administered before coronavirus exposure. In highly endemic situations in which kittens are infected at a young age, vaccination at 16 weeks of age may be too late to prevent infection.

Equine Infectious Anemia

EIAV is caused by a lentivirus. Following recovery from the first attack of clinical disease characterized by anemia, fever, thrombocytopenia, weight loss, and depression, horses may remain healthy for weeks or months. However, three or four relapses at 2- to 8-week intervals may occur before the horse either develops a chronic wasting disease or becomes clinically normal. Each episode of disease tends to be milder than the previous one. The fevers are lower and the anemia less severe. EIAV, like other lentiviruses, undergoes random mutation, and new, antigenically different variants are produced. The elimination of these variants is determined by the presence of neutralizing antibodies and cytotoxic T cells. As variant strains of the virus are produced, the infected horse makes neutralizing antibodies to that variant, and as a result, the viremia ends. Variants of the EIA virus, however, appear rapidly and randomly. The appearance of a new non-neutralizable variant leads to a clinical relapse. After the virus has undergone several of these mutations and the horse has responded to them all, the neutralizing antibody spectrum of the horse's serum becomes very broad, and viremia drops to a low level. Large amounts of tissues may then have to be examined to isolate the virus.

In addition to evading the immune response through antigenic variation, EIAV is associated with significant immunologically mediated tissue damage. The red cells of viremic horses adsorb circulating EIAV onto their surface. Antibodies and complement then bind to the virus, as a result of which the red cells are cleared from the circulation more rapidly than normal. Infected horses may also develop a membranoproliferative glomerulonephritis as a result of immune complex deposition on glomerular basement membranes. Horses infected with EIAV have unusually low levels of IgG3, although their circulating lymphocytes appear to be unaffected and respond normally to mitogens such as phytohemagglutinin. The macrophage receptor for equine infectious anemia virus has been designated equine lentivirus receptor-1. It is a member of the family of TNF receptor proteins.

Porcine Respiratory and Reproductive Syndrome

The porcine respiratory and reproductive syndrome virus (PRRSV) is caused by a single-stranded, positive-sense RNA virus belonging to the family Arteriviridae. It infects pigs and causes a syndrome characterized by reproductive failure, infertility, abortions, anorexia, and secondary pneumonia. The virus replicates in macrophages and dendritic cells. (It kills M-DCs and suppresses the activities of P-DCs.) It shows a special preference for alveolar macrophages and, as a result of their destruction, leads to an increase in secondary enzootic pneumonia. When PRRSV infects neonatal piglets, it causes a great increase in B cell activity. The piglets present with polyclonal B cell activation, autoimmunity (antibodies specific for Golgi antigens and dsDNA), grossly enlarged lymph nodes, and hypergammaglobulinemia (a 100- to 1000-fold increase in IgG; a 10- to 100-fold increase in IgM and IgA). The immunoglobulins produced are not directed against PRRSV, and the B cell proliferative response is not purely polyclonal. The antibodies produced are derived from a limited number of dominant B cell clones. They are not neutralizing antibodies. It is speculated that the virus produces some form of B cell superantigen. Affected pigs also show a decrease in CD4+ T cells and an increase in CD8+ cells after several weeks. Cell-mediated responses and virus-neutralizing antibodies to PRRSV do not develop for about 4 weeks as a result of the loss of CD4 cells. Because of this immunosuppression, PRRSV may cause persistent infections lasting for up to 6 months. The levels of IL-1, IL-6, TNF-α, and IFN-α are upregulated earlier and to a greater extent in pigs infected with a highly pathogenic strain of PRRSV than in pigs infected with less virulent strains. These cytokines are produced by pulmonary septal and alveolar macrophages. The high levels of these cytokines may reduce adaptive immune responses to this virus. PRRSV infects mature dendritic cells. This infection reduces the expression of CD80/86 as well as MHC class II molecules and increases their production of IL-10.

Canine Distemper

Canine distemper is caused by a negative-sense, single-stranded RNA morbillivirus related to measles and rinderpest. Although the virus affects many organs, one of its prime targets is the lymphoid system. The virus invades lymphocytes through its receptor CD150 (also called signaling lymphocyte activation molecule, or SLAM) and then induces apoptosis of CD4+ T cells. Thus in canine distemper there is a viremia-associated loss of CD4+ T cells due to lymphoid cell apoptosis. As a result, there is lymphoid organ depletion and leucopenia. The viral H protein binds to SLAM, followed by cell entry. SLAM expression is then upregulated. Since SLAM is also expressed on dendritic cells and activated macrophages, antigen presentation may also be affected. As a result of CDV infection, lymphocytes are depleted in spleen, lymph nodes, and tonsils. Thymic atrophy occurs with a reduction in Hassall's corpuscles. There is a complete loss of secondary follicles. The bone marrow, in contrast, is minimally affected. The most affected lymphocyte populations are CD4+ T, CD8+ T, and CD21+ B cells. Subsequent regeneration of the lymphoid organs leads to a recovery of double-negative T cell subsets. The numbers of CD5- and immunoglobulin-positive cells remain reduced. The CDV N-protein interacts with FcγR (CD32) to suppress IL-12 production and B cell maturation. This leads to reduced plasma cell formation and immunoglobulin production. Even after CDV has cleared, affected dogs remain profoundly immunosuppressed.

CDV also causes a demyelinating leukoencephalomyelitis. This is a two-stage process. The initial lesion is probably due to direct viral activity, but this is followed by plaque progression that is triggered by a strong Th1 response and the production of proinflammatory cytokines (IL-6, IL-8, IL-12, and TNF-α). Thus the damage may be secondary to excessive macrophage function and bystander mechanisms. Cytotoxic CD8+ cells may also contribute to the loss of myelin.

Some Antiviral Vaccines

Because of the lack of antiviral drugs, vaccination is the only effective method for the control of most viral diseases in domestic animals. As a result, the development of viral vaccines is, in many ways, more advanced than the development of their bacterial counterparts. It has, for example, proved relatively easy to attenuate many viruses so that effective vaccines containing modified live virus (MLV) derived from tissue culture are readily available.

As discussed in Chapter 24, MLV vaccines are usually good immunogens, but their use may involve certain risks. The most important problem encountered is residual virulence. One serious example of this was the development of clinical rabies in some dogs and cats following administration of older strains of MLV rabies vaccine. Some strains of infectious bovine rhinotracheitis and equine herpesvirus-1 vaccines may cause abortion when given to pregnant cows or mares, respectively, and MLV bluetongue vaccines may cause disease in fetal lambs if given to pregnant ewes (Chapter 21). More commonly, the residual virulence in these vaccines causes a mild disease. Thus intraocular or intranasal rhinotracheitis or calicivirus vaccines may cause a transient conjunctivitis or rhinitis in cats. MLV infectious bursal disease vaccines, some canine parvovirus-2 vaccines, and some bovine viral diarrhea vaccines can cause a mild immunosuppression.

Transient side effects such as these, which may otherwise be regarded as inconsequential, can be of major significance in the broiler chicken industry, where even a minor slowing in growth can have major economic results. Two strains of infectious bronchitis vaccine are available. The Massachusetts strain is mildly pathogenic but a good immunogen, whereas the Connecticut strain is nonpathogenic but a poor immunogen. It is common, therefore, in order to minimize complications, to use the Connecticut strain for primary vaccination and, if boosters are required, to use the Massachusetts strain subsequently. Similarly, of the two major vaccine strains of Newcastle disease, the LaSota strain is a good immunogen but may provoke mild adverse reactions. In contrast, the B1 strain is considerably milder but is less immunogenic, especially if given in drinking water. In other situations, birds may be primed with the very mild G2 Newcastle disease strain. Then, in the face of severe challenge, they may be boosted with a relatively virulent live vaccine.

Because of problems of this nature, persistent attempts have been made to minimize residual virulence in vaccines. One method involves the use of temperature-sensitive (ts) mutants. Ts strains of BHV-1, for example, will grow only at temperatures a few degrees lower than normal body temperature. When this organism is administered intranasally, it is able to colonize the relatively cool nasal mucosa but is unable to invade the rest of the body. Thus the vaccine can stimulate local immunity without incurring the risk for a systemic invasion. (It also has the advantage that its activity is not blocked by maternal immunity.) Some vaccine viruses may persist in vaccinated animals and cause a prolonged carrier state. Although this is a problem largely associated with herpesviruses, concerns have been expressed that the widespread use of MLV vaccines may serve to seed viruses into animal populations and that untoward consequences may develop in the future. This is a threat not to be taken lightly.

An alternative approach to overcoming the problems caused by MLV involves the increasing use of inactivated and subunit vaccines. Excellent inactivated vaccines are available against diseases such as foot-and-mouth disease, equine herpesvirus-4 (rhinopneumonitis), pseudorabies, feline panleukopenia, feline herpes (rhinotracheitis), and rabies. A genetically engineered subunit vaccine directed against the gp70 envelope antigen of feline leukemia virus is also available. At their best, these vaccines confer immunity comparable in strength and duration to that induced by MLV vaccines, with the assurance that they are free of residual virulence.

Serology of Viral Diseases

Tests to Detect and Identify Viruses

Historically, serological tests were used to identify the presence of viruses within tissues The tests commonly employed for this purpose included fluorescent antibody tests, enzyme-linked immunosorbent assay (ELISA), hemagglutination inhibition, virus neutralization, complement fixation, and gel precipitation. The precise tests employed depended on the nature of the unknown virus. The development of the polymerase chain reaction (PCR) has made many of these techniques obsolete. Exquisitely sensitive, the PCR can be used to detect viral DNA. A reverse transcriptase PCR can be used to detect RNA viruses. The PCR is best suited for use in well-equipped laboratories. For animal-side testing or in situations in which the equipment is not available, a more suitable technique for the detection of viral antigen or antiviral antibodies is the membrane filter ELISA test (Chapter 41). This test has the advantage that both positive and negative controls can be incorporated with the test serum in one well. In addition to serum, whole blood, plasma, or saliva may be employed as a source of antigen or antibody.

If the precise location of a virus needs to be determined in, for example, infected tissues, immunofluorescence or enzyme-linked immunohistochemical techniques may be employed. Specific antibodies can be used to enrich virus suspensions before electron microscopy. For example, a fecal sample may be centrifuged, leaving a clear supernatant that contains a small number of many different viruses. After sonication to break up clumps, antibody specific for the virus of interest is added to the supernatant, and after a brief incubation, the fluid is centrifuged again. Virus particles clumped by antibody are spun to the bottom, where they can be removed and examined by electron microscopy after negative staining (Figure 26-13). The antibody, by clumping only the virus of interest, renders it much easier to see by electron microscopy, and the presence of visible antibody within the virus clumps provides direct confirmation of the identity of the virus.

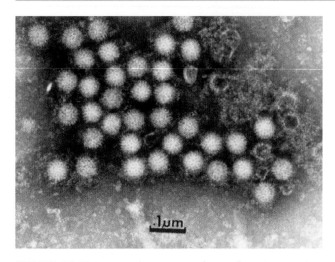

FIGURE 26-13 Immunoelectron microscopy of porcine rotavirus clumped by convalescent antiserum. Original magnification ×130,500. (Courtesy Dr. L. Saif.)

Tests to Detect and Identify Antiviral Antibodies

In general, the most widely employed techniques for detecting antibodies to viruses are hemagglutination inhibition, indirect ELISA, immunofluorescence, gel diffusion, Western blotting, complement fixation, and virus neutralization. The first four of these are technically simple and are thus preferred. The complement fixation test and the virus neutralization tests are complex, restricting the circumstances in which they may be used. The virus neutralization tests are also extremely specific, which as discussed earlier tends to reduce their value as screening tests.

For sources of additional information, please visit http://evolve.elsevier.com/tizard/immunology/

Immunity to Parasites

Key Points

- Parasites, by definition, are able to evade their host's immune response for at least sufficient time for the parasite to reproduce.
- In general antibody-mediated immune responses protect against extracellular protozoa, whereas cell-mediated responses control intracellular protozoa.
- Protozoan parasites employ some very sophisticated techniques to ensure their survival in the face of an animal's immune response.
- Helminth parasites have a unique ability to trigger Th2 responses and immunoglobulin E (IgE) production. IgE may have evolved as an antiparasite antibody.
- Parasitic worms have a thick cuticle that protects them against damage caused by most protective cells. However, eosinophils appear to be uniquely able to damage and kill helminths.
- Immunity to parasitic arthropods such as ticks and biting flies also appears to be a property of the Th2 responses. However, although immune responses can reduce arthropod feeding and reproduction, they rarely kill the arthropods.

Infectious diseases, as pointed out earlier, rarely result from the deliberate activities of a malicious microorganism. In most cases, disease occurs because of the host's reaction to the infection or because the invader inadvertently causes damage to its host. Well-adapted parasites do not make these mistakes. They have evolved in such a way that their presence in the host is scarcely noticed. They exploit the host's resources without causing irreparable damage or triggering an effective defensive response. Parasitic infections caused by protozoan parasites or helminths may be noticed only by production losses. Indeed, in many cases, the presence of parasites comes to our attention only when they are present in unusually large numbers or when they damage critical organs by accident. Sometimes, of course, a parasite may deliberately cause disease. For instance, the protozoan parasite *Toxoplasma gondii* causes its rodent hosts to become slow, confused and fearless so that they are more readily eaten by cats, its alternative host.

A consistent feature of all parasite infestations however, is that they block or significantly delay the innate and adaptive defenses of their host so that they may persist for sufficient time to reproduce. Some parasites may simply delay their destruction until they complete a single life cycle. Other well-adapted parasites may contrive to survive for the life of their host protected from immunological attack by sophisticated and specific evasive strategies (Figure 27-1).

In contrast to the acute, short-lived infections caused by bacteria and viruses, infections by parasitic protozoa or helminths are long-lasting. Ideally, a successful parasite will regulate a host's immune responses, selectively suppressing these to permit parasite survival, while at the same time allowing other responses to proceed and thus preventing the death of the host from other infections. In addition, many parasites make use of the host's metabolic or control pathways for their own purposes. Epithelial growth factor and IFN-γ can enhance the growth of *Trypanosoma brucei,* whereas IL-2 and GM-CSF promote the growth of *Leishmania amazonensis.* The sharing of cytokines by host and parasites in this way reflects the long history of their association and their success in adapting to a parasitic lifestyle. It is evident that these parasites must have evolved very effective mechanisms to prevent immunological destruction.

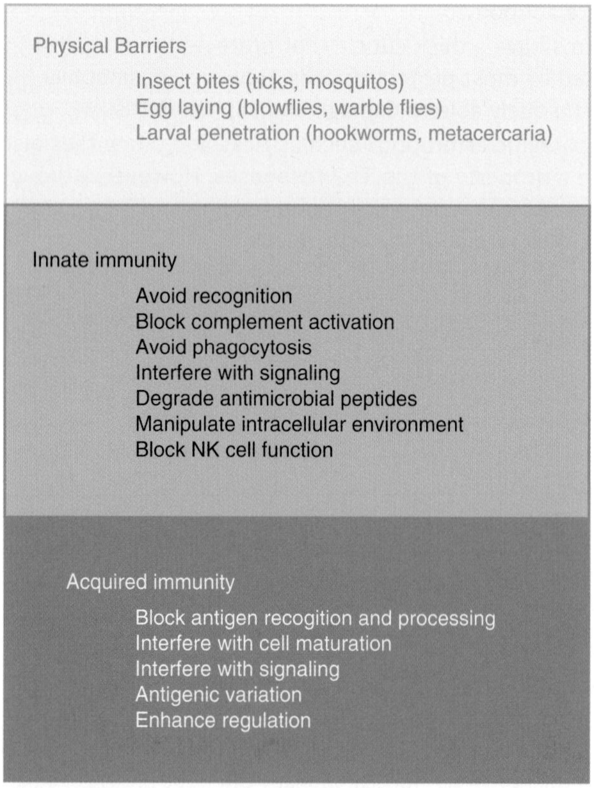

Immunity to Protozoa

Innate Immunity

The mechanisms of innate resistance to protozoa are similar to those that prevent bacterial and viral invasion, although species influences are of much greater significance. For example, *T. brucei, Trypanosoma congolense,* and *Trypanosoma vivax* do not cause disease in the wild ungulates of East Africa but will kill domestic cattle, presumably as a result of lack of mutual adaptation. Similarly, the coccidia are extremely host specific; for example, *Toxoplasma gondii* tachyzoites can infect any species of mammal, but their coccidian stages affect only felids (e.g., cats).

These species differences are reflected by more subtle genetic influences within breeds. Thus some breeds of African cattle, most notably N'Dama, are resistant to infection by pathogenic trypanosomes. This "trypanotolerance" results from selection of the most resistant animals over many generations and results in a greater ability to control infection as well as resistance to the pathological effects of the parasite. The γ/δ T cells of N'Dama are much more responsive to trypanosome antigens than are the γ/δ T cells of non-native cattle. Trypanotolerant animals produce more IL-4 and less IL-6 than susceptible animals. At the same time trypanotolerant animals show neither the severe anemia nor the production loss seen in susceptible cattle. Trypanotolerant animals produce high levels of IgG against *T. congolense* cysteine protease. Since this enzyme contributes to the pathology of infection, these antibodies may partially account for their tolerance.

Adaptive Immunity

Like other invaders, protozoa stimulate both antibody- and cell-mediated immune responses. In general, antibodies control parasites in blood and tissue fluids, whereas cell-mediated responses are directed largely against intracellular parasites.

Serum antibodies directed against protozoan surface antigens may opsonize, agglutinate, or immobilize them. Antibodies together with complement and cytotoxic cells may kill them, and some antibodies (called ablastins) may inhibit their division. In genital infections of humans due to *Trichomonas vaginalis,* a local IgE response is stimulated. This triggers an allergic reaction that increases vascular permeability, permitting IgG antibodies to reach the site of infection and immobilize and eliminate the organisms.

In babesiosis the infective stages of the organisms (sporozoites) invade red blood cells. Infected red cells incorporate *Babesia* antigens into their membranes. These in turn induce antibodies that opsonize the red cells and cause their removal by phagocytosis. Infected red cells may also be destroyed by antibody-dependent cell-mediated responses. Macrophages

---

Physical Barriers

Insect bites (ticks, mosquitos)
Egg laying (blowflies, warble flies)
Larval penetration (hookworms, metacercaria)

Innate immunity

Avoid recognition
Block complement activation
Avoid phagocytosis
Interfere with signaling
Degrade antimicrobial peptides
Manipulate intracellular environment
Block NK cell function

Acquired immunity

Block antigen recogition and processing
Interfere with cell maturation
Interfere with signaling
Antigenic variation
Enhance regulation

FIGURE 27-1 Evasion of the immune response is critical to parasite survival. Some of the many ways by which parasites evade immune destruction or exclusion are shown.

and cytotoxic lymphocytes can recognize the *Babesia* antigen-antibody complexes on the surface of infected erythrocytes. T cell cytotoxicity may be important early in infection when the number of infected erythrocytes is small.

Intracellular parasites use many different and unique strategies to invade cells and inhibit intracellular killing. Most gain entry to a cell by employing host-mediated processes such as phagocytosis or induced uptake. Apicomplexans such as *Toxoplasma* and *Cryptosporidium,* however, actively penetrate cells using a system of adhesion-based motility called "gliding." Once inside, these parasites reside in specially modified vacuoles. Protective immunity against apicomplexan protozoa, such as *Cryptosporidium, Eimeria, Neospora, Plasmodia,* and *Toxoplasma* species, is generally mediated by Th1 responses. For example, *T. gondii* is an obligate intracellular parasite whose tachyzoites grow within cells, especially macrophages (Figure 27-2). The parasites produce perforin-like molecules that permeabilize the cell membrane and permit the tachyzoites to escape and invade other cells. They penetrate these cells by "gliding" through a molecular junction in the cell membrane and do not trigger proper phagosome formation or maturation. *Toxoplasma* tachyzoites are therefore not destroyed since their "parasitophorous vacuoles" do not mature and fuse with lysosomes. *Toxoplasma* can grow inside cells in an environment free of antibodies, oxidants, or lysosomal enzymes. *Toxoplasma*-infected dendritic cells are attacked and killed by perforins from natural killer (NK) cells. However, the released parasites can then invade the NK cells! These infected NK cells, in contrast, are not effectively targeted by other NK cells.

The production of IL-12 and IFN-γ is essential for the early control of *Toxoplasma* infection. The toxoplasma actin-binding protein profilin is the ligand for TLR11. TLR11 on dendritic cells signals through the MyD88 pathway stimulating IL-12 and IFN-γ production. *T. gondii* cyclophilin also stimulates

IL-12 production from dendritic cells through CCR5. The IL-12 and IFN-γ in turn trigger a strong Th1 response. Some antibodies are produced that, together with complement, destroy extracellular organisms and prevent its spread between cells (Figure 27-3). This response, however, has little or no influence on the intracellular forms of the parasite. The intracellular organisms are only destroyed by the IL-12-dependent Th1 response. Activated Th1 cells secrete IFN-γ in response to *Toxoplasma* ribonucleoproteins. This IFN-γ activates macrophages, permitting lysosome-vacuole fusion and killing the intracellular organisms. In addition, cytotoxic T cells can destroy *Toxoplasma* tachyzoites and *Toxoplasma*-infected cells on contact. *T. gondii* tachyzoites, however, may convert into a cyst form containing bradyzoites. The cysts are weakly immunogenic and do not stimulate inflammation. It is possible that this cyst stage is not recognized as foreign. As a result, the cysts persist indefinitely within tissues.

Th1-mediated responses resulting in the activation of macrophages are important in many protozoan diseases in which the organisms are resistant to intracellular destruction. One of the most significant destructive pathways in M1 cells is the production of nitric oxide (NO). Nitrogen radicals formed by the interaction of NO with other oxidants are lethal for many intracellular protozoa. However, protozoa are also experts in surviving within macrophages; for example, *Leishmania, Toxoplasma,* and *Trypanosoma cruzi,* can migrate into safe intracellular vacuoles by blocking phagosome maturation. *Leishmania* and *T. cruzi* can suppress the production of oxidants or cytokine production, whereas *T. gondii* can promote macrophage apoptosis. *T. gondii* tachyzoites can inhibit proinflammatory cytokine production by preventing nuclear translocation of NF-κB.

In *Theileria parva* infection (East Coast fever) of cattle, sporozoites can invade α/β and γ/δ T cells, as well as B cells. The parasite then activates NF-κB by continuously phosphorylating its inhibitor proteins Iκ-Bα and Iκ-Bβ (Chapter 8). The NF-κB thus persists, maintains the cell in an activated state, and prevents its apoptosis. The activated cells produce both IL-2 and IL-2R. As a result, a loop is established, by which infected cells secrete IL-2, which in turn stimulates their growth. As *Theileria* schizonts develop within lymphocytes, the infected cells enlarge and proliferate. Since the parasite divides synchronously with its host cell, there is a rapid increase in parasitized cells resulting in overwhelming infection and death. Some animals, however, may recover from infection and become solidly immune. In these animals, CD8+ T cells can kill infected lymphocytes by recognizing parasite antigens in association with MHC class I molecules. In susceptible animals, the parasites interfere with MHC class I expression.

Infection of chickens or mammals with *Eimeria* oocysts generally leads to strong, species-specific immunity that can prevent reinfection. This immune response inhibits the growth of trophozoites, the earliest invasive stage, within intestinal epithelial cells. This growth inhibition is reversible since the arrested stages can be transferred to normal animals and complete their development uneventfully. Studies in mice suggest

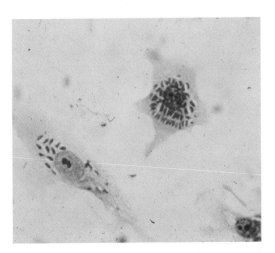

FIGURE 27-2 Mouse macrophages containing healthy, growing tachyzoites of *Toxoplasma gondii*. After an immune response develops, these cells become activated and acquire the ability to destroy ingested tachyzoites.

(Courtesy Dr. C.H. Lai.)

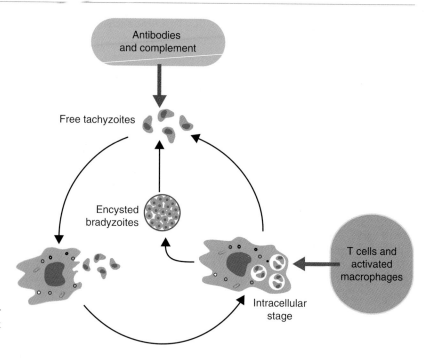

FIGURE 27-3 The points in the life cycle of *Toxoplasma gondii* at which the immune system can exert a controlling influence.

that resistance to primary infection is mediated by multiple cell-mediated mechanisms that involve CD4+ T cells and their cytokines IL-12 and IFN-γ, macrophages, and NK cells. In contrast, resistance to secondary challenge is mediated by CD8+ T cells. In chickens, IFN-γ , tumor necrosis factor-α (TNF-α), and transforming growth factor-β (TGF-β), as well as intraepithelial CD8+ α/β T cells, appear to be essential for anticoccidial immunity. It is interesting to note that *Eimeria*-susceptible chickens express much more IL-10 in their intestines than do resistant chickens, both constitutively and after infection. Given that IL-10 promotes a Th2 bias, it is likely that this is the cause of reduced resistance in susceptible birds.

For many years it was thought that a common feature of many protozoan infections was *premunition,* a term used to describe resistance that is established after the primary infection has become chronic and is only effective if the parasite persists in the host. It was believed, for example, that only cattle actually infected with *Babesia* were resistant to clinical disease. If all organisms were removed from an animal, resistance was believed to wane immediately. Studies have shown that this is not entirely true. Cattle cured of *Babesia* infection by chemotherapy are resistant to challenge with the homologous strain of that organism for several years. Nevertheless, the presence of infection does appear to be mandatory for protection against heterologous strains. Babesiosis is also of interest since splenectomy of infected animals will result in clinical disease. The spleen not only serves as a source of antibodies in this disease but also removes infected erythrocytes. Splenic macrophages and dendritic cells trigger a Th1 response involving both NK cells and γ/δ T cells. They also generate NO. The absence of NO in splenectomized animals permits the disease to reappear.

Leishmaniasis The importance of immunity in determining the course and nature of a protozoan disease is best seen in canine leishmaniasis. Canine leishmaniasis is caused by *Leishmania infantum* or its New World synonym *Leishmania chagasi* and transmitted by biting sandflies. When the promastigote forms of this parasite are injected by a sandfly into the skin of dogs, they are rapidly phagocytosed by neutrophils. When the neutrophils undergo apoptosis, the parasites are released and then engulfed by macrophages and dendritic cells in which the organisms differentiate into amastigotes. *Leishmania* amastigotes are obligate intracellular parasites. They divide within the macrophages until the cells rupture, and the released organisms are then phagocytosed by neighboring cells. Depending on the degree of host immunity, the parasites may be restricted to the skin (cutaneous disease); alternatively, infected dendritic cells may migrate to lymph nodes or enter the circulation and lodge in the internal organs, leading to disseminated visceral disease. Although infection is widespread in endemic areas, most dogs are resistant to *Leishmania,* and only 10% to 15% develop visceral disease.

Macrophages are the main host cells for *Leishmania* and the effector cells for parasite killing. Parasites divide within the phagolysosomes of infected macrophages. Their resistance to intracellular destruction is a result of multiple mechanisms. (One study of 245 macrophage genes showed that 37% were suppressed by *Leishmania* infection). *Leishmania* lipophosphoglycan delays phagosome maturation, preventing the production of NO and inhibiting macrophage responses to cytokines. The parasite also reduces the antigen-presenting ability of macrophages by suppressing major histocompatibility complex (MHC) class II expression. As a result of their persistence, the parasites trigger chronic inflammation. Initially characterized by granulocyte invasion, this is followed by macrophages, lymphocytes, and NK cells that collectively form granulomas.

The clinical signs of leishmaniasis are directly linked to the immune response of the infected dog. In susceptible animals, the organisms may spread from the skin to the local lymph node, spleen, and bone marrow within a few hours. In resistant dogs, the parasites remain restricted to the skin and draining lymph node and either remain healthy or develop a mild, self-limited disease. These resistant dogs mount a weak antibody response but a strong and effective Th1 response. They may have low antibody titers, but they produce IFN-γ in response to parasite antigens, generate type I granulomas, mount strong delayed hypersensitivity responses, and eventually destroy the parasites. Resistance to *Leishmania* has a strong genetic component; for example, Ibizian hounds appear to be resistant to this parasite. There is also an association between resistance and certain MHC class II alleles as well as some Slc11a1 (Nramp) alleles in dogs (see Box 6-1).

Susceptible dogs, in contrast, mount a Th2 response characterized by high antibody levels but poor cell-mediated immunity. These differences have been attributed to the activities of IL-10–producing regulatory T cells. In addition, the parasite may actively suppress transcription of the *IL-12* gene, ensuring that a Th2 response predominates. Chronic, progressive disease develops in susceptible dogs. Parasite-laden macrophages accumulate, but the organism continues to multiply. These macrophages spread throughout the body, resulting in disseminated infection. Dogs develop severe generalized nodular dermatitis, granulomatous lymphadenitis, splenomegaly, and hepatomegaly. They show polyclonal (occasionally monoclonal) B cell activation involving all four IgG classes, as well as hypergammaglobulinemia, and they develop lesions associated with type II and type III hypersensitivity. Thus excessive immunoglobulin production can lead to development of an immune-mediated hemolytic anemia, thrombocytopenia, and the production of antinuclear antibodies. Glomerulonephritis, uveitis, and synovitis may result from chronic immune complex deposition, leading to renal failure and death. Significantly elevated antihistone antibodies are a feature of dogs with *Leishmania*-associated glomerulonephritis. There is a positive correlation between the levels of these antihistone antibodies and the urine protein-to-creatinine ratio since these antibodies increase the probability of developing glomerulonephritis.

Evasion of the Immune Response

Despite their antigenicity, parasitic protozoa survive within their host by using multiple evasion mechanisms acquired over many millions of years of evolution. For example, *T. gondii* can avoid neutrophil attachment and phagocytosis. *T. parva* invades and destroys T cells. Other protozoa such as the trypanosomes may promote the development of suppressive regulatory cells or stimulate the B cell system to exhaustion. *Plasmodium falciparum* can suppress the ability of dendritic cells to process antigen.

Parasite-induced immunosuppression may promote parasite survival. For example, *Babesia bovis* is immunosuppressive for cattle. As a result, its host vector, the tick *Boophilus microplus*, is better able to survive on infected animals. Infected cattle have more ticks than noninfected animals, and the efficiency of transmission of *B. bovis* is enhanced. It must be pointed out, however, that parasite-induced immunosuppression may kill the host as a result of secondary infection, so it is not always beneficial to the parasite. Death in bovine trypanosomiasis is commonly due to bacterial pneumonia or sepsis following immunosuppression.

In addition to immunosuppression, protozoa have evolved two other effective evasive techniques. One involves becoming less antigenic, and the other involves the ability to alter surface antigens rapidly and repeatedly. An example of a nonantigenic organism is the bradyzoite stage of *T. gondii*, which, as mentioned previously, does not appear to stimulate a host response. Some protozoa may mask themselves with host antigens. Examples of these include *Trypanosoma theileri* in cattle and *Trypanosoma lewisi* in rats, both nonpathogenic trypanosomes that survive in the bloodstream because they are covered by host serum proteins and are not regarded as foreign. *T. brucei*, a pathogenic trypanosome of cattle, may also adsorb host serum proteins or soluble red cell antigens, reducing its antigenicity.

Although reduced antigenicity may be considered the ultimate evasive technique, many protozoa, especially the trypanosomes, successfully employ repeated antigenic variation. If cattle are infected with the pathogenic trypanosomes *T. vivax*, *T. congolense*, or *T. brucei* and their parasitemia measured at regular intervals, the numbers of circulating organisms are found to fluctuate greatly. Periods of high parasitemia alternate regularly with periods of low or undetectable parasitemia (Figure 27-4). Serum from infected animals contains antibodies against trypanosomes isolated before bleeding but not against those that develop subsequently. Each period of high parasitemia corresponds to the expansion of a population of trypanosomes with a new surface glycoprotein antigen. The

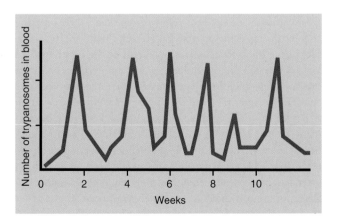

FIGURE 27-4 The time course of *Trypanosoma congolense* parasitemia in an infected calf. Each parasitemic peak represents the development of a new, antigenically original population of organisms.

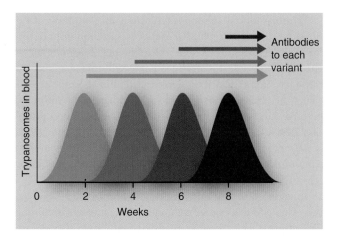

FIGURE 27-5 A schematic diagram showing how repeated antigenic variation accounts for the cyclical parasitemia observed in African trypanosomiasis. Each peak represents the growth of a new antigenic variant.

elimination of this population by antibodies leads to a rapid fall in parasitemia. Among the survivors, however, some parasites express new surface glycoproteins and grow without hindrance. As a result, a fresh population arises to produce yet another period of high parasitemia (Figure 27-5). This cyclical fluctuation in parasite levels, with each peak reflecting the appearance of a new population with new surface glycoproteins, can continue for many months.

The major surface antigens of these trypanosomes are known as variant surface glycoproteins (VSGs). These are the antigens targeted by host antibodies. The VSGs produced early in trypanosome infections tend to develop in a predictable sequence. However, as the infection progresses, the production of VSGs becomes more random. The VSGs form a thick coat on the surface of the trypanosome. When antigenic change occurs, the VSGs in the old coat are shed and replaced by an antigenically different VSG. Analysis indicates that these trypanosomes possess about 200 *VSG* genes, with an additional 1600 silent genes, of which two thirds are pseudogenes. Antigenic variation occurs as a result of repeated DNA breaking and repair, replacing an active *VSG* gene with one from the silent gene pool. Since only a small part of the tightly packed VSG is exposed to host antibodies, it is not even necessary for the complete molecule to change. Replacement of exposed epitopes by gene conversion is sufficient for effective variation (Chapter 17). Early in infections, complete *VSG* gene replacement occurs. Later on, partial replacement and point mutations can create new antigenic specificities. In some cases, the expressed *VSG* gene can be constructed as a mosaic from several archival pseudogenes. The potential for recombination-based variation is therefore absolutely enormous.

Trypanosomiasis is not the only protozoan infection in which variation of surface antigens occurs. It has also been recorded in infections by *B. bovis,* the plasmodia, and the intestinal parasite *Giardia lamblia.*

Since parasitic protozoa must evade the immune responses, it is not surprising that they preferentially invade immunosuppressed individuals. Organisms that are normally controlled by the immune response, such as *T. gondii* or *Cryptosporidium bovis,* can grow and produce severe disease in immunosuppressed animals. For this reason, acute toxoplasmosis and cryptosporidiosis commonly occur in humans immunosuppressed for transplantation purposes or for cancer therapy and in those infected with human immunodeficiency virus (HIV).

Adverse Consequences

The immune responses against protozoa may cause hypersensitivity reactions that contribute to disease. Type I hypersensitivity is a feature of trichomoniasis and results in local irritation and inflammation in the genital tract. Type II cytotoxic reactions are of significance in babesiosis and trypanosomiasis, in which they contribute to the anemia. In babesiosis, red cells express parasite antigens on their surfaces and are thus recognized as foreign and eliminated by hemolysis and phagocytosis. In trypanosomiasis, either fragments of disrupted organisms or possibly preformed immune complexes bind to red cells and provoke their elimination, causing anemia. Immune complex formation on circulating red cells is not the only problem of this type in trypanosomiasis. In some cases, excessive immune complex formation can lead to vasculitis and glomerulonephritis (type III hypersensitivity; see Chapter 30). Immune complex lesions are a marked feature of visceral leishmaniasis, as described previously.

Trypanosome infections may trigger an enormous increase in IgM-secreting cells so that very high levels of IgM are found in the blood of infected animals. Some of these antibodies are directed against autoantigens. These include rheumatoid factor–like molecules, and antibodies against thymocytes, single-stranded DNA, red cells, and platelets. In *T. congolense*–infected cattle, these polyclonally stimulated B cells are BoCD5+. As pointed out earlier, CD5+ B1 cells are of a different lineage to conventional B2 cells (Chapter 15). The mechanism of this polyclonal B cell activation is unknown.

It is probable that a type IV hypersensitivity reaction contributes to the inflammation that occurs when *Toxoplasma* cysts break down and release fresh tachyzoites. Extracts of *T. gondii* (toxoplasmin), if administered intradermally to infected animals, will cause a delayed hypersensitivity response (Figure 27-6).

Vaccination

Successful vaccination against protozoan infections of domestic animals is currently limited to coccidiosis, babesiosis, leishmaniasis, giardiasis, and theileriosis.

Several live coccidial vaccines are given to poultry. These vaccines typically contain multiple species and strains of coccidia. Some consist of virulent, drug-sensitive organisms administered repeatedly in very low doses (trickle infection). Other vaccine strains have been attenuated by repeated passaging through eggs, or they have been selected for precocity.

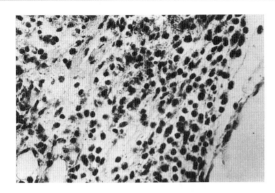

FIGURE 27-6 The characteristic mononuclear cell infiltration of a delayed hypersensitivity reaction in the skin of a mouse following an intradermal injection of an extract of *Toxoplasma gondii* (toxoplasmin).

(Courtesy Dr. C.H. Lai.)

Precocious strains mature very rapidly and, as a result, have less time to replicate and are thus less virulent. All of these vaccines provide solid immunity to coccidia when applied carefully under good rearing conditions. Nevertheless, the dose of coccidia vaccine must be carefully controlled, and the vaccines must be harvested from the feces of infected birds. Vaccinated birds shed oocysts that are transmitted to other birds in a flock. Because of regional strain variation, vaccination with a specific suspension of live oocysts may not be effective in protecting against field strains in all locations.

A commercial vaccine is available to protect dogs and cats against *Giardia duodenalis*. The vaccine contains disrupted cultured *Giardia* trophozoite extracts administered subcutaneously and protects experimentally challenged dogs and cats against infection and clinical disease.

Effective vaccines are available against leishmaniasis. The most effective consist of purified *Leishmania* fractions. These include a glycoprotein-enriched fraction also called the fucose-mannose ligand. Not only does this vaccine prevent the development of the disease, but it may also serve as an immunotherapeutic agent, producing clinical improvement in dogs with disseminated disease. An alternative vaccine containing excretory and secretory products of *L. infantum* promastigotes with a muramyl dipeptide adjuvant also appears to work well. Experimental vaccines, including killed vaccines and DNA vaccines, have shown encouraging results.

Babesia vaccines consist of tick-borne organisms that parasitize red cells and cause anemia. Many factors contribute to the resistance of animals against babesiosis, including genetic factors (Zebu cattle are more resistant to disease than European cattle) and age (cattle show a significant resistance to babesiosis in the first 6 months of life). Animals that recover from acute babesiosis are resistant to further clinical disease. It is therefore possible to infect young calves when they are still relatively insusceptible to disease, so that they become resistant to reinfection. The organisms employed for this procedure are first attenuated by repeated passage through splenectomized calves and then administered to recipient animals in whole blood. As might be anticipated, the side effects of this type of controlled infection may be severe, and chemotherapy may be required to control them. The transfer of blood from one calf to another may also trigger the production of antibodies against the foreign red cells. These antibodies complicate any attempts at blood transfusion in later life and may provoke hemolytic disease of the newborn (Chapter 29). In a slightly different approach, cattle can be made resistant to East Coast fever (*T. parva* infection) by infecting them with virulent sporozoites and treating them simultaneously with tetracycline.

Since a primary infection with *T. gondii* will confer strong protective immunity on an animal, protective immunization is a real possibility. A live *Toxoplasma* vaccine containing the S48 incomplete strain has been used successfully for the control of toxoplasmosis in sheep. The strain was developed by prolonged passage in laboratory mice and has lost the ability to develop bradyzoites or to initiate the sexual stages of the life cycle in cats. It produces protection against a severe challenge for at least 18 months. Unfortunately, the vaccine has a shelf life of only 7 to 10 days and can infect people.

Immunity to Helminths

Helminths, like protozoa, have adapted to a parasitic existence and so, of necessity, must have evolved to overcome or evade the immune responses. Parasitic helminths are therefore not maladapted pathogens but rather are fully adapted obligate parasites whose very survival depends on reaching some form of accommodation with the host. Helminths do not replicate within a host; unlike protozoa, the number of helminths present in an individual will be no more than the number that has gained access to the host. Consequently, they usually cause only mild or subclinical disease. As a rule, they cause morbidity but not mortality. Only when helminths invade a host to which they are not fully adapted or in unusually large numbers does acute lethal disease occur. Indeed, one consistent feature of intestinal nematode infestations is the very wide variation in parasite load within an animal population. Most animals harbor a few worms, but a few animals harbor a lot of worms. The size of the parasite burden in a host is controlled by genetic factors and by the host's response to these parasites. Some animals may be predisposed to a heavy infection as a result of genetic, behavioral, nutritional, or environmental factors.

Innate Immunity

Innate factors that influence helminth infestations include not only host-derived effects but also the influence of other parasites within the same host. The presence of adult worms in the intestine may delay the further development of larval stages of the same species within tissues. For example, calves infected with *Cysticercus bovis* show increased resistance to further infestation by this parasite. Similarly, lambs can acquire resistance to *Echinococcus granulosus* so that multiple dosing with large numbers of ova does not result in the development of massive worm burdens. The original dose of ova may stimulate rejection of subsequent doses. Interspecies competition among helminths for mutual habitats and nutrients in the intestinal tract will also influence the numbers, location, and composition of an animal's helminth population.

Innate factors of host origin that influence helminth burdens include the age, sex, and most important, the genetic background of the host. The influence of age and sex on helminth burdens appears to be largely hormonal. In animals whose sexual cycle is seasonal, parasites tend to synchronize their reproductive cycle with that of their hosts. For instance, ewes show a "spring rise" in fecal nematode ova, which coincides with lambing and the onset of lactation. Similarly, the development of helminth larvae in cattle in early winter tends to be inhibited until spring in a phenomenon called hypobiosis. The larvae of *Toxocara canis* may migrate from an infected bitch to the liver of the fetal puppy, resulting in a congenital infection. Once born, the infected pups can reinfect their mother by the more conventional fecal-oral route.

An example of genetically mediated resistance to helminths is seen in the superior resistance of sheep with hemoglobin A to *Haemonchus contortus* and *Teladorsagia circumcincta* compared with sheep with hemoglobin B. The reasons for this are unclear, but sheep with HbA mount a more effective self-cure reaction and a better immune response to many other antigens as well. Another example is the enhanced resistance to *Cooperia oncophora* seen in Zebu cattle compared with European cattle. In many cases, resistance to parasites is MHC linked. Thus cattle possessing BoLA-Aw7 and A36 tend to have low fecal egg counts, whereas animals with Aw3 tend to have high fecal egg counts. Some BoLA haplotypes may also be associated with high antibody levels against *Ostertagia*. The SLA complex has been defined in miniature swine, and its effects on parasite immunity have been assessed. In one study there was a 50% lower muscle larval burden in *Trichinella spiralis*–infected *cc* minipigs compared with pigs with the *dd* or *aa* haplotype. Minipigs carrying at least one copy of the *a* allele showed an enhanced ability to kill encysted muscle larvae—47% of pigs carrying the *a* allele responded to *Trichinella* compared with 8% of pigs that lacked this allele. The response was characterized by a predominance of lymphocytes and macrophages in the cellular reaction around each larva.

Chitinases are the enzymes that degrade chitin. Chitin is abundant in helminth cuticles and arthropod exoskeletons, and chitinases play a role in resistance to helminth and arthropod parasites. Chitinases are produced by mast cells, macrophages, and neutrophils. Some members of the mammalian chitinase family may lack enzyme activity. Nevertheless they may bind to helminth cuticles and serve as opsonins or chemoattractants.

Adaptive Immunity

Helminths present the immune system with a challenge. Most parasitic worms migrate through the tissues as larval forms and eventually reach the intestine or lungs, where they develop into adults. Clearly, the mechanisms that destroy these migrating larvae in the tissues must be very different from those that attack large adult worms in the intestine or airways. In general, larvae or adult worms within tissues are attacked by specialized inflammatory responses that tend to employ eosinophils as the attacking cells. Adult worms attached to mucosal surfaces are expelled by IgE and cytokine-mediated mechanisms. In the case of tissue larvae, the body seeks to destroy the invaders. In the case of mucosal adults, expulsion is the desired effect.

Humoral Immunity

Th2-mediated responses are the normal responses to parasitic helminths. Experimentally, mice that expel their parasites mount a predominantly Th2 response. Mice that cannot control their worm burden and become chronically infected mount a Th1 response.

Because nematodes trigger Th2 responses, IgE levels and eosinophil numbers are usually elevated in parasitized animals. Many helminth infestations are associated with the characteristic signs of type I hypersensitivity, including eosinophilia, edema, asthma, and urticarial dermatitis. For example, pigs infested with *Ascaris suum* show cutaneous allergic reactions to injected parasite antigens, as well as degranulation of intestinal mucosal mast cells. Lungworms such as *Metastrongylus* induce a strong IgE response. In addition, many helminth infections, such as oesophagostomiasis, ancylostomiasis, trichinosis, strongyloidiasis, taeniasis, and fascioliasis, are accompanied by a positive passive cutaneous anaphylaxis (PCA) reaction to worm antigens (Chapter 28). Th2 cytokines also have a direct effect on worm populations. For example, mice that cannot produce IL-4 or IL-13 are much more susceptible to *Trichuris muris* than normal mice. If IL-4 is neutralized by administration of specific antibodies or if IL-12 is administered, mice lose their ability to expel worms and become chronically infected. Likewise, if TNF-α is neutralized, the mice also lose their ability to expel the worms. On the other hand, neutralization of the Th1 cytokines IFN-γ or IL-18 enables chronically infected mice to expel their parasites rapidly. Whether an animal mounts a Th1 or Th2 response depends on the dendritic cells that process the antigen. This in turn appears to depend on the way in which antigen encounters dendritic cells and the set of TLRs activated by the antigen.

Immunity to Tissue Helminths

Migrating larvae and some adult worms such as schistosomes migrate through tissues where they can be attacked by inflammatory cells and molecules. Unlike bacteria or protozoa, however, larval worms have a thick cuticle that protects their vulnerable hypodermal plasma membrane. As larvae develop and undergo periodic molts, a damaged cuticle can be shed to be replaced with a new one. Likewise these cuticles cannot be penetrated by the terminal complement complex or by T cell perforins. If the immune system is to successfully combat these larvae, it must either employ cells that can destroy the intact cuticle or attack them through weak spots on their surface such as their digestive tract. Thus macrophages and eosinophils are the key destroyers of migrating larvae. Both possess FcγR (CD23) and can therefore bind to IgE-coated parasites and kill them. In cats infected with the filarial worm *Brugia pahangi*, those animals with high levels of parasite-specific IgE can kill adult worms. In contrast, cats that fail to mount a high IgE response permit adult filaria to survive. Macrophages that bind to helminth larvae through IgE become M1 cells with increased lysosomal enzymes, oxidant production, IL-1, leukotrienes, prostaglandins, and platelet-activating factor. These cells are capable of causing parasite destruction.

If the migrating worm cannot be killed, at least it can be walled off. One feature of these Th2-mediated responses to migrating larvae is the production of alternatively activated macrophages or M2 cells. M2 cells produce arginase. Arginase acts on its substrate arginine to produce ornithine that is further metabolized to proline, polyamines, and urea. Proline and the polyamines are substrates for collagen synthesis and can induce fibroblast proliferation. The type 2 granulomas that develop around tissue helminths such as schistosomes appear to be driven by arginase from M2 cells.

Mammals will eventually develop limited immunity to tissue helminths after several months. One parasite, *Ostertagia ostertagi*, is an exception. Cattle remain susceptible to reinfection by *Ostertagia* for many months, and immunity that can inhibit the production of viable larvae is not seen until an animal is more than 2 years old. It is not surprising that this is the most economically important bovine parasite.

Eosinophils and Parasite Destruction

Eosinophils are attracted to tissue helminths by chemoattractants released by degranulating mast cells (see Figure 28-17). Cytokines such as IL-5 from Th2 cells also mobilize bone marrow eosinophils, releasing large numbers of eosinophils into the circulation. Many chemokines such as the eotaxins (CCL11, CCL24, and CCL26) also attract eosinophils (Figure 27-7). Invading parasites may induce two waves of eosinophil migration. The first wave provoked by mast cell or parasite-derived products, the second by IL-5 and other cytokines from Th2 cells. Purified eosinophils exposed to *Strongyloides* antigens significantly increased their expression of CD69 and MHC class II molecules and became antigen-presenting cells. These antigen-presenting eosinophils are highly effective in initiating Th2 responses against worm antigens.

Eosinophils employ Fc receptors through which they can bind to antibody-coated parasites, degranulate, and release their granule contents directly onto the worm cuticle (Figure 27-8). These contents include oxidants, nitric oxide, and enzymes such as lysophospholipase and phospholipase D. Major basic protein, the crystalline core of the eosinophil specific granules can damage the cuticles of schistosomula, *Fasciola*, and *Trichinella*. Eosinophil cationic protein and eosinophil neurotoxin are ribonucleases that are lethal for helminths. It is important to point out, however, that eosinophils may not be effective against all parasites. Some larval parasites may evade destruction. For example, larvae of *Toxocara canis*, exposed to eosinophils simply shed their outer coat together with the attached cells. Eosinophil granules released from cells

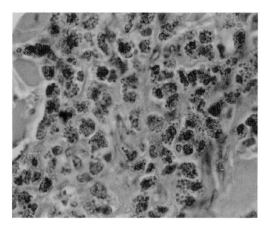

FIGURE 27-7 Photomicrograph of a lesion in horse skin caused by allergy to migrating parasitic helminth larvae. The granular cells are eosinophils, and their presence indicates the occurrence of a type I hypersensitivity reaction.

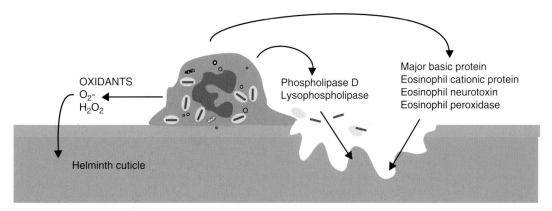

FIGURE 27-8 Some of the molecules released from eosinophils that cause damage to the cuticle of parasitic helminths.

can function within tissues. These free granules express membrane receptors for IFN-γ, and for the chemokine eotaxin. These receptors are functional and stimulate the granules to secrete their contents. Thus eosinophil granules function autonomously to contribute to the tissue changes mediated by these cells.

There has long been a debate over the precise roles of eosinophils in nematode immunity. For example, both *Teladorsagia circumcincta* and *Haemonchus contortus*, two major parasitic nematodes, produce chemoattractants for eosinophils, whereas the free-living nematode *Caenorhabditis elegans* does not. This suggests that some nematodes actively encourage eosinophil recruitment. Perhaps local tissue damage caused by eosinophils provides a suitable microenvironment for parasite invasion. Many nematodes are damaged or killed by eosinophil toxic products, supporting the idea that eosinophils serve a protective function, but when *Trichinella spiralis* survival was studied in mice lacking eosinophils, it was found that the *T. spiralis* larvae in the muscles of these mice died in much larger numbers compared with wild-type mice. The larval death correlated with increased IFN-γ and decreased IL-4 production. In this case, at least, eosinophils may provide an environment that promotes parasite survival rather than destruction.

Although the IgE-dependent eosinophil-mediated response is probably the most significant mechanism of resistance to larval helminths, other immunoglobulins may also play a protective role. The mechanisms involved include antibody-mediated neutralization of larval proteases, blocking of the anal and oral pores of larvae by immune complexes (Figure 27-9) and prevention of molting and inhibition of larval development by antibodies directed against exsheathing antigens. Antibodies to the enzyme glutathione S-transferase protect against *Fasciola hepatica* in sheep. Other enzymes may be blocked by antibodies acting against adult worms, stopping egg

production, or interfering with worm development (Figure 27-10). Thus female *Ostertagia ostertagi* worms fail to develop vulvar flaps when grown in immune calves. Similarly, spicule morphology may be altered in *Cooperia* males from immune hosts.

Immunity to Adult Helminths

Adult parasitic worms in the intestine or respiratory tract attach to the mucosa only by their mouth. They are however bathed in a complex mixture of enzymes, IgA, and mucus, whereas their feeding end and alimentary tract encounter effector cells, cytokines, antibodies, and complement. γ/δ T cells in the intestinal epithelium may be activated by the presence of intestinal worms without the necessity of conventional antigen processing. On first contact with nematodes, these intraepithelial γ/δ T cells produce IL-4 and IL-25. These cytokines activate Th2 cells to produce IL-4 and IL-13. These cytokines in turn stimulate mucus production by goblet cells and the production of IgE.

IgE plays a key role in controlling adult worm burdens on mucosal surfaces. This is seen in the self-cure reaction in sheep infected with gastrointestinal nematodes, particularly *H. contortus*. While embedded in the intestinal and abomasal mucosa, these worms secrete multiple proteins (Figure 27-11). Some

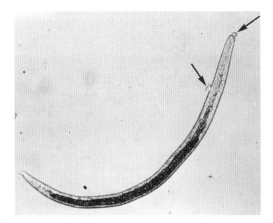

FIGURE 27-9 A *Toxocara canis* larva after incubation in specific antiserum. Serum antibodies bind and precipitate antigens in the saliva and excretions of this larva. This precipitate may block these pores and kill the larva. The immune precipitates at the oral and excretory pores are indicated by *arrows*.

(Courtesy Dr. D.H. DeSavigny.)

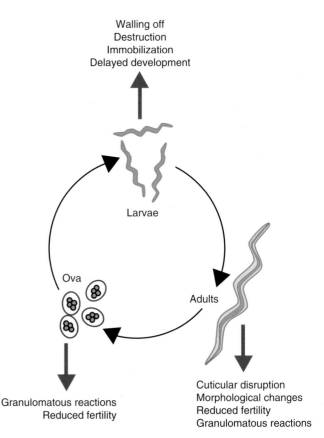

FIGURE 27-10 Some effects of the immune responses on the stages of helminth development.

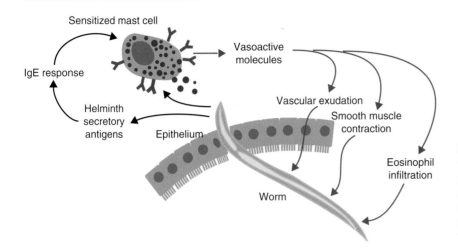

FIGURE 27-11 The mechanisms involved in the self-cure reaction against intestinal helminths. In essence, the animal mounts an allergic response to the salivary antigens of attached nematodes. This acute inflammatory response causes the worms to detach from the intestinal wall and pass out in the feces.

serve as damage-associated molecular patterns (DAMPs) and promote innate responses, whereas others are effective antigens and trigger Th2 responses with high IgE levels. The IgE binds to mast cell receptors (Chapter 28). The combination of helminth antigens with mast cell–bound IgE triggers mast cell degranulation and the release of vasoactive molecules, cytokines such as IL-13 and IL-33, and proteases. These molecules stimulate vigorous smooth muscle contraction and increase vascular permeability. The Th2 cytokine IL-13 promotes parasite expulsion by stimulating epithelial cell proliferation. Presumably the rapid epithelial cell turnover acts as an "epithelial elevator" to assist in expelling the parasites. IL-33 also induces the expulsion of adult worms. Expulsion of worms is accompanied by mucosal mast cell infiltration, intestinal eosinophilia, elevated serum IgE, and elevated parasite-specific IgG1 levels.

The violent contractions of the intestinal muscles and the increase in the permeability of intestinal capillaries, leading to an efflux of fluid into the intestinal lumen (a leaky gut), can result in dislodgment and expulsion of many worms. In sheep that have just undergone self-cure, IgE antibody levels are high, and experimental administration of helminth antigens will result in acute anaphylaxis, confirming the role of type I hypersensitivity in this phenomenon. A similar reaction is seen in fascioliasis in calves, in which peak PCA antibody titers coincide with expulsion of the parasite.

Variations Among Worms Tissue helminths may be thought of as xenografts. That is, grafts between individuals of two different species. The intensity of the graft rejection process can vary between different hosts and between different worms. Inbred mouse strains differ in their ability to expel intestinal nematodes such as *T. muris*. Since inbred mice are genetically homogeneous, these variations in resistance to *T. muris* must be due to differences among the worms. Is it possible that some individual worms can trigger DC1 responses, whereas others trigger DC2 responses? We know that strains of these parasites differ in their ability to trigger Th1 and Th2 responses. This may be due to manipulation of the immune response by each

worm. For example, *T. muris* can produce a molecule related to IFN-γ that suppresses Th2 responses and so enhances worm survival. Alternatively, these differences may be due to parasite dose. Thus low-level infestations of *T. muris* provoke a Th1 response, and the parasites persist. If higher doses of parasites are administered, mice mount Th2 responses and expel the parasites. Therefore a threshold of infection is likely critical for the development of resistance.

Cell-Mediated Immunity

As pointed out previously, worm antigens preferentially stimulate Th2 responses, and Th1 responses may be of little protective benefit. Nevertheless, cytotoxic T cells may attack helminths that are deeply embedded in the intestinal mucosa or undergoing tissue migration. Cell-mediated immune reactions have been shown to occur in *Trichinella spiralis* and *Trichostrongylus colubriformis* infections. In the former, immunity can be transferred to normal animals by lymphoid cells, and infected animals show delayed hypersensitivity reactions to worm antigens. In vitro tests for cell-mediated immunity such as cytokine production and lymphocyte proliferation are also positive in these infections. In the case of *T. colubriformis*, immunity can be transferred to normal animals from immune ones by both cells and serum, and the site of worm attachment is subjected to a massive lymphocyte infiltration (see Box 27-1). Lymphocytes from sheep infected with *H. contortus* will release cytokines and divide in response to worm antigen, and it has been shown that immunity to this organism can be adoptively transferred to syngeneic sheep by lymphocytes.

Live cysts of the tapeworm *Taenia solium* trigger a Th2 response and thus IgE production. However, after the cysts die, they stimulate a Th1 response and granuloma formation. Biopsies show IL-12, IL-2, and IFN-γ associated with granulomas surrounding dying tapeworm cysts. It may be that the Th1 response occurs only when the parasite can no longer modulate the host's immune response.

Sensitized T cells attack helminths by two mechanisms. First, the development of delayed hypersensitivity attracts

□ Box 27-1 | **Specialized Antihelminth Cells**

Type II immunity encompasses the antibody-mediated responses required for protection against helminths. This type of response is normally mediated by Th2 cells secreting three major cytokines: IL-4, IL-5, and IL-13. The sources of these three cytokines were investigated in mice experimentally infected with the nematode *Nippostrongylus brasiliensis,* and the investigators found that the IL-13 did not come from Th2 cells but rather from a new population of mononuclear cells called nuocytes. Nuocytes expand in response to the type II–inducing cytokines IL-25 and IL-33. Nuocytes are found in the spleen, mesenteric lymph nodes, and bone marrow of naïve mice, where they constitute less than 0.2% of the cells. They show none of the characteristic markers found in other leukocytes but are MHC class II positive. It remains to be seen whether they truly represent a new leukocyte population.

Neill DR, Wong SH, Bellosi A, et al: Nuocytes represent a new innate effector leukocyte that mediates type-2 immunity, *Nature* 464:1367–1370, 2010.

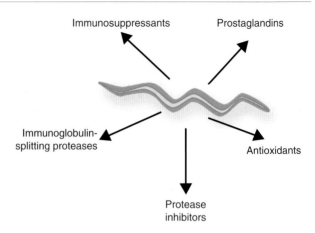

FIGURE 27-12 Some methods by which migrating helminth larvae evade host defenses.

mononuclear cells to the site of larval invasion and renders the local environment unsuitable for growth or migration. Second, cytotoxic lymphocytes may cause larval destruction. Thus treatment of experimental animals with bacille Calmette-Guérin (BCG) vaccine, a treatment that stimulates T cells (Chapter 39), inhibits the metastases of hydatid cysts (*Echinococcus granulosus*). In these treated animals, the space that surrounds the cysts may be filled with large lymphocytes. It is also common to observe large lymphocytes adhering firmly to migrating nematode larvae in vivo.

In tapeworm infestations in which the parasite cyst (metacestode) grows within the host, the parasite must obtain protein for nourishment. However, the cysticerci of *Taenia ovis* actually grow larger in the presence of immune serum than nonimmune serum. The parasites possess Fc receptors, and it is possible that host immunoglobulins may feed the parasite. Since cyst fluid contains lymphocyte mitogens, it has also been suggested that these might stimulate immunoglobulin production that can then be used by the parasite.

The complexity of resistance to helminths is well demonstrated in sheep bred for resistance to *H. contortus.* Compared with susceptible sheep, there are differences in B cell function; resistant sheep have significantly more IgA- and IgG1-containing cells. There is also evidence for differences in T cell function because resistant sheep respond better to a T-dependent antigen such as ovalbumin, and treatment of resistant lambs with a monoclonal antibody to CD4 completely blocks their resistance to *H. contortus.* Mucosal mast cell numbers and tissue eosinophilia are also reduced in these treated sheep. In contrast, depletion of CD8+ cells has no effect on resistance. In general, resistant sheep have higher eosinophil numbers, and curiously, these resistant sheep are calmer than susceptible sheep!

Evasion of the Immune Response

Although there are multiple mechanisms whereby animals resist helminth infection, it is obvious, even to a casual observer, that these defenses are not very effective. Successfully adapted parasitic helminths can survive and function in the presence of a fully functional host immune system. In general, helminths are most vulnerable to immunological attack while migrating through tissues. Thus most evasive strategies work at the larval stage. Given the great diversity of helminth species and reproductive strategies, it is reasonable to point out that they employ a very great diversity of immunoevasive strategies as well.

Evasion of Innate Responses

Brugia malayi secretes serpins that inhibit neutrophil serine proteases. *E. granulosus* secretes an elastase inhibitor that blocks neutrophil attraction by C5a or platelet-activating factor (PAF). Many helminths express surface antioxidants such as superoxide dismutase, glutathione peroxidase, and glutathione S-transferase, which can neutralize the host's respiratory burst and protect their surfaces from oxidation (Figure 27-12). A secreted antioxidant from *F. hepatica* called peroxiredoxin causes alternative activation of bovine macrophages resulting in high arginase activity, low nitric oxide, low IFN-γ, and high IL-10 production. This, plus elevated IL-4, IL-5 and IL-13 production, promotes Th2 responses.

Many parasites interfere with the complement system. For example, schistosomes can neutralize the alternative complement pathway by inserting decay accelerating factor (CD55) from their host into their outer lipid bilayer. Tapeworms can secrete sulfated proteoglycans, which activate complement in the tissue fluid. Calreticulin is a molecule that can bind and block the activities of C1q. Parasites such as *Necator americanus* and *H. contortus* secrete calreticulin homologs that also bind C1q and block its activities.

Evasion of Acquired Responses

Helminths become progressively less antigenic as they evolve in the presence of a functioning immune system. Presumably, natural selection favors the survival of parasites with reduced antigenicity. *H. contortus* is much less antigenic in sheep, its natural host, than in rabbits, which it does not normally infect. Sheep therefore respond to fewer *H. contortus* antigens than do rabbits.

Helminths living within tissues may reduce their antigenicity by adsorbing host antigens onto their surface and masking parasite antigens. This occurs in *T. solium* infestations in swine, in which the parasites are coated with IgG. It is probable that the worm has an Fc receptor. Cysticerci can also adsorb MHC molecules to their surface.

Another mechanism of immune evasion is the use of sequential antigenic variation. Although helminths have not evolved a system as complex as that seen in trypanosomiasis, gradual antigenic variation is recognized. The cuticular antigens of *T. spiralis* larvae change after each molt. Even during their growth phase, these larvae change the expression of surface antigens. Some parasites such as *Fasciola hepatica* shed their glycocalyx and hence their surface antigens when exposed to antibodies.

Some parasites interfere with antigen processing. Macrophages from schistosome-infested animals are incompetent antigen-presenting cells. Filarial worms secrete inhibitors that block macrophage proteases. *Taenia taeniaeformis* secretes taeniastatin, a protease inhibitor that inhibits neutrophil chemotaxis, complement activation, T cell proliferation, and IL-2 production.

Immunosuppression is a consistent feature of parasitized animals. This may be due to the production of immunosuppressive molecules or to redirection of immune responses toward Treg cell production and tolerance. *F. hepatica* secretes proteases that destroy immunoglobulins. These proteases can generate Fab fragments that can bind and mask parasite antigens. In addition, *F. hepatica* tegumental protein suppresses production of IFN-γ and IL-12 by acting directly on dendritic cells and possibly suppressing signaling by NF-κB.

Many helminths suppress host immunity by promoting the production of Treg cells and IL-10-secreting B cells. These suppressive effects may also reduce Th17-mediated inflammation. Because *F. hepatica* infestation is such a strong inducer of Th2 responses, it can adversely affect an animal's ability to mount Th1 responses and interfere with diagnostic tests such as the whole blood IFN-γ assay used in the diagnosis of bovine tuberculosis. Sheep infected with *H. contortus* may become specifically suppressed so that they are unreactive to *H. contortus*, even though they remain responsive to unrelated parasites. *Ostertagia ostertagi* and *Trichostrongylus axei* infestations depress calf lymphocyte responses to mitogens. *Oesophagostomum radiatum* secretes molecules that inhibit the responses of lymphocytes to antigens and mitogens. In other helminth infections, such as trichinosis, infected animals are nonspecifically immunosuppressed. This immunosuppression is reflected in a lowered resistance to other infections, a poor response to vaccines, and prolongation of skin graft survival.

Vaccination

It is not surprising, considering the poor host response to parasitic worms and the availability of cheap and effective anthelmintics, that antihelminth vaccines are not widely available. Nevertheless, the emergence of anthelmintic resistance and environmental concerns raised by excessive chemical use have resulted in an increased interest in antiparasite vaccines. Vaccine use is predicated on the assumption that a host's immune response can control or prevent an infestation. This is not always obvious in helminth infestations, and traditional vaccines may be of little use. Despite this, a recombinant *T. ovis* vaccine has been produced that can induce protective immunity in sheep. This vaccine contains a cloned oncosphere antigen (To45W) with a saponin-based adjuvant. It stimulates a response that prevents parasite penetration of the intestinal wall. The vaccine provides protective immunity for at least 12 months, and up to 98% of naturally challenged lambs are protected. Similar single-antigen recombinant vaccines have been shown to be highly effective against *E. granulosus* in sheep.

Effective protection against some helminths has also been obtained by the use of live irradiated organisms. The most important of these is the vaccine used to protect calves against pneumonia caused by the lungworm *Dictyocaulus viviparus*. In this vaccine, second-stage larvae hatched from ova in culture are exposed to 40,000 R X-irradiation, and two doses of these larvae are then fed to calves. The larvae can penetrate the calf's intestine, but since they are unable to develop to the third stage, they never reach the lung and are thus nonpathogenic. During their exsheathing process, the larvae stimulate the production of antibodies that can block reinfection. The efficiency of this vaccine depends very much on timing and on the size of the challenge dose since even vaccinated calves may show mild pneumonic signs if placed on grossly infected pastures.

The major helminth antigens are of two types, soluble excretory-secretory products and antigens bound to the parasite surface (somatic antigens). Important secretory products include periredoxin, annexins, galectins, heat shock proteins, HMGB homologs, and S100 homologs. The immunodominant antigens of nematodes are polyprotein allergens and antigens that act as lipid-binding proteins. Another important somatic antigen is the enzyme γ-glutamyl transpeptidase. Some somatic antigens, such as those in the parasite gut, are hidden since they are not normally exposed to the host's immune response and may therefore be potential candidates for vaccines. For example, experimental vaccination of lambs and kids against the intestinal aminopeptidase of *H. contortus* (called H11) has resulted in significant drops in parasite numbers and fecundity.

Cattle mount protective responses against *Fasciola* infections. These are especially effective against single high doses but are less efficient against low-level trickle infections of the type likely to be encountered in the field. Animals may be protected against fascioliasis by the use of defined parasite antigens, such as fatty acid–binding protein, glutathione S-transferase, cathepsin L proteases, and liver fluke hemoglobin. Irradiated parasites may induce immunity, as may crude parasite extracts.

In general, the use of helminth vaccines has not been widely accepted. There is reluctance on the part of farmers to change established control procedures, especially when the major financial burden of these infestations is borne by others.

Immunity to Arthropods

When arthropods such as ticks or mosquitos bite an animal, they inject saliva. This saliva contains digestive enzymes that assist the parasite in obtaining its blood meal. The saliva also contains components designed to minimize host responses. For example, arthropod saliva contains kininases that destroy bradykinin, which mediates pain and itch, and histamine-binding proteins, which have a similar effect. Anticomplement proteins are found in the saliva of many different tick species. For example, the saliva of the tick *Ixodes scapularis* contains a protein that regulates the alternative complement pathway. It displaces properdin and enhances the degradation of C3bBb convertase. As a result, host scratching and grooming responses are minimized.

The saliva of the tick, *Ixodes ricinus*, impairs the maturation and antigen-presenting abilities of dendritic cells in culture. Administration of tick saliva to mice inhibits the migration of dendritic cells from inflamed skin to draining lymph nodes and decreases the ability of these dendritic cells to present antigen to T cells. Furthermore these treated dendritic cells failed to promote Th1 and Th17 responses while promoting Th2 responses. All these effects serve to promote the prolonged attachment and feeding of ticks.

Because some salivary proteins are antigenic, they would be expected to induce immune responses that impair a parasite's ability to feed. Ticks, however, have evolved immunosuppressive and anti-inflammatory countermeasures that permit them to feed more effectively. Tick saliva impairs macrophage function and suppresses T cell responses to mitogens, as well as production of IL-1β and the Th1 cytokines IFN-γ and IL-2. It suppresses NK cell activity and macrophage nitric oxide production. Saliva from the ticks *Dermacentor andersoni* and *I. ricinus* increases production of the Th2 cytokines IL-4 and IL-10. A tick saliva immunosuppressor binds specifically to T cell CD4 and blocks antigen-induced signaling and T cell responses. Saliva from *I. ricinus* also inhibits host B cell proliferation. A salivary protein from *I. scapularis* inhibits the proliferation of B cells exposed to the Osp proteins from the Lyme disease bacterium *Borrelia burgdorferi* but has no effect on T cells. It is abundantly clear that ticks have evolved many mechanisms to prevent immunological attack while they are feeding.

Host immune responses to injected arthropod saliva are of three types. Some salivary components are of low molecular weight and cannot function as normal antigens. They may, however, bind to skin proteins such as collagen and then act as haptens, stimulating Th1 responses. On subsequent exposure, these haptens induce a delayed hypersensitivity reaction. Other salivary antigens may bind to epidermal Langerhans cells and induce cutaneous basophil hypersensitivity, a Th1 response associated with the production of IgG antibodies and a basophil infiltration. If these basophils are destroyed by antibasophil serum, resistance to biting arthropods is reduced. The third type of response to arthropod saliva is a Th2 response, leading to IgE production and type I hypersensitivity. This response may induce severe local inflammation in the skin, leading to pain or pruritus. Each of these three types of response may modify the skin in such a way that the feeding of the offending arthropod is impaired and the animal becomes a less attractive source of food. Unfortunately, natural selection and evolution ensure that the biting arthropod is well able to withstand such responses. (These hypersensitivities are discussed further in Chapter 28.)

Demodectic Mange

The mange mite *Demodex folliculorum* is a normal symbiont commonly present in hair follicles and only occasionally causes disease. When demodectic mange does occur, the inflammatory reaction around mites and mite fragments contains mononuclear cells with a few plasma cells. The infiltrating lymphocytes tend to be CD8+ T cells. Type II granuloma formation may occasionally occur. The presence of cytotoxic T cells suggests that this is a type IV hypersensitivity reaction, perhaps a form of allergic contact dermatitis. The T cells may also be directed against mite antigens and reflect a defensive response by the host, whereas the absence of eosinophils and edema in the lesion suggests that type I hypersensitivity is relatively unimportant. It is of interest to note that immunosuppressive agents such as antilymphocyte serum, azathioprine, or prolonged steroid therapy predispose animals to the development of demodectic mange. Animals with generalized demodicosis have normal neutrophil function and respond normally to vaccines or other foreign proteins. Nevertheless their T cell response to mitogens such as phytohemagglutinin and concanavalin A is depressed. This is a progressive suppression, and it tends to increase in severe cases. If the T cells of dogs with demodicosis are washed free of serum, they regain their ability to respond to mitogens. Serum from these animals is also able to suppress the proliferation of T cells from normal animals.

Flea Bite Dermatitis

Biting fleas secrete saliva into the skin wound. Some of the components of flea saliva are of low molecular weight and act as haptens after binding to dermal collagen As a result, a local type IV hypersensitivity reaction characterized by a mononuclear cell infiltration occurs. In some sensitized animals, this type IV reaction is gradually replaced over a period of months by a type I reaction, and the mononuclear cell infiltration gradually changes to an eosinophil infiltration. (A similar series of events has been recorded in sarcoptic mange in pigs.) The immune response mounted by flea-allergic animals is protective. Thus fleas produce fewer eggs on flea-allergic cats than on flea-naïve cats. Flea-allergic cats also appear to remove more fleas by grooming than do flea-naïve animals. Experimental vaccines containing the major antigens from the cat flea midgut have been able to reduce flea populations on dogs, and the female fleas recovered from these immunized animals produced significantly fewer eggs. This suggests that vaccination may eventually be effective in controlling flea populations.

Likewise success has been achieved with a recombinant salivary gland protein vaccine to disrupt blood-feeding by horn flies (*Haematobia irritans*). It reduced blood meal size and delayed egg development in flies feeding on vaccinated animals.

Tick Infestation

It has been observed that ticks on nonimmune animals are larger than those on immune animals. Although the nature of this resistance is unclear, it has been suggested that local hypersensitivity reactions to tick saliva may restrict the blood flow to the tick, reduce its food supply, and stunt its growth. It is possible to immunize guinea pigs with tick homogenates and show that ticks feeding on these animals have reduced fecundity. Although vaccination against salivary antigens is unlikely to be very effective in conferring effective immunity against blood feeding arthropods, there is an alternative approach. Since many of the arthropods of veterinary importance take the blood of their host into their digestive tract, it follows that they will also take up immunoglobulins, complement components, and cells. This suggests that if an animal were immunized with internal antigens from the tick, this could cause local damage. These internal antigens have been called "hidden" or "concealed" antigens since under normal circumstances the host would not usually encounter them. Vaccines made against

antigens from the intestine of the tick *B. microplus* can inhibit tick reproduction. Indeed, a recombinant tick vaccine based on such a recombinant antigen, Bm86, is available in Australia and Central America. The antibodies produced bind to the brush border of tick intestinal cells, inhibit endocytosis, and prevent the tick from engorging fully. Thus the digestive processes are impaired, and the tick experiences starvation, loss of fecundity, and weakness and may disengage from its host. As a result, the number of ticks on vaccinated animals is reduced.

Hypoderma Infestation

Unlike the arthropods described previously, the larvae of the warble flies (*Hypoderma bovis* and *Hypoderma lineatum*) actually migrate through body tissues. These larvae are therefore in somewhat the same position as migrating helminth larvae—they must effectively survive or evade the host's xenograft response. In fact, the first instar larvae of these flies do not trigger significant inflammation and are also immunosuppressive. Hypodermin A, the protease secreted by these larvae, can inhibit responses to mitogens and reduce IL-2 production, probably by destroying cell surface receptors. Vaccination with a cloned *Hypoderma* protein has effectively protected cattle against subsequent infestations.

Immune defenses also play a role in preventing invasion by other skin-penetrating arthropods. Body strike results from infestation of sheep skin with the larvae of the fly *Lucilia cuprina*. Sheep can be bred for low and high resistance to body strike. The resistant sheep have greater numbers of IgE-positive B cells in their skin than do susceptible sheep. Resistant sheep also mount a greater inflammatory response and produce more fluid exudate when injected with larval excretory and secretory products. On the other hand, larval proteases inhibit complement activation and degrade immunoglobulins.

For sources of additional information, please visit http:// evolve.elsevier.com/tizard/immunology/

28

Type I Hypersensitivity

Key Points

- Type I hypersensitivities, also called immediate hypersensitivity, are mediated by immunoglobulin E (IgE) attached to mast cells.
- Disease is caused by the release of inflammatory molecules from mast cells following the binding of antigens to IgE.
- The clinical signs of allergic disease depend in large part on the route by which antigens (allergens) enter the body.
- Massive systemic release of inflammatory molecules by mast cells may give rise to allergic anaphylaxis. In this syndrome, animals may collapse and die rapidly as a result of the contraction of critical smooth muscles such as those lining the bronchi.
- Animals commonly suffer from allergies to foods, inhaled antigens, vaccines, or drugs.
- In many cases, especially in the dog, these allergies may manifest as intense pruritus.
- Treatment may include epinephrine for allergic anaphylaxis, corticosteroids for local inflammation, and desensitizing injections of allergen for prolonged control. The most satisfactory solution is to prevent exposure to the offending allergens.

Type I hypersensitivity reactions are a form of acute inflammation that results from the interaction of antigens with mast cell–bound IgE. This leads to the release of mast cell granule contents (Figure 28-1). The granule contents in turn cause acute inflammation. The benefits of this type of inflammation are unclear, but it is of major clinical significance in veterinary medicine (Box 28-1).

Induction of Type I Hypersensitivity

All animals are exposed to environmental antigens in food and inhaled air. Most normal animals respond to these antigens by producing IgG or IgA antibodies, and there is no obvious clinical consequence. Some animals, however, may respond to environmental antigens by mounting an exaggerated Th2 response and produce excessive amounts of IgE antibodies. It is these animals that develop type I hypersensitivity reactions or allergies. The excessive production of IgE is called atopy, and affected individuals are said to be atopic. The development of atopy and type I hypersensitivity depends on the interaction of genes and environmental factors. The genetics of atopy and allergy are complex. If both parents are atopic, most of their offspring will also be atopic and will suffer from allergies. If only one parent is atopic, the percentage of atopic offspring varies. There is also a breed predisposition to atopy in dogs. For example, atopic dermatitis is most commonly observed in Terriers (Bull, Welsh, Cairn, West Highland White, Scottish), Dalmatians, and Irish Setters, although nonpurebred dogs may

□ **Box 28-1 | Nomenclature**

IgE mediates immediate hypersensitivity reactions, so called because they develop within seconds or minutes after exposure to antigen. This type of hypersensitivity reaction is also commonly called an allergy. Antigens that stimulate allergies may be called allergens. If an immediate hypersensitivity reaction is systemic and life-threatening, it is called allergic anaphylaxis or anaphylactic shock. Sometimes an animal may have a reaction that is similar to allergic anaphylaxis but is not immunologically mediated. This type of reaction is described as anaphylactoid.

also be affected. The heritability of atopic dermatitis in Labrador and Golden Retrievers is estimated to be a relatively high 0.47. In horses, high levels of IgE are associated with certain ELA-DRB haplotypes.

Environmental factors such as childhood infections also influence the development of atopic diseases in humans. Children who have had multiple infections when young appear to be less likely to develop allergies than those not exposed to such infections. On the other hand, contact with allergens on the first day of life predisposes puppies to develop significantly higher IgE levels than puppies sensitized at 4 months of age. As discussed in Chapter 22, there is a growing belief that the development of the immune system, and especially a tendency to develop allergies, is regulated by the intestinal microflora. It is possible that the great increase in allergic disease observed

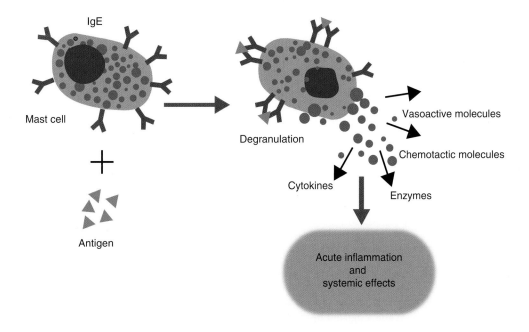

FIGURE 28-1 The mechanism of type I hypersensitivity reactions. Numerous biologically active molecules are released by mast cells and basophils when antigen cross-links two IgE molecules on the mast cell surface. Some are produced immediately. Others may be synthesized within minutes or hours.

in developed countries is influenced by changes in the micro-flora brought about by changes in diet or antibiotic use.

Normal animals infested by parasitic worms and insects also tend to produce large amounts of IgE. It is believed that the IgE response may have evolved specifically to counteract these organisms. Chitin, the biopolymer that confers structural rigidity to fungi, insects, and helminths, induces the accumulation of cells such as eosinophils and basophils in tissues and may be a key trigger of some of these allergic reactions. Indeed, the self-cure reaction seen in parasitized sheep has long been the only well-characterized beneficial feature of type I hypersensitivity. It is of interest to note that atopic and parasitized dogs may have reduced IgA levels, an observation supporting the concept that a deficiency of IgA may predispose to a compensatory increase in IgE production (Chapter 22).

Immunoglobulin E

IgE is an immunoglobulin of conventional four-chain structure and is about 200 kDa in size (see Figure 16-7). It is found in serum in exquisitely small quantities (9 to 700 μg/mL in dogs), and its half-life there is only 2 days. Most of the body's IgE is firmly bound to Fcε receptors on tissue mast cells, where it has a half-life of 11 to 12 days. Some IgG subclasses may also bind to mast cell receptors and mediate type I hypersensitivity reactions. For example, IgG4 is associated with atopic dermatitis in the dog. However, the affinity of these subclasses for mast cells is much lower than that of IgE, and they are of much less clinical significance.

Immunoglobulin E Production

Atopic individuals are predisposed to generate Th2 cells. The Th2 cells produce interleukin-4 (IL-4), IL-5, and IL-13. These cytokines, together with co-stimulation from CD40, trigger B cell IgE synthesis. IL-4 is also produced in significant amounts by stimulated mast cells. This mast cell–derived IL-4 may alter the helper cell balance and enhance yet more Th2 cell production and IL-4 release (Figure 28-2). Some allergic humans overexpress IL-4, leading to excessive Th2 cell activity and enhanced IgE production.

Immunoglobulin E Receptors

There are two types of IgE receptors: high-affinity FcεRI and low-affinity FcεRII (CD23). There are two forms of FcεRI. One form is found on mast cells, basophils, neutrophils, and eosinophils. This form consists of four chains, one α, one β, and two γ chains ($\alpha\beta\gamma_2$) (Figure 28-3). The α chain binds IgE, the β chain stabilizes the complex, and the γ chains serve as signal transducers. (This same γ chain is also a signal transducer in FcγRI, FcγRIII, and γ/δ TCR.) The affinity of FcεRI for IgE is very high (10^{-10} M), so they bind almost irreversibly. The presence of FcεRI ensures that mast cells are constantly coated with IgE.

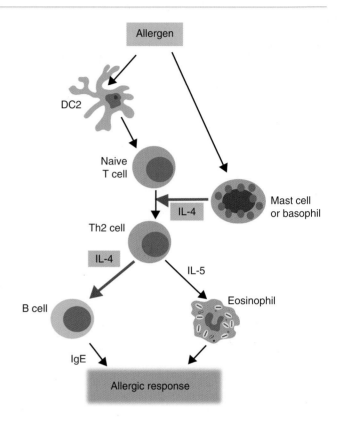

FIGURE 28-2 The role of IL-4 in induction of IgE responses. IL-4 is produced by Th2 cells. Once released, it promotes the development of more Th2 cells, which are major sources of this cytokine and promote IgE responses. The degranulation of mast cells also releases IL-4, which further promotes this reaction. NK cells may serve as an initial source of IL-4. The response to IL-4 is inhibited by IFN-γ and IL-12.

The second form of FcεRI consists of three chains: one α and two γ chains ($\alpha\gamma_2$). It is found on antigen-presenting dendritic cells and monocytes. When an antigen binds to IgE and the complex binds to this receptor, it is ingested and treated as exogenous antigen. The expression of FcεRI on antigen-presenting cells is enhanced by IL-4 from Th2 cells. Thus a positive feedback loop (the allergy loop) develops (Figure 28-4). The antigen processing cells present antigen more effectively to Th2 cells. The Th2 cells then secrete IL-4 and enhance IgE production.

The second IgE receptor, FcεRII (CD23), is a selectin found on B cells, natural killer (NK) cells, macrophages, dendritic cells, eosinophils, and platelets. In addition to binding IgE, FcεRII also binds to the complement receptor CR2 (CD21) (Figure 28-5). Thus B cells expressing FcεRII will bind CR2 on other B cells, T cells, and dendritic cells. By binding B cells to dendritic cells, FcεRII enhances B cell survival and promotes IgE production.

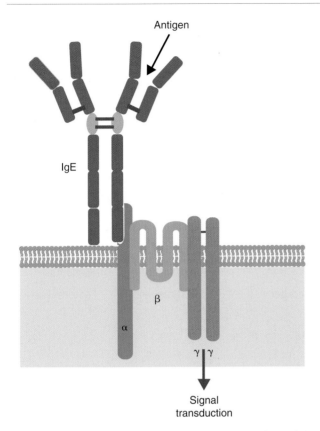

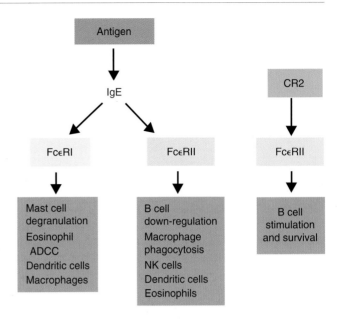

FIGURE 28-5 The combination of the Fcε receptors with their ligands stimulates many different responses in mast cells depending on the nature of these stimuli.

FIGURE 28-3 The structure of FcεRI. This tetrameric form of this receptor containing two γ chains is found on mast cells and basophils.

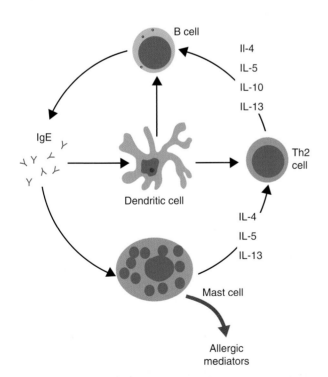

FIGURE 28-4 The allergy loop. Dendritic cells express trimeric FcεRI and as a result can bind antigen-IgE complexes. This antigen, once processed, stimulates Th2 responses. These Th2 cells in turn secrete cytokines, which further promote the IgE response.

Mast Cells

Mast cells have long been known to play a key role in allergic diseases. They also play a major role in innate immunity. Because they are located close to body surfaces as well as their ability to release proinflammatory molecules within seconds, mast cells serve as sentinel cells. They are covered by an array of receptors that permit them to react in response to many different stimuli. For example, they release inflammatory molecules in response to microbial invasion or tissue damage (Chapter 3). This release normally occurs in a controlled manner and ensures that the severity and type of inflammation are appropriate to the body's immediate needs.

Structure and Location

Mast cells are large, round cells (15 to 20 μm in diameter) scattered throughout the body in connective tissue, under mucosal surfaces, in the skin, and around nerves (Figure 28-6). They are found in greatest numbers at sites in the body exposed to potential invaders such as under the skin or in the intestine and airways. In these locations they are located close to blood vessels, where they can regulate blood flow and influence cellular migration. They are easily recognizable because their cytoplasm is densely packed with large granules that stain very strongly with dyes such as toluidine blue. These granules often mask the large, bean-shaped nucleus (Figure 28-7). (Mast cells are so called because, being full of granules, they were considered to be "well-fed cells" [German *Mastzellen*]).

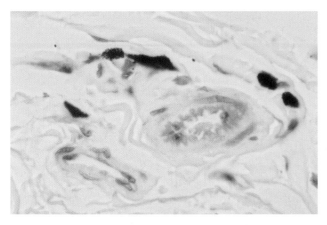

FIGURE 28-6 A section of canine skin stained to show mast cells. The mast cells stain intensely because of the heparin in their cytoplasmic granules.

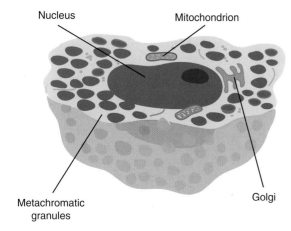

FIGURE 28-7 The structural features of a connective tissue mast cell. The term *metachromatic* simply means that the granules stain intensely.

Life History

Mast cells originate from myeloid stem cells in the bone marrow. Their precursors emigrate to tissues, where they mature and survive for several weeks or months. In rodents, mast cells from connective tissue and skin and from the intestinal mucosa differ both chemically and structurally (Table 28-1). For example, connective tissue and skin mast cells are rich in histamine and heparin, whereas intestinal mast cells contain chondroitin sulfate and have little histamine in their granules. Although connective tissue mast cells remain at relatively constant levels, mucosal mast cells can proliferate. It has been suggested that the mucosal mast cells respond specifically to invasion by parasitic worms.

Mast cells play a key role in inflammation because when they encounter invading microorganisms they degranulate, releasing their granules into the tissues. Their granules then release molecules that cause acute inflammation. Many different stimuli can trigger mast cell degranulation. The best recognized of these involves IgE. IgE and antigen together can

□ Table 28-1 | Comparison of Two Major Types of Mast Cell

	MUCOSAL MAST CELLS	CONNECTIVE TISSUE MAST CELLS
Structure	Few, variable-sized granules	Many uniform granules
Size	9 to 10 μm diameter	19 to 20 μm diameter
Proteoglycan	Chondroitin sulfate	Heparin
Histamine	1.3 pg/cell	15 pg/cell
Life span	<40 days	>6 months
Location	Intestinal wall, lung	Peritoneal cavity, skin

trigger mast cell degranulation and generate allergic diseases. However, allergies are but a special type of inflammation. Numerous other signals can activate mast cells, including cytokines, chemokines, chemical agents, physical stimuli, insect and animal venoms, and viruses. Many damage-associated molecular patterns (DAMPs), including the defensins, anaphylatoxins, neuropeptides, adenosine, and endothelins (small peptides from endothelial cells), also trigger mast cell degranulation.

Mast cells express diverse pattern-recognition receptors (PRRs) that permit them to recognize pathogens. These include TLR1, TLR2, TLR3, TLR4, TLR6, TLR7, and TLR9 and a mannose receptor (CD48). The expression of and the response to TLR ligands may differ between populations and locations. Mast cells also possess receptors for some complement components. Triggering their TLRs causes mast cells to release different mixtures of mediators. Thus bacterial peptidoglycans acting through TLR2 stimulate histamine release, whereas lipopolysaccharides acting through TLR4 do not. Mast cells can use their receptor sets to distinguish between different pathogens and release a select combination of cytokines, chemokines, and other inflammatory mediators, depending the nature of the stimulus.

Response of Mast Cells to Antigen

Although there are numerous ways by which mast cells can be activated, the best studied of these is mediated by IgE bound to FcεRI on the surface of mast cells (Figure 28-8). A mast cell coated in this way is primed to bind antigen. The mast cell can reside in tissues, with its attached IgE acting like a mine in a minefield. If an antigen encounters the mast cell and cross-links two bound IgE molecules, the mast cell is triggered to release its granules and their contents into the surrounding tissues.

This triggering of granule exocytosis is initiated when an antigen molecule cross-links two FcεRI and activates several tyrosine kinases. These, in turn, activate phospholipase C,

leading to the production of diacylglycerol and inositol triphosphate. These mediators then increase intracellular calcium and activate more protein kinases. These protein kinases phosphorylate myosin in the cytoskeleton and make the granules move to the cell surface. Granule membranes then fuse with the plasma membrane, and their contents are released into the extracellular fluid (Figure 28-9).

Cross-linking of two FcεRI by an antigen also activates phospholipase A, which acts on membrane phospholipids to produce arachidonic acid. Other enzymes then convert the arachidonic acid to leukotrienes and prostaglandins (see Figure 3-6). Finally, the protein kinases promote transcription and expression of genes coding for many different cytokines as well as the genes for cyclooxygenases and lipoxygenase.

These mast cell responses are extremely rapid. For example, degranulation occurs within seconds after antigen binds to IgE (Figure 28-10). Because the release is rapid and extensive, sudden acute inflammation develops. Degranulated mast cells do not die but, given time, will regenerate their granules. In normal inflammation, mast cells may release their inflammatory mediators relatively slowly in a process called piecemeal degranulation.

The degranulation of mast cells is the central event in the development of allergic (type I hypersensitivity) reactions. The contents of these granules consist of a mixture of potent proinflammatory molecules (Chapter 3). It is now recognized that

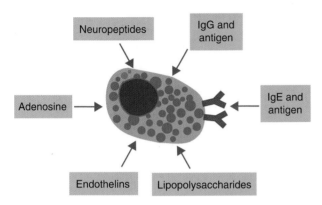

FIGURE 28-8 Some of the stimuli that make mast cells degranulate. Antigen bound through IgE causes rapid complete degranulation. The other stimuli shown cause a more gradual, piecemeal degranulation. Thus in normal inflammatory responses, the degree of mast cell degranulation is tailored to local defensive needs.

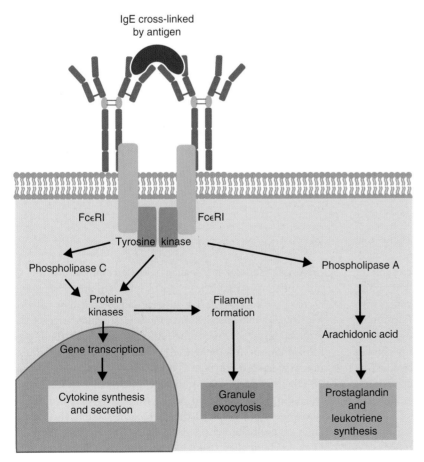

FIGURE 28-9 A simplified view of mast cell signal transduction. The process is triggered by cross-linking two bound IgE molecules with antigen. The combined signal eventually leads to degranulation (granule exocytosis), leukotriene and prostaglandin synthesis, and cytokine production.

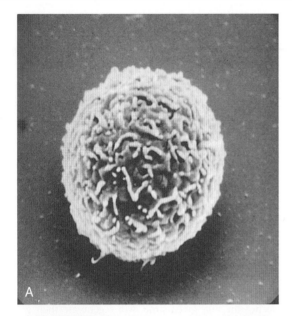

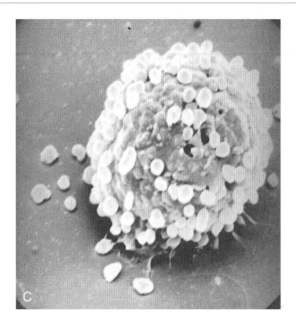

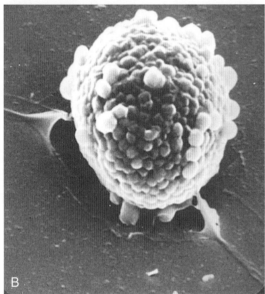

FIGURE 28-10 Scanning electron micrographs. **A,** A normal rat mast cell. **B,** A sensitized mast cell fixed 5 seconds after exposure to antigen. **C,** A sensitized mast cell fixed 60 seconds after exposure to antigen. Original magnification ×3000.

(From Tizard IR, Holmes WL: Degranulation of sensitised rat peritoneal mast cells in response to antigen, compound 48-80 and polymyxin B. A scanning electron microscope study, *Int Arch Allergy Appl Immunol* 46:867–879, 1974.)

there are distinct granule subsets within mast cells and that these different subsets may be released under different conditions. Some granules in mouse mast cells contain serotonin or cathepsin D, whereas others contain histamine and tumor necrosis factor-α (TNF-α). Different stimuli associated with specific isoforms of membrane fusion proteins determine which granule subsets are exocytosed and thus which mediators are released. The significance of this lies in the possibility that different clinical forms of allergy may be determined by the granule subset released. Some less typical allergic manifestations may be a result of the release of the contents of different granule subsets. Likewise, appropriate treatment of allergies may differ according to the mixture of inflammatory mediators released.

Mast Cell–Derived Mediators

Mast cell granules are loaded with a complex mixture of inflammatory mediators, enzymes, and cytokines. Triggering of receptor-bound IgE by antigen causes the mast cells to degranulate and release stored molecules, which triggers the productions of new mediators. All these molecules (both preformed and newly synthesized) generate the acute inflammation characteristic of type I hypersensitivity response (Figure 28-11). The most important include histamine, serotonin, prostaglandins, and the leukotrienes. Mast cells secrete multiple cytokines, chitinases, and the chemokine CCL3. These cytokines are proinflammatory or promote Th2 responses, or both. High levels of these cytokines are found in tissue fluids in

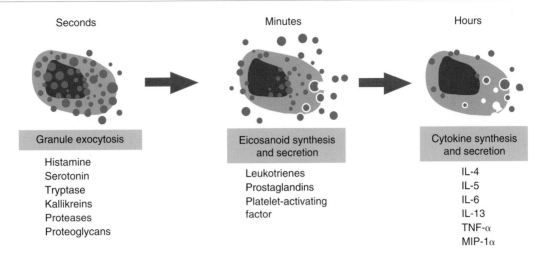

FIGURE 28-11 The soluble mediators released from degranulating mast cells. These fall into three categories: molecules released from exocytosed granules, lipids (eicosanoids) synthesized within minutes, and proteins synthesized over several hours.

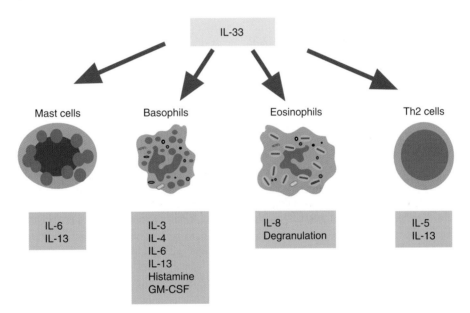

FIGURE 28-12 The biological properties of interleukin-33. This cytokine stimulates the production of inflammatory cytokines and chemokines from many different cell types. It is probably therefore a major mediator of type I hypersensitivity.

allergic reactions. It is no coincidence that mast cells also produce and secrete chitinases. Chitin is characteristically found in insects, fungi, and helminths, and the production of chitinases supports the suggestion that allergic reactions may have evolved to combat these invaders. Chitin itself is a key allergen in some helminth infections.

During infection, mast cells also release small heparin-containing granules that also contain a cytokine mixture. They are especially rich in TNF-α. These particles are carried in the afferent lymph to draining lymph nodes, where they trigger changes in cell behavior. The presence of heparin stabilizes the TNF-α so that it persists for a long time after delivery to a lymph node.

Interleukin-33

IL-33 is a member of the IL-1 family that plays an important role in inflammation and promotes Th2 responses leading to allergies (Figure 28-12). Unlike IL-1 and IL-18, it is produced as an active 18-kDa molecule that does not require cleavage of a precursor. It is produced by smooth muscle cells, epithelial cells, fibroblasts keratinocytes, dendritic cells, and activated macrophages. IL-33 also escapes when cells undergo necrosis and has similar activities to HMGB1. In the presence of IgE, IL-33 binds to a receptor on mast cells, basophils, and Th2 cells. When bound to mast cells, it induces their degranulation and so triggers acute anaphylaxis in the absence of antigen.

IL-33 cannot mediate this degranulation alone. The mast cells must be sensitized by prior exposure to IgE. It also activates basophils and induces basophil differentiation from bone marrow cells.

IL-33 is elevated in humans suffering anaphylactic shock and in atopic human tissues. It is found in high concentrations in the lungs of humans with severe asthma. IL-33 is mainly produced on mucosal surfaces in the lungs and intestine. It stimulates mucus overproduction and goblet cell hypertrophy. IL-33 also plays a role in rheumatoid arthritis by stimulating the release of mast cell inflammatory mediators. Endothelial cells are the major source of IL-33 in affected joints. It is possible that IL-33 is a key mediator of other forms of atopic disease such as atopic dermatitis as well as an activator of mast cells in acute cellular injury.

Regulation of Mast Cell Degranulation

Mast cells express two surface receptors for catecholamines called the α and β adrenoceptors. These G-protein–linked receptors have opposing effects. Molecules that stimulate the α adrenoceptors (such as norepinephrine and phenylephrine) or block the β adrenoceptors (such as propranolol) enhance mast cell degranulation (Table 28-2). In contrast, molecules that stimulate β receptors or block α receptors inhibit mast cell degranulation. β Stimulators include isoproterenol, epinephrine, and salbutamol and are widely used in the treatment of allergies. β Receptor blockers enhance mast cell degranulation and promote allergies. Some respiratory pathogens such as *Bordetella pertussis* and *Haemophilus influenzae* can cause β blockade. As a result, the airways of infected animals are more likely to become severely inflamed because of mast cell degranulation. These infections may also predispose animals to the development of respiratory allergies.

Regulation of the Response to Mast Cell Mediators

The α and β adrenoceptors are found not only on mast cells but also on secretory and smooth muscle cells throughout the body. α Stimulators cause vasoconstriction and may be of use treating severe allergic reactions, reducing edema, and raising blood pressure. β Stimulators mediate smooth muscle relaxation and may therefore reduce the severity of smooth muscle contraction. Pure α and β stimulators are of only limited use in the treatment of allergic diseases because each alone is insufficient to counteract all the effects of mast cell–derived factors. Epinephrine (or adrenaline), on the other hand, has both α and β adrenergic activity. In addition to causing vasoconstriction in skin and viscera, its β effects cause smooth muscle to relax. This combination of effects is well suited to combat the vasodilation and smooth muscle contraction produced in type I hypersensitivity. Ideally, epinephrine should be available whenever potential allergens are administered to animals.

Mast Cells in Infections

Mast cells play important roles in both antimicrobial and antiparasite immunity. They can respond within seconds or minutes to microbial invasion. They possess a large array of PRRs as well as being able to recognize antigen indirectly through their Fc receptors. Lipopolysaccharide stimulation of mast cell TLR4 can induce cytokine production in the absence of degranulation. Increased vascular permeability due to mast cell–derived mediators promotes the inflammatory process. They also release preformed antimicrobial peptides such as the cathelicidins. Mast cell tryptase and chymases have antibacterial and antiparasite activity. Neutrophils are attracted by mast cell–derived leukotrienes.

Late-Phase Reaction

When antigen is injected into the skin of an allergic animal, two waves of inflammation occur. There is an immediate acute inflammatory response that occurs within 10 to 20 minutes as a result of the release of the preformed mast cell mediators. This is followed several hours later by a second wave called the late-phase reaction, which peaks at 6 to 12 hours and then gradually diminishes. This late-phase reaction is characterized by redness, edema, and pruritus. It is believed that this late reaction results from the release of inflammatory mediators by T cells, endothelial cells, neutrophils, and macrophages attracted by mast cell chemotactic factors. Th17 cells may play a role in this late process (Chapter 20).

Basophils

The least numerous granulocytes, the basophils, are so called because their cytoplasmic granules stain intensely with basic dyes, such as hematoxylin (Figure 28-13). Basophils constitute about 0.5% of blood leukocytes. They are not normally found outside the bloodstream but may enter tissues under the influence of some T cell–derived chemokines. Basophil granules contain a complex mixture of vasoactive molecules similar to that found in mast cells. The importance of the role of basophils relative to that of mast cells in acute systemic anaphylaxis is unclear. Basophils are relatively uncommon cells in blood,

▫ **Table 28-2** | Effects of Stimulating α and β Adrenoceptors

SYSTEM	α RECEPTOR STIMULATION OR β BLOCKADE	β RECEPTOR STIMULATION OR α BLOCKADE
Mast cells	Enhances degranulation	Suppresses degranulation
Smooth muscle	Contracts	Relaxes
Blood vessels	Constricts	Dilates

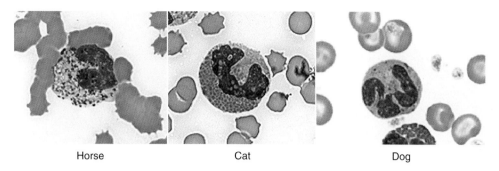

FIGURE 28-13 Photomicrographs of peripheral blood basophils from a horse, a cat, and a dog. These cells are about 10 μm in diameter; all were photographed at the same magnification. Giemsa stain.

(Courtesy Dr. M.C. Johnson.)

whereas mast cells are numerous in tissues. Both cell types contribute to systemic anaphylaxis. In mice, basophils and mast cells develop from a common stem cell.

Basophils possess FcεRI receptors and so bind IgE. Antigens binding to this IgE will induce basophil degranulation and the release of vasoactive mediators. Basophils can also mediate IgG-mediated systemic anaphylaxis since they possess FcγRs and bind IgG-containing immune complexes. Basophils release platelet-activating factor (PAF), a lipid, in response to IgG1-mediated stimulation. PAF is about 10,000 more effective than histamine in increasing vascular permeability. Thus there are two distinct pathways in mouse anaphylaxis: one mediated by basophils and one mediated by mast cells. Although mast cells induce acute inflammation, basophils probably mediate more chronic allergic states such as chronic allergic dermatitis. This may be of relevance to those situations in domestic animals in which there appears to be little relationship between IgE levels and the severity of allergic diseases. Perhaps these animals also use a basophil-IgG1 pathway.

Basophils can initiate allergen- and helminth-driven CD4+ Th2 responses by functioning as antigen-presenting cells. Basophils can capture antigen through FcR-bound antibodies. When activated, they produce IL-4 and IL-6, and some basophils also express MHC class II. They can endocytose, process, and present soluble antigens but not particulate antigens. IL-4 and IL-6 drive Th2 differentiation and as a consequence promote IgE responses.

Eosinophils

Tissues undergoing type I hypersensitivity reactions characteristically contain large numbers of eosinophils. These cells are attracted to sites of mast cell degranulation, where they degranulate and release their own biologically active molecules. Eosinophils may be considered the terminal effector cells of the allergic response.

Eosinophils are polymorphonuclear cells, slightly larger than neutrophils, with cytoplasmic granules that stain intensely with the red dye eosin (Figure 28-14). They originate in the bone marrow and spend about 30 minutes circulating in the

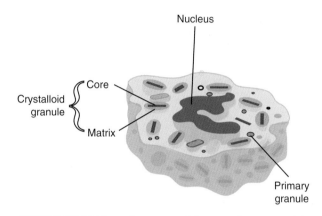

FIGURE 28-14 The major structural features of an eosinophil.

bloodstream before migrating into the tissues, where they have a half-life of about 12 days. The proportion of eosinophils among the blood leukocytes varies greatly since it is affected by the presence of parasites. Normal values range from 2% in dogs to about 10% in cattle.

Eosinophils contain two types of granules (Figures 28-15 and 28-16). Their small, primary granules contain arylsulfatase, peroxidase, and acid phosphatase. Their large crystalloid granules have a core of major basic protein (MBP) surrounded by a matrix containing eosinophil cationic protein (ECP), eosinophil peroxidase (EPO), and eosinophil-derived neurotoxin (EDN).

Eosinophil Activation

Three mechanisms are involved in mobilizing eosinophils (Figure 28-17). First, both Th2 cells and mast cells produce IL-5, and the chemokines known as eotaxins that stimulate the release of eosinophils from the bone marrow. Thus Th2 cells mobilize eosinophils at the same time that they stimulate IgE responses. Second, these eosinophils are attracted to sites of mast cell degranulation by molecules such as the eotaxins, histamine and its breakdown product imidiazoleacetic acid, leukotriene B$_4$, 5-hydroxytryptamine (5-HT), and PAF.

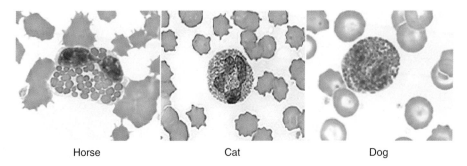

Horse   Cat   Dog

FIGURE 28-15 Photomicrographs of peripheral blood eosinophils from a horse, a cat, and a dog. Each cell is about 12 µm in diameter. Giemsa stain.

(Courtesy of Dr. M.C. Johnson.)

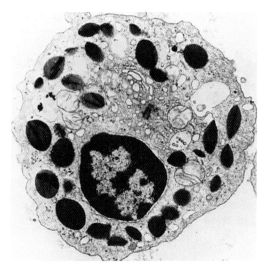

FIGURE 28-16 A transmission electron micrograph of a rabbit eosinophil.

(Courtesy Dr. S. Linthicum.)

◻ Table 28-3 ┃ Major Cytokines Produced in Type I Hypersensitivity Reactions

MAST CELLS	BASOPHILS	EOSINOPHILS
IL-3	IL-4	IL-1α
IL-4	IL-6	IL-3
IL-5		IL-4
IL-6		IL-5
IL-13		IL-6
IL-16		GM-CSF
IL-22		TNF-α
IL-25		TGF-β
GM-CSF		
TNF-α		

Activated eosinophils are especially attracted by CXCL8 (IL-8) complexed to IgA. Third, some common allergens directly activate eosinophils, stimulating their chemotaxis and upregulating CR3 expression. Once they reach sites of mast cell degranulation, eosinophils are activated by these same molecules. The mobilization and activation of eosinophils enhance their ability to kill parasites and support the belief that the major function of the IgE-mediated responses is the control of helminth parasites (Chapter 27). Activated eosinophils express MHC class II molecules and can serve as antigen-presenting cells.

Eosinophil Degranulation and Mediators

Although eosinophils can phagocytose small particles, they are much more suited to extracellular destruction of large parasites since they can degranulate into the surrounding fluid. Eosinophils may release their granules by exocytosis or, more commonly, undergo piecemeal degranulation. In this process small vesicles bud off the secondary granules and are released into the extracellular tissues. This degranulation occurs in response to IgE-coated parasites, antigen-bound IgE, many chemokines, PAF, and C5a. Once released into the tissues, eosinophil granules can function autonomously as independent structures capable of secreting granule proteins in response to IFN-γ or CCL11.

Eosinophil granules contain a mixture of inflammatory and toxic mediators, including cationic proteins, peroxidase, and MBP (Figure 28-18). Eosinophils also produce lipid mediators such as leukotrienes and PAF. Particles bound to eosinophil receptors trigger a powerful respiratory burst. The eosinophil peroxidase uses bromide in preference to chloride, thus producing OBr⁻. The peroxidase generates nitric oxide and nitrotyrosine, both potent oxidizing agents. Eosinophil granule proteins can kill helminths and bacteria and are important mediators of tissue pathology. They all, for example, damage respiratory epithelium. The production by eosinophils of multiple Th2 cytokines (Table 28-3) as well as indoleamine dioxygenase inhibits local Th1 responses and ensures that a "Th2 environment" is maintained in regions of eosinophil accumulation. Eosinophils can produce their own CCL5 and CCL11 so that additional eosinophils can be attracted to the inflammatory focus.

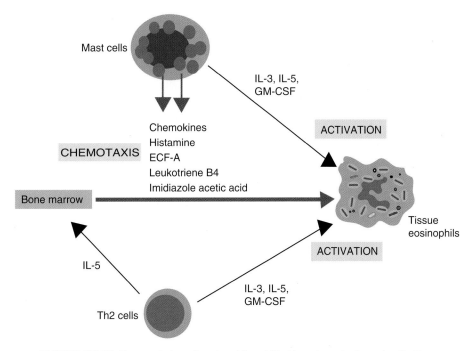

FIGURE 28-17 The regulation of eosinophil mobilization, chemotaxis, and activation.

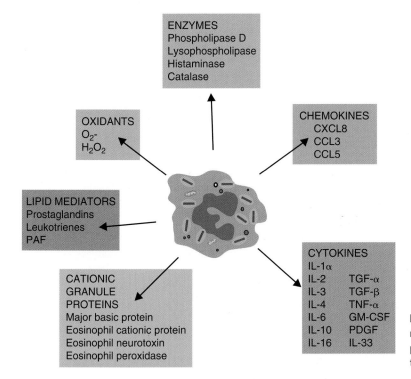

FIGURE 28-18 Eosinophils release a complex array of molecules that contribute to the acute inflammatory process. It is clear that on balance, eosinophils exacerbate the inflammation triggered by mast cells.

Mast cells and eosinophils interact extensively. Thus eosinophil-derived basic proteins activate mast cells to release histamine. Mast cells in turn release eosinophil chemotactic agents, activate eosinophils, and enhance the expression of eosinophil receptors. Mast cells can synthesize and secrete IL-3, IL-5, and GM-CSF, all of which promote eosinophil degranulation, growth, and survival.

Other Cells

Although it has long been accepted that immediate hypersensitivity results from the IgE-mediated degranulation of mast cells, it has recently been shown that fatal anaphylaxis may be induced in mast cell–deficient mice! Analysis indicates that this is mediated by IgG acting through FcγRIV on platelets and neutrophils. Their role in allergies in other species is unclear.

Clinical Type I Hypersensitivity

The clinical signs of type I hypersensitivity result from the abrupt and excessive release of inflammatory mediators from mast cells, basophils, and eosinophils. The severity and location of these responses depend on the number and location of these cells; this, in turn, depends on the degree of sensitization of an animal, the amount of antigen involved, and its route of administration. In its most extreme form, antigen administered rapidly to a sensitized animal will cause generalized mast cell degranulation and massive mediator release. If the rate of release of vasoactive molecules from these mast cells exceeds its ability to adjust to the rapid changes in the vascular system, an animal will undergo allergic anaphylaxis and may die.

Allergic Anaphylaxis

Allergic anaphylaxis is a severe, life-threatening systemic hypersensitivity reaction. Its clinical signs (Table 28-4) are determined by organ system involvement, which differs among the major domestic animals. Many of the symptoms result from smooth muscle contraction in the bronchi, gastrointestinal tract, uterus, and bladder.

The major shock organs of horses are the lungs and the intestine. Bronchial and bronchiolar constriction leads to coughing, dyspnea, and eventually apnea. On necropsy, severe pulmonary emphysema and peribronchiolar edema are commonly seen. In addition to the lung lesions, edematous hemorrhagic enterocolitis may cause severe diarrhea. The major mediators of anaphylaxis in horses are probably histamine and serotonin.

In cattle the major shock organ is the lung. Allergic anaphylaxis is characterized by profound systemic hypotension and pulmonary hypertension. The pulmonary hypertension results from constriction of the pulmonary vein and leads to pulmonary edema and severe dyspnea. The smooth muscle of the bladder and intestine contract, causing urination, defecation, and bloating. The main mediators of anaphylaxis in cattle are serotonin, kinins, and the leukotrienes. Histamine is of lesser importance. Dopamine enhances histamine and leukotriene release from the lung, thus exerting a form of positive feedback. Because of the anticoagulant properties of heparin from mast cells, blood from animals experiencing anaphylaxis may not coagulate. In cattle, in contrast to the other species, β stimulants such as isoproterenol potentiate histamine release from leukocytes, whereas α stimulants such as norepinephrine inhibit histamine release. In addition, epinephrine potentiates histamine release in the bovine. The significance of these anomalous effects is unclear.

▢ Table 28-4 ǀ Anaphylaxis in the Domestic Species and Humans

SPECIES	SHOCK ORGANS	SYMPTOMS	PATHOLOGY	MAJOR MEDIATORS
Horse	Respiratory tract Intestine	Cough Dyspnea Diarrhea	Emphysema Intestinal hemorrhage	Histamine Serotonin
Ruminants	Respiratory tract	Cough Dyspnea Collapse	Lung edema Emphysema Hemorrhage	Serotonin Leukotrienes Kinins Dopamine
Swine	Respiratory tract Intestine	Cyanosis Pruritus	Systemic hypotension	Histamine
Dog	Hepatic veins	Collapse Dyspnea Diarrhea Vomiting	Hepatic engorgement Visceral hemorrhage	Histamine Leukotrienes Prostaglandins
Cat	Respiratory tract Intestine	Dyspnea Vomiting Diarrhea Pruritus	Lung edema Intestinal edema	Histamine Leukotrienes
Human	Respiratory tract	Dyspnea Urticaria	Lung edema Emphysema	Histamine Leukotrienes
Chicken	Respiratory tract	Dyspnea Convulsions	Lung edema	Histamine Serotonin Leukotrienes

In sheep, pulmonary signs predominate in allergic anaphylaxis as a result of constriction of the bronchi and pulmonary vessels. Smooth muscle contraction also occurs in the bladder and intestine with predictable results. The major mediators of type I hypersensitivity in sheep are histamine, serotonin, leukotrienes, and kinins.

In pigs, allergic anaphylaxis is largely the result of systemic and pulmonary hypertension, leading to dyspnea and death. In some pigs the intestine is involved, whereas in others no gross intestinal lesions are observed. The most significant mediator identified in this species is histamine.

Dogs differ from the other domestic mammals in that the major shock organ is not the lung but the liver, specifically the hepatic veins. Dogs undergoing allergic anaphylaxis show initial excitement followed by vomiting, defecation, and urination. As the reaction progresses, dogs collapse with weakness and depressed respiration, become comatose, convulse, and die within an hour. On necropsy, the liver and intestine are massively engorged, perhaps holding up to 60% of the animal's total blood volume. All these signs result from occlusion of the hepatic vein due to a combination of smooth muscle contraction and hepatic swelling. This results in portal hypertension and visceral pooling, as well as a decrease in venous return, cardiac output, and arterial pressure. Identified mediators include histamine, prostaglandins, and leukotrienes.

In cats, the major shock organ is the lung. Cats undergoing allergic anaphylaxis show vigorous scratching around the face and head as histamine is released into the skin. This is followed by dyspnea, salivation, vomiting, incoordination, collapse, and death. Necropsy reveals bronchoconstriction, emphysema, pulmonary hemorrhage, and edema of the glottis. The major mediators in the cat are histamine and the leukotrienes.

Specific Allergic Conditions

Although allergic anaphylaxis is the most dramatic and severe type I hypersensitivity reaction, it is more common to observe local allergic reactions, the sites of which are referable to the route of administration of antigens. For example, inhaled antigens (allergens) provoke inflammation in the upper respiratory tract, trachea, and bronchi, resulting in fluid exudation from the nasal mucosa (hay fever) and tracheobronchial constriction (asthma). Aerosolized antigen will also contact the eyes and provoke conjunctivitis and intense lacrimation. Ingested antigens may provoke diarrhea and colic as intestinal smooth muscle contracts violently. If sufficiently severe, the resulting diarrhea may be hemorrhagic. Antigen reaching the skin causes local dermatitis. The reaction is erythematous and edematous and is described as an urticarial type (*Urtica dioica* is the name of the "stinging nettle," a plant that has hollow stinging hairs that inject histamine into the skin when touched) (Figure 28-19). Urticarial lesions are extremely pruritic; consequently, scratching may mask the true nature of the lesion.

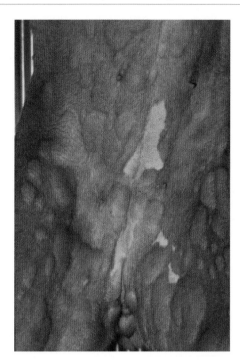

FIGURE 28-19 Severe urticaria in a boxer stung by three wasps. (Courtesy Dr. G. Elissalde.)

Hygiene Hypothesis

Many aspects of allergic reactions resemble the reactions induced by intestinal helminths or biting insects. Both involve Th2 activation and the production of IgE. This has led to the concept that the immune system in allergic individuals is somehow tricked into reacting to innocuous antigens as if they were parasites. Reactions to parasites decline once the invader has gone. In allergies, however, the reactions persist, suggesting a defect in immunoregulatory pathways. It has been hypothesized that the current allergy epidemic in children is due to a lack of appropriate antigenic stimulation in childhood, the so-called hygiene hypothesis (Chapter 22). As living standards improve, exposure to pathogens is reduced. Young children with even minor infections are routinely treated with antibiotics. Since these infections normally promote a strong Th1 response, in their absence Th2 responses predominate. A version of this theory suggests that changes in the commensal population of the gut as a result of Western diets may also modulate the Th1/Th2 balance. Thus the intestinal microbiota may exert a significant influence on allergy development. There is some evidence suggesting that the composition of the "normal" flora of the upper respiratory tract may also determine the development of asthma.

Milk Allergy

Jersey cattle may become allergic to the α casein of their own milk. Normally, this protein is synthesized in the udder, and provided that the animals are milked regularly, nothing untoward occurs. If milking is delayed, however, the increased intramammary pressure forces milk proteins into the bloodstream. In allergic cattle, this may result in reactions ranging from mild discomfort with urticarial skin lesions to acute anaphylaxis and death. Prompt milking can treat the condition, although some seriously affected animals may have to go for several lactations without drying off because of the severe reactions that occur on cessation of milking.

Food Allergy

About 2% of food protein is absorbed from the intestine as peptide fragments large enough to be recognized as foreign. This antigen may travel in the blood and reach mast cells in the skin within a few minutes. It has been claimed that up to 30% of skin diseases in dogs are due to allergic dermatitis and that responses to ingested allergens may account for 1% of cutaneous disease in dogs and cats, although their true prevalence is unknown. The clinical consequences of food allergies are seen both in the digestive tract and on the skin.

It is important not to confuse *food allergy,* an immunologically mediated reaction to food allergens, with *food intolerance.* The American Academy of Allergy and Immunology has defined *food intolerance* as "those adverse reactions to foods that are not immunologically mediated." These reactions can include food idiosyncrasies, in which an animal responds abnormally to a food; metabolic reactions, in which a food component affects the metabolism of the animal; pharmacological reactions, in which some food components may act like drugs; and food poisoning, in which the adverse reaction is caused by a toxin or organism.

Only about 10% to 30% of dogs with food allergies have gastrointestinal problems. The intestinal reaction may be mild, perhaps showing only as an irregularity in the consistency of the feces, or it may be severe, with vomiting, cramps, and violent, sometimes hemorrhagic diarrhea occurring soon after feeding. Most dogs show cutaneous symptoms, and these may be indistinguishable from atopic dermatitis. Skin reactions to dietary antigens in dogs are classified as cutaneous adverse skin reactions since the immunological mechanisms involved are unclear. About half of affected dogs have a nonseasonal pruritic dermatitis. The skin reactions are usually papular and erythematous and may involve the feet, eyes, ears, and axillae or perianal area. The lesion itself is highly pruritic and is commonly masked by self-inflicted trauma and secondary bacterial or yeast infections. This pruritus tends to respond poorly to corticosteroids, suggesting that it may not be a true type I hypersensitivity reaction. In chronic cases the skin may be hyperpigmented, lichenified, and infected, leading to a pyoderma. A chronic pruritic otitis externa may also develop. The foods involved vary but are usually protein-rich such as dairy products, wheat meal, fish, chicken, beef, or eggs. In pigs, fishmeal and alfalfa have been incriminated. Immunoblot analysis of serum from dogs that are allergic to beef and cow's milk showed that they produce IgE against bovine IgG heavy chains. Thus, IgG is a major allergen in cow's milk. A second major antigen in lamb and beef extracts has been identified as phosphoglucomutase. Analysis of skin T cell populations in these dogs shows that CD8+ T cells predominate and that gene expression of IL-4, IL-13, and FoxP3 is increased. Food allergies have been reported in the horse but are uncommon. Wild oats, white clover, and alfalfa have been recognized as allergens in this species.

The most reliable test for suspected food allergies is to remove all potential allergens and then feed a hypoallergenic diet. These elimination diets usually contain meat and carbohydrates from sources to which the animal is unlikely to have been exposed. Examples include mutton, duck, venison, or rabbit with brown rice or potato. An alternative solution is to feed a hydrolyzed diet that contains smaller and less allergenic protein fragments. Several commercial hypoallergenic diets are available to facilitate this diagnosis. These diets may be supplemented by adding other ingredients until the allergen is identified by a recurrence of clinical signs. Treatment involves eliminating the responsible food after correctly identifying it. The development of food allergies may be significantly promoted by the presence of nematode parasites. Parasitized cats develop significantly higher levels of antibodies to food antigens. Most importantly they develop higher levels of IgE antibodies, suggesting that the presence of parasitic worms in the intestine may provoke food allergies.

Allergic Inhalant Dermatitis and Atopic Dermatitis

In dogs and cats, allergy to inhaled environmental antigens commonly results in the development of allergic inhalant dermatitis. Terriers and Dalmatians appear to be predisposed to this, but any breed may be affected. Animals may present with the allergic triad: face rubbing, axillary pruritus, and foot licking, although skin lesions may be found anywhere on the body. The specific lesions are secondary to the intense pruritus and vary from acute erythema and edema to chronic secondary changes including crusting, scaling, hyperpigmentation, lichenification, and pyoderma. Some animals may have otitis externa or conjunctivitis. The cutaneous inflammatory infiltrate contains mast cells, γ/δ T cells, dendritic cells, low numbers of eosinophils and neutrophils, and few B cells. Depending on the source of allergen, the atopy may be seasonal. Hypersensitivity to a single allergen is uncommon, and most animals develop multiple sensitivities. Diagnosis is based on history and identification of the offending antigens by direct skin testing. Canine allergic inhalent dermatitis may be treated by corticosteroids or by hyposensitization therapy. Antihistamines and nonsteroidal antiinflammatory drugs seem to help some of the time, although leukotrienes likely play an important role in this disease (Box 28-2).

Nasolacrimal urticaria (hay fever) is an uncommon manifestation of respiratory allergy in dogs and cats. Pollens usually provoke a rhinitis and conjunctivitis characterized by a profuse watery nasal discharge and excessive lacrimation. If the allergenic particles are sufficiently small, they may reach the bronchi or bronchioles, where the resulting reaction can

□ Box 28-2 | **Interleukin-31**

Chronic itching is one of the most important and distressing features of atopic skin disease. It is mediated by mediators released by resident skin cells. These mediators bind directly to itch-specific receptors (pruriceptors) that are linked to specific areas of the brain. Itch mediators include histamine, some prostaglandins and leukotrienes, some neuropeptides, and IL-31. IL-31, when released into the skin of mice, causes intense itching similar to that seen in atopic dermatitis. Mice that overexpress IL-31 develop skin lesions resembling atopic dermatitis, and conversely, mice with natural atopic dermatitis overexpress IL-31 in their skin lesions. In humans with atopic dermatitis or allergic contact dermatitis, the level of IL-31 mRNA is higher in atopic skin lesions than in normal skin. IL-31 also activates bronchial epithelial cells and plays a major role in respiratory allergies. It is produced by both Th2 cells and mast cells in response to antimicrobial peptides such as β-defensins and cathelicidins. Thus it is possible that IL-31 plays a central role in atopic dermatitis.

□ Box 28-3 | **Atopic Dermatitis Phenotypes**

It has long been recognized that the development of canine atopy is determined in part by genetic factors. Not only the development of this disease but also its clinical phenotype vary between breeds. Careful clinical evaluation has recognized several different disease phenotypes that differ in such features as age of onset, the presence of hot spots, gastrointestinal disorders, flexural dermatitis, and the distribution of the skin lesions. Some breeds may develop lesions in specific areas. Thus French Bulldogs develop lesions in the axillae, eyelids, and flexural surfaces. German Shepherds, in contrast, tend to develop lesions in the elbows, hind limbs, and thorax. Since dog breeds often represent genetically homogeneous populations with their own set of genes and mutations, it is perhaps unsurprising that they differ in their atopic phenotype.

Wilhem S, Kovalik M, Favrot C: Breed-associated phenotypes in canine atopic dermatitis, *Vet Dermatol* 22:143–149, 2011.

cause bronchoconstriction, wheezing, and recurrent asthma-like paroxysmal dyspnea. It should be noted that Basenji dogs have unusually sensitive airways and experience a disease similar to humans with asthma. Cats are also recognized as suffering from asthma manifested by paroxysmal wheezing, dyspnea, and coughing. Although its pathogenesis has not been clarified, asthmatic cats respond well to corticosteroids and inhaled bronchodilators as well as allergen avoidance. It is of interest to note that there is a concordance between asthma in cats and in their owners, suggesting the involvement of similar allergens.

A familial allergic rhinitis characterized by extreme nasal pruritus, violent sneezing, dyspnea, mucoid nasal discharge, and excessive lacrimation has been observed in cattle. Depending on the allergen, it may be seasonal. The antigens involved are inhaled and come from a variety of plant and fungal sources. Diagnosis may be confirmed by skin testing. Nasal granulomas may form in chronically affected cattle. These consist of numerous polypoid nodules, 1 to 4 mm in diameter, situated in the anterior nasal mucosa. The nodules contain large numbers of mast cells, eosinophils, and plasma cells.

Atopic dermatitis is a chronic, multifactorial syndrome characterized by chronically inflamed and itchy skin. It is very common in humans and dogs (as many as 15% are affected) and has been recognized in cats, horses, and goats.

The International Task Force on Canine Atopic Dermatitis has listed eight diagnostic criteria for this disease:

1. The disease mainly occurs in indoor dogs.
2. Disease onset occurs before the animal is 3 years of age.
3. Animals develop a corticosteroid-responsive pruritus.
4. This pruritus is initially without obvious lesions.
5. The pruritus eventually affects the front feet.
6. The ear pinnae are affected next.
7. The ear margins are affected next.
8. The dorsolumbar area remains unaffected.

Any combination of five criteria from this set will diagnose atopic dermatitis with a sensitivity of 85% and a specificity of 79% (Chapter 41).

Canine atopic dermatitis has a major breed predilection, being most common in Retrievers, Setters, Terriers, Beagles, Cocker Spaniels, Boxers, Bulldogs, and Shar-Peis. Both susceptibility and protective gene loci have been identified in dogs. It is commonly associated with reactions to environmental allergens such as molds; tree, weed, and grass pollens (especially pollens that are small and light and are produced in very large quantities); house dust mites (*Dermatophagoides farinae* and *Dermatophagoides pteronyssinus*); animal danders; and the yeast *Malassezia pachydermatis*. However, the etiology of atopic dermatitis is complex, and not all cases are associated with IgE antibodies to environmental antigens (Box 28-3).

In humans it has been suggested that the initial lesion in atopic dermatitis is a defect in epithelial cells leading to barrier dysfunction and that the immunological lesions may be secondary. It is believed that defects in a skin barrier protein filaggrin increase skin water loss and its susceptibility to irritation. Filaggrin is a filament-associated protein involved in cross-linking keratin fibers in epidermal cells. The loss of its barrier function would permit allergens to penetrate the skin and sensitize animals. SNPs within the canine filaggrin gene have been associated with some forms of canine atopic dermatitis.

Atopic dogs commonly present with pruritus. Initially there are no obvious skin lesions, but this progresses to diffuse erythema. Chronic licking and scratching lead to hair loss, papules, scaling, and crusting. Hyperpigmentation and lichenification may occur. Skin lesions occur most commonly on front feet, the ventral abdomen, and in the inguinal and axillary regions. Many affected dogs have otitis externa. Dogs may also develop focal "hot spots." The cellular infiltrate within these lesions contains increased numbers of mast cells, dendritic cells, Langerhans cells, macrophages, and γ/δ T cells. There are small numbers of eosinophils and neutrophils and very few B cells. Secondary bacterial or yeast infections complicate the disease. Depending on the inducing allergen, the disease may be seasonal and relapsing. Once it starts, it tends to get progressively more severe unless treated.

Atopic dermatitis is provoked by environmental, food, and respiratory allergens that enter animals by the oral, respiratory, or percutaneous routes. The importance of the latter route is reflected by the frequency of lesions on contact areas such as the feet, and ears. Affected animals commonly show positive skin test responses to intradermally injected allergens. However, serological assays that measure IgE antibodies to the offending allergens rarely correlate with disease severity or the levels of IgE in the skin and are of limited usefulness. Blood IgE levels may drop to undetectable levels, whereas levels in skin and skin reactivity remain high. (A phenomenon probably related to the very short half-life of IgE.) The many false-negative serologic results probably reflect the fact that the immunological reactions such as the presence of reactive Th2 cells are largely restricted to areas of affected skin. Affected skin contains more IL-4, IFN-γ, TNF-α, and IL-2 and less TGF-β compared to healthy skin.

Allergen avoidance is the best treatment. Specific immunotherapy gives good responses in up to 80% of cases, but secondary infections such as bacterial or yeast (*Malassezia*) infections or flea infestations must also be controlled. Topical therapy such as bathing with emollient shampoos helps considerably. Antihistamines are of limited usefulness but may be of benefit in mild cases. Diets enriched in the omega-3 fatty acids eicosapentaenoic acid and docosahexaenoic acid may be beneficial when fed to dogs with chronic allergic dermatitis. Omega-3 (fish) oil or omega-6 (evening primrose) oil probably promote the synthesis of antiinflammatory eicosanoids (see Box 39-1).

Certain drugs have demonstrated some evidence of efficacy in the treatment of canine atopic dermatitis. These include tacrolimus, topical triamcinolone, oral corticosteroids, and oral cyclosporine. The effective dose of prednisolone may be significantly reduced by the use of an oral essential fatty acid supplement.

Allergies to Vaccines and Drugs

An IgE response may result from the administration of any antigen, including vaccines. It is most likely to occur in vaccines that contain trace amounts of fetal calf serum, gelatin, or casein. Severe allergies have been associated with the use of killed foot-and-mouth disease, rabies, and contagious bovine

pleuropneumonia vaccines in cattle. IgE responses may also occur following administration of drugs. Most drug molecules are too small to be antigenic, but many can bind to host proteins and then act as haptens. Penicillin allergy, for example, may be triggered either by therapeutic exposure or by ingestion of penicillin-contaminated milk. The penicillin molecule is degraded in vivo to several compounds; the most important of these contains a penicilloyl group. This penicilloyl group can bind to proteins and provoke an immune response. In sensitized animals, injection of penicillin may cause acute systemic anaphylaxis or milder forms of allergy. Feeding of penicillin-contaminated milk to these animals can lead to severe diarrhea. Allergies to many drugs, especially antibiotics and hormones, have been reported in the domestic animals. Even substances contained in leather preservatives used in harnesses, in catgut sutures, or compounds such as methylcellulose or carboxymethylcellulose used as stabilizers in vaccines may provoke allergies.

Allergies to Parasites

The beneficial role of the IgE–mast cell–eosinophil system in immunity to parasitic worms was first observed in the self-cure phenomenon (Chapter 27). Helminths preferentially stimulate IgE responses, and helminth infestations are commonly associated with many of the signs of allergy and anaphylaxis; for example, animals with tapeworms may show respiratory distress or urticaria. Anaphylaxis may be provoked by rupture of a hydatid cyst during surgery or through transfusion of blood from a dog infected with *Dirofilaria immitis* to a sensitized animal.

Allergies are also commonly associated with exposure to arthropod antigens. Insect stings account for many human deaths each year as a result of acute anaphylaxis following sensitization to venom. Anaphylaxis can also occur in cattle infested with the warble fly (*Hypoderma bovis*). The pupae of this fly develop under the skin on the back of cattle after the larvae have migrated through the tissues from the site of egg deposition on the hind leg. Because the pupae are so obvious, it is tempting to remove them manually. Unfortunately, if they rupture during this process, the release of coelomic fluid may provoke lethal anaphylaxis.

In horses and cattle, hypersensitivity to insect bites may cause an allergic dermatitis variously called Gulf Coast itch, Queensland itch, and sweet itch. The insects involved include midges (*Culicoides* species), black flies (*Simulium* species), stable flies (*Stomoxys calcitrans*), mosquitoes, and stick-tight fleas (*Echidnophaga gallinacea*). If animals are allergic to antigens in the saliva of these insects, biting results in the development of urticaria accompanied by intense pruritus. The itching may provoke severe self-mutilation with subsequent secondary infection that may mask the original allergic nature of the lesion. It is interesting to note that IgE sensitization of skin mast cells is common in clinically healthy horses exposed to *Culicoides* midges, so allergic disease is not an inevitable result of exposure and sensitization.

Animals do not inevitably respond to arthropod allergens with a type I hypersensitivity. Thus, responses to *Demodex* mites and to flea saliva may be cell mediated (type IV hypersensitivity, Chapter 31). Flea-bite allergic dermatitis is the single most important allergic skin disease. There is no breed or gender predisposition, but atopic animals as well as those exposed to fleas on an intermittent basis tend to get more severe disease. Continual exposure to fleas at an early age appears to result in hyposensitization. Pruritus is a consistent feature, as is a history of flea infestation. Affected animals, in addition to the characteristic clinical signs, show a reaction to intradermally injected flea antigen. Most sensitive animals will respond within a few minutes, but up to 30% may show a delayed reaction at 24 to 48 hours. Hyposensitization therapy has not been shown to be successful in treating flea allergy. Flea allergy can be successfully treated only by total flea control.

Eosinophilic Granuloma Complex

The eosinophilic granuloma complex comprises a confusing group of diseases associated with various types of skin lesions (ulcer, plaque, granuloma) in cats. Although their cause is unknown, they have been associated with flea or food allergies or atopic dermatitis. The presence of eosinophils in skin is often associated with the development of pathological lesions. Thus when purified ECP or EDN are injected into guinea pig or rabbit skin, they disrupt skin integrity and cause inflammation. The ECP produces ulcers, whereas the EDN produces cellular exudates. Purified EPO and MBP-1 produce induration and erythema. The activities of these proteins can explain the development of lesions in eosinophil-associated skin diseases.

A seasonal form of eosinophilic lesion has been associated with mosquito bites. This may present as scattered individual crusted papules. The eosinophilic plaques in the skin are intensely pruritic. As a result, the lesions may be masked by self-inflicted trauma and secondary bacterial infection. Histologically they are associated with a local mast cell and eosinophil infiltration, as well as an eosinophilia. Eosinophilic granulomas, in contrast, are not pruritic, and they present as a line of raised pink plaques. Some may present as scattered individual crusted papules. Linear eosinophilic ulcers (sometimes called indolent or rodent ulcers) are commonly located in the oral cavity or on the lips. Removal of the offending allergen may result in clinical improvement, and corticosteroid treatment is usually of benefit. The linear form and indolent ulcers may be difficult to treat and may require more aggressive therapy. An idiopathic hypereosinophilic syndrome has been described in humans, cats, and dogs. It is characterized by a prolonged, unexplained eosinophilia, the infiltration of many organs with eosinophils, organ dysfunction (affecting especially the heart, but also the lungs, spleen, liver, skin, bone marrow, gastrointestinal tract, and central nervous system), and death. An eosinophilic enteritis may result from canine hookworm infestation.

Diagnosis of Type I Hypersensitivity

The term *hypersensitivity* is used to denote inflammation that occurs in response to normally harmless material. For example, animals normally do not react to antigens injected intradermally. If, however, a hypersensitive animal is given an intradermal injection of allergen, it will provoke inflammation. Vasoactive molecules are released within minutes to produce redness (erythema) as a result of capillary dilation, as well as circumscribed edema (a wheal) due to increased vascular permeability. The reaction may also generate an erythematous flare due to arteriolar dilation caused by a local axon reflex. This wheal-and-flare response to an allergen reaches maximal intensity within 30 minutes and then disappears within a few hours. A late-phase reaction sometimes occurs 6 to 12 hours after intradermal injection as a result of the release of mediators by eosinophils and neutrophils.

Intradermal skin testing using very dilute aqueous solutions of allergens has been widely used for the diagnosis of allergies, especially canine atopic dermatitis. Following injection, the site is examined for an inflammatory response. The results obtained must be interpreted carefully since both false-positive and false-negative responses may occur. For example, the concentration of antigen in commercial skin testing solutions may be too low. Dogs may be up to 10 times less sensitive than humans to intradermal allergens such as pollens, fungi, or danders. False-positive reactions may be due to the presence of preservatives in allergen solutions. Results of skin testing are affected by steroid treatment. The mixture of allergens used for intradermal skin testing commonly includes allergens from trees, grasses, fungi, weeds, danders, feathers, house dust mites, and insects. Intradermal skin testing is less commonly performed in cats because they fail to develop a significant wheal, and the reaction is therefore difficult to evaluate.

An experimental technique used to detect IgE antibodies is called the passive cutaneous anaphylaxis (PCA) test. In this test, dilutions of test serum are injected at different sites into the skin of a normal animal. After waiting 24 to 48 hours, the antigen solution is administered intravenously. In a positive reaction, each injection site will show an immediate inflammatory response. The injected antibodies may remain fixed in the skin for a very long period. In the case of the calf, this may be up to 8 weeks. Because it is sometimes difficult to detect very mild inflammatory responses, they can be made more visible by injecting the test animal intravenously with Evans blue dye. The dye binds to serum albumin and does not normally leave the bloodstream. At injection sites where vascular permeability is increased, the dye-labeled albumin enters the tissue fluid and forms a striking blue patch (Figure 28-20).

Serological methods of measuring the level of specific IgE in body fluids include the RAST (radioallergosorbent test), Western blotting, and ELISA (Chapter 41). These are not subject to clinical bias, but there has been a poor correlation between the results obtained by serology or skin testing and

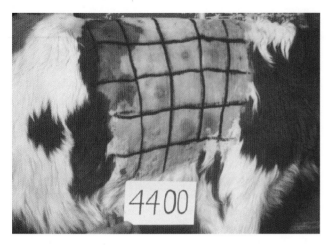

FIGURE 28-20 PCA reactions in a calf. Several different sera were tested for PCA activity on the flank of a normal calf.

(Courtesy Dr. P. Eyre.)

clinical severity. There is also a poor correlation between ELISA results and intradermal testing. Serological assays are especially prone to a high level of false-positive results (low specificity). A negative ELISA will generally rule out atopy. Best results are obtained by testing for individual allergens rather than groups of allergens. The reasons for this poor correlation between direct IgE measurements and in vivo methods such as skin testing are debatable but probably reflect the fact that the skin microenvironment is much more complex than in the bloodstream. Heavily parasitized dogs may have elevated IgE levels, and this may result in false-positive serological results. It is also possible that immunoglobulins of classes other than IgE may contribute to the development of allergic dermatitis in the dog. For these reasons many veterinary dermatologists prefer skin testing.

Treatment of Type I Hypersensitivity

By far the most satisfactory treatment of allergic disease is avoidance of exposure to the allergen. Other treatments such as allergen-specific immunotherapy may also be used. This has the potential to induce stable, long-term remissions, but is not a substitute for avoidance. The principal indications for drug therapy include short-term temporary relief either while waiting to begin immunotherapy or while waiting for it to take effect. Drugs may also be useful for relief of transient recurrences or in animals in which immunotherapy is not possible. Many different drugs are available to treat type I hypersensitivity, although veterinarians tend to employ only a few of these. Corticosteroids are most commonly used to reduce the

irritation and inflammation associated with the acute allergic response. These drugs can suppress all aspects of inflammation by inhibiting NF-κB and blocking the production of inflammatory mediators (Chapter 3). Corticosteroids have a considerable palliative effect on chronic type I hypersensitivities, but it is important to remember that these steroids can have serious side effects. They can be immunosuppressive and increase susceptibility to infection (Chapter 39).

The β stimulants include epinephrine, isoprenaline, and salbutamol; α antagonists include methoxamine and phenylephrine. All have been used extensively in humans and are available for use in animals. Epinephrine is the most important drug used to treat anaphylaxis. It is rapidly absorbed following intramuscular injection and thus can rapidly reverse the clinical signs of shock. Another group of drugs widely employed in the treatment of type I hypersensitivity reactions are the specific pharmacological inhibitors. These drugs, by mimicking the structure of the active mediators, competitively block specific receptors. Thus H1 antihistamines such as diphenhydramine can effectively inhibit the activities of histamine. However, since histamine is but one of a large number of mast cell–derived mediators, antihistamines possess limited effectiveness in controlling hypersensitivity diseases in animals.

A multifaceted approach has been recommended for the treatment of atopic dermatitis. Acute flares may be treated with a combination of skin baths and topical corticosteroids, with oral corticosteroids and antibiotics as needed. Skin hygiene should be improved as much as possible. The severity of the pruritus may be reduced with combinations of antiinflammatory drugs. These include oral and topical corticosteroids and calcineurin inhibitors such as oral cyclosporine and topical tacrolimus. Allergen-specific immunotherapy should be offered when feasible.

Allergen-Specific Immunotherapy

Allergies may be controlled by allergen-specific immunotherapy. This involves administering gradually increasing quantities of an allergen to the animal in order to reduce the severity of subsequent allergic disease. Multiple controlled studies have shown that this therapy is effective in humans. It appears to be most effective for the treatment of allergic rhinitis (hay fever), asthma, and allergies to insect stings. Its effectiveness is less clear in the treatment of food allergies and allergic dermatitis. In veterinary medicine multiple open studies have suggested that this therapy is effective in the treatment of atopic dermatitis, although few randomized controlled trials have been published.

Immunotherapy injections promote IgG rather than IgE production and reduce the recruitment of inflammatory cells. In humans, this reduces mast cell and eosinophil numbers in the lung, as well as the infiltration of CD4+ T cells and eosinophils in the skin. It induces a shift in the dominant helper cell

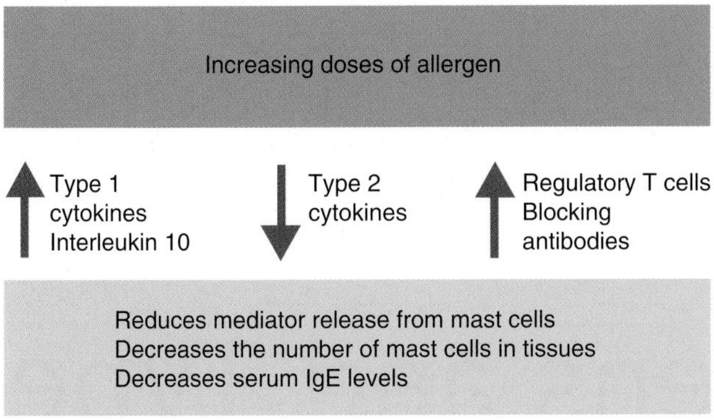

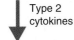

Increasing doses of allergen

↑ Type 1 cytokines Interleukin 10

↓ Type 2 cytokines

↑ Regulatory T cells Blocking antibodies

Reduces mediator release from mast cells
Decreases the number of mast cells in tissues
Decreases serum IgE levels

FIGURE 28-21 The principles of allergen-specific immunotherapy. Increasing doses of allergen promote a Th1 response, while at the same time reducing the Th2 response and regulating antibody production.

response from Th2 to Th1 (Figure 28-21). For example, the IFN-γ/IL-4 ratio is low in atopic dogs, indicating a Th2 cytokine profile. After immunotherapy, the ratio rises, IFN-γ levels increase, and the balance shifts toward a Th1 response. This IFN-γ reduces the effects of Th2 cells on IgE antibody synthesis and shift allergen-specific immunoglobulin production from IgE to IgG. Immunotherapy may also induce dendritic cell production of IL-12 and IL-18, and promote Th1 responses. It also stimulates Tregs to produce IL-10, inhibiting IgE production, mast cell activation, and histamine and leukotriene release.

In immunotherapy, small amounts of dilute aqueous solutions of antigen are administered. The first injections contain very little allergen. Over a number of weeks, the dose is gradually increased. If an animal's allergy is of the seasonal type, the course of injections should be timed to reach completion just before the anticipated antigen exposure. It has been estimated that up to 80% of dogs have a good to excellent response to this procedure. This includes clinical improvement and a reduction in the amount of medication required. It may take several months before the benefits of immunotherapy become apparent. Cats may respond even better than dogs. On the other hand, horses with hypersensitivity to biting flies have a poor response to immunotherapy .

For sources of additional information, please visit http://evolve.elsevier.com/tizard/immunology/

29

Red Cell Antigens and Type II Hypersensitivity

Key Points

- Type II hypersensitivity, also called cytotoxic hypersensitivity, occurs when antibodies (and complement) destroy normal cells.
- The destruction of transfused red blood cells when administered to a mismatched recipient is an example of type II hypersensitivity. The resulting disease is due to the lysis of the transfused red cells by antibodies and complement.
- Mothers may become sensitized by their fetus during pregnancy and make antibodies against fetal red cells. These antibodies, if ingested in colostrum, may cause destruction of a newborn animal's red cells. This is called hemolytic disease of the newborn.
- Some vaccines may induce anti-MHC antibodies in cows. If ingested in mother's colostrum, these antibodies may cause a lethal pancytopenia in their calves.
- Some drugs may bind to blood cells and make them targets of antibodies in a type II hypersensitivity reaction.

Red cells, like nucleated cells, express cell surface molecules that can act as antigens. However, unlike the major histocompatibility complex (MHC) molecules, red cell surface antigens are not involved in antigen processing, although they do influence graft rejection (allografts between blood group–incompatible animals are rapidly rejected.) Most red cell surface antigens are either glycoproteins or glycolipids and are integral functional components of the cell membrane. For example, the ABO antigens in humans are anion and glucose transporter proteins, whereas the antigens of the M and C systems of sheep red cells are associated with the membrane potassium pump and amino acid transport, respectively.

If blood is transfused from one animal to another, genetically different individuals, the red cell antigens will stimulate an antibody response in the recipient. These antibodies cause the rapid elimination of the transfused red cells as a result of intravascular hemolysis by complement and of extravascular destruction through opsonization and removal by the mononuclear phagocyte system. Cell destruction by antibodies in this way is classified as a type II hypersensitivity reaction.

Blood Groups

The antigens expressed on the surface of red blood cells are called blood group antigens or erythrocyte antigens (EAs). There are many different blood group antigens, and they vary in their antigenicity, some being more potent and therefore of greater importance than others. The expression of blood group antigens is controlled by genes and inherited in conventional fashion. For each blood group system, there exists a variable number of alleles. (If blood group alleles are invariably inherited together in groups of two or more, they are called phenogroups.) The alleles, in turn, control a variable number of EAs. The complexity of erythrocyte blood group systems varies greatly. They range from simple systems like the L system of cattle, which consists of two alleles controlling a single antigen, to the highly complex B system of cattle. The B system contains several hundred alleles or phenogroups that, together with the other cattle blood groups, may yield millions of unique blood group combinations. Although most blood group antigens are integral cell membrane components, some are soluble molecules found free in serum, saliva, and other body fluids and passively adsorbed onto red cell surfaces. Examples of such soluble antigens include the J antigens of cattle, the R antigens of sheep, the A antigens of pigs, and the DEA 7 antigens of dogs.

Animals may possess antibodies against foreign blood group antigens even though they may never have been exposed to foreign red cells. For example, J-negative cattle have anti-J antibodies in their serum, and A-negative pigs have anti-A antibodies. These "natural" antibodies (or isoantibodies) are derived not from previous contact with foreign red cells but from exposure to cross-reacting epitopes that are commonly encountered in nature (see Figure 9-8). Many blood group antigens are also common structural components of plants, the intestinal microbiota, protozoa, or helminths. The presence of these natural antibodies is not, however, a uniform phenomenon, and not all blood group antigens are accompanied by the production of natural antibodies to their alternative alleles.

Blood Transfusion and Incompatible Transfusions

Blood is easily transfused from one animal to another. If the donor red cells are identical to those of the recipient, no immune response results. If, however, the recipient possesses preexisting antibodies to donor red cell antigens, they will be attacked immediately. These preexisting antibodies are usually of the immunoglobulin M (IgM) class. When these antibodies bind red cell antigens, they may cause agglutination or

hemolysis, or stimulate opsonization and phagocytosis of the transfused cells. In the absence of preexisting antibodies, the transfused red cells will stimulate an immune response in the recipient. The transfused cells will circulate until antibodies are produced and will then be eliminated. A second transfusion with identical foreign cells results in their immediate destruction.

The rapid destruction of large numbers of foreign red cells can lead to serious illness. The severity of transfusion reactions ranges from a mild febrile response to rapid death and depends mainly on the amount of incompatible blood transfused. Early recognition of a problem may avert the most severe consequences. The most severe reactions occur when large amounts of incompatible blood are transfused to a sensitized recipient. This results in complement activation and hemolysis of the transfused cells. Large amounts of free hemoglobin escape, resulting in hemoglobinemia and hemoglobinuria. Large numbers of lysed red cells may trigger blood clotting and disseminated intravascular coagulation. Complement activation also results in anaphylatoxin production, mast cell degranulation, and the release of vasoactive molecules and cytokines. These molecules provoke circulatory shock with hypotension, bradycardia, and apnea. The animal may show sympathetic responses such as sweating, salivation, lacrimation, diarrhea, and vomiting. This may be followed by a second stage in which the animal is hypertensive, with cardiac arrhythmia as well as increased heart and respiratory rates.

If a reaction is suspected, the transfusion must be stopped immediately. It is important to maintain urine flow with fluids and a diuretic because accumulation of hemoglobin in the kidneys may cause renal tubular destruction. Recovery follows elimination of the foreign red cells.

Transfusion reactions can be almost totally prevented by prior testing of the recipient's serum for antibodies against the donor's red cells. The test is called cross-matching. Blood from the donor is centrifuged and the plasma discarded. The red cells are then resuspended in saline and recentrifuged. This washing procedure is repeated (usually three times), and eventually a 2% to 4% suspension of red cells in saline is made. These donor red cells are mixed with recipient serum and then incubated at 37° C for 15 to 30 minutes. If the red cells are lysed or agglutinated by the recipient's serum, no transfusion should be attempted with those cells. It is occasionally found that the donor's serum may react with the recipient's red cells. This is not of major clinical significance because transfused donor antibodies are rapidly diluted within the recipient. Nevertheless, blood giving such a reaction is best avoided.

Hemolytic Disease of the Newborn

Female animals may become sensitized to foreign red cells not only by incompatible blood transfusions given for clinical purposes but also by leakage of fetal red cells into their bloodstream through the placenta during pregnancy. In sensitized females, these anti–red cell antibodies may then be concentrated in their colostrum. When a newborn animal suckles, these colostral antibodies are absorbed through the intestinal wall and reach its circulation. These antibodies, directed against the blood group antigens of the newborn, cause rapid destruction of their red cells. The resulting disease is called hemolytic disease of the newborn (HDN) or neonatal isoerythrolysis.

Four conditions must be met for HDN to occur: The young animal must inherit a red cell antigen from its sire that is not present in its mother. The mother must be sensitized to this red cell antigen. The mother's response to this antigen must be boosted repeatedly by transplacental hemorrhage or repeated pregnancies. Finally, a newborn animal must ingest colostrum containing high-titered antibodies to its red cells.

Blood Groups, Blood Transfusion, and Hemolytic Disease in Domestic Animals

All mammals possess red cell antigens that can affect blood transfusions and on occasion cause HDN in newborn animals (Table 29-1). Although historically they were named alphabetically in order of their discovery, there is a growing tendency to add the prefix EA (erythrocyte antigen) to reduce confusion with MHC antigens.

□ **Table 29-1 | Domestic Animal Blood Groups**

SPECIES	BLOOD GROUP SYSTEMS	SEROLOGY
Horse	EAA, C, D, K, P, Q, U	Agglutination Hemolytic
Bovine	EAA, B, C, F, J*, L, M, R*, S, Z, T′	Hemolytic
Sheep	EAA, B, C, D, M, R*	Hemolytic Agglutination (D only)
Pig	EAA*, B, C, D, E, F, G, H, I, J, K, L, M, N, O, P	Agglutination Hemolytic Antiglobulin
Dog	DEA 1.1, 1.2, 3, 4, 5, 6, 7*, 8	Agglutination Hemolytic Antiglobulin
Cat	AB	Agglutination Hemolytic

*Soluble blood group substances.

Horses

Horses possess seven internationally recognized blood group systems (EAA, EAC, EAD, EAK, EAP, EAQ, and EAU.) Some, such as EAC, EAK, and EAU, are simple, one-factor, two-allele, two-phenotype systems. On the other hand, the EAD system is very complex, with at least 25 alleles identified to date. Their major significance lies in the fact that HDN in foals is relatively common (Figure 29-1). In mules, in which the antigenic differences between dam and sire are great, about 8% to 10% of foals may be affected. In thoroughbreds and standardbreds, the prevalence is considerably less, ranging from 0.05% to 2% of foals. This is despite of the fact that in up to 14% of pregnancies, the mare and the stallion have incompatible red cells.

HDN may occur in foals from mares that have been sensitized by previous blood transfusions or by administration of vaccines containing equine tissues. Most commonly, however, mares are sensitized by exposure to fetal red cells as a result of repeated pregnancies. The mechanism of this sensitization is unclear, but fetal red cells are assumed to gain access to the maternal circulation as a result of transplacental hemorrhage. Mares have been shown to respond to fetal red cells as early as day 56 after conception. The greatest leakage probably occurs during the last month of pregnancy and during foaling as a result of the breakdown of placental blood vessels.

Maternal sensitization is usually minimal following a first pregnancy. However, if repeated pregnancies result in exposure to the same red cell antigens, the maternal response will be boosted. Hemolytic disease is therefore usually only a problem in mares that have had several foals. The most severe form of the disease results from the production of antibodies directed against the Aa antigen of the EAA system. Anti-Qa (EAQ system) produces a less severe disease of slower onset. All in all, 90% of clinical cases are attributable to anti-Aa and -Qa, although other minor antigens, such as Pa, Ab, Qc, Ua, Dc, and Db, have also been implicated. Mares that lack Aa and Qa are therefore most likely to produce affected foals. Pregnant mares may also produce antibodies to Ca (EAC system), but these are rarely associated with clinical disease. Indeed preexisting antibodies to Ca may reduce sensitization by Aa. The presence of this anti-Ca in a mare may eliminate foal red cells that enter her bloodstream and prevent further sensitization.

Antibodies produced by mares do not cross the placenta but reach the foal through the colostrum. Affected foals are therefore born healthy but sicken several hours after suckling. The severity of the disease is determined by the amount of antibody absorbed and by the sensitizing antigen. The earliest signs are weakness and depression. The mucous membranes of affected foals may be pale and may eventually show a distinct jaundice. Some foals sicken by 6 to 8 hours and die from shock so rapidly that they may not have time to develop jaundice. More commonly the disease presents as lethargy and weakness between 12 and 48 hours of age, although it may be delayed for as long as 5 days. Icterus of the mucous membranes and sclera is consistent in foals that survive for at least 48 hours.

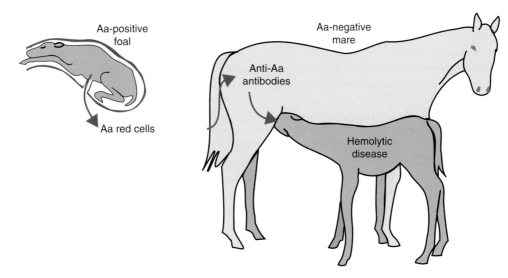

FIGURE 29-1 The pathogenesis of hemolytic disease of the newborn in foals. In the first stage, fetal lymphocytes leak into the mother's circulation and sensitize her. In the second stage, these antibodies are concentrated in colostrum and are then ingested by the suckling foal. These ingested antibodies enter the foal's circulation and cause red cell destruction.

Hemoglobinuria, although uncommon, is diagnostic in a newborn foal. As a result of anoxia, some foals in the terminal stages of the disease may convulse or become comatose. The most common causes of death in these foals are liver failure, brain damage, and bacterial sepsis.

Hemolytic disease is readily diagnosed by clinical signs alone. Hematological examination is of little diagnostic use but may be of assistance in indicating appropriate treatment. Definitive diagnosis requires that immunoglobulin be demonstrated on the surface of the red cells of the foal. In the case of anti-Aa or anti-Qa, addition of a source of complement (fresh normal rabbit serum) causes rapid hemolysis. If hemolytic disease is anticipated, the serum of a pregnant mare may be tested for antibodies by an indirect antiglobulin test. By using red cells from horses with a major sensitizing blood group, it is possible to show that the antibody titer increases significantly in the month before parturition when sensitization is occurring.

A test that may be useful for detecting the presence of antierythrocyte antibodies in colostrum is the jaundiced foal agglutination test. This involves making serial dilutions of colostrum in saline. A drop of anticoagulated foal blood is added to each tube, and the tubes are centrifuged so that the red cells form pellets at the bottom. In the presence of antibodies, the cells clump tightly, and the pellets remain intact when the tubes are emptied. Nonagglutinated red cells, in contrast, flow down the side of the tube. Concentrated colostrum is viscous and tends to induce rouleaux formation that mimics agglutination. However, if the mare's blood is used as a negative control, this can be accounted for. The foal's blood should also be diluted in saline to ensure that the foal has not already absorbed antibodies and that false-positive results are not obtained.

Mildly affected foals, with a packed cell volume (PCV) of 15% to 25% and a red cell count greater than 4×10^6, will continue to nurse. Those with a PCV of less than 10% will stop nursing and become recumbent. Marked icterus is suggestive of HDN in foals, but mild icterus may be seen in septicemia despite the fact that septic foals are not anemic.

The prognosis of uncomplicated hemolytic disease is good provided the condition is diagnosed sufficiently early and the appropriate treatment instituted rapidly. Management of HDN includes prevention of further antibody absorption, adequate nutrition, oxygen therapy, fluid and electrolyte therapy, and maintenance of the acid-base balance. Warmth, adequate hydration, and antimicrobial therapy are also critically important. In acute cases, blood transfusion is necessary. A red cell count of less than $3 \times 10^6/\mu L$ or a PCV of less than 15% warrants a blood transfusion. Transfused equine red cells have a half-life of only 2 to 4 days, so transfusion is only a temporary life-saving measure. Compatible blood may be difficult to find because of the high prevalence of Aa and Qa in the normal equine population. A donor should not only be Aa or Qa negative but should also lack antibodies to these antigens. Exchange transfusion, although efficient, requires a donor capable of providing at least 5 L of blood as well as a double intravenous catheter and an anesthetized foal. A much simpler procedure that avoids many difficulties is transfusion of washed cells from the mare. About 3 to 4 L of blood is collected in sodium citrate and centrifuged, after which the plasma is discarded. The red cells are washed once in saline and transfused slowly into the foal. The blood is usually given in divided doses about 6 hours apart. Milder cases of hemolytic disease may require only careful nursing.

If hemolytic disease is anticipated as a result of either a rising antibody titer or the previous birth of a hemolytic foal, stripping off the mare's colostrum and giving the foal colostrum from another mare may prevent its occurrence. The foal should not be allowed to suckle its mare for 24 to 36 hours. Once suckling is permitted, the foal should only be allowed to take small quantities at first and should be observed carefully for adverse side effects.

Neonatal thrombocytopenia has been recorded in the foal. Immunoglobulins can be identified on the foal's platelets, and antibodies to these platelets can be found in the mare's serum.

Serological Testing Horse blood groups may be identified by agglutination, hemolytic, and antiglobulin tests. Each blood group system has a preferred test system. The complement used in the hemolytic test comes from rabbits, but it must be absorbed before use to remove any antihorse antibodies.

Cattle

Eleven blood group systems—EAA, EAB, EAC, EAF, EAJ, EAL, EAM, EAR′, EAS, EAT′, and EAZ—have been identified in cattle. Two of these (EAB and EAJ) are of the greatest importance. The EAB blood group system is one of the most complex systems known since it is estimated to contain more than 60 different alleles. These alleles are not inherited independently but rather in combinations called phenogroups. Because of the complexity of the EAB system, it is practically impossible to obtain absolutely identical blood from any two unrelated cattle. Indeed, it has been suggested that the complexity of the EAB system is such that there exist sufficient different antigenic combinations to provide a unique identifying character for each bovine in the world. Naturally, such a system provides an ideal method for the accurate identification of individual animals, and many breed societies use blood grouping to check the identity of registered animals. The EAC system is also complex, with 10 alleles combining to form about 90 phenogroups.

The J antigen is a lipid found free in body fluids and passively adsorbed onto red cells. It is absent from the red cells of newborn calves but is acquired within the first 6 months of life. J-positive cattle are of two types. Some possess J antigen in high concentration, and this may be detected both on their red cells and in serum. Other animals may have low levels of J in serum, and it is detected only with great difficulty on red cells. (It is probable that a secretor gene controls the expression of J in cattle). J-negative cattle, lacking the J antigen completely, may possess natural anti-J antibodies, although the level of these antibodies shows a marked seasonal variation, being highest in the summer and fall. Because of the presence of these antibodies, transfusion of J-positive red cells into J-negative recipients may result in a transfusion reaction even in the absence of known previous sensitization.

HDN in calves is rare but has resulted from vaccination against anaplasmosis or babesiosis. Some of these vaccines contain red cells from infected calves. In the case of *Anaplasma* vaccines, for example, the blood from a large number of infected donors is pooled, freeze-dried, and mixed with adjuvant before being administered to cattle. The vaccine against babesiosis consists of fresh, infected calf blood. Both vaccines cause infection and, consequently, the development of immunity in recipients. They may also stimulate the production of antibodies against blood group antigens of the EAA and EAF systems. Cows sensitized by these vaccines and then mated with bulls carrying the same blood groups can transmit colostral antibodies to their calves, which may then develop hemolytic disease.

The clinical signs of HDN in calves are related to the amount of colostrum ingested. Calves are usually healthy at birth but begin to show symptoms from 12 hours to 5 days later. In acute cases, death may occur within 24 hours after suckling, with the animals developing respiratory distress and hemoglobinuria. On necropsy, these calves have severe pulmonary edema, splenomegaly, and dark kidneys. Less severely affected animals develop anemia and jaundice and may die during the first week of life. The red cells of affected calves have antibodies on their surface (detected by an antiglobulin test) and may sometimes be lysed by the addition of complement in the form of fresh normal rabbit serum. Death is due to disseminated intravascular coagulation as a result of activation of the clotting system by red cell ghosts.

Serological Testing Bovine blood groups are detected by hemolytic tests. Washed red cells are incubated in specific antisera, and rabbit serum is used as a source of complement.

Bovine neonatal pancytopenia Beginning in 2007, multiple outbreaks of an unexplained hemorrhagic disease of newborn beef calves have been reported from many countries in Western Europe. It is called bovine neonatal pancytopenia. Affected calves show sudden-onset bleeding, including nasal hemorrhage, petechiation on mucus membranes, internal bleeding and excessive bleeding from minor wounds such as injection or ear-tag sites. These calves may die within 48 hours of disease onset. Clinical investigation shows a profound pancytopenia, including a thrombocytopenia, anemia, and leucopenia. The bone marrow may be completely aplastic. Mortality may be as high as 90% in clinically affected calves but there are clearly many subclinical cases as well. Since the disease only occurs in suckled calves and develops within hours of suckling, it appears to result from the consumption of colostrum. Studies have now shown that the colostrum of cows known to produce affected calves contains antibodies directed against the surface MHC class I antigens of neonatal leukocytes and bone marrow stem cells. These antibodies are not present in the serum or colostrum of cows producing healthy calves. The antibodies mediate phagocytosis of blood cells since they bind both the α chain of MHC class I antigens and β2-microglobulin.

Epidemiologic analysis has traced the cause of this disease to use of a specific bovine virus diarrhea vaccine (BVD) in cows. This vaccine contains inactivated cytopathogenic BVDV grown on bovine kidney cells. A potent, oil-in-water adjuvant containing Quil A is added (Chapter 23). Immunization with the vaccine or the kidney cells alone induces high levels of anti-MHC alloantibodies in cattle. These antibodies, if transferred to calves via colostrum bind to leukocytes and bone

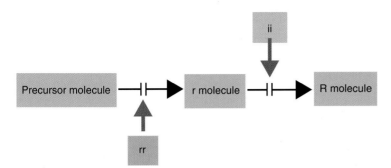

FIGURE 29-2 The regulation of expression of EAR blood group antigens in sheep. The *I* gene controls expression of the EAR system.

marrow stem cells and so induce pancytopenia and bone marrow destruction. Not all calves born from mothers that received this specific vaccine develop pancytopenia. The reasons for this are unknown but perhaps depend upon the mother's MHC class I haplotype.

Sheep

The blood groups of sheep resemble those of cattle. Six blood group systems (EAA, EAB, EAC, EAD, EAM, and EAR) are currently recognized. The ovine equivalent of bovine EAB is also termed EAB and, like the bovine system, is complex, containing at least 52 different alleles. Sheep also possess an ovine equivalent of the bovine EAJ system, called the EAR system. Two soluble antigens are found in this system, R and O, coded for by alleles R and r. The production of R and O substances is controlled by a gene called *I* and its recessive allele i. If a sheep is homozygous for i, it expresses neither R nor O antigens. This interaction between the I/i genes and the R-O system is called an epistatic effect (Figure 29-2). R and O antigens are soluble antigens found in the serum of II or Ii sheep and are passively adsorbed onto red cells. Natural anti-R antibodies may be found in R-negative sheep. Sheep also fall into two groups according to whether their red cells have high or low potassium levels. This is regulated by the EAM blood group system. The Mb antigen is an inhibitor of potassium transport.

Serological Testing Sheep blood groups are detected by hemolytic tests. One exception to this rule is the EAD system, which is detected by agglutination.

Pigs

Sixteen pig blood group systems have been identified (EAA to EAP). Of these, the most important is the EAA system. The EAA system, like the human ABO system, controls the expression of two carbohydrate antigens, A and O, through the use of glycosyltransferases. Their expression is regulated by a gene called *S* (secretor) with two alleles S and s. In the homozygous recessive state (ss), this gene can prevent the production of the A and O substances (Figure 29-3). As a result, the amount of these antigens bound to red cells in these animals is reduced to an undetectable level (Box 29-1). A and O substances, like

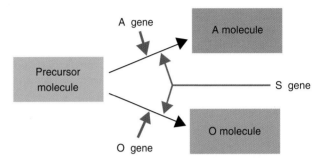

FIGURE 29-3 The production of A or O blood group substances by a pig requires the presence of the *S* gene. Pigs that lack this gene (ss animals) produce neither of these blood group substances.

□ **Box 29-1 | Inheritance of the EAA Blood Group System in Pigs**

In pigs, the expression of the EAA blood group is regulated by two gene loci. One locus, the A locus, contains two alleles, A and O, of which A is dominant. The other, the S locus, also contains two alleles, S and its recessive allele s. The S locus controls the expression of the A system so that A or O blood groups can only be expressed if the animal carries at least one S gene. Possible genotypes are, therefore, AA, AO, and OO, as well as SS, Ss and ss. These may be combined thus:

- Animals that are AASS, AASs, AOSS, or AOSs will have A red cells.
- Animals that are OOSS or OOSs will have O red cells.
- Animals that are AAss, Aoss, or Ooss will express neither A nor O and so will have "null" red cells.

J in cattle and R and O in sheep, are not true red cell antigens but rather are soluble carbohydrates found in serum and passively adsorbed onto red cells after birth. Natural anti-A antibodies may occur in A-negative pigs, and transfusion of A-positive blood into such an animal may cause transient collapse and hemoglobinuria.

HDN in piglets formerly occurred as a result of the use of hog cholera vaccine containing pig blood. This vaccine consisted of pooled blood from viremic pigs inactivated with the dye crystal violet. Sensitization of sows by this vaccine led to the occasional occurrence of hemolytic disease of their off-spring. There appeared to be a breed predisposition to this disease, which was most commonly seen in the offspring of Essex and Wessex sows. Affected piglets did not necessarily show clinical disease, although their red cells were sensitized by antibody. Other piglets showed rapidly progressive weakness and pallor of mucous membranes preceding death, and those animals that survived longest showed hemoglobinuria and jaundice. The severity of the reaction did not appear to be directly related to the anti–red cell antibody titer in the piglet serum. Since the withdrawal of all live hog cholera virus vaccines, the problems associated with their use have disappeared.

True HDN has also been recorded in the pig. The antibodies responsible are usually directed against antigens of the EAE system. In addition to the development of hemolytic anemia in newborn piglets, the presence of antibodies to platelet antigens may cause a thrombocytopenia. This is seen clinically as a bleeding problem on tail docking and a tendency to bruise easily (neonatal purpura). On blood smears, the platelets may be clumped, and antiglobulin testing of them will yield a positive result. Deprivation of colostrum in an attempt to prevent piglets from absorbing anti–red cell antibodies may result in the newborn animals being highly susceptible to infection.

Serological Testing Pig blood groups are detected by agglutination, hemolytic, and antiglobulin tests.

Dogs

In dogs, eight red cell antigens are internationally recognized (DEA 1.1, 1.2, 3, 4, 5, 6, 7, 8), but five others have been described. (An older nomenclature called them by the traditional alphabetic system, A, Tr, B, C, D, F, J, K, L, M, and N.) Most of these appear to be inherited as simple mendelian dominants. Only the DEA 1 antigens are sufficiently antigenic to be of clinical significance. These include both alleles 1.1 and 1.2. About 60% of dogs express a DEA 1 antigen. Naturally occurring antibodies to DEA 1.1 and 1.2 do not occur. Antibodies to DEA 7 may occur in 20% to 50% of DEA 7–negative dogs. Antibodies to DEA 3 and 5 are found in about 10% of negative dogs, but these are usually of low titer and not of clinical significance. Therefore, it is recommended that canine blood donors be negative for DEA 1.1, 1.2, 3, 5, and 7. More than 98% of the canine population is DEA 4 positive. A universal donor would be an animal negative for all the DEA groups except DEA 4. Unless the blood type of the recipient is known, universal donor blood should only be used and a cross-match performed on all recipients. In practice, the most important canine blood type is DEA 1.1. About 33% to 45% of the dog population is DEA 1.1 positive, and in general these dogs can be considered to be universal recipients. Dogs that are DEA 1.1 negative can also be considered to be universal donors. DEA 1.1–positive blood should never be transfused into a DEA 1.1–negative dog. If so, the recipient will become sensitized to DEA 1.1, and high-titered antibodies will be produced. Subsequent transfusion of positive blood into such an animal could lead to a severe reaction. Similarly, if a negative bitch is sensitized by incompatible transfusions and mated to a positive dog, hemolytic disease may occur in her puppies. Natural HDN in dogs is extremely rare. It occurs when a DEA 1.1–negative breeding bitch is transfused with DEA 1.1–positive blood and subsequently bred to a DEA 1.1–positive male. The puppies develop a hemolytic anemia after 3 to 10 days.

The DEA 7 system (Tr system) is a soluble antigen system antigenically related to the human A, cattle J, sheep R, and pig A systems. Two antigens belong to the system—Tr and O. An epistatic secretor gene controls their expression. Anti–DEA 7 occurs naturally in some DEA 7–negative dogs. When healthy female dogs with a prior history of pregnancies were examined, the only alloantibodies detected were directed against DEA 7. However, the prevalence of these antibodies was similar in dogs with a prior history of pregnancy and control dogs. This suggests that pregnancy does not sensitize dogs to alloantigens and that females with a prior pregnancy can be employed as blood donors.

A blood group antigen called Dal has been identified on the basis of antibodies produced in Dalmatians following blood transfusion. Presumably some Dalmatians lack this antigen, which is present in other dog breeds.

Serological Testing Agglutination at 4° C and hemolytic and antiglobulin tests have been used for the detection of canine blood groups. The source of complement can be either fresh dog or rabbit serum. There are several commercial blood typing kits available for dogs. One is a card agglutination test that uses monoclonal DEA 1.1 antibodies to detect positive dogs. The other is an immunochromatographic technique (Chapter 41). This test uses a monoclonal antibody against DEA 1.1 to detect the antigen in a blood sample.

Cats

In cats, only one major blood group system, the AB system, has been reported. The AB antigens are glycolipids. Cats may be A, B, or AB. A is completely dominant over B. About 75% to 95% of cats are A positive, about 5% to 25% are B positive, and less than 1% are AB. However, this distribution differs among countries and among different purebred cat breeds. In the United States more than 99% of domestic short-hair and long-hair cats are type A, whereas in the United Kingdom only about 40% of short-hair breeds are type A. Severe transfusion reactions have been described in group B cats that received very small quantities of group A blood since 95% of B cats possess IgM anti-A. (Interestingly, only about 35% of A cats possess anti-B, and it is of the IgG and IgM classes and of much lower titer.) If completely matched blood is transfused into cats, its half-life is about 4 to 5 weeks. If, however, group B blood is transfused into cats of blood group A, its half-life is only a few days. If group A blood is transfused into a cat of blood group B, its half-life is just over 1 hour. It is this very rapid destruction that results in severe clinical reactions. Thus a group B cat given as little as 1 mL of group A blood will go into shock, with hypotension, apnea, and atrioventricular block, within a few minutes. Cross-matching is essential in this species.

Occasionally, hemolytic transfusion reactions occur between AB blood group–matched cats. These appear to be due to natural antibodies against a blood group antigen called Mik. Its mode of inheritance is undefined.

HDN has been recorded in Persian and related (Himalayan) breeds but is very rare. It occurs in kittens from queens of blood group B bred to sires of blood group A. The queens subsequently develop high-titered anti-A antibodies. Although healthy at birth, these kittens develop severe anemia as a result of intravascular hemolysis. Affected kittens show depression and possibly hemoglobinuria. Necropsy may reveal splenomegaly and jaundice. Antibodies to the sire's and the kitten's red cells are detectable in the queen's serum.

Serological Testing Agglutination and immunochromatographic tests are used for feline blood typing. Serum from type B cats has strong anti-A activity. Anti-B reagents can use the lectin from *Triticum vulgaris* (wheat germ) or increasingly, monoclonal antibodies. The agglutination tests can be performed in several different formats, such as in tubes, on cards, in matrix gels, or on glass slides. Results are comparable. (Matrix gel agglutination relies on performing the agglutination test on top of a viscous gel layer. Nonagglutinated red cells will sink through the gel, whereas agglutinated cells will remain on top.)

Humans

In humans, HDN is due almost entirely to immunization of the mother against the antigens of the Rhesus (Rh) system (now classified as CD240). The condition is, or should be, of historical interest only because a very simple but effective technique is available for its prevention. This depends on preventing an Rh-negative mother from reacting to the Rh-positive fetal red cells that escape from the placenta into her circulation at birth. Strong human anti-Rh globulin is obtained from male volunteers and given to mothers at risk soon after birth. It acts by specifically inhibiting the B cell response to that antigen (Chapter 20). Routine use of this material therefore prevents maternal sensitization, antibody production, and hemolytic disease. The use of a similar system in the domestic mammals is unnecessary because deprivation of colostrum is sufficient to prevent the disease.

Parentage Testing

Under some circumstances it is necessary to confirm the parentage of an animal. One way of doing this is by examining the blood group antigens of an animal and its alleged parents (Table 29-2). The method is based on the principle that since blood group antigens are inherited, they must be present on the red cells of one or both parents. If a blood group antigen

□ **Table 29-2 | Use of Blood Groups to Assign Paternity**

	BLOOD GROUP				
	DEA 1.1	**DEA 1.2**	**DEA 6**	**DEA 7**	**DEA 8**
Sire 1 ?	+	+	−	+	−
Sire 2 ?	+	+	−	−	+
Dam	−	−	+	+	−
Puppy 1	+	+	−	+	−
2	+	+	−	+	−
3	−	−	−	+	+*
4	−	−	+	+	−

*This puppy possesses DEA 8, which could not have come from sire 1 or its dam. Sire 1 could not have sired this litter.
Courtesy Dr. D. Colling.

is present in a tested animal but absent from both its putative parents, parentage must be reassigned. Similarly, if one parent is homozygous for a specific blood group antigen, this antigen must inevitably appear in the offspring. However, it must be recognized that blood typing procedures can only exclude, never prove, parentage.

Hemophagocytic Syndrome

Hemophagocytic syndrome is a disorder of activated macrophages associated with multiple cytopenias in the blood. These cytopenias result from hemophagocytosis and probably reflect excessive phagocytic activity by macrophages. The syndrome has been described in humans, dogs, and cats. In humans it may be either inherited or acquired. In dogs, the syndrome has been reported as secondary to infectious, neoplastic, or immune-mediated diseases. Diagnostic criteria include the presence of pancytopenia or bicytopenia and the presence of greater than 2% hemophagocytic macrophages in a bone marrow aspirate. Most of these dogs have an underlying disease. About one third of canine cases are associated with immune-mediated diseases such as lupus or immune-mediated thrombocytopenia. These animals are commonly anemic, neutropenic, and thrombocytopenic, and it may be argued that autoantibodies opsonized the blood cells leading to their phagocytosis. Other affected dogs suffer from infectious diseases such as pyometra, pleuritis, ehrlichiosis, blastomycosis, or Lyme disease. In some cases affected dogs recover once their underlying infection is treated. The disease is also associated with some neoplastic diseases such as malignant lymphoma or myelodysplastic syndrome. Canine hemophagocytic syndrome may also occur in the absence of any obvious associated disease. Affected dogs are anemic, neutropenic, thrombocytopenic, febrile, anorexic, and lethargic. In humans this syndrome results from a natural killer (NK) cell deficiency or as a result of excessive macrophage activation resulting from oversecretion of Th1 cytokines.

Type II Hypersensitivity Reactions to Drugs

Red cells may be destroyed in drug hypersensitivities by three mechanisms. First, the drug and antibody may combine directly and activate complement, and red cells will be destroyed in a bystander effect as activated complement components bind to nearby cells.

Second, some drugs may bind to cell surface glycoproteins. For example, penicillin, quinine, L-dopa, aminosalicylic acid, and phenacetin may bind to red cells. Since these cells are then modified, they may be recognized as foreign and eliminated by antibodies, resulting in hemolytic anemia. Penicillin-induced hemolytic anemia is not uncommon in horses. These conditions can be suspected based on recent treatment with penicillin and improvement when its use is discontinued. It may also be possible to detect antibodies against penicillin or penicillin-coated red cells in these animals. Sulfonamides, phenylbutazone, aminopyrine, phenothiazine, and possibly chloramphenicol may cause agranulocytosis by binding to granulocytes, and phenylbutazone, quinine, chloramphenicol,

and sulfonamides can result in a thrombocytopenia as they bind to platelet surface glycoproteins. If the cells from animals experiencing these reactions are examined using a direct antiglobulin test, antibody may be demonstrated on their surface. If these antibodies are eluted, they can be directed not against the blood cells but against the offending drug.

Third, drugs such as the cephalosporins may modify red cell membranes in such a way that the cells passively adsorb antibodies and then are removed by phagocytic cells.

Type II Hypersensitivity in Infectious Diseases

Just as drugs can be adsorbed onto red cells and render them immunologically foreign, so too can bacterial antigens such as the lipopolysaccharides, viruses such as equine infectious anemia virus and Aleutian disease virus, bacteria such as *Anaplasma*, and protozoa such as the trypanosomes and *Babesia*. These altered red cells are regarded as foreign and are either lysed by antibody and complement or phagocytosed by mononuclear phagocytes. Clinically severe anemia is, therefore, characteristic of all these infections.

For sources of additional information, please visit http://evolve.elsevier.com/tizard/immunology/

30

Immune Complexes and Type III Hypersensitivity

Key Points

- When antigens and antibodies combine, they form immune complexes. Immune complexes can trigger severe inflammation when deposited in large amounts in tissues. This type of inflammation is classified as type III hypersensitivity.
- Local deposition of immune complexes in the lungs following inhalation of antigenic dusts causes hypersensitivity pneumonitis.
- Immune complexes formed in the bloodstream are deposited in the glomeruli of the kidney and cause membranoproliferative glomerulonephritis.
- Type III hypersensitivity is a feature of many viral diseases, especially if the virus is not neutralized by antibodies and large amounts of immune complexes are generated as a result.

Immune complexes formed by the combination of antibodies with antigen activate the classical complement pathway. When these immune complexes are deposited in tissues, the activated complement generates chemotactic peptides that attract neutrophils. The accumulated neutrophils may then release oxidants and enzymes, causing acute inflammation and tissue destruction. Lesions generated in this way are classified as type III or immune complex–mediated hypersensitivity reactions.

Classification of Type III Hypersensitivity Reactions

The severity and significance of type III hypersensitivity reactions depend, as might be expected, on the amount and site of deposition of immune complexes. Two major forms of reaction are recognized. One form includes local reactions that develop when immune complexes form within tissues. The second form results when large quantities of immune complexes form within the bloodstream. This can occur, for example, when an antigen is administered intravenously to an immune recipient. Immune complexes generated in the bloodstream are deposited in glomeruli in the kidney, and the development of glomerular lesions (glomerulonephritis) is characteristic of this type of hypersensitivity. If the complexes bind to blood cells, anemia, leukopenia, or thrombocytopenia may also result. Complexes may also be deposited in blood vessel walls to cause a vasculitis or in joints to cause arthritis.

It might reasonably be pointed out that the combination of an antigen with antibody always produces immune complexes. However, the occurrence of clinically significant type III hypersensitivity reactions results from the formation of excessive amounts of these immune complexes. For example, several grams of an antigen are needed to sensitize an animal, such as a rabbit, in order to produce experimental type III reactions. Minor immune complex–mediated lesions probably develop relatively frequently following an immune response to many antigens, without causing clinically significant disease.

Local Type III Hypersensitivity Reactions

If an antigen is injected subcutaneously into an animal that already has a very high level of antibodies in its bloodstream, acute inflammation will develop at the injection site within several hours. This is called an Arthus reaction after the scientist who first described it. It starts as a red, edematous swelling; eventually local hemorrhage and thrombosis occur; and if severe, it culminates in local tissue destruction.

The first events observed following antigen injection are neutrophil adherence to vascular endothelium followed by their emigration into the tissues. By 6 to 8 hours, when the

reaction has reached its greatest intensity, the injection site is densely infiltrated by large numbers of these cells (Figure 30-1). As the reaction progresses, destruction of blood vessel walls results in hemorrhage and edema, platelet aggregation, and thrombosis. By 8 hours, mononuclear cells appear in the lesion, and by 24 hours or later, depending on the amount of antigen injected, they become the predominant cell type. Eosinophils are not a significant feature of this type of hypersensitivity.

The fate of the injected antigen can be followed if is labeled with a fluorescent dye. The antigen first diffuses from the injection site through tissue fluid. When small blood vessels are encountered, the antigen diffuses into the vessel walls, where it encounters the circulating antibodies. Immune complexes form and are deposited between and beneath vascular endothelial cells. Complement components activated by the classical pathway will be deposited here as well.

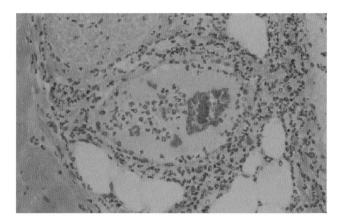

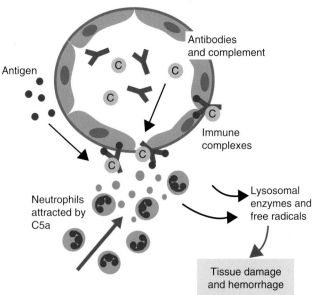

FIGURE 30-1 The mechanisms of an Arthus reaction as well as a histological section of an Arthus reaction in the skin of a cat 6 hours after intradermal inoculation of chicken red blood cells.

(Courtesy Dr. A. Kier.)

Immune complexes formed in tissues must be removed. The first step involves binding to Fc and complement receptors on cells. The most widespread of these Fc receptors is FcγRIIa expressed on macrophages. Immune complexes binding to these receptors stimulate production of nitric oxide, leukotrienes, prostaglandins, cytokines, and chemokines. Immune complexes also bind to mast cells through FcγRIII and trigger them to release their vasoactive molecules. Among the molecules released by mast cells are chemotactic factors and proteases that activate complement, cytokines, kinins, and lipid mediators. All these mediators promote inflammation by acting on vascular endothelium and stimulating neutrophil adherence and emigration.

Immune complexes activate complement and generate the chemotactic peptide C5a (Figure 30-2). Neutrophils, attracted by C5a and mast cell–derived chemokines, emigrate from the blood vessels, adhere to immune complexes, and promptly phagocytose them. Eventually the immune complexes are digested and destroyed. During this process, however, proteases and oxidants are released into the tissues. When neutrophils attempt to ingest immune complexes attached to structures such as basement membranes, they secrete their granule contents directly into the surrounding tissues. Neutrophil proteases disrupt collagen fibers and destroy ground substances, basement membranes, and elastic tissue. Normally tissues contain antiproteinases that inhibit neutrophil enzymes. However, neutrophils can subvert these inhibitors by secreting OCl⁻. The OCl⁻ destroys the inhibitors and allows tissue destruction to proceed.

Although it has long been assumed that immunoglobulin molecules do not themselves damage antigens, recent evidence has shown that they can kill microorganisms and cause tissue damage. When provided with singlet oxygen from phagocytic neutrophils, antibodies catalyze the production of oxidants

such as ozone. This ozone kills not only bacteria but also nearby cells. Biopsy specimens from Arthus reactions contain detectable amounts of ozone!

Neutrophil proteases also act on C5 to generate C5a, which promotes further neutrophil accumulation and degranulation. Other enzymes released by neutrophils make mast cells degranulate or generate kinins. As a result of all this, inflammation and destruction of blood vessel walls result in the development of the edema, vasculitis, and hemorrhage characteristic of an Arthus reaction.

Although the classical direct Arthus reaction is produced by local administration of an antigen to hyperimmunized animals, any technique that deposits immune complexes in tissues will stimulate a similar response. A reversed Arthus reaction can therefore be produced if antibodies are administered intradermally to an animal with a high level of circulating antigen. Injected, preformed immune complexes, particularly those containing a moderate excess of an antigen, will provoke a similar reaction, although, as might be anticipated, there is less involvement of blood vessel walls, and the reaction is less severe. A passive Arthus reaction can be produced by giving antibody intravenously to a nonsensitized animal, followed by an intradermal injection of an antigen, and real enthusiasts can produce a reversed passive Arthus reaction by giving antibody intradermally followed by intravenous antigen.

Although it is unusual for pure hypersensitivity reactions of only a single type to occur under natural conditions, there are some diseases in the domestic animals in which type III reactions play a major role. Experimentally, Arthus reactions are usually produced in the skin since that is the most convenient site at which to inject the antigen. However, local type III reactions can occur in many tissues, with the precise site depending on the location of the antigen.

Blue Eye

Blue eye is a condition seen in a small proportion of dogs that have been either infected or vaccinated with live canine adenovirus type 1 (see Figures 26-8 and 26-9). These animals develop an anterior uveitis leading to corneal edema and opacity. The cornea is infiltrated by neutrophils, and virus-antibody complexes are present in the lesion. Blue eye develops about 1 to 3 weeks after the onset of infection and usually resolves spontaneously as the virus is eliminated.

Hypersensitivity Pneumonitis

Type III hypersensitivity reactions may occur in the lungs when sensitized animals inhale antigens. For example, cattle housed during the winter are exposed to dust from hay. Normally, these dust particles are relatively large and are deposited in the upper respiratory tract, trapped in mucus, and eliminated. If, however, hay is stored when damp, bacterial growth and metabolism will result in heating. As a result of this warmth, thermophilic actinomycetes will grow. One of the most important of these thermophilic actinomycetes is

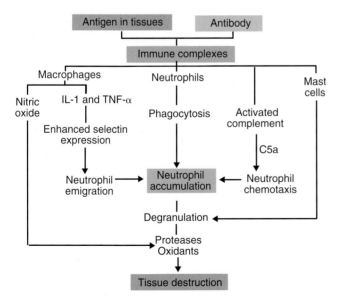

FIGURE 30-2 Some of the mechanisms involved in the pathogenesis of the Arthus reaction.

Saccharopolyspora rectivirgula, an organism that produces large numbers of very small spores (1 μm diameter). On inhalation, these spores can penetrate as far as the alveoli. If cattle are fed moldy hay for long periods, constant inhalation of *S. rectivirgula* spores will result in sensitization and in the development of high-titered antibodies to *S. rectivirgula* antigens in serum. Eventually inhaled spore antigens will encounter antibodies within the alveolar walls, and the resulting immune complexes and complement activation will cause a pneumonia (or pneumonitis), the basis of which is a type III hypersensitivity reaction.

The lesions of hypersensitivity pneumonitis consist of an acute alveolitis together with vasculitis and exudation of fluid into the alveolar spaces (Figure 30-3). The alveolar septa may be thickened, and the entire lesion is infiltrated with inflammatory cells. Since many of these cells are eosinophils and lymphocytes, it is obvious that the reaction is not a pure type III reaction. Nevertheless, examination of the lungs of affected cattle by immunofluorescence demonstrates deposits of immunoglobulin, complement, and antigen. In animals inhaling small amounts of an antigen over a long period, proliferative bronchiolitis and fibrosis may be observed. Clinically, hypersensitivity pneumonitis presents as a pneumonia occurring between 5 and 10 hours after acute exposure to grossly moldy hay. The animal may have difficulty breathing and develop a severe cough. In chronically affected animals, the dyspnea may be continuous. The most effective method of managing this condition is by removing the source of the antigen. Administration of steroids may be beneficial.

A hypersensitivity pneumonitis also occurs in farmers chronically exposed to *S. rectivirgula* spores from moldy hay and is called farmer's lung. Many other syndromes in humans have an identical pathogenesis and are usually named after the source of the offending antigen. Thus pigeon breeder's lung arises following exposure to the dust from pigeon feces, mushroom grower's disease is due to hypersensitivity to inhaled spores from actinomycetes in the soil used for growing mushrooms, and librarian's lung results from inhalation of dusts from old books! Hay sickness is a hypersensitivity pneumonitis seen in horses in Iceland that is probably an equine equivalent of farmer's lung.

Equine Respiratory Disease Two forms of chronic respiratory disease occur in horses. Recurrent airway obstruction (RAO) is seen in older horses, and inflammatory airway disease (IAD) is seen in horses of any age. Both are forms of chronic bronchiolitis associated with exposure to molds and other allergens in dusty stable air.

RAO occurs most obviously in horses that inhale large amounts of organic dusts such as those generated in dusty stables. It includes obstructive pulmonary disease seen in stabled horses and summer pasture-associated obstructive pulmonary disease. RAO is defined as a severe debilitating disease characterized by coughing and an increased breathing effort due to cholinergic bronchospasm, airway hyperreactivity, and neutrophil and mucus accumulation in the airways. Characteristically horses with RAO suffer from respiratory difficulty even while at rest.

RAO is probably a hypersensitivity disease associated with an enhanced Th2 response, although there is also limited evidence for a Th1 or mixed response. Some studies suggest that RAO is simply a nonspecific response to endotoxin-like molecules. Horses with these syndromes may show positive skin reactions to intradermal inoculation of actinomycete and fungal extracts (such as *Rhizopus nigricans, Candida albicans, S. rectivirgula, Aspergillus fumigatus,* or *Geotrichum deliquescens*). Some horses react to mite extracts. There is no evidence of IgE involvement in RAO. There is evidence for a genetic predisposition.

Affected horses may respond to aerosol challenge with extracts of these organisms by developing respiratory distress. Clinical signs may resolve on removal of the moldy hay and reappear on reexposure. However, there is little correlation between skin test results and severity of disease. Affected animals usually have large numbers of neutrophils or eosinophils in their small bronchioles and high titers of antibodies to equine influenza in their bronchial secretions. The significance of the latter is unclear. High concentrations of the chemokine CXCL8 (interleukin-8 [IL-8]) are found in the bronchoalveolar washings of affected animals. Exposure of cultured equine bronchial epithelial cell cultures to hay dust or lipopolysaccharide increases IL-8, CXCL2, and IL-1β expression. It has been suggested that continuous prolonged activation of bronchoalveolar epithelial cells by dust particles and air-borne endotoxins leads to excessive production of neutrophil chemotactic chemokines. These neutrophils then cause damage by producing proteases, peroxidases, and oxidants.

Removal of clinically affected horses to air-conditioned stalls results in improvement of the disease, but this is reversed if the horses are returned to dusty stables. In some cases, RAO

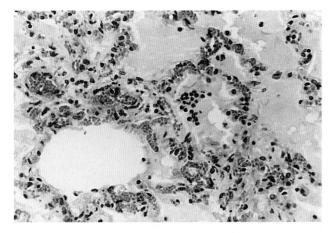

FIGURE 30-3 A histological section of the lung from a cow that died suddenly 24 hours after being fed moldy hay. The alveoli are full of fluid, and the alveolar walls are thickened and inflamed. This acute alveolitis is probably due to a hypersensitivity reaction to inhaled actinomycete spores. Original magnification ×400.

(Courtesy Dr. B.N. Wilkie.)

may persist even when horses are moved to low dust environments, probably as a result of airway remodeling.

IAD affects up to 30% of young horses in training. Although commonly linked to bacterial or viral infections, in many cases no infectious agent can be isolated. Horses with IAD show poor performance, exercise intolerance, and coughing. There is evidence of nonseptic inflammation detected by cytological evaluation of bronchiolar lavage fluid. Excessive airway mucus is apparent. Unlike RAO, the disease is not clinically apparent at rest. The pathogenesis is unknown, but like RAO, IAD is associated with inhalation of organic dusts and aeroallergens.

Staphylococcal Hypersensitivity

Staphylococcal hypersensitivity is a pruritic pustular dermatitis of dogs. Skin testing with staphylococcal antigens suggests that types I, III, and IV hypersensitivity may be involved. The histological findings of neutrophilic dermal vasculitis suggest that the type III reaction may predominate in some cases.

Generalized Type III Hypersensitivity Reactions

If an antigen is administered intravenously to animals with circulating antibodies, immune complexes form in the bloodstream. These immune complexes are normally removed by binding to either erythrocytes or platelets, or if very large, they are removed by the mononuclear phagocyte system (Figure 30-4). If, however, complexes are produced in excessive amounts, they are deposited in the walls of blood vessels, especially medium-sized arteries, and in vessels where there is a physiological outflow of fluid such as glomeruli, synovia, and the choroid plexus (Figure 30-5). An example of this type of hypersensitivity is serum sickness.

Serum Sickness

Many years ago, when the use of antisera for passive immunization was in its infancy, it was observed that wounded soldiers who had received a very large dose of equine antitetanus serum developed a characteristic reaction about 10 days later. This reaction, called serum sickness, consisted of a generalized vasculitis with erythema, edema, and urticaria of the skin; neutropenia; lymph node enlargement; joint swelling; and proteinuria. The reaction was usually of short duration and subsided within a few days. A similar reaction can be produced experimentally in rabbits by administration of a large intravenous dose of antigen. The development of sickness coincides with the formation of large amounts of immune complexes in the circulation as a result of the immune response to circulating antigens (Figure 30-6). The experimental disease may be acute if it is caused by a single, large injection of an antigen; or chronic, if caused by multiple small injections. In either case, animals develop glomerulonephritis and arteritis (Figure 30-7).

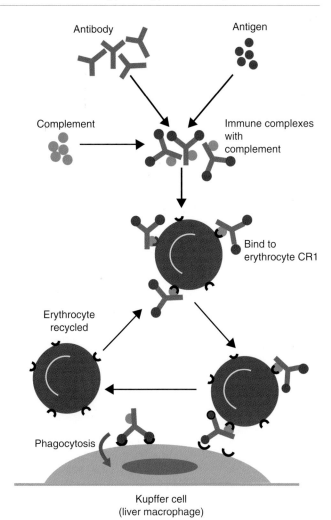

FIGURE 30-4 In primates, immune complexes are removed by binding to complement receptors on red blood cells. They are then carried to the liver, where they are transferred to Kupffer cells for phagocytosis. In the absence of complement components, significant accumulation of immune complexes occurs in tissues. In other mammals immune complexes bind to receptors on platelets.

Glomerulonephritis

When immune complexes are deposited in the glomeruli, they cause basement membrane thickening and stimulate glomerular cells to proliferate. Any or all of the three glomerular cell populations—epithelial cells, endothelial cells, and mesangial cells—can proliferate. The lesion is therefore called membranoproliferative glomerulonephritis (MPGN). If immune complexes are deposited only in the mesangium, mesangial cell proliferation will result in a mesangioproliferative glomerulonephritis. MPGN lesions are classified into three types based on their histopathology and pathogenesis (Figure 30-8).

Type I Membranoproliferative Glomerulonephritis
Type I MPGN is caused by immune complex deposition in glomerular vessels. These complexes usually penetrate the vascular endothelium, but not the basement membrane, and are

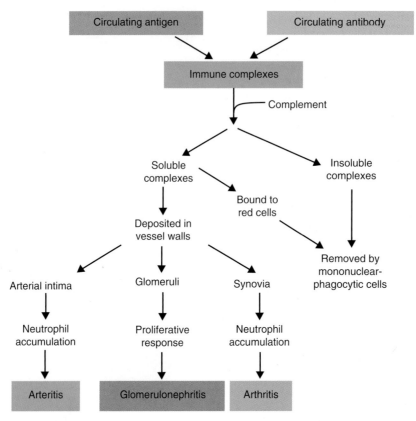

FIGURE 30-5 The mechanisms involved in the pathogenesis of acute serum sickness.

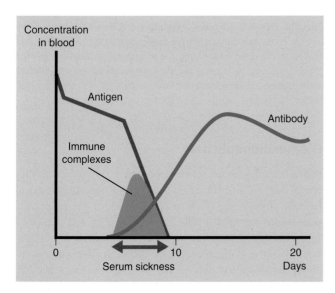

FIGURE 30-6 The time course of acute serum sickness. The appearance of the disease coincides with the generation of immune complexes in the bloodstream.

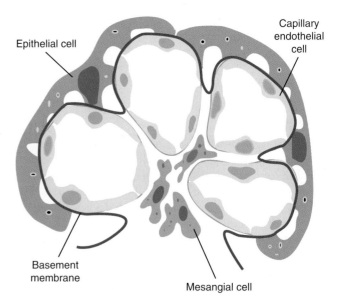

FIGURE 30-7 The structure of a typical glomerulus. Immune complexes may be deposited on either side of, or within, the glomerular basement membrane.

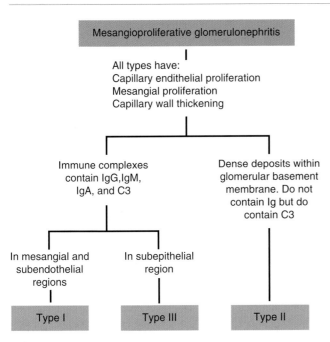

FIGURE 30-8 A classification of different forms of membranoproliferative glomerulonephritis.

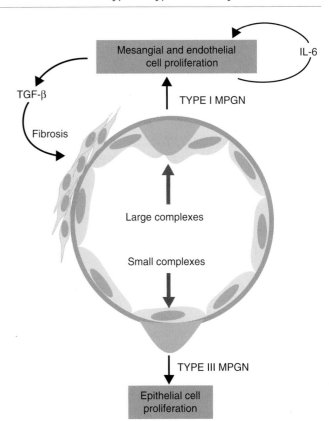

FIGURE 30-9 The pathogenesis of different forms of immune complex–mediated glomerulonephritis. Remember, however, that more than one type of lesion may be present in an animal at the same time.

therefore trapped on the inside, where they stimulate endothelial cell swelling and proliferation (Figure 30-9). If an animal is given repeated injections of small doses of an antigen over a long period, continued damage to the glomerular cells by immune complexes leads to production of transforming growth factor-β (TGF-β). This cytokine stimulates nearby cells to produce fibronectin, collagen, and proteoglycans. This results in a thickening of the basement membrane to form the so-called wire loop lesion (also called a membranous glomerulonephritis). Alternatively, the immune complexes may be deposited in the mesangial region of glomeruli. Mesangial cells are modified smooth muscle cells. As such they can release cytokines and prostaglandins and ingest immune complexes. They respond to these immune complexes by proliferation and production of IL-6 and TGF-β. The IL-6 stimulates autocrine growth of the mesangial cells. The TGF-β stimulates production of extracellular matrix. This glomerulonephritis eventually interferes with glomerular function. By immunofluorescence, it can be shown that lumpy aggregates of immune complexes are deposited in capillary walls and on the epithelial side of the glomerular basement membrane (Figure 30-10).

Type II Membranoproliferative Glomerulonephritis

Type II MPGN (or dense deposit disease) is similar to the type I disease in that there is endothelial and mesangial proliferation. However, it is characterized by the presence of homogeneous, dense deposits within the glomerular basement membrane (in the lamina densa) rather than on its surface (see Figure 7-18). The deposits may contain C3 but not immunoglobulin. Type II MPGN results from uncontrolled complement activation and is seen in factor H deficiency in pigs (Chapter 7).

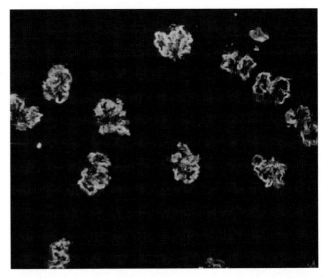

FIGURE 30-10 A fluorescent micrograph of a section of kidney from a Finnish-Landrace lamb with immune complex–mediated glomerulonephritis. The labeled antisheep globulin reveals the presence of "lumpy-bumpy" deposits characteristic of type I membranoproliferative glomerulonephritis in many glomeruli.

(From Angus KW, Gardiner AC, Morgan KT, et al: Mesangiocapillary glomerulonephritis in lambs. II. Pathological findings and electron microscopy of the renal lesions, J Comp Pathol 84:319–330, 1974.)

Type III Membranoproliferative Glomerulonephritis

Type III MPGN is a variant of type I MPGN. It differs from typical type I disease by the presence of immune complexes on both the endothelial and epithelial sides of the basement membrane. It is believed that very small immune complexes penetrate the basement membrane and are deposited where they stimulate epithelial cell swelling and proliferation. If excessive, these proliferating cells may fill the glomerular space to form epithelial crescents. A single case of unknown cause has been described in a cat.

Clinical Features of Glomerulonephritis

Type I MPGN develops when prolonged antigenemia persists in the presence of antibodies. It is therefore characteristic of chronic viral diseases such as equine infectious anemia, infectious canine hepatitis, Aleutian disease of mink, and African swine fever; parasitic diseases such as leishmaniasis; and chronic bacterial diseases such as Lyme disease and ehrlichiosis (Table 30-1). Clinically it should be suspected in an animal with proteinuria without evidence of infection, although definitive diagnosis requires a renal biopsy and histological evaluation. Type I MPGN has also been reported in dogs with pyometra, chronic pneumonia, distemper encephalitis, acute pancreatic necrosis, and bacterial endocarditis. In animals with tumors, large amounts of antigen may be shed into the bloodstream and give rise to a type I MPGN. This is, for example, a feature of feline leukemia. It has also been reported in animals with lymphosarcomas, osteosarcomas, and mastocytomas. Circulating immune complexes and renal lesions have been found in dogs with systemic lupus erythematosus (Chapter 36), discoid lupus, generalized demodicosis, and recurrent staphylococcal pyoderma. Some cases may be due to deficiencies of complement components. As a result of these deficiencies, removal of immune complexes is impaired, and they accumulate in glomeruli. Many cases of type I MPGN develop in the absence of an obvious predisposing cause.

The presence of immune complex lesions within glomeruli stimulates neutrophils, mesangial cells, macrophages, and platelets to release thromboxanes, nitric oxide, and platelet-activating factor. These increase basement membrane permeability to macromolecules so that plasma proteins, especially albumin, are lost in the urine. This loss, if severe, may exceed the ability of the body to replace the protein. As a result, albumin levels drop, the plasma colloid osmotic pressure falls, fluid passes from blood into tissue spaces, and the animal may become edematous and ascitic. The loss of fluid into tissues results in a reduction of blood volume, a compensatory increase in secretion of antidiuretic hormone, increased sodium retention, and accentuation of the edema. The decreased blood volume also results in a drop in renal blood flow, reduction in glomerular filtration, retention of urea and creatinine, azotemia, and hypercholesterolemia. Although all these may occur

□ **Table 30-1** | Infectious Diseases with a Significant Type III Hypersensitivity Component

ORGANISM OR DISEASE	MAJOR LESION
Erysipelothrix rhusiopathiae	Arthritis
Mycobacterium johnei	Enteritis
Streptococcus equi	Purpura
Staphylococcus aureus	Dermatitis
Borrelia burgdorferi	Glomerulonephritis
Ehrlichiosis	Glomerulonephritis
Canine adenovirus-1	Uveitis, glomerulonephritis
Canine adenovirus-2	Glomerulonephritis
Feline leukemia	Glomerulonephritis
Feline infectious peritonitis	Peritonitis, glomerulonephritis
Aleutian disease	Glomerulonephritis, anemia, arteritis
Hog cholera	Glomerulonephritis
African swine fever	Glomerulonephritis
Bovine virus diarrhea	Glomerulonephritis
Equine viral arteritis	Arteritis
Equine infectious anemia	Anemia, glomerulonephritis
Visceral leishmaniasis	Glomerulonephritis
Dirofilaria immitis	Glomerulonephritis

as a result of immune complex deposition in glomeruli, the development of this nephrotic syndrome is not inevitable. In fact, the clinical course of these conditions is extremely unpredictable, with some animals showing a progressive deterioration in renal function and others showing spontaneous remissions. Many animals may be clinically normal despite the presence of immune complexes in their glomeruli, and immune complexes are commonly observed in old, apparently healthy dogs, horses, and sheep. The most common initial signs are anorexia, weight loss, and vomiting. Polyuria and polydipsia occur when about two thirds of glomeruli are destroyed. Azotemia occurs when 75% are destroyed. Development of nephrotic syndrome (proteinuria, hypoproteinemia, edema, or ascites) only occurs in about 15% of affected dogs but in up to 75% of affected cats. Some dogs become hypertensive. Thromboembolic disease may also develop. Because of the unpredictable occurrence of spontaneous remissions, it is difficult to judge the effects of treatment. It has been usual to treat affected animals with corticosteroids and immunosuppressive drugs, but the rationale and effectiveness of this treatment are open to question except when the glomerulonephritis is associated with concurrent autoimmune disease such as systemic lupus erythematosus. Recently encouraging responses have been obtained with angiotensin-converting enzyme inhibitors (captopril) and experimental thromboxane synthase inhibitors. Protein restriction may help reduce the clinical signs of renal failure. If the glomerulopathy is secondary, clearly the underlying cause should be treated. The glomerular lesion is not inflammatory, and although the lesion in primary immune complex glomerulonephritis contains immunoglobulins, there is no evidence to suggest that it is caused by hyperactivity of the immune system. Steroid treatment of rabbits with experimental immune complex disease has been shown to exacerbate the condition.

Immunoglobulin A Nephropathy

By far the most important cause of renal failure in humans is IgA nephropathy. In this form of type I MPGN, patients have elevated serum IgA, and IgA-containing immune complexes are deposited in the mesangial region. The resulting cellular proliferation and glomerulonephritis can lead to renal failure. The cause of IgA nephropathy is unknown. IgA deposits can be found in the glomeruli of up to 35% of some human populations and up to 47% of dogs. In these dogs, the IgA is deposited in the mesangial and paramesangial areas and is associated with mesangial proliferation. Dogs with enteritis or liver diseases showed the highest incidence of glomerular IgA deposition. A slightly different condition has also been described in dogs aged 4 to 7 years. The animals developed a type III MPGN with mild hematuria, proteinuria, and hypertension. IgA-containing immune complexes formed in both the subepithelial and subendothelial locations. IgA nephropathy has also been described in pigtailed macaques (*Macaca nemestrina*).

Swine Glomerulopathy

Spontaneous type I MPGN is observed in pigs. It is especially common in Japan, where it appears to be due to deposition of immune complexes containing IgG (and IgA) antibodies against *Actinobacillus pleuropneumoniae*. In other cases, it may be secondary to chronic virus infections such as hog cholera or African swine fever. Occasionally, however, proliferative glomerulonephritis develops spontaneously. In most cases epithelial crescent formation suggests that the proliferating cells are epithelial in origin. However, occasional membranoproliferative lesions are observed as well. There is usually strong staining for C3 and weaker staining for IgM using immunofluorescence assays. Pigs rarely have IgG or IgA deposits. Affected pigs are relatively young (<1 year). There is a high prevalence of gastric ulcers in affected animals, but whether this is related is unclear. An inherited complement factor H deficiency in Yorkshire pigs results in the development of a lethal type II MPGN called porcine dense deposit disease (Chapter 7).

Dirofilariasis

Some dogs heavily infected with the heartworm *Dirofilaria immitis* develop glomerular lesions and proteinuria. The lesions include thickening of the glomerular basement membrane with minimal endothelial or mesangial proliferation. Since IgG1-containing deposits may be found on the epithelial side of the basement membrane (type III MPGN), it has been suggested that immune complexes formed by antibodies to heartworm antigens provoke these lesions. Other investigators dispute the immune complex nature of this condition and claim that the lesions develop in response to the physical presence of microfilariae in glomerular blood vessels. The fact that infected dogs may develop amyloidosis (Chapter 6) suggests that they mount a significant immune response to the worms.

Finnish-Landrace Glomerulopathy

Some lambs of the Finnish-Landrace breed die within a few weeks of age as a result of renal failure due to a type I MPGN. The lesions develop in utero and are present at birth. The glomerular lesions are similar to those seen in chronic serum sickness, with mesangial cell proliferation and basement membrane thickening (Figure 30-11). In extreme cases epithelial cell proliferation may result in epithelial crescent formation. Neutrophils may be present in small numbers within glomeruli, and the rest of the kidney may exhibit diffuse interstitial lymphoid infiltration and necrotizing vasculitis. Deposits

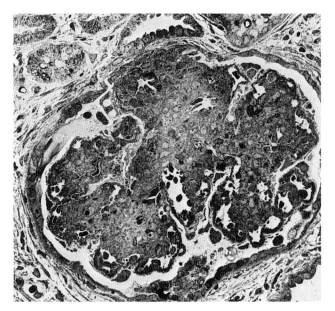

FIGURE 30-11 A thin section of glomerulus from a Finnish-Landrace lamb with type I membranoproliferative glomerulonephritis. The primary lesion in this case is mesangial proliferation with some basement membrane thickening.

(From Angus KW, Gardiner AC, Morgan KT, et al: Mesangiocapillary glomerulonephritis in lambs. II. Pathological findings and electron microscopy of the renal lesions, *J Comp Pathol* 84:319–330, 1974.)

containing IgM, IgG, and C3 are found in the glomeruli and choroid plexus, and serum C3 levels are low. The lesions are therefore probably produced as a result of immune complex deposition within these organs, although the nature of the inducing antigen is unknown.

Canine Glomerulopathy

C3 deficiency inherited as an autosomal recessive condition has been described in Brittany Spaniels (Chapter 7). Many of these dogs develop type I MPGN, which may lead to renal failure. The lesions are typical with mesangial proliferation, thickening of the glomerular capillary wall, and deposition of electron-dense deposits in the mesangium and subendothelial space. The deposits contain both IgG and IgM. A familial glomerulopathy has been observed in Bernese Mountain Dogs. It is associated with MPGN and interstitial nephritis.

Other Immune Complex– Mediated Lesions

Purpura Hemorrhagica

Two to four weeks after an acute *Streptococcus equi* infection (or vaccination against *S. equi*), horses may develop urticaria, followed by severe subcutaneous edema, especially involving the limbs, and the development of hemorrhages in the mucosa and subcutaneous tissues. Affected horses are anorexic and depressed and have a high fever. Immune complexes containing *S. equi* antigens (M-protein or R-protein) may be found in the bloodstream of affected animals. These immune complexes cause an acute vasculitis as well as a type I MPGN with resulting proteinuria and azoturia. Other triggers of purpura hemorrhagica in the horse include infections with *Corynebacterium pseudotuberculosis*, *Rhodococcus equi*, equine influenza virus, and equine herpesvirus type 1. In some cases it develops in the absence of any obvious infection. Horses usually recover if aggressively treated with systemic glucocorticosteroids.

Pigs may also suffer from sporadic cases of an immune complex–mediated thrombocytopenic purpura syndrome. The animals have thrombocytopenia, anemia, excessive bleeding, and membranoproliferative lesions in their glomeruli. The cause is unknown.

Dietary Hypersensitivity

If an antigenic milk replacer, such as soy protein, is fed to very young calves before the development of ruminal function, the foreign antigen may be absorbed and stimulate antibody formation and a type III hypersensitivity. As a result, the calves become unthrifty and lose weight. However, the precise pathogenesis of this condition is unclear. A small proportion of calves develop an IgE response and a type I hypersensitivity.

Polyarthritis

Immune complexes can be readily found in the blood and synovial fluid of animals with rheumatoid arthritis and in many with osteoarthritis. In rheumatoid arthritis, they are believed to have a major role in the etiologic progression of disease. Their role in osteoarthritis is unclear, but they may be a secondary result of local trauma. Important examples of this type of arthritis are the nonerosive polyarthritides seen in foals and puppies and described in Chapter 36.

Drug Hypersensitivities

In the previous chapter, it was pointed out that if a drug attached itself to a cell such as an erythrocyte, the immune response against the drug could lead to elimination of the cell. A similar reaction may occur through type III hypersensitivity reactions if immune complexes bind to host cells. In this case, the cells are recognized as opsonized and are removed by phagocytosis. As might be predicted, if immune complexes bind to erythrocytes, anemia results; if they bind to platelets, thrombocytopenia and purpura result. Binding to granulocytes leads to a granulocytopenia and, consequently, recurrent infection. Severe skin reactions may follow deposition of antibody-drug complexes in the blood vessels of the dermis. However, in many cases, it is difficult to distinguish between the toxic effects of a drug and type III hypersensitivity unless specific antibodies can be eluted from affected cells.

For sources of additional information, please visit http:// evolve.elsevier.com/tizard/immunology/

31

Type IV Hypersensitivity: Delayed Hypersensitivity

□ **Key Points**

- Some antigens, when injected into the skin, induce a slowly developing inflammatory response called delayed, or type IV, hypersensitivity.
- Delayed hypersensitivity reactions are mainly mediated by T cells and natural killer (NK) cells.
- A good example of delayed hypersensitivity is the reaction of tuberculous cattle to intradermal injection of tuberculin. This tuberculin response provides a convenient diagnostic test for tuberculosis.
- A different form of type IV hypersensitivity occurs in allergic contact dermatitis. This is a slowly developing inflammatory response that occurs when reactive chemicals bind to skin cells and trigger T cell responses.
- In vitro assays for cell-mediated immunity generally focus on detecting secreted cytokines or measuring cell division induced by exposure to antigens.
- In vivo assays generate a biological response such as the development of a delayed hypersensitivity skin reaction or the rejection of an allograft.

Certain antigens, when injected into the skin of sensitized animals, provoke an inflammatory response at the injection site after a delay of 12 to 24 hours. Since these "delayed" hypersensitivity reactions can only be transferred from sensitized to normal animals by lymphocytes, they must be cell mediated. Delayed hypersensitivity reactions are classified as type IV hypersensitivities and result from interactions among the injected antigen, antigen-presenting cells, and T cells. An important example of a delayed hypersensitivity reaction is the tuberculin response. This is an inflammatory response that develops in the skin of an animal infected with tuberculosis following intradermal injection of tuberculin. Delayed hypersensitivity reactions can be considered a specialized form of inflammation directed against organisms that are resistant to elimination by conventional responses.

The Tuberculin Reaction

Tuberculin is the name given to extracts of mycobacteria used to skin-test animals in order to identify those suffering from tuberculosis. Several types of tuberculin have been employed for this purpose. The most important is purified protein derivative (PPD) tuberculin, prepared by growing organisms in synthetic medium, killing them with steam, and filtering. The PPD tuberculin is precipitated from this filtrate with trichloroacetic acid, washed, and resuspended in buffer ready for use. Thus PPD tuberculin is a crude antigen mixture. Its major antigenic component is probably the heat-shock protein (HSP) 65. Many of its proteins are shared among different mycobacterial species, thus ensuring that tests that use PPD tuberculin are relatively nonspecific. It is possible to increase the specificity of the tuberculin test with a defined mycobacterial protein such as early secretory antigenic target-6 (ESAT-6). ESAT-6 is a mycobacterial protein of unknown function that is recognized strongly by T cells. However, the reactions induced by very pure proteins tend to be minimal and require greater amounts of antigen to induce a satisfactory response.

When tuberculin is injected into the skin of a normal animal, there is no apparent response. On the other hand, if it is injected into an animal infected with mycobacteria, a delayed hypersensitivity response occurs. In these animals, a red, indurated (hard) swelling develops at the injection site. The inflammation begins after 12 to 24 hours, reaches its greatest intensity by 24 to 72 hours, and may persist for several weeks before fading gradually. In very severe reactions, tissue destruction and necrosis may occur at the injection site. The lesion is infiltrated with mononuclear cells (lymphocytes, macrophages), although neutrophils are present in the first hours of the reaction (Figure 31-1).

The tuberculin reaction is mediated by T cells. When an animal is infected with *Mycobacterium tuberculosis*, the organisms are readily phagocytosed by macrophages. Some of this mycobacterial antigen triggers a Th1 response and generates memory cells. These memory T cells will respond to injected mycobacterial antigens such as tuberculin. Since a positive tuberculin test can be elicited many years after exposure to an antigen, some of these memory T cells must be very long lived.

When tuberculin is injected intradermally, it is taken up by Langerhans cells, which then migrate to the draining lymph node (Figure 31-2). Here they present antigen to memory T cells that respond by generating Th1 effector cells. The circulating Th1 cells recognize the antigen when they encounter it in the skin and accumulate around the antigen deposit. By 12 hours in cattle, the injection site is infiltrated with T cells. (In humans and mice, α/β T cells tend to predominate, whereas in sheep and cattle, γ/δ, WC1 T cells predominate.) There are no B cells in the lesion.

The γ/δ T cells recruit other Th1 lymphocytes and macrophages to the site. The Th1 cells secrete interferon-γ (IFN-γ), interleukin-2 (IL-2), and IL-16. The first two act on endothelial cells to increase expression of adherence molecules. IL-2 stimulates production of the chemokines CXCL8, CCL5, and XCL1, which attract and activate more T cells. IL-16 attracts CD4+ T cells. The macrophages also release serotonin and chemokines such as CXCL1 and CCL2, which attract basophils. Basophil-derived serotonin (in rodents) or histamine (in humans) causes yet more inflammation and enhances migration of mononuclear cells into the lesion. The T cell–derived chemokines CCL2 and CCL3 can induce mast cell degranulation, whereas some CD4+ T cells can activate mast cells directly through MHC class II–bound antigen.

T cell–derived chemokines cause inflammation and attract even more T cells. Most of these new T cells are not specifically sensitized to the inducing antigen. Only a very small proportion, perhaps 5%, of the lymphocytes seen in a delayed hypersensitivity reaction are specific for the antigen. Most are attracted nonspecifically by XCL1 (lymphotactin). By 60 to 72 hours, the predominant lymphocytes are $\alpha/\beta+$, CD4+, and CD8+. Macrophages accumulate in the lesion attracted by CXCL8 and may be activated by IFN-γ. Some of the tissue damage in intense delayed hypersensitivity reactions may be due to the release of proteases and oxidants from these activated macrophages. The macrophages ingest and eventually destroy the injected antigen. This, plus the appearance of regulatory cells in the lesion, permits the tissues to return eventually to normal.

Cutaneous Basophil Hypersensitivity

Sometimes, basophils predominate in a delayed hypersensitivity reaction (Figure 31-3). This type of reaction, called cutaneous basophil hypersensitivity (CBH), can be transferred between animals with antibody, with purified B cells, or even with T cells. CBH is therefore mediated by several different mechanisms. CBH occurs in chickens in response to intradermal Rous sarcoma virus, in rabbits in response to schistosomes,

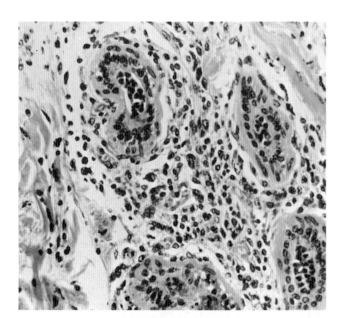

FIGURE 31-1 A histological section of a positive tuberculin reaction in bovine skin. Note the perivascular mononuclear cell infiltration as well as the lack of neutrophils or edema.

(From Thomson RG: *General veterinary pathology*, Philadelphia, 1978, WB Saunders.)

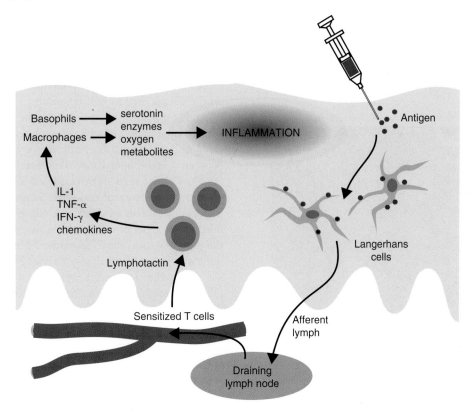

FIGURE 31-2 A schematic diagram depicting the mechanism of a delayed hypersensitivity reaction.

and in humans with allergic contact dermatitis and renal allograft rejection. CBH reactions may contribute to the development of flea allergy dermatitis in dogs.

Tuberculin Reactions in Cattle

Because a positive tuberculin reaction occurs only in animals that have, or have had, tuberculosis, skin testing may be used to identify animals affected by this disease. Indeed, the tuberculin test has provided the basis for all tuberculosis eradication schemes that involve the detection and subsequent elimination of infected animals.

Skin testing of cattle may be performed in several ways (Table 31-1). The simplest is the single intradermal (SID) test. In this test, 0.1 mL of PPD tuberculin derived from *M. tuberculosis* or *Mycobacterium bovis* is injected into one caudal fold (the folds of skin underneath the tail), and the injection site is examined 72 to 96 hours later. A comparison is easily made between the injected and the uninjected folds, and a positive reaction consisting of a firm lump or marked discoloration at the injection site is readily detected.

In the United States, two separate tests are performed. Thus two injections of tuberculin are made—one into the mucocutaneous junction of the vulva and the other into a caudal fold; in other countries, tuberculin is normally injected into the skin on the side of the neck. The neck site is more sensitive than the caudal folds, but restraint of the animal may be more difficult, and good injection technique is critical.

The advantage of the SID test is its simplicity. Its main disadvantage is that because of cross-reactions, it cannot distinguish between tuberculosis and infection by related mycobacteria such as *Mycobacterium avium* and *Mycobacterium avium paratuberculosis*, or the *Nocardia* group of organisms. A second disadvantage is that some animals react positively to the test but on necropsy do not have detectable tuberculosis lesions. The reasons for this are unclear but may be false positives resulting from exposure to nonpathogenic environmental mycobacteria such as *Mycobacterium phlei*.

False-negative SID tests may occur in animals with advanced tuberculosis, in animals with very early infection, in animals that have calved within the preceding 4 to 6 weeks, in very old cows, and in animals tested during the preceding 1 to 10 weeks. The lack of reaction (anergy) seen in advanced cases of tuberculosis is also seen in clinical Johne's disease and appears to be due to the presence of an IgG antibody that prevents T cells from reacting with antigen. There is also evidence for the involvement of regulatory cells in anergy. Repeated short-interval tuberculin testing leads to desensitization associated with elevated IL-10 and decreased IL-1β responses. (It does not influence IFN-γ responses.) Because of these defects in the SID, several modifications of this test have been developed. The comparative cervical test, for example, involves intradermal inoculation of both avian and bovine tuberculins. Each tuberculin is injected into the side of the neck at separate sites, and these sites are examined 72 hours later. In general, if the avian tuberculin site shows the greatest reaction, the animal is considered to be infected with *M. avium* or *M. avium paratuberculosis*. On the other hand, if the *M. bovis* site shows a significantly greater reaction, then it is believed that the animal is infected with *M. bovis* or *M. tuberculosis*. This test is useful when a high prevalence of avian tuberculosis or Johne's disease is anticipated. PPD from *M. bovis* is more specific in cattle than *M. tuberculosis*, giving less cross-reaction with *M. avium* as well as being more appropriate for use in cattle, and is therefore preferred. In practice, the comparative test has a sensitivity of 90% (10% false negatives) and a specificity of greater than 99% (<1% false positives); however, this depends on the criteria used to read the results.

Anther modified tuberculin test is the short thermal test, in which a large volume of tuberculin solution is given subcutaneously, and the animal is examined for a rise in temperature between 4 and 8 hours later. (Presumably the tuberculin acts on T cells that then provoke the release of IL-1 and other cytokines from macrophages.) The Stormont test relies on the increased sensitivity of a test site, which occurs after a single injection; it is performed by giving two doses of tuberculin at the same injection site 7 days apart. Both tests are relatively sensitive. As a result, they may be used in postpartum cows as well as for the testing of heavily infected animals. Repeated tuberculin testing results in a period of decreased reactivity and the induction of antibodies against *M. bovis* antigen HSP 70.

Tuberculin Reactions in Other Animals

Tuberculin skin testing has never been a widely employed procedure in domestic animals other than cattle, so information on these is scanty. Nevertheless, it appears that the ability of different species to mount a classic tuberculin reaction varies greatly. In pigs and cats, for example, the tuberculin test is unreliable, being positive for only a short period following infection. In pigs and dogs, the best test is an SID test given in the skin behind the ear, whereas in cats, the short thermal test is probably best. In sheep and goats, the antigen is usually given in the anal fold, but the results are usually unreliable in these species as well. Horses appear to be unusually sensitive to tuberculin, and the dose used must be reduced accordingly. Nevertheless, the results obtained do not always correlate well with the disease status of the animal. In birds, good reactions may be obtained by inoculating tuberculin into the wattle or wing web.

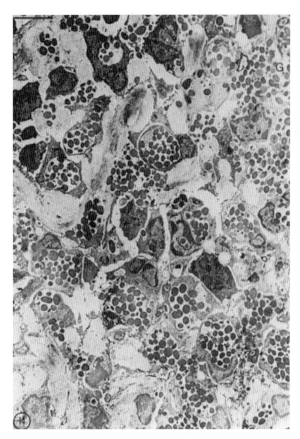

FIGURE 31-3 A section of guinea pig skin 18 hours after attachment of a tick in an animal sensitized by prior infestation with tick larvae. The skin is infiltrated with large numbers of basophils.

(From McLaren D, Worms MJ, Askenase PW: Cutaneous basophil associated resistance to ectoparasites (ticks). Electron microscopy of *Rhipicephalus appendiculatus* larval feeding sites in actively sensitised guinea pigs and recipients of immune serum, *J Pathol* 139:291, 1983.)

□ Table 31-1 | Tuberculin Tests Used in Cattle

TEST	USE	ADVANTAGES	DISADVANTAGES
Single intradermal	Routine testing	Simple	Prone to false positives Poor sensitivity
Comparative	When avian TB or Johne disease is prevalent	More specific than SID	More complex than SID
Short thermal	Use in postpartum animals and in infected animals	High efficiency	Time-consuming Risk for anaphylaxis
Stormont	Use in postpartum animals and in advanced cases	Very sensitive and accurate	Three visits required May sensitize an animal

Johnin Reactions

Animals infected with *M. avium* var. *paratuberculosis*, the cause of Johne's disease, may develop a delayed hypersensitivity reaction following intradermal inoculation of an extract of this organism called johnin. Johnin can be used in a single intradermal test but, like tuberculin, may give a negative result in animals with clinical disease. An intravenous johnin test is positive in these cases and may be a preferable alternative to the SID test. In this test the antigen is administered intravenously, and the animal's temperature is noted 6 hours later. A rise in temperature of 1° C or neutrophilia is considered a positive result. These tests are probably of limited usefulness in individual animals but may help identify infected herds.

Other Skin Tests

Positive delayed hypersensitivity skin reactions may be obtained in any infectious disease in which cell-mediated immunity has a significant role. Thus extracts of *Brucella abortus* have been used from time to time in attempts to diagnose brucellosis. These include brucellin, a filtrate of a 20-day broth culture, and brucellergen, a nucleoprotein extract. Because these preparations may induce antibodies to brucella, they cannot be employed in areas where eradication is monitored by serological tests. In glanders of horses, a culture filtrate of the organism *Burkholderia mallei*, termed mallein, is used for skin testing. Mallein can be used in either a short thermal test or an ophthalmic test. An ophthalmic test, also occasionally employed in tuberculosis, is performed by dropping the antigen solution into an eye. Transient conjunctivitis develops if the test is positive. Another method of testing for glanders is the intrapalpebral test. In this test, mallein is injected into the skin of the lower eyelid, where a positive reaction results in swelling and ophthalmia.

Intradermal skin testing with microbial extracts is also employed in the diagnosis of many fungal diseases; thus histoplasmin is used for histoplasmosis, coccidioidin for coccidioidomycosis, and so on. In these cases, the tests are not very specific, and the test procedure may effectively sensitize the tested animal, causing it to become serologically positive. This problem also arises when toxoplasmin is used in attempts to diagnose toxoplasmosis (see Figure 27-6).

Pathological Consequences of Type IV Hypersensitivity

Tubercle Formation

Although the tuberculin reaction induced by intradermal inoculation is artificial in that antigen is administered by injection, a similar inflammatory response occurs if living tubercle bacilli lodge in tissues and sensitize an animal. However, *M. tuberculosis* is resistant to intracellular destruction until M1 macrophages are activated by Th1 cells (Chapter 18), and dead organisms are very slowly removed because they contain large quantities of poorly metabolized waxes. As a result, the reaction to whole organisms is prolonged, and macrophages accumulate in very large numbers. Many of these macrophages ingest the bacteria but fail to prevent its growth and so die. Other macrophages fuse to form multinucleated giant cells. After 4 to 5 weeks of infection, microscopic granulomas enlarge and coalesce. The lesion that develops around invading tubercle bacilli therefore consists of a mass of caseous (cheesy!) debris containing both living and dead organisms surrounded by a layer of fibroblasts, lymphocytes, and macrophages, which in this location are called epithelioid cells (Chapter 25). The entire lesion is a type 1 granuloma called a tubercle (Figure 31-4). The mycobacteria are unable to multiply within the necrotic tissue because of its low pH and lack of oxygen. Nevertheless some bacteria may survive in a dormant state. If the host mounts an adequate immune response of the correct (Th1) type, this may be sufficient to control the infection. However, if immunity is insufficient or inappropriate (e.g., a Th2 response), the organisms may escape from the tubercle and spread to local lymph nodes and nearby tissues. When the response is inadequate, the multiplying organisms continue to spread, and the resulting lung damage, together with liquefaction of the caseous center of the tubercle, leads to rapidly progressive disease.

During the early stages of granuloma formation, macrophages are highly motile and provide the pathogen with fresh cells to infect. These infected macrophages die but then recruit uninfected macrophages to the site of infection. They phagocytose old macrophages and their bacterial contents. This

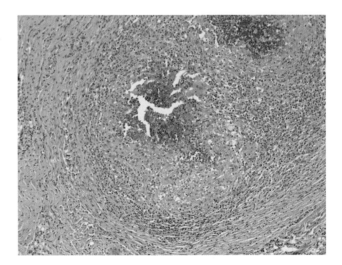

FIGURE 31-4 A histological section from the lymph node of a cow infected with *Mycobacterium bovis* showing a small tubercle. The dark central mass is caseous material. It is surrounded by layers of macrophages and lymphocytes and walled off by fibroblasts.

(Courtesy Dr. John Edwards.)

process leads to the efficient spread and expansion of the bacterial population. Thus virulent mycobacteria exploit the process by which macrophages promote tissue repair.

Allergic Contact Dermatitis

If reactive chemicals are painted onto the skin, they may bind to skin proteins, and the resulting complexes are processed by Langerhans cells in the dermis (Figure 31-5). Depending on the antigen, the Langerhans cells may bind the antigen directly to MHC molecules on the cell surface or process the hapten internally into a complete antigen. The Langerhans cells then migrate to draining lymph nodes through afferent lymphatics and present the antigen to T cells. While presenting the antigen, the Langerhans cells secrete large amounts of IL-12, IL-18, and IL-23 that activate both Th1 and Th17 cells. The Th1 cells in turn both produce large amounts of IFN-γ and promote the activities of cytotoxic T cells. Following exposure to an antigen in sensitized animals, macrophages and lymphocytes infiltrate the dermis by 24 hours. Eventually, the cytotoxic T cells kill the altered cells, resulting in the development of intraepithelial vesicles. This inflammatory reaction presents as an intensely pruritic skin disease called allergic contact dermatitis. In addition to α/β T cells, other cell types, such as γ/δ T cells, B-1 cells, and NK T cells, may be involved in the reaction. The reaction is moderated by IL-10 produced by mast cells.

Recent studies have demonstrated that contact dermatitis can be readily induced in mice that lack all types of lymphocytes except NK cells! In addition, contact dermatitis appears to be antigen specific insofar as primed animals mount a much stronger response than unprimed animals. This appears to be a property of a subpopulation of NK cells. These NK cells can survive for at least 28 days in mice and form a memory cell

population. These results clearly are at variance with our previous ideas about the antigenic specificity of NK cells and their role in immunity. It is also of interest to note that contact dermatitis will not occur in skin that lacks functional nerve fibers. Clearly allergic dermatitis has a complex and poorly understood etiology.

The chemicals that induce allergic contact dermatitis are usually highly reactive molecules that combine chemically with skin proteins to act as haptens; they include formaldehyde, picric acid, aniline dyes, plant resins and oils, organophosphates, some topical medications such as neomycin, and salts of metals such as nickel and beryllium (Figure 31-6). Thus, allergic contact dermatitis can occur on pathologists' fingers as a result of exposure to formaldehyde; on the ears of dogs treated with neomycin for otitis externa; on the foot pads, scrotum, and ventral abdomen of dogs on exposure to some carpet dyes and deodorizers; on parts of the body exposed to the oils (urushiol) of the poison ivy plant (*Rhus radicans*); and around the neck of animals as a result of exposure to dichlorvos (2,2-dichlorovinyldimethylphosphate) in flea collars (Box 31-1). Severe lesions may develop on the teats of dairy cattle as a result of a contact dermatitis to a component of the rubber in a milking machine (N-isopropyl-N-phenyl diamine). Allergic contact dermatitis involving the muzzle of dogs has been reported to result from sensitivity to components of plastic food bowls. Some dogs, instead of developing the more usual type I hypersensitivity to pollen proteins, experience an allergic contact dermatitis as a result of a type IV hypersensitivity to pollen resins. It is unusual for allergic contact dermatitis to affect the haired areas of the skin unless the allergen is in a liquid. Thus allergic contact dermatitis to shampoo components may result in total-body involvement. The period required for sensitization ranges from 6 months to several years. Calcium cyanamide (CaCN₂) is a widely used

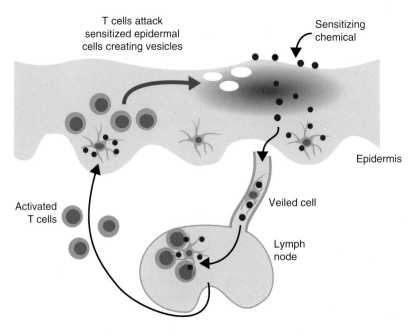

FIGURE 31-5 The pathogenesis of allergic contact dermatitis.

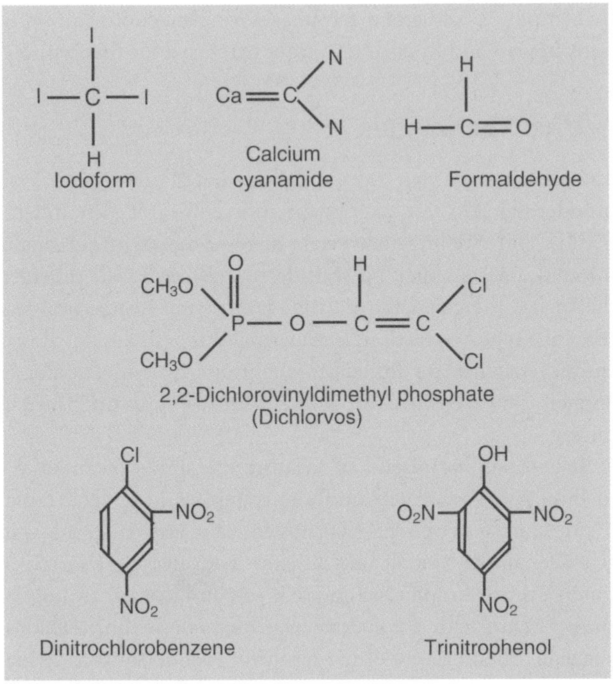

FIGURE 31-6 Some of the simple chemicals that can cause allergic contact dermatitis.

□ **Table 31-2 | Comparison of the Major Forms of Allergic Dermatitis**

	ATOPIC DERMATITIS	ALLERGIC CONTACT DERMATITIS
Pathogenesis	Type I hypersensitivity	Type IV hypersensitivity
Clinical signs	Hyperemia, urticaria, pruritus	Hyperemia, vesiculation, alopecia, erythema
Distribution	Face, nose, eyes, feet, perineum	Hairless areas, usually ventral abdomen and feet
Major allergens	Foods and pollens, fleas, inhaled allergens	Reactive chemicals, dyes in contact with skin
Diagnosis	Intradermal testing, immediate response	Delayed response on patch testing
Pathology	Eosinophilic infiltration, edema	Mononuclear cell infiltration, vesiculation
Treatment	Steroids, antihistamines, hyposensitization	Steroids

□ **Box 31-1 | Sources of Contact Allergens in Animals**

Insecticides in flea collars
　In sprays
　In dips
Wood preservatives
Floor waxes
Carpet dyes
Some pollens
Dermatological drugs (creams, ointments)
Leather products
Paints
House plants

nitrogenous fertilizer. It has also been used to reduce *Escherichia coli* levels in bedding. Dairy cattle have developed severe dermatitis on contact with calcium cyanamide spread on the floor of a cattle shed to prevent mastitis. A patch test using calcium cyanamide induced significant contact dermatitis in affected cattle.

The lesions of allergic contact dermatitis vary in severity, ranging from a mild erythema to a severe erythematous vesiculation. However, because of the intense pruritus, self-trauma, excoriation, ulceration, and secondary staphylococcal pyoderma often mask the true nature of the lesion. If the exposure

to the allergen persists, hyperkeratosis, acanthosis, and dermal fibrosis may eventually occur. Histologically, the lesion is marked by a mononuclear cell infiltration and vacuolation of skin cells under attack by cytotoxic T cells (Table 31-2).

Allergic contact dermatitis is diagnosed by removal of the suspected antigen and by patch testing. In "closed" patch tests, suspected allergens are used to impregnate gauze swabs that are then attached to the shaved skin with tape. After 48 to 72 hours the dressing is removed and the areas in contact with the swabs examined. A positive reaction is indicated by local erythema and vesiculation. Closed patch tests may be impractical for some dogs and cats. An "open" patch test may therefore be employed. In this procedure, a solution of the suspected allergen is applied to shaved normal skin and the area examined daily for up to 5 days. Identification of the offending allergen and its avoidance by the animal are the optimal therapies for allergic contact dermatitis. Hyposensitization therapy is not effective. Steroids are used in acute cases, with antibiotics to control secondary infections.

Stevens-Johnson Syndrome

Three related mucocutaneous disorders—erythema multiforme, Stevens-Johnson syndrome, and toxic epidermal necrolysis—are well recognized in humans and have been diagnosed in dogs and cats. The three diseases are characterized by lesions of increasing severity. Erythema multiforme is characterized by patchy skin loss and low morbidity; Stevens-Johnson syndrome is more severe but involves less than 10% of the body surface; toxic epidermal necrolysis is much more serious, with affected individuals losing more than 30% of their epidermis. Mortality is high. The three conditions however, overlap considerably. Stevens-Johnson syndrome and toxic epidermal necrolysis are believed to involve a T cell–mediated hypersensitivity to drugs. Erythema multiforme is not associated with drug administration. Affected animals develop vesicles, shed large areas of epidermis, and develop skin ulcers as a result of widespread keratinocyte apoptosis. The apoptosis is believed to result from drugs or their metabolites binding to the epidermal cells and upregulating CD95L expression as well as the production of soluble CD95L and granulysin, triggering their destruction by cytotoxic T cells. (Intradermal inoculation of granulysin solutions in mice at a concentration found in blister fluid results in the development of lesions mimicking Stevens-Johnson syndrome.) Skin lesions are infiltrated mainly by CD8+ T cells and fewer CD4+ cells. Many different drugs may trigger these responses, but common inducers in dogs include trimethoprim-potentiated sulfonamides, β-lactam antibiotics, penicillin, and cephalexin. Beginning about 14 days after drug exposure, the skin begins to blister and slough. Animals develop generalized illness, including dyspnea, vomiting, fever, and weight loss. In dogs, sloughing of the epidermis occurs over the nasal planum, the footpads, and the oral, pharyngeal, nasal, conjunctival, and preputial mucosa. Fluid loss leads to electrolyte imbalances, whereas life-threatening secondary infections are common. Biopsy specimens show extensive epidermal cell death.

Treatment involves immediate withdrawal of the offending drug followed by symptomatic treatment, including fluid replacement. Corticosteroids should be avoided since they increase the animal's susceptibility to skin infections and worsen the prognosis. Antibiotics should only be administered if skin infections occur. Intravenous administration of high doses of human immunoglobulins have been used successfully to treat this disease in dogs. It is believed that these immunoglobulins block CD95/CD95-ligand interactions and prevent keratinocyte apoptosis (Chapter 39).

Measurement of Cell-Mediated Immunity

Although diagnostic immunology is based largely on the detection of serum antibodies, measurement of cell-mediated immune responsiveness in animals may be desirable under some circumstances. For example, in determining the effectiveness of a vaccine, one must take into account that serum antibody levels may not truly reflect the degree of immunity possessed by an animal. Animals without detectable antibodies may possess significant cell-mediated immunity. The term cell-mediated immunity encompasses a diverse set of mechanisms

that employ T cells and macrophages for protection. Currently, both in vivo and in vitro techniques are used for this purpose.

In Vivo Techniques

The simplest in vivo test of cell-mediated immunity is an intradermal skin test such as the tuberculin test. The inflammation and swelling that occur in response to intradermally injected antigens may be considered cell mediated, provided that it has the characteristic time course and histological features of a type IV reaction. Intradermal skin tests are not always convenient, they are difficult to quantitate, and injection of an antigen may sensitize an animal, thus preventing further testing.

It is sometimes useful to measure the ability of an animal to mount cell-mediated immune responses in general rather than response to one specific antigen. One way to do this is to give the animal a small skin allograft and measure its survival time. A much simpler technique is to paint a small area of the animal's skin with a contact sensitizer such as dinitrochlorobenzene. The intensity of the resulting allergic contact dermatitis provides a rough estimate of the animal's ability to mount a cell-mediated immune response.

If the T cell–stimulating lectin phytohemagglutinin is injected intradermally, it provokes a local tissue reaction with many features of a delayed hypersensitivity response. In pigs, for example, this reaction is characterized by infiltration with γ/δ+, CD4−, CD8−T cells. This is a very convenient and rapid method of assessing an animal's ability to mount a cell-mediated response without the need for first sensitizing the animal to an antigen. However, the response to phytohemagglutinin is nonspecific, and its interpretation may be difficult.

In Vitro Techniques

In vitro tests are designed to measure the antigen-specific activation and proliferation of T cells. These also include their cytotoxic activities and their production of cytokines. All of these tests require that T cells be grown in cell culture; therefore few are useful for use in the field.

To measure T cell proliferation in response to an antigen, a suspension of purified peripheral blood lymphocytes from the animal to be tested is mixed with the antigen and cultured for 48 to 96 hours (Figure 31-7). Twelve hours before harvesting, thymidine labeled with the radioactive isotope tritium is added to the cultures. Normal, nondividing lymphocytes do not take up thymidine, but dividing cells do because they are actively synthesizing DNA. Thus if the T cells are proliferating, they will take up the tritiated thymidine, and their radioactivity provides a measure of this proliferation. The greater the response of the cells to an antigen, the greater will be their radioactivity. The ratio of the radioactivity in the stimulated cultures to the radioactivity in the controls is called the stimulation index. A related technique is to measure the proliferation of lymphocytes in response to mitogenic lectins (Box 13-2).

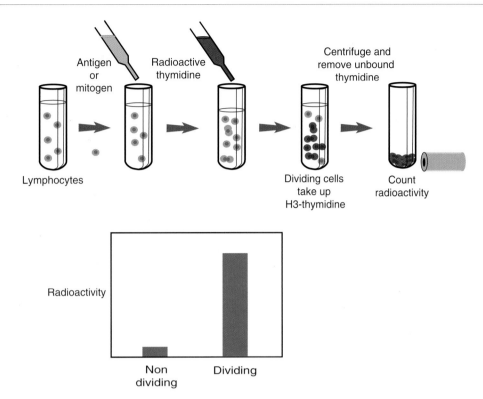

FIGURE 31-7 The measurement of cell proliferation by detecting the uptake of tritiated thymidine. Cells are stimulated to divide by specific antigen or a mitogen. The thymidine is incorporated into the DNA of the dividing cells. The uptake is simply measured by the radioactivity of the cells.

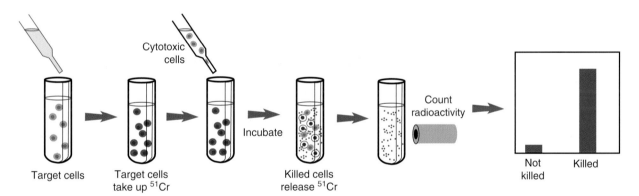

FIGURE 31-8 The measurement of cell death by detecting the release of chromium-51 by dying cells. This release may be triggered by cytotoxic T cells or NK cells.

The intensity of the lymphocyte proliferative response, as measured by tritiated thymidine uptake, provides an estimate of the reactivity of an animal's lymphocytes.

Radioactive tritium may be replaced in proliferation assays by a simple colorimetric enzyme assay. Methylthiazoldiphenyltetrazolium bromide (MTT) is a pale yellow compound that serves as a substrate for active mitochondrial enzymes. The enzymes change the MTT color to dark blue. The intensity of this color change is a measure of the number of living cells in a culture. In proliferation assays, the number of living cells increases, and this can be measured colorimetrically. The test is sufficiently sensitive to quantify the increase in T cell numbers triggered by antigen or mitogens.

To measure T cell–mediated cytotoxicity, it is necessary to have a simple method of measuring cell death. This is usually based on the fact that living cells take up and retain chromium ions, but if the cell dies, the chromium is released into the extracellular fluid. Radioactive sodium chromate (^{51}Cr) may be used in this way to label target cells (Figure 31-8). Lymphocytes from an immune animal are mixed in an appropriate ratio with ^{51}Cr-labeled target cells. The mixture is then incubated for 4 to 24 hours at 37° C. At the end of this time, the cell suspension is centrifuged and the presence of free ^{51}Cr in the supernatant measured. The amount of chromium released is related directly to the number of target cells killed. The amount of chromium released in the absence of cytotoxic cells must also

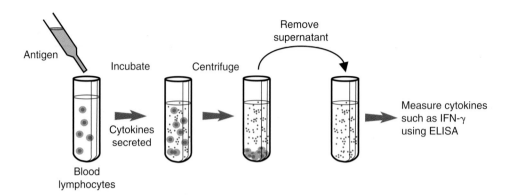

FIGURE 31-9 The release of IFN-γ by peripheral blood lymphocytes following exposure to tuberculin or to purified mycobacterial antigens This technique can be used for the diagnosis of tuberculosis in cattle and deer. Tuberculin PPD is added to blood, and the mixture is incubated for 24 to 48 hours. The plasma is then removed and assayed for any interferon produced.

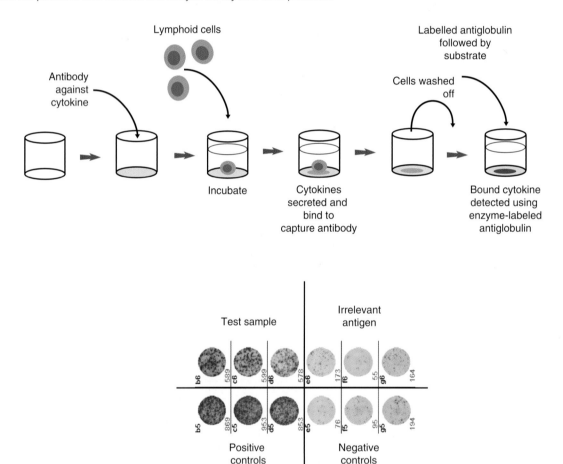

FIGURE 31-10 The principles of the ELISpot assay. The photograph shows the IFN-γ response of bovine peripheral blood mononuclear cells exposed to a defined *Anaplasma marginale* antigen.

(Courtesy Dr. W. Mwangi.)

be measured and subtracted from that released in the presence of cytotoxic cells to obtain a true reading.

A third in vitro assay is the measurement of cytokine release by T cells. One important example of this technique involves measuring the release of IFN-γ by peripheral blood lymphocytes following exposure to tuberculin or to purified mycobacterial antigens (Figure 31-9). This method has been developed

as an alternative or supplement to the tuberculin test for the diagnosis of tuberculosis in cattle and deer. It involves adding tuberculin PPD to heparinized blood and incubating the mixture for 24 to 48 hours at 37° C. The plasma is then removed and assayed for any interferon produced, either by means of a simple bioassay or preferably by use of a sandwich enzyme-linked immunosorbent assay (ELISA) employing monoclonal antibodies. Three "antigens" are commonly used: no antigen (negative control), *M. bovis* PPD, and *M. avium* PPD. The *M. avium* PPD is used to detect false-positive cross-reactions. Purified, recombinant mycobacterial proteins such as ESAT-6 can reduce the incidence of false-positive results even further. This technique has advantages over conventional tuberculin tests in that it does not sensitize the animal under testing by injection of antigen. In addition, the animal does not have to be held for several days for the test to be read. It is also much simpler than other in vitro tests for cell-mediated immunity. The assay is at least as sensitive as the single intradermal test and, if purified recombinant mycobacterial proteins are employed, is highly specific. (Its sensitivity is about 85%, and its specificity is as high as 90% to 99%). Positive results are obtained earlier than by skin testing. However, it does appear to detect tuberculosis in a slightly different population of animals than the skin test. It has also been successfully used to diagnose Johne's disease in sheep.

It is possible to use a variation of a sandwich ELISA assay (Chapter 41) to determine the frequency of cytokine-secreting cells. (Figure 31-10). In the enzyme-linked immunospot (ELISpot) assay, a capture-antibody directed against the cytokine of interest is coated on the bottom of plastic tissue culture wells. The cells to be tested are cultured on this surface and exposed to the antigen of interest. If the cells respond by secreting the cytokine of interest, it will bind to nearby capture-antibodies. Once the culture period is completed, the presence of this bound cytokine can be detected by a conventional sandwich ELISA using specific detection antibody and enzyme-labeled antiglobulin. This results in the development of a pattern of colored spots that each correspond to the location of a cytokine-secreting cell. These spots can be counted and the frequency of specific cytokine-producing cells determined. This assay can also be used to quantitate cytotoxic cells by detecting granzyme or perforin production.

Although all of the assays described previously can be used to measure at least some aspects of cell-mediated immunity, none provides a complete picture. The investigator may of course simply be interested in the response to a single antigen or organism. In these cases, either a skin test or an in vitro assay may be appropriate. This is best exemplified by the tests available for the diagnosis of tuberculosis. In vitro tests are also useful if the time course of a cell-mediated immune response is to be examined. Repeated testing can be performed simply by obtaining more lymphocytes. If, on the other hand, an investigator wishes to obtain an overview of an animal's abilities in this area, one of the nonspecific in vivo assays may be more appropriate. These can be useful, for example, in assessing immune function in young animals thought to be immunodeficient. However, it is important to point out that in these animals, a complete hematological examination should be performed before more complex assays are considered. It is also prudent to measure the important lymphocyte subpopulations by flow cytometry. An animal that has no T cells is unlikely to mount any sort of cell-mediated response.

For sources of additional information, please visit http://evolve.elsevier.com/tizard/immunology/

Organ Graft Rejection

□ Key Points

- Organ grafts between two unrelated individuals of the same species are called allografts.
- Allografts are rejected by the recipient as a result of immune responses directed against donor blood group antigens and histocompatibility antigens.
- The response to donor histocompatibility antigens causes acute rejection and is mainly mediated by cytotoxic T cells attacking graft vascular endothelium.
- Chronic rejection and rejection directed against donor blood groups are mainly antibody mediated.
- Bone marrow stem cell allografts given to immunosuppressed recipients can attack the recipient and cause graft-versus-host disease.
- Some allografts, such as those from the cornea, are not readily rejected.
- The fetus can be considered an allograft but is not rejected as a result of multiple immunosuppressive mechanisms acting at the maternal-placental interface.

Although the immune response first attracted the attention of scientists because of the body's ability to fight infections, the observation that animals reject foreign organ grafts led to a much broader view of the immune system in that it indicated that the immune system had a surveillance function. The rejection of a foreign organ graft simply reflects the role of the immune system in identifying and destroying "abnormal" cells.

Grafting of Organs

Advances in surgery have permitted the transfer of many tissues or organs between different parts of the body or between different individuals. When moved to a different part of an animal's own body, such transplants do not trigger an immune response. This type of graft within an individual is called an autograft (Figure 32-1). Examples of autografting include the

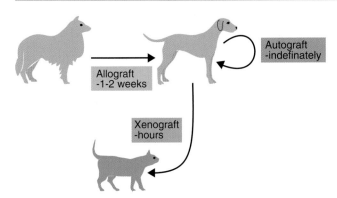

FIGURE 32-1 The differences among autografts, allografts, and xenografts.

use of skin to cover a burn in plastic surgery and the use of a segment of vein to bypass blocked cardiac arteries. Since autografts do not express foreign antigens, they do not trigger an immune response.

Isografts are grafts transplanted between two genetically identical individuals. Thus a graft between identical (monozygotic) twins is an isograft. Similarly, grafts between two inbred mice of the same strain are isografts and present no immunological difficulties. Since the animals are identical, the immune system of the recipient does not differentiate between the graft and normal body cells.

Allografts are transplanted between genetically different members of the same species. Most grafts performed on animals or humans for therapeutic reasons are of this type because tissues are obtained from a donor who is usually unrelated to the graft recipient. Because the major histocompatibility complex (MHC) and blood group molecules on the allograft are different from those of their host, allografts induce a strong immune response that causes graft rejection. This rejection process must be suppressed if the grafted organ is to survive.

Xenografts are organ grafts transplanted between animals of different species. Thus, the transplant of a baboon heart into a human infant is a xenograft. Xenografted tissues differ from their host both biochemically and immunologically. As a result, they can provoke a rapid, intense rejection response that is very difficult to suppress.

Clinical grafting in domestic animals is a recent procedure. However, renal allografting is now routine in dogs and cats, and bone marrow allografts promise to be very useful in some forms of tumor therapy. It is unlikely that cadaveric allografting will become important in veterinary medicine. Most current organ grafts are obtained from healthy donor animals. This raises significant ethical issues as to whether it is appropriate to subject a donor animal to major surgery in order to provide an organ for another animal. Although the benefits of allografting to the recipient are obvious, it is unclear how the donor animal might benefit. Unlike human donors driven by altruism, an animal donor is given no choice in the matter. It is possible, however, to justify organ donation if thereby an animal would be saved from inevitable euthanasia and if the

donor could be provided with a good home. For this reason, many animal transplantation centers require that the donor animal be adopted and cared for by the owner of the recipient animal.

Allograft Rejection

The identification and destruction of foreign molecules are central to the body's defense. Allografted organs represent a major source of these foreign molecules. They include not only antigens such as the foreign blood group glycoproteins and MHC molecules expressed on the grafted cells, but also any endogenous antigens presented on the MHC class I molecules of these same cells. The mechanisms of allograft rejection are basically the same irrespective of the organ grafted, and both antibodies and T cells participate in the rejection of allografts.

Histocompatibility Antigens

When an organ is transplanted into a genetically dissimilar animal, the recipient will mount an immune response against many different antigens in and on the cells of the allograft. These are called histocompatibility antigens. Three types of histocompatibility antigens are of major importance in stimulating graft rejection. These are the MHC class I molecules, the MHC class II molecules, and the major blood group molecules. All are expressed on the surface of the graft cells, but their distribution varies. MHC class I antigens are found on almost all nucleated cells. The major blood group antigens are found both on red cells and nucleated cells. MHC class II antigens, in contrast, have a restricted distribution that varies among mammals (Chapter 11). For example, in rats and mice, MHC class II molecules are expressed only on the professional antigen-presenting cells (APCs): macrophages, dendritic cells, and B cells. In other species, such as humans and pigs, MHC class II molecules are also expressed on the endothelium of renal arteries and glomeruli, the sites where host cells first make contact with the graft. These MHC class II molecules are recognized as foreign and trigger the rejection process. It is interesting to note that, as a result of these differences, it is much easier to prolong renal allograft survival in laboratory rodents than in humans or pigs.

As would be expected, grafts that differ minimally from the recipient will generally survive longer than grafts that are highly incompatible. When blood group A-O-compatible pigs are given renal allografts, median survival is about 12 days for MHC-unmatched grafts, 25 days for grafts compatible for MHC class I alone, 32 days for grafts compatible for MHC class II alone, and 80 days for grafts compatible for both class I and class II (Figure 32-2). When dogs are given MHC-unmatched renal allografts, the grafts survive for about 10 days. Completely matched allografts in dogs survive for about 40 days. A more impressive result is obtained with canine liver grafts, which survive for about 8 days in unmatched animals and for 200 to 300 days in DLA-matched recipients.

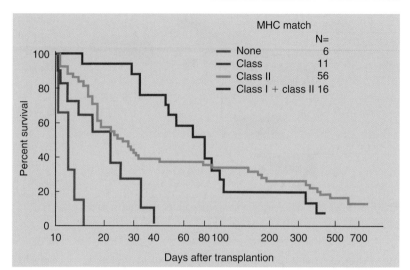

FIGURE 32-2 Survival time of organ allografts between SLA-incompatible minipigs clearly depends on the degree of MHC compatibility between donor and host.

(From Pescovitz MD, Thistlethwaite JR Jr, Auchincloss H Jr, Ildstad ST, Sharp TG, Terrill R, Sachs DH. Effect of class II antigen matching on renal allograft survival in miniature swine. *J Exp Med.* 1984,160:1495-1508.)

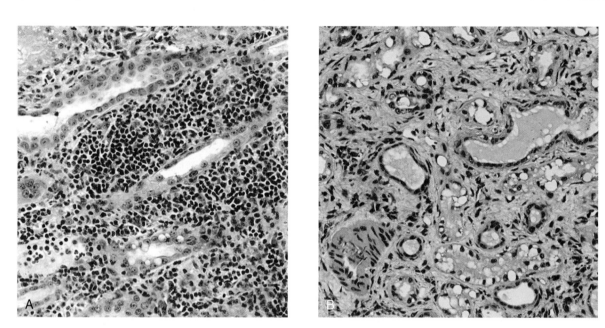

FIGURE 32-3 A, Section of a canine kidney that had been acutely rejected and as a consequence is densely infiltrated with lymphocytes. **B,** Section of a kidney that has undergone chronic allograft rejection. In this case the section shows interstitial fibrosis with tubular atrophy and a mild lymphocytic infiltration.

(Courtesy Dr. A.E. Kyles.)

The failure of MHC and blood group–compatible grafts to survive indefinitely is a result of the cumulative effects of many other minor antigenic differences. For example, skin grafts from male donors placed on histocompatible females are usually rejected, although the reverse is not the case. This is because male cells carry an antigen coded for by genes on the Y chromosome called the H-Y antigen.

During the acute rejection process, the grafted tissue gradually becomes infiltrated with cytotoxic T cells, which cause progressive damage to the endothelial cells lining small blood vessels (Figure 32-3). The T cells roll along the endothelial surface and bind using leukocyte function-associated antigen-1 (LFA-1). T cell–mediated damage releases chemokines that attract more T cells into the graft. Cellular destruction,

stoppage of blood flow, hemorrhage, and death of the grafted organ follow thrombosis of these vessels. The blood vessels of second organ grafts become blocked even more rapidly as a result of the action of antibodies and complement on the vascular endothelium. This secondary reaction is specific for any graft from the original donor or from a donor syngeneic with the first. It is not restricted to any particular site or to any specific organ since MHC and blood group molecules are present on most nucleated cells.

In practice it is usually not difficult to ensure that the donor and recipient have identical major blood group antigens. MHC compatibility is much harder to achieve because MHC polymorphism ensures that individuals differ widely in their MHC haplotype. In general, the more closely donor and recipient are related, the less will be their MHC difference. For this reason it is preferable that grafts be obtained from a recipient's parents or siblings. If this is not possible, a donor must be selected at random and the inevitable rejection responses suppressed by drugs such as cyclosporine or tacrolimus (Chapter 39).

Renal Allografts

Clinical Allograft Rejection

Renal allograft rejection is of major clinical importance in humans and has been widely studied in animals. It therefore serves as a good example of the allograft response. Rejection may occur at any time after transplantation. In humans, in whom a great deal of experience with transplantation has been gained, four distinct clinical rejection syndromes are recognized. *Hyperacute rejection* occurs within 48 hours after grafting. Rejection occurring up to 7 days after grafting is called *accelerated rejection*. Rejection after 7 days is called *acute rejection*. *Chronic rejection* develops several months after grafting. It is unclear whether a similar classification is useful in animals.

When kidneys are allografted, the blood supply to the transplanted kidney is established at the time of transplantation. The graft and host cells come into contact almost immediately. In an unsensitized host, a primary immune response is mounted, and renal allografts are only rejected after at least 10 days and possibly much longer. In sensitized animals in which the immune system is already primed, hyperacute rejection occurs, and the graft is destroyed within days or even hours without ever becoming functional. Acute rejection should be suspected when the recipient shows a rapidly rising blood creatinine associated with an enlarged, painful kidney accompanied by signs of depression, anorexia, vomiting, proteinuria, hematuria, and ultrasonography showing an enlarged, hypoechoic kidney. In contrast, chronic rejection should be suspected if the creatinine and urea levels rise gradually, and this is associated with proteinuria, microscopic hematuria, and a small, hyperechoic kidney. It is also associated with a slow loss of renal function and tends to be related to with interstitial fibrosis and proliferation of vascular endothelium. Renal biopsy is necessary to confirm rejection.

Pathogenesis of Allograft Rejection

The allograft rejection process is directed against the dominant antigens on the cells of the graft. The MHC molecules tend to trigger a T cell–mediated rejection response, whereas the blood group antigens tend to trigger antibody formation. The rejection process may be divided into two stages. First, the host's lymphocytes encounter the antigens of the graft and trigger a response. Second, cytotoxic T cells and antibodies from the host enter the graft and destroy graft cells (Figure 32-4).

Innate Mechanisms Damage to the graft as a result of surgical trauma and ischemia followed by reperfusion upregulates MHC expression and generates cytokines and inflammatory mediators that attract neutrophils and macrophages into the graft. If large quantities of damage-associated molecular patterns (DAMPs) such as high mobility group box protein-1 (HMGB1) are generated, they will activate toll-like receptors and other pattern-recognition receptors. An increase in expression of MICA molecules on graft endothelial cells can activate natural killer (NK) cells. Complement components such as C5a and C3a may also activate APCs within the graft.

Adaptive Mechanisms Donor antigens are presented to the T cells of the recipient by APCs. The graft recipients may be sensitized by a direct pathway in which recipient T cells circulating through the graft encounter antigens presented by donor APCs. These donor APCs may also carry antigens to draining

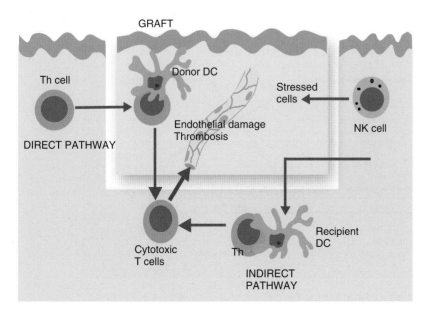

FIGURE 32-4 Some of the mechanisms involved in the rejection of an allograft (see text for details).

lymph nodes and the spleen. Alternatively, recipients may be sensitized when their own APCs circulate through the graft and encounter and process donor antigens (the indirect pathway). The direct pathway operates early in the rejection process but is replaced by the indirect pathway once donor APCs have been destroyed. In humans, the direct pathway is responsible for the vigorous immune response that occurs in acute rejection, whereas the indirect pathway is more important in chronic rejection. Although macrophages and dendritic cells are important APCs, donor B cells and tubular epithelial and endothelial cells can also process antigen, and they can migrate to lymphoid organs where they activate recipient T cells.

In laboratory rodents, MHC class II molecules are expressed on professional APCs. In these species the intensity of graft rejection is related to the number of donor B cells, macrophages, and dendritic cells transplanted within the graft. Removal of these cells by careful flushing of the graft before surgery or by pretreatment of the donor with cytotoxic drugs greatly reduces the intensity of the rejection process. In other mammals in which MHC class II molecules are also expressed on vascular endothelial cells, these "passenger" cells are of less significance.

The APCs that process donor MHC molecules migrate to the draining lymph node and activate other T cells. The paracortical regions of lymph nodes draining a graft therefore contain dividing lymphocytes. The number of these cells is greatest about 6 days after grafting and declines rapidly once the graft has been rejected. In addition to these signs of an active T cell–mediated immune response, germinal center formation occurs in the cortex, and plasma cells accumulate in the medulla, indicating that antibody formation is also occurring. In a conventional immune response, only one cell in 10^5 to 10^6 T cells can respond to a specific antigen. In graft rejection, however, there may be 1% to 10% of responding T cells since these cells have low activation thresholds for foreign MHC molecules.

The activated Th1 cells produce interleukin-2 (IL-2) and interferon-γ (IFN-γ) and so activate cytotoxic T cells and NK cells. The NK cells produce more IFN-γ and tumor necrosis factor-α (TNF-α) that activates macrophages and additional NK cells. The cytotoxic CD8+ T cells recognize the foreign peptides bound to recipient MHC class I molecules and kill any target cell they encounter. Donor MHC class II molecules trigger an immune response in two ways. First, because they are foreign proteins, they are processed as endogenous antigens. Second, they may directly bind to recipient T cell receptors (TCRs) and trigger cytotoxicity.

IL-2 and IFN-γ not only promote cytotoxic T cell activity but also enhance the expression of MHC molecules on the cells of the graft. During allograft rejection, therefore, MHC expression is increased, and the graft becomes an even more attractive target for cytotoxic T cells.

Although cytotoxic T cells are of major importance in acute allograft rejection, B cells, eosinophils, and macrophages also play a significant role in hyperacute and chronic rejection (Figure 32-5). Hyperacute rejection occurs when the recipient has preexisting antibodies to graft MHC or blood groups. These bind to graft vascular endothelial cells, activate complement by the classical pathway, and cause endothelial cell lysis. The damaged endothelial cells trigger platelet deposition as well as multiple chemokines and cytokines, especially IL-1β, CXCL8, and CCL2. These attract leukocytes as well, and the damage results in thrombosis and infarction. Anti-MHC antibodies also play a major role in secondary rejection, in which they activate the classical complement pathway and mediate antibody-dependent cytotoxic cell activity.

Graft Destruction Once activated, cytotoxic T cells reach the graft through the bloodstream. They bind and destroy vascular endothelium and other accessible cells through caspase-mediated apoptosis. As a result of this damage, hemorrhage, platelet aggregation, thrombosis, and stoppage of blood flow

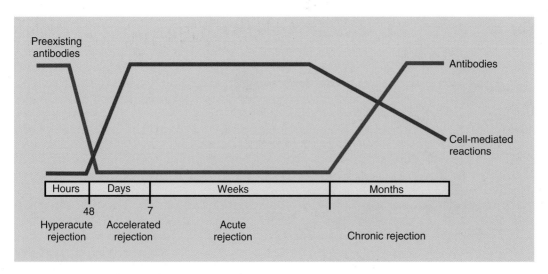

FIGURE 32-5 Role of antibodies and cell-mediated immunity in different allograft rejection syndromes.

occur. The grafted tissue dies because of the failure of its blood supply. CD4+ T cells that enter the graft may release cytotoxic cytokines such as TNF-α. This triggers apoptosis in endothelial cells. Invading cytotoxic T cells can also cross the basement membrane and cause apoptosis of renal tubular cells. Activated macrophages releasing proinflammatory cytokines impair graft function and intensify T cell–mediated rejection.

Prevention of Allograft Rejection

In preventing allograft rejection, the transplantation surgeon seeks to induce the minimal level of immunosuppression to prevent rejection while not making the recipient more susceptible than necessary to infection. Dogs mount very strong allograft responses, and kidney allografts are rejected in 6 to 14 days in untreated animals. Unrelated dogs with renal allografts show about 50% 1-year survival when treated with azathioprine, prednisolone, and cyclosporine. Survival is considerably enhanced by a simultaneous bone marrow allograft from the donor animal or by treatment with rabbit antidog thymocyte serum. In practice, median survival times of 8 months can be achieved, with some animals surviving for longer than 5 years. Dogs have significant perioperative mortality, and two thirds experience recurrent acute infections, especially respiratory tract infections with *Bordetella bronchiseptica* and urinary tract infections. Newer immunosuppressive agents such as leflunomide (Chapter 39) show promise of vastly improving the prognosis for canine renal allografting.

Cats that receive renal allografts without immunosuppression die in 8 to 34 days. Immunosuppressive therapy involves the use of prednisolone and cyclosporine possibly supplemented with ketoconazole. (The ketoconazole suppresses cyclosporine metabolism in the liver and prolongs its half-life.) The therapy can begin 2 days before surgery so that cyclosporine levels are optimum when the graft is introduced. Six-month survival of treated cats ranges from 59% to 70%, whereas 3-year survival ranges from 40% to 50%. The longest survival time reported for cats receiving renal allografts is 8 years. These figures are gradually improving as experience grows. Long-term complications include acute or chronic rejection and opportunistic infections. (Infection is the second most important cause of death or euthanasia after acute rejection.) Acute rejection can occur at any time, especially if cyclosporine levels fall below the therapeutic range. Chronic allograft rejection (graft vascular disease) due to progressive arterial arteriosclerosis may cause ischemic graft destruction. It is not responsive to immunosuppressive therapy.

In some circumstances, such as when a dog has maintained functioning renal allografts for several years, immunosuppressive therapy may be reduced gradually and eventually discontinued as graft acceptance becomes complete. It is probable that the immunosuppressive drugs gradually eliminate antigen-sensitive cells. Once their numbers are sufficiently low, the large mass of grafted tissue may be sufficient to establish and maintain tolerance.

Skin Allografts

Although the mechanisms of rejection are similar among different tissues, minor differences are observed in the process. For example, if a skin graft is placed on an animal, it takes several days for blood vessels and lymphatic connections to be established between the graft and the host. Only when these connections are made can host cells enter the graft and commence the rejection process. The first sign of rejection is a transient neutrophil accumulation around the blood vessels at the base of the graft. This is followed by infiltration with mononuclear cells (lymphocytes and macrophages) that eventually extends throughout the grafted skin. The first signs of tissue damage are observed in the capillaries of the graft, whose endothelium is destroyed. As a result, the blood clots, blood flow stops, and tissue death follows. The presence of Langerhans cells in the epidermis significantly enhances the antigenicity of skin allografts. In a secondary reaction, host blood vessels usually do not have time to grow into a skin graft since a destructive mononuclear cell and neutrophil infiltration rapidly develops in the graft bed.

Liver Allografts

It was originally reported that a high percentage of liver allografts between outbred pigs were accepted without immunosuppression. However, these pigs were not genetically defined, and the degree of MHC mismatching was unclear. When liver allografts are made between genetically defined miniature pigs with known MHC differences, it is found that their speed of rejection is similar to that observed with kidney or skin allografts. Liver graft rejection in dogs tends to occur fairly slowly. This inhibition of liver allograft rejection appears to be due to the production of indoleamine 2,3-dioxygenase (IDO) by hepatocytes. IDO destroys the amino acid tryptophan. Since tryptophan is essential for Th1 responses, its absence within the grafted liver is highly immunosuppressive.

Cardiac Allografts

Acute rejection of canine heart allografts is associated with massive lymphocytic infiltration and myocyte damage leading to rapid graft destruction. If, however, the rejection process is slowed for some reason, the pathological process in the chronically rejected organ changes. In these cases, lymphocytes and antibodies directed against vascular smooth muscle cells stimulate vascular rejection. T cells and macrophages release a chemokine cascade that activates vascular smooth muscle and endothelial cells. The resulting smooth muscle cell growth and inflammation lead to obliteration of the blood vessel lumen and eventually cardiac failure (Figure 32-6). This graft arteriosclerosis (or graft vascular disease) results from the growth-stimulating effects of both T cell–derived cytokines and

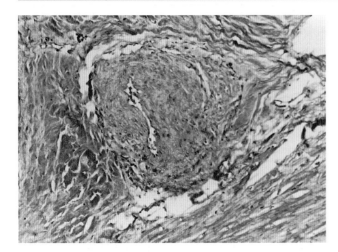

FIGURE 32-6 A section of coronary artery from a canine cardiac allograft. There is severe narrowing of the lumen as a result of smooth muscle cell proliferation, an example of graft vascular disease. Original magnification ×100.

(Courtesy Olaf Penn.)

antibodies. A similar lesion is seen in renal allografts undergoing chronic rejection.

Corneal Allografts

Certain areas of the body, such as the anterior chamber of the eye, the cornea, the thymus, the testes, and the brain, are immune-privileged sites. As a result, grafts made into these sites may not be rejected. In humans, for example, 90% of first-time corneal allografts survive without tissue typing or immunosuppressive drugs. These sites are privileged because the body rigorously controls inflammation in their critical tissues. Several mechanisms are involved in this. They have an impermeable blood-tissue barrier, lack dendritic cells, express low levels of MHC class I and II molecules, and may contain high levels of immunosuppressive molecules such as IDO, transforming growth factor-β (eyes and testes), neuropeptides (eyes), complement inhibitors (eyes), and corticosteroids (testes). Molecules found in normal aqueous humor also block innate immune mechanisms. They block NK cell lysis, inhibit neutrophil activation by CD95L, suppress nitric oxide production by activated macrophages, and interfere with alternative complement activation. The eye and testes are also unique in that they express very high levels of CD95L (Fas ligand). As a result, any CD95+ T cells that enter these organs will bind to CD95L and be killed by apoptosis.

Bone Allografts

Bone cortical allografts are used to repair severe nonreconstructible diaphyseal fractures as well as to reconstruct defects created by the resection of tumors. Rejection of bone

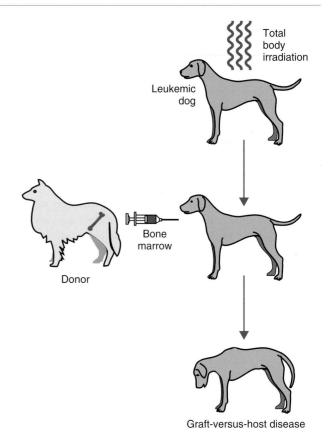

FIGURE 32-7 Induction of graft-versus-host disease in dogs that have received a bone marrow allograft.

allografts is rarely a problem, probably because of the absence of soft tissues in the graft. Unfortunately, long-term bone allografts have a high incidence of mechanical failure because the graft is resorbed before it is replaced. Joints may be successfully transplanted in horses provided that such joints have been previously frozen.

Bone Marrow Allografts

High-dose, total-body irradiation may be administered to dogs to completely destroy tumors such as leukemias. Unfortunately, such treatment also destroys bone marrow stem cells, and these must be replaced by a bone marrow allograft. The new hematopoietic stem cells restore bone marrow function (Figure 32-7). The recipient dog must first be conditioned by total-body irradiation or chemotherapy with cyclophosphamide. This creates space for the growing transplanted cells, reduces the intensity of the rejection process, and, in leukemic animals, destroys all tumor cells. Marrow is aspirated from the long bones of the donor and administered intravenously to the recipient. Hematopoietic stem cells migrate from the blood to the bone marrow. An optimal dose is about 2×10^8 allogeneic bone marrow cells per kilogram of body weight for matched recipients. The success rate of this procedure is relatively low. There was a 20% success rate with untreated mismatched canine marrow allografts but a

90% success rate with treated matched allografts. In a successfully engrafted dog, it takes about 30 days for the granulocytes to return to normal, but the lymphocytes take about 200 days to recover. Marrow survival is not generally enhanced by treatment with single immunosuppressive agents, but combinations such as mycophenolate mofetil plus cyclosporine or methotrexate plus cyclosporine can result in the development of stable canine bone marrow chimeras.

Graft-Versus-Host Disease

If healthy lymphocytes are injected into the skin of an allogeneic recipient, the lymphocytes attack the host cells and cause local acute inflammation. Provided the recipient has a functioning immune system, this graft-versus-host (GVH) reaction is not serious because the recipient can destroy the foreign lymphocytes and thus terminate the reaction. If, however, the recipient cannot reject the grafted lymphocytes because it has been immunosuppressed or is otherwise immunodeficient, the grafted cells may cause uncontrolled destruction of the host's tissues and, eventually, death. Thus GVH disease occurs in bone marrow allograft recipients who have been effectively immunosuppressed by total-body irradiation or cyclophosphamide treatment.

The lesions generated in GVH disease depend on MHC differences between donor and recipient. When they differ only in the MHC class I molecules, the disease is caused by cytotoxic T cells that attack all the nucleated cells of the host. This leads to a wasting syndrome characterized by bone marrow destruction leading to pancytopenia, aplastic anemia, loss of T and B cells, and hypogammaglobulinemia. Lymphocytes infiltrate the intestine, skin, and liver and secrete TNF-α, that causes mucosal destruction and diarrhea, skin and mouth ulcers, liver destruction, and jaundice.

If donor and recipient differ in MHC II, both graft and host CD4+ T helper cells may be stimulated. The production of Th2-derived cytokines may lead to immunostimulation, autoantibody formation, and even a syndrome resembling systemic lupus erythematosus and polyarthritis (Chapter 36). (This is called autoimmune GVH disease and may be treated with antibodies against IL-4.)

In practice, pure class I or class II disparities rarely occur naturally. Thus in dogs GVH disease can either be an acute disease causing death within 4 weeks of transplantation or prolonged and chronic. The major target organs are the skin, liver, gastrointestinal tract, and lymphoid system. The first clinical signs are exudative ear lesions, scleral injection, hyperkeratosis, alopecia, skin atrophy, and generalized erythema seen by 10 days (Figure 32-8). Jaundice and diarrhea frequently occur, as does inflammation of the eyes, nose, and oral mucous membranes. An antiglobulin-positive hemolytic anemia may also develop. The immunosuppressive drug methotrexate, together with monoclonal antilymphocyte antibodies, may be used to suppress GVH disease.

It is of interest to note that bone marrow transplantation in cats that previously received immunosuppressive irradiation

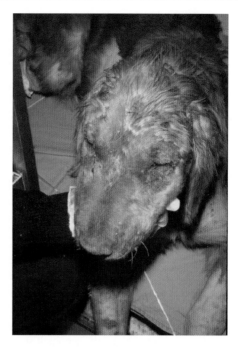

FIGURE 32-8 Very severe cutaneous erythematous lesions on the face of a dog suffering from graft-versus-host disease as a result of a bone marrow allograft.

(Courtesy Dr. C.K. Harris.)

or cyclosporine is a very successful procedure and that GVH disease is not a major problem in this species.

Xenografts

Although humans currently receive organs from dead human donors, the demand for organ grafts greatly exceeds the supply. It is possible that xenografting from nonhuman donors would eliminate this shortage. Unfortunately, xenografts are usually rejected within a few hours. The pathology of hyperacute xenograft rejection includes extensive hemorrhage and thrombosis brought about by massive destruction of endothelial cells. This allows blood cells to escape while exposing the underlying basement membrane to platelets.

Concordant xenografts are those between two closely related mammals such as between a chimpanzee and a human. In these cases rejection is largely mediated by cellular reactions. In discordant xenografts (those between unrelated mammals such as from a pig to a human), rejection is mediated largely by humoral mechanisms. In practice, concordant human xenografting from other primates such as chimpanzees or baboons is impractical because of the difficulty in providing large numbers of donor animals. Pigs, however, may be more practical sources of organs. They breed rapidly, and their organs are of an appropriate size. Unfortunately pig organs trigger a severe discordant xenograft rejection response in humans mediated by natural anticarbohydrate antibodies. Humans and Old

World monkeys lack the enzyme α1,3-galactosyltransferase and therefore do not make carbohydrates or glycoproteins with the α1,3-galactosyl linkage (Gal α1-3Gal). Because humans are exposed to this structure on many bacteria, we make high levels of antibodies to the Gal α1-3Gal epitope. Indeed more than 2% of total human immunoglobulin M (IgM) and IgG consists of antibodies to this epitope. The αGal epitope, on the other hand, is found in pig glycoproteins. If a pig organ is grafted into a human, these antibodies bind to graft cells, activate the classical complement pathway, and lyse cells. A second mechanism that contributes to hyperacute rejection is activation of the alternate complement pathway as a result of the failure of human complement factor H to prevent assembly of the alternate C3 convertase on the surface of pig cells. A third mechanism results from the species-specific activity of complement control proteins. Thus the natural inhibitors of complement such as CD46, CD55, and CD59 found on pig cells cannot control the activation of human complement. Transgenic pigs have been produced that express these human complement inhibitors on their cells and do not trigger hyperacute rejection on grafting. Should the xenograft survive attack by these natural antibodies and complement, it is still susceptible to delayed attack from induced antibodies and from antibody-dependent, cell-mediated cytotoxicity mediated through NK cells and monocytes. Many barriers are yet to be overcome if pig organs are ever to be routinely used as human organ transplants.

One other point relevant to xenografting is that donor animals may carry viruses that could cause disease in a severely immunosuppressed recipient or, even worse, recombine with human viruses to create new and potentially hazardous pathogens. These xenograft-derived infections (xenozoonoses) are of special concern if primates are used as organ donors. These animals are known to carry viruses such as simian immunodeficiency virus and herpes B virus that can infect humans. Pigs possess an endogenous retrovirus that has the ability to infect some human cell lines in tissue culture, although it is not known to cause human disease.

Allografts and the Reproductive System

Sperm

Allogeneic sperm can successfully and repeatedly penetrate the female reproductive tract without provoking graft rejection. The reason for this is that seminal plasma is immunosuppressive. Sperm exposed to this fluid are nonimmunogenic, even after washing. Prostatic fluid, one of the immunosuppressive components of seminal plasma, also inhibits complement-mediated hemolysis. In cattle, the immunosuppressive components of seminal plasma are proteins of less than 50 kDa and 150 kDa. Nevertheless, occasional cases of infertility resulting from the production of antisperm antibodies in the uterus do occur.

Pregnancy

When mammals evolved to become viviparous and the fetus developed inside its mother's uterus, a significant immunological problem had to be overcome. The fetus could not be rejected like an allograft even though it possesses paternal MHC molecules and its trophoblast lodges deep in the uterine wall. In a normal pregnancy the fetus establishes and maintains itself despite these MHC differences. The uterus is not a privileged site since grafts of other tissues, such as skin, in the uterine wall are readily rejected. Likewise, a mother may make antibodies against fetal blood group antigens, and these can destroy fetal red blood cells either in utero, as in primates, or following ingestion of colostrum, as occurs in other mammals (Chapter 29). Nevertheless, allograft rejection does not occur.

In general, pregnancy is associated with a strong skewing of the mother's immune system in favor of Th2 responses and a reduction in Th1 responses. (This raises the interesting concept that infections that promote a strong Th1 response might reverse this skewing, compromise pregnancy, and lead to abortion. This would certainly apply to protozoan infections such as toxoplasmosis, *Neospora caninum* infection, and brucellosis.)

The immunological destruction of the fetus and its trophoblast is prevented by the combined activities of many different immunosuppressive mechanisms acting at the maternal-fetal interface (Figure 32-9). First, no polymorphic MHC molecules are expressed on preimplantation embryos or oocytes. Likewise MHC class Ia or class II molecules are not expressed on the cell layer of the trophoblast in contact with maternal tissues. Cytokines that usually enhance MHC expression, such as IFN-γ, have no effect on trophoblast cells. The absence of MHC should permit trophoblast cells to avoid destruction by cytotoxic T cells but make them susceptible to attack by NK cells. This is prevented, however, by expression of the nonpolymorphic class Ib molecules HLA-G and HLA-E. These molecules prevent attack on the trophoblast by NK cells while the NK cells control invasion of the uterine wall by the trophoblast. Thus there is a balance between MHC class Ib expression on the trophoblast and NK cells in the uterine wall that together regulates trophoblast growth and invasion. The NK cells in the placenta are of a distinct subtype called uNK cells. uNK cells called endometrial gland cells have been described in rodents, bats, pigs, and horses.

Regulatory T (Treg) cells play an important role in preventing fetal rejection. Estrogen treatment and pregnancy both induce FoxP3 protein and may help support this regulation. It has been demonstrated that trophoblast cells secrete IDO, which blocks Th1 responses and promotes apoptosis. Inhibitors of IDO permit maternal rejection of allogeneic fetuses in mice. Treg cells upregulate IDO expression in dendritic cells. In addition, IDO induces trophoblast HLA-G expression, suggesting that these molecules interact to maintain pregnancy. In humans substantial numbers of maternal T cells cross the placenta to reside in fetal lymph nodes. This induces Treg cells that suppress fetal antimaternal immunity.

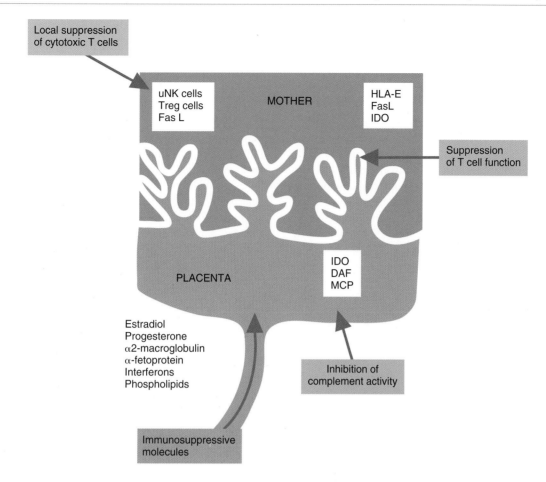

FIGURE 32-9 Some of the immunosuppressive factors that prevent rejection of the fetus by the mother's immune system.

Galectins regulate immune responses by binding to cell surface carbohydrates (glycans). One subfamily of these galectins are specifically expressed in the placenta of primates, especially in the syncytiotrophoblast, the placental layer that contacts the fetal cells. These specific galectins induce apoptosis in T cells. Thus they serve as local immunosuppressive agents that reduce the danger of maternal immune attacks on the fetus.

Although the mechanisms described previously minimize maternal sensitization by allogeneic fetal cells, cytotoxic T cells or antibodies do develop during pregnancy. We know that a pregnant mother may mount an immune response to her fetus. For example, in the pregnant mare, placental cells invade the uterine wall to form structures called endometrial cups. These in turn stimulate a strong immune response against paternal MHC antigens around day 60 of gestation. As a result, the cups are surrounded by large numbers of CD4+ and CD8+ T cells, macrophages, and plasma cells. This eventually leads to degeneration of the endometrial cups around 120 days of pregnancy. Despite these responses, the pregnancy is unaffected. It is possible that these are Th2 responses dominated by IL-10 production that does not threaten the pregnancy rather than Th1 responses that may lead to fetal rejection.

Up to 90% of pregnant mares make antibodies to foal MHC class I molecules. Similar antibodies develop in multiparous sheep and cattle. In some mouse strains, up to 95% of pregnant animals make antibodies against fetal MHC molecules. Up to 40% of women make antibodies to fetal MHC molecules after giving birth. The presence of these antibodies has no adverse effect on the course of the pregnancy. On the contrary, the maternal immune response may actually stimulate placental function. In mice, hybrid placentas are larger than the placentas of inbred animals, and females tolerant to paternal antigens have smaller placentas than intolerant females. Other studies show that mothers sensitized to paternal MHC molecules have better fetal survival. This may be due to the stimulatory effect of IL-3 and granulocyte-macrophage colony-stimulating factor (GM-CSF) from maternal T cells on trophoblast growth. It is of interest to note that in cattle there is a clear association between retention of the placenta and its MHC class I haplotype. MHC class I compatibility between a mother and her calf increases the risk for a retained placenta, whereas MHC class II compatibility has no effect. It has been suggested that the expulsion of the placenta after birth may be due, at least in part, to an allograft response.

Some antibodies made by the mother against fetal antigens may coat placental cells, preventing their destruction by maternal T cells. This blocking antibody can be eluted from the placenta and shown to suppress other cell-mediated immune reactions against paternal antigens, such as graft rejection.

Absence of this blocking antibody accounts for some cases of recurrent abortion in women. Nevertheless it can also be shown that totally immunodeficient mice can have successful pregnancies. CD55 (DAF) is incorporated in the trophoblast at the fetomaternal interface and also protects it against complement attack.

The fetus does not depend entirely on maternal mechanisms for its protection. The placenta is a source of many immunosuppressive factors, including estradiol and progesterone and possibly also chorionic gonadotropin. In addition, some pregnancy-associated glycoproteins, including α_2-macroglobulin, α-fetoprotein, the major protein in fetal serum and placental interferons, have immunosuppressive properties. In mammals, unique interferons (IFN-ω in humans, horses, and dogs; IFN-τ in ruminants; and IFN-γ and IFN-δ in pigs) from the embryonic trophoblast act as signaling proteins between the embryo and mother during early development. These interferons may also inhibit lymphocyte activities. Amniotic fluid is rich in immunosuppressive phospholipids.

Despite the previous discussion, if the antigenic differences between the mother and her fetus are very great, then pregnancy may not go to completion. Studies on xenogeneic hybridization of two different mouse species show that the embryos develop until midgestation and are then attacked and destroyed by maternal lymphocytes. Similarly, donkey embryos transferred to horse mares are destroyed by large numbers of maternal lymphocytes.

Mild immunosuppression is a consistent feature of late pregnancy and the early postpartum period. Pregnant animals may have minor deficiencies in cell-mediated immune reactivity to nonfetal antigens. Dairy cows experience a periparturient depression in neutrophil function and reduced T cell cytotoxicity and cytokine production. This suppression appears to be mediated by CD8+ T cells. In mares, blood lymphocyte responses to mitogens drop from 4 weeks before to 5 weeks after parturition. NK cell activity in pigs drops at the end of gestation to reach a low point 2 to 3 weeks after parturition. Ewes in late pregnancy may show a reduction of some immunoglobulin classes such as IgG1. This may be due to alterations in helper T cell function or, more plausibly, to diversion of the IgG1 into the mammary gland to produce colostrum. This suppression may be significant in parasitized animals, in which the immune response barely controls the parasite. Similarly, immunosuppression may permit *Demodex* mite populations to rise in pregnant or lactating bitches and aid in the transmission of mites to their puppies.

Parturition can be considered to be mediated in part by a sterile inflammatory response following invasion of the uterus by large numbers of leukocytes, especially macrophages, neutrophils, and T cells, late in pregnancy. These in turn release an array of cytokines, proteases (especially collagenases), prostanoids, and chemokines. These cytokines in turn stimulate uterine stromal cells to amplify the process; and the collagenases remodel collagen, weakening fetal membranes, soften the cervix, and increase the contractility of the myometrium, leading to fetal expulsion. After delivery, the uterus involutes as most of the leukocytes leave or are destroyed.

For sources of additional information, please visit http:// evolve.elsevier.com/tizard/immunology/

Resistance to Tumors

□ Key Points

- Cancer cells may differ antigenically from normal body cells. As a result they may trigger an immune response. This immune response, however, may not be very strong.
- Because cancer cells can mutate as they grow, those cells that survive may be selected for their lack of antigenicity.
- The most important mechanism of destruction of spontaneous tumors probably involves killing by natural killer (NK) cells. NK cells recognize and attack target cells that fail to express major histocompatibility (MHC) class I molecules.
- Under some circumstances, cytotoxic T cells, activated macrophages, or antibodies may also attack cancer cells.
- Failure of antitumor immunity involves not only tumor cell selection but also the activities of regulatory T cells and blocking antibodies.
- It has proved very difficult to devise effective, consistent antitumor immunotherapy. This may involve administration of cytokines or antibodies or active immunization using vaccines against tumor antigens.
- Many tumors are profoundly immunosuppressive.

Normal cellular functions depend on the careful regulation of cell division. When cells multiply, it is essential that they do so only as and when required. Unfortunately, as a result of mutations triggered by chemicals, radiation, or viruses, cells may occasionally break free of the constraints that regulate cell division. A cell that is proliferating in an uncontrolled fashion will give rise to a growing clone of cells that eventually develops into a tumor or neoplasm. If these cells remain clustered together at a single site, the tumor is said to be benign. Benign tumors can usually be removed by surgery. In some cases, however, tumor cells break off from the main tumor mass and are carried by the blood or lymph to distant sites, where they lodge and continue to grow. This form of tumor is said to be malignant. The secondary tumors that arise in these distant sites are called metastases. Surgical treatment of malignant tumors may be very difficult because it may be impossible to remove all metastases. Malignant tumors are subdivided according to their tissue of origin. Tumors arising from epithelial cells are called carcinomas; those arising from mesenchymal cells, such as muscle, lymphoid, or connective tissue cells, are called sarcomas. A leukemia is a tumor derived from hematopoietic stem cells.

The essential difference between a normal cell and a tumor cell is a loss of control of cell growth as a result of multiple mutations. These mutations may also result in tumor cells expressing abnormal proteins on their surface.

Tumors as Allografts

When organ transplantation became a common procedure as a result of the development of potent immunosuppressive drugs, it was found that patients with prolonged graft survival were many times more likely to develop certain cancers than were nonimmunosuppressed individuals. It was also observed that some immunodeficient patients had an increased tendency to develop malignant tumors. It was therefore suggested that the immune system was responsible for the prevention of cancer. From this suggestion the immune surveillance theory emerged. This theory held that the body constantly produces neoplastic cells but that in a healthy individual the immune system rapidly recognizes and eliminates these cells. The theory suggested that progressive cancer would result if the cancer cells somehow evaded recognition by T cells.

The immune surveillance theory soon ran into problems. Common human cancers such as those of the lung or breast do not develop more frequently in immunodeficient individuals. Likewise, nude (*nu/nu*) mice, although T cell deficient, are no more susceptible than normal mice to chemically induced or spontaneous tumors (Chapter 37). Finally, it became clear that many tumor antigens induce tolerance in a manner similar to normal self-antigens. Thus most evidence has failed to support the idea that the immune system distinguishes between tumor cells and normal, healthy cells.

Notwithstanding this, there are situations in which the immune system can recognize and kill cancer cells. For example, some immunodeficient mouse strains, which are "cleaner" subjects than nude mice, show an increased prevalence of spontaneous cancer. (Nude mice have some persistent T and B cell function and intact innate defenses.) These include recombinase-activating gene (*RAG*) knockout mice that cannot produce functional T or B cells and *STAT-1* knockout mice that lack both adaptive and innate responses by being unresponsive to interferon-γ (IFN-γ). RAG knockout mice suffer from an increased incidence of spontaneous tumors of the intestinal epithelium, whereas *RAG/STAT-1* knockout mice develop mammary cancers.

It is perhaps therefore more appropriate to think of the immune system as "immunoediting" cancers. Under some circumstances the immune system can indeed eliminate some cancer cells. If, however, the cancer cells evade destruction, they may survive indefinitely or be selected by the immune responses to produce new tumor cell variants. Eventually, however, some of these variants may escape any control by the immune system and grow to produce clinical cancers.

If a metastasizing tumor does not invade lymphoid organs, it may escape immune surveillance. On the other hand, tumors that invade lymph nodes can be divided into strongly and weakly immunogenic types. Strongly immunogenic tumors elicit a strong T cell response following processing by dendritic cells. Weakly immunogenic tumors tend to grow as walled-off nodules that may not be processed in sufficient amounts to trigger immune responses. These are the most common tumors in humans. It is possible that tumor cells that trigger inflammation in tissues trigger dendritic cell activation and processing. On the other hand, tumors that fail to generate inflammation may simply be ignored by the immune system. Alternatively, it is possible that the antigens of the tumor may be tolerated by the immune system. If successful tumor therapy is to be achieved, these two states must be distinguished.

Most humans who develop "spontaneous" cancer have a normal immune system. Immunosuppressed individuals such as allograft recipients and patients with AIDS develop a very different spectrum of cancers from that of the general population. The only cancers to which they are at greater risk are those caused by viruses, such as Kaposi's sarcoma. Immunosuppressed individuals are at no more likely than the general population to develop the common cancers, such as those of breast, lung, or colon.

Although the original surveillance hypothesis has had to be drastically modified, it is clear that under some circumstances the immune system may destroy tumor cells and that this response may be enhanced to protect an individual against some cancers. However, there is a great difference between the strong and effective cell-mediated immune response triggered by foreign organ grafts and the much weaker responses to the antigens associated with tumor cells.

The outcome of the interaction between a tumor cell and the immune system can thus have one of three results: first, elimination of the cancer; second, cancer equilibrium whereby the more immunogenic cells are destroyed but permitting the less immunogenic cells to survive (immunoediting); or third,

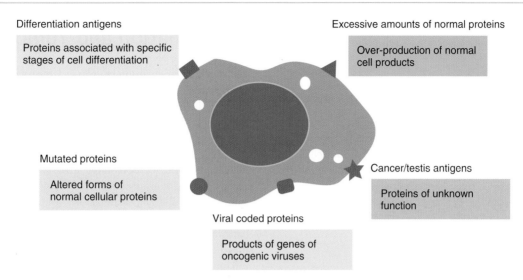

FIGURE 33-1 Some of the great variety of new antigens that may appear on the surface of tumor cells and provoke an immune response.

tumor escape, whereby the tumor cells are unaffected by any immune responses they may trigger.

Tumor Antigens

Spontaneous cancer cells develop as a result of multiple mutations in regulatory genes. These mutations may generate molecules that are unique to the tumor cells (tumor-specific antigens) or, more commonly, abnormal or unusual molecules (tumor-associated antigens). To distinguish between normal and tumor cells, host T cells must recognize tumor cell antigens. Five major types of tumor antigen have been identified. First, there are differentiation antigens associated with specific stages in the development of a cell type. For example, some tumor cells may express the products of developmental genes that are turned off in adult cells and are normally only expressed early in an individual's development. These proteins are called oncofetal antigens. Examples include tumors of the gastrointestinal tract that produce a glycoprotein called carcinoembryonic antigen (CEA; also called CD66e), normally found only in the fetal intestine. The presence of detectable amounts of CEA in serum may indicate the presence of a colon or rectal adenocarcinoma. α-Fetoprotein produced by hepatoma cells is normally found only in the fetal liver. Likewise, squamous cell carcinoma cells may possess antigens normally restricted to fetal liver and skin. These oncofetal antigens are usually poor immunogens and do not provoke protective immunity. However, their detection in blood may be useful for diagnosis and for monitoring the progress of the tumor.

Second, there are mutated forms of normal cellular proteins. For example, melanoma cells may express the products of mutated oncogenes on their surface (Figure 33-1). Some tumor antigens are recognized because they are abnormally glycosylated. Chemically induced tumors may express mutated surface antigens unique to the tumor and not to the inducing chemical (Figure 33-2). Because carcinogenic chemicals can produce many different mutations, tumors induced by a single

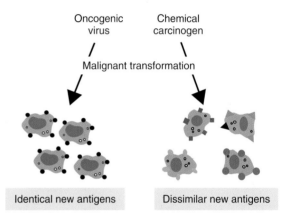

FIGURE 33-2 Although oncogenic viruses induce tumor cells with identical new antigens, chemical carcinogens induce tumor cells with a great variety of new antigens.

chemical in different animals may be antigenically different. Even within a single chemically induced tumor mass, antigenically distinct subpopulations of cells exist. As a result, immunity to one chemically induced tumor does not prevent growth of a second tumor induced by the same chemical.

Third, normal proteins are produced in excessive amounts. A good example is the production of prostate-specific antigen (PSA) by prostate carcinomas of humans. PSA is a protease exclusively produced by the prostate epithelium. Increased blood levels of this protein indicate excessive prostate activity. One cause of this is the growth of a carcinoma.

Fourth, cancer/testis (CT) antigens are a group of tumor antigens only expressed in the testes and in various malignancies. Their function is unknown.

Fifth, tumors caused by viruses express antigens characteristic of the inducing virus or of other endogenous retroviruses. These antigens, although coded for by a viral genome, are not part of a virion. Examples include the FOCMA antigens found on the neoplastic lymphoid cells of cats infected with feline leukemia virus and Marek's tumor-specific antigens found on

Marek's disease tumor cells in chickens. (Both of these are virus-induced, naturally occurring, T cell tumors.)

Immunity to Tumors

If tumor cells express unusual antigens, why are they not regarded as foreign and attacked by the immune system? The main problem appears to be that the abnormal molecules are not appropriately presented to the cells of the immune system, especially cytotoxic T cells. Nevertheless, on occasion, tumor cells may be attacked by NK cells, cytotoxic T cells, activated macrophages, or antibodies (Figure 33-3). It is likely that the most important of these attackers are NK cells.

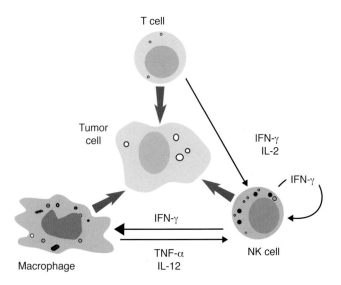

FIGURE 33-3 The three major cell types that participate in tumor cell destruction and the role of interferon in stimulating that activity.

Inflammation and Tumors

The tumor microenvironment plays a large part in determining the behavior of a tumor. The tumor cells communicate extensively with nearby cells. Among the most important of these are fibroblasts and inflammatory cells. As a result, the elimination of tumor cells by immune mechanisms is determined in part by the presence of inflammation. Inflammatory diseases increase the risk for developing many types of cancer; conversely, the use of nonsteroidal antiinflammatory drugs reduces tumor susceptibility (Figure 33-4). Mutations in oncogenes such as *ras* and *myc* are closely linked to the inflammatory pathways. Inflammatory cytokines, chemokines, and cells are present in the microenvironment of early tumors. Blocking of inflammatory mediators, key transcription factors, or inflammatory cells decreases the incidence and spread of cancer. Conversely, adoptive transfer of inflammatory cells may promote tumor development. More than half of the mass of a tumor may consist of supporting cells, including fibroblasts, macrophages, and vascular endothelial cells. Cancers cannot spread and metastasize without the support of these cells. The process by which these stromal cells are recruited is closely related to inflammation. Inflammatory cytokines, such as tumor necrosis factor-α (TNF-α), and macrophages are often required for tumor development and spread.

Cancer and inflammation are linked by two pathways. The intrinsic pathway is activated by mutations leading to neoplasia. These include the activation of various oncogenes, chromosomal rearrangements, or the inactivation of tumor suppressor genes. Cells transformed in this way generate transcription factors, produce inflammatory mediators, and generate an inflammatory microenvironment around tumor cells. The extrinsic pathway involves the development of inflammation by inflammatory or infectious disease. Toll-like receptor

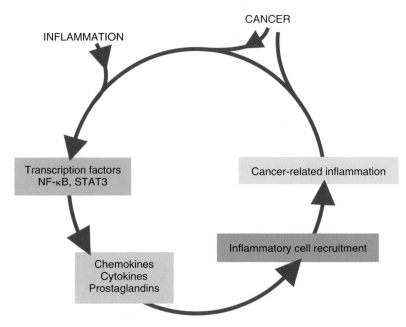

FIGURE 33-4 The mechanisms of inflammation also promote tumor formation.

(TLR) ligands or interleukin-1β (IL-1β) generate transcription factors such as NF-κB by acting through the MyD88 pathway. These transcription factors may be generated not only in inflammatory cells but also in any nearby tumor or stromal cells. NF-κB is an important endogenous tumor promoter. It stimulates inflammatory cytokine production and promotes the survival of tumor cells by reducing expression of the anti-apoptotic gene *bcl-2* (Chapter 18).

Tumor cells exploit signals from their microenvironment. Stromal cells such as fibroblasts, macrophages, and endothelial cells can all generate IL-6, a cytokine that promotes tumor growth and angiogenesis. Inflammatory cells such as macrophages, mast cells, and tumor-infiltrating lymphocytes can promote tumor growth by remodeling tissues, stimulating angiogenesis and suppressing immune responses. This polarization may result from the activities of regulatory T (Treg) cells within the tumors secreting transforming growth factor-β (TGF-β) and IL-10.

Cellular Defenses

Natural Killer Cells

Natural killer (NK) cells are the subject of Chapter 19. These are cytotoxic cells that respond to abnormal or stressed cells without prior priming and belong to the innate immune system. They have two major types of receptors: inhibitory receptors that can recognize the presence of major histocompatibility complex (MHC) class I molecules on a target cell surface and in so doing are prevented from killing their targets; and activating receptors that can recognize the presence of certain stress-induced proteins on cell surfaces and as a result are activated and kill their targets. Thus NK cells effectively kill two types of cellular targets: cells that fail to express MHC class I molecules and cells that express certain stress-related proteins. Both conditions commonly apply to cancer cells. As a result, NK cells play a key role in the destruction of tumors.

Cytotoxic T Cells

Peptides from the products of mutated genes or abnormally expressed cellular proteins may be expressed and presented to T cells. As a result, lymphocytes from some tumor-bearing animals may kill tumor cells cultured in vitro. For example, a protein called cyclin B1 that regulates mitosis is barely expressed in normal cells but overexpressed in many tumors, where it can stimulate T cell cytotoxicity.

Macrophage-Mediated Immunity

In some experimental systems, macrophages may have antitumor activities. This is especially true of M1 macrophages activated by exposure to IFN-γ. These M1 cells secrete cytotoxic molecules, including potent oxidants. Nonspecific activation of macrophages by bacillus Calmette-Guérin (BCG) or

Propionibacterium acnes results in enhanced production of IL-1 or TNF-α and subsequent enhancement of helper T cell and NK cell activity. IL-1 has a cytostatic effect on some tumors, and TNF-α may have potent antitumor activity. Unfortunately, malignant tumors may inhibit macrophage activation, and the macrophages of tumor-bearing animals may be of the M2 phenotype.

Antibody-Mediated Immunity

Antibodies to tumor cells are found in many tumor-bearing animals; for instance, about 50% of dogs with lymphosarcomas have serum antitumor antibodies. These antibodies may, together with complement, lyse free tumor cells within the bloodstream. Antibodies are not effective in destroying the cells in solid cancers.

Failure of Immunity to Tumor Cells

The fact that tumors are so readily induced and are so relatively common testifies to the inadequacies of the immunological protective mechanisms. Studies of tumor-bearing animals have indicated several mechanisms by which immune systems fail to reject tumors.

Immunosuppression

It is commonly observed that tumor-bearing animals are immunosuppressed. This suppression is most clearly seen in animals with lymphoid tumors; for example, tumors of B cells tend to suppress antibody formation, whereas tumors of T cell origin suppress cell-mediated immune responses and NK cell activity. Mechanisms of immunosuppression can include defects in antigen recognition, in co-stimulation, and in cytokine production. Immunosuppression in animals with chemically induced tumors is due in part to production of immunosuppressive molecules such as prostaglandins by tumor cells or tumor-associated macrophages. The presence of actively growing tumor cells represents a severe protein drain on an animal. This protein loss may also be immunosuppressive.

Some tumor-derived molecules may redirect macrophage activities so that they promote tumor growth. Thus tumor-derived IL-4, IL-6, IL-10, TGF-β, prostaglandin E_2, and macrophage colony-stimulating factor can deactivate or suppress the activation of macrophages and Th1 responses. TGF-β can convert antitumor effector cells into Treg cells. Many tumors produce indolamine 2,3-dioxygenase (IDO), a potent immunosuppressive agent and a suppressor of NK cell function (Chapter 20).

Tumor cells can suppress macrophage cytokine production and circumvent macrophage cytotoxicity. Tumors may also evade T cell responses as a result of their failure to trigger inflammation and other innate responses. Interferon-induced signaling is impaired in the B and T cells of many patients with cancer. Once tumors have effectively immunosuppressed the host, they enter the escape phase during which their growth is uncontrolled.

Lymphocyte phenotypes have been measured in normal and tumor-bearing dogs. In addition to having higher leukocyte counts than normal dogs, tumor-bearing animals tend to show reduced numbers of CD4 and CD8 T cells. This decline in T cell numbers increases as the disease progresses. Tumor-bearing dogs may also have elevated plasma IL-6 and α_1-acid glycoprotein levels relative to normal animals.

CD95 Ligand Expression CD95 ligand (CD95L) is normally expressed on both cytotoxic T cells and NK cells. When it binds to the death receptor CD95 on target cells, it triggers their apoptosis. CD95L, however, also has been detected on some leukemic T cells and NK cells, colon adenocarcinoma cells, melanomas, and hepatocellular carcinomas. Since cytotoxic T cells may also express CD95, it is possible that cytotoxicity may work in reverse and that these CD95L+ tumor cells may kill the T cells. At the same time, these cancer cells may downregulate their own CD95 so that they become resistant to cell-mediated cytotoxicity. It is interesting to note that the anticancer drug doxorubicin enhances expression of both CD95 and CD95L on tumor cells and may permit these molecules to interact with T cells, thus killing themselves by apoptosis. Some tumor cells such as those in lung carcinomas may secrete decoy receptors for CD95L. These decoy receptors bind to CD95L and prevent it from binding to CD95. Thus tumor cells that downregulate CD95 while upregulating their decoy receptor expression may be resistant to T cell cytotoxicity.

Regulatory Cells Much of the immunosuppression seen in tumor-bearing individuals may be due to the activities of regulatory cell populations. These suppressor cells may be CD8+ Treg cells, IL-10-secreting Th2 cells, M2 macrophages, or even B cells. Enhanced regulatory cell activity can be detected in humans with osteogenic sarcomas, thymomas, myelomas, and Hodgkin's disease and in many tumor-bearing animals. FoxP3+CD4+ Treg cells may be increased in the blood and tumor-draining lymph nodes of dogs with cancer. Thus in normal dogs, FoxP3+ cells constitute about 5% of blood T cells and 10% of lymph node T cells. In tumor-bearing dogs, however, they may constitute as many as 7.5% in blood and 17% in tumor-draining lymph nodes. Dogs with osteosarcomas were shown to have elevated Treg cells (CD4+, CD25+) and fewer CD8 cells in blood, lymph nodes, and tumors. The CD8/Treg ratio was significantly lower in tumor-bearing dogs, and dogs with the greatest decrease had a shorter survival time. Treg numbers in blood are also raised in dogs with carcinomas. The CD8/Treg ratio is decreased in dogs with T cell lymphomas implying that tumor-bearing dogs may be immunosuppressed by Tregs and that inhibition of Treg activity may promote antitumor immunity.

Myeloid-Derived Suppressor Cells Myeloid-derived suppressor cells (MDSC) are immature myeloid cells that normally generate macrophages and dendritic cells. They inhibit T cell responses by blocking activation of the T cell receptor (TCR) by secreting peroxynitrite. Peroxynitrite causes nitrate addition to TCR and thus inactivates these receptors. MDSCs also produce arginase that impairs T cell function by reducing expression of CD3ζ. Vascular endothelial growth factor (VEGF) promotes MDSC production by blocking dendritic cell maturation. IL-1β also promotes MDSC production. MDSCs may also cause immunosuppression by promoting the switch from M1 to M2 cells.

Blocking Antibodies Although tumor cells may be antigenic and stimulate a protective cell-mediated immune response, antibodies may have an opposite effect. Thus serum from tumor-bearing animals may cause the tumors of other animals to grow even faster, a phenomenon called enhancement. This serum may also inhibit T cell cytotoxicity. Many tumors release large quantities of cell surface antigen into the bloodstream, and this may bind to cytotoxic T cells, saturating their antigen receptors and blocking their ability to bind to target cells. Alternatively, blocking antibodies may be produced. These are non–complement-activating, antitumor antibodies that can bind and mask tumor antigens on cell surfaces and protect the tumor cells from attack by cytotoxic T cells. In general, the presence or absence of blocking antibodies correlates well with the state of progression of a tumor.

Tumor Cell Selection

Tumor cells do not usually become malignant in a single step. Rather, they gradually become malignant over a long period, going from benign to malignant in a process called tumor progression. The process occurs through a series of mutations that switch genes on and off. These mutations do not necessarily alter the immunogenicity of tumor cells or do so in small steps. Immunogenicity may not alter until the cells are irreversibly committed to malignancy. Thus there are two selection mechanisms by which tumor cells can evade the host's immune response and so enhance their own survival. One is "sneaking through," the process by which malignant cells may not trigger an immune response until the tumor has reached a size at which it cannot be controlled by the host. Thus in experimental tumors, small numbers of tumor cells may grow after subcutaneous inoculation, although large numbers may not. It may be that the tumor cells may not reach lymph nodes and trigger an immune response until the tumor burden is too large to be controlled. Even a very small tumor may contain an enormous number of cells. For example, a 10-mm tumor contains about 10^9 cells. The second mechanism, tumor cell selection, reflects the fact that tumor cells that have mutated in such a way as to be antigenically different from the host will induce a strong immune response and be eliminated without leading to disease. Surviving tumor cells must therefore be selected for their lack of antigenicity and their inability to stimulate an immune response. To this extent, therefore, tumors that do develop have, by definition, already beaten the immune system.

Administration of a potent carcinogen to mice will result in many of them developing lethal tumors. Some mice, however, will survive. These animals have dormant tumors kept under control by the immune system. Subsequent immunosuppressive therapy may activate these dormant tumors. The control of dormant tumors is mediated by Th1 cells.

Tumor Immunotherapy

Immunotherapy may be either active or passive. In active immunotherapy, the patient's own immune system is stimulated to respond to the tumor. In passive immunotherapy, immune cells or their products are administered.

Active Immunotherapy

Three general approaches have been used in attempts to cure or modify tumor growth through immunotherapy (Box 33-1). The simplest is to stimulate the immune system nonspecifically (Figure 33-5). Any improvement in an animal's immune abilities will tend to enhance its resistance to tumors, although a cure may be expected only if the tumor mass is small or is surgically excised. The most widely used immune stimulant is the attenuated strain of *Mycobacterium bovis*, BCG. This organism activates macrophages and stimulates cytokine release, thus promoting T cell activity. It may be given systemically or injected directly into the tumor mass. Most positive results from the use of BCG have come from studies on human patients with melanomas or bladder cancer. Direct injection of BCG into skin melanoma metastases may cause complete regression, not only of the injected lesion but also, occasionally, of uninjected skin metastases. However, visceral metastases usually remain unaffected. BCG enhances survival or remission in some leukemias, and its direct intravesicular application in human bladder cancer gives complete or partial response rates of up to 70%. However, BCG can cause severe lesions at the site of injection and, occasionally, systemic hypersensitivity. Other immunostimulants that have been employed include *P. acnes*, levamisole, and various mixed bacterial vaccines.

Many investigators have also studied the effects of vaccinating a patient with tumor cells or antigens. This approach has worked best in human melanoma patients, in whom several different antigen preparations are undergoing clinical trials. Because many tumors can evade the immune response, it is usual to treat the tumor cells in an attempt to enhance their antigenicity. Thus, irradiated, neuraminidase-treated, or glutaraldehyde-treated cells have been used in experimental tumor vaccines.

Passive Immunotherapy

Cytokine Therapy Many attempts have been made to treat human cancer patients with isolated cytokines but with limited success. Interferons, for example, are only effective against certain selected tumors. Thus 70% to 90% of patients with hairy cell leukemia treated with IFN-α show complete or partial remission. The antitumor activities of TNF-α are synergistic with the interferons. On the other hand, administration of IL-2 to melanoma and renal cell cancer patients induces partial or complete remission in only 15% to 20% of cases.

One major difficulty in cytokine therapy has been their toxicity. For example, when given at pharmacological doses, TNF-α produces clinical signs similar to those induced by

---

□ Box 33-1 | **Some of the Approaches to Tumor Immunotherapy**

Nonspecific Immune Stimulation

Microbial products (e.g., bacille Calmette-Guérin, *Propionibacterium acnes*, yeast glucans, levamisole)

Complex carbohydrates (glycans)

Cytokines (interferons, tumor necrosis factor, interleukin-2, interleukin-4)

Lymphokine-activated killers (natural killer cells, T cells, tumor-infiltrating lymphocytes)

Passive Immunization

Monoclonal antibodies against tumor antigens (alone or conjugated to toxins)

Active Immunization

Chemically modified tumor cells

DNA vaccination against related antigens in another species

Vaccination against oncogenic viruses (feline leukemia, Marek's disease)

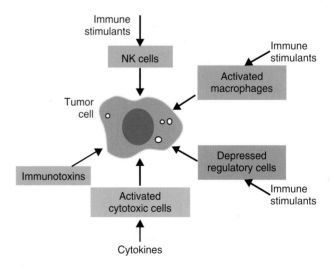

FIGURE 33-5 Some of the ways in which the immune system can be stimulated to mount a protective response to tumors.

endotoxin. IL-2 is also extremely toxic. In low doses, it induces fever, chills, nausea, and weight gain as well as a capillary leak syndrome resulting in massive pulmonary edema. IL-2 also produces anemia, thrombocytopenia, and eosinophilia. Patients may also develop a severe, very itchy rash, neuropsychiatric changes, and endocrine abnormalities. Thus IL-2 is a hazardous protein and has limited usefulness when used alone. Preliminary trials of IL-4 have shown similar toxic effects. Nevertheless it is important to note that local application of IL-2 may produce useful results. For example, relatively low doses of recombinant human IL-2 when injected locally into papillomas or carcinomas of the vulva in cattle induced remissions in 83% of treated animals. Some complete regressions were observed. IL-2 therapy produced 63% complete remissions in cattle with ocular squamous cell carcinomas.

T Cell Therapy Autologous lymphocytes grown and expanded in the presence of IL-2 for 4 days develop cytotoxic properties. Injection of these activated cells, called lymphokine-activated killer (LAK) cells, into mice with experimental lung tumors can lead to cancer remission. A combination of LAK cells and IL-2 has given encouraging results when administered to human cancer patients.

LAK cells from blood include about 40% NK cells and 60% T cells. The activated NK cells are mainly CD3+, CD16+, and CD56+. They release LAK-1, a cytotoxic protein, as their effector molecule. LAK cells have been induced in both cat and dog (Figure 33-6). Cell supernatants rich in IL-2 derived from concanavalin A–stimulated feline blood lymphocytes kill feline leukemia virus–transformed tumor cells. Recombinant human IL-2 stimulates the cytotoxic activity of canine blood lymphocytes.

In an attempt to obtain even better results in humans, tumors have been surgically removed from cancer-bearing patients; then the lymphocytes within these tumors were removed and cultured in the presence of IL-2 for 4 to 6 weeks so that their numbers grow significantly. These tumor-infiltrating lymphocytes recognize and infiltrate only the tumors from which they come. Returned with IL-2 to the donor patients, they have produced remissions in about one third of patients. The most encouraging results have been obtained in patients with melanomas and those with colorectal and kidney cancer. Unfortunately, the chemokine environment within many tumors ensures that these may be predominantly Th2 cells. The resulting inflammatory responses may therefore promote rather than inhibit tumor growth.

Limited success has been obtained in treating melanoma in gray horses by immunotherapy. For example, administration of a plasmid expressing IL-13 directly into metastases produced significant regression in 60% of cases and appeared to be safe. In dogs with melanomas, plasmids containing DNA coding for the herpesvirus thymidine kinase suicide gene were able to sensitize transfected cells to ganciclovir. (Ganciclovir is a potent antiherpesvirus drug.) The treatment induced substantial regression. A similar therapy given in association with a subcutaneous autologous killed cancer vaccine appeared to work well in a horse.

Antibody Therapy Despite the risk for enhancement by blocking antibodies, some successes have been achieved by the use of monoclonal antibodies against tumor antigens. Monoclonal antibodies can be used to destroy tumors, either when given alone or when complexed to highly cytotoxic drugs or potent radioisotopes, which they carry directly to the tumor cells. A monoclonal antibody against canine T cells (CL/MAb231) has yielded encouraging results when used to manage lymphomas in dogs. It greatly increased life expectancy following two cycles of L-asparaginase-vincristine-cyclophosphamide-doxorubicin chemotherapy to bring the lymphoma into remission. The monoclonal antibody is given for 5 days, beginning 3 weeks after the conclusion of chemotherapy.

Immunoprevention

In contrast to the techniques described previously, most of which have met with only limited success, there are established successful techniques for vaccination against tumor viruses. These include such effective vaccines against viral antigens such as hepatitis B and human papillomavirus, the causes of hepatocellular carcinoma and cervical cancer, respectively. The most important of these in veterinary medicine are the vaccines against feline leukemia in cats. These vaccines usually contain high concentrations of the major viral antigens, and immunity is almost entirely directed against viral glycoproteins. Other important vaccines are those directed against Marek's disease, a T cell tumor of chickens caused by a herpesvirus. The immune response evoked by these vaccines has two components. First, humoral and cell-mediated responses act directly on the virus to reduce the quantity available to infect cells. Second, an immune response is provoked against virus-coded antigens on the surface of tumor cells. Both the antiviral and antitumor immune responses act synergistically to protect the birds.

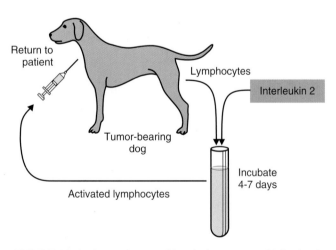

FIGURE 33-6 The production of lymphokine-activated killer (LAK) cells by incubation of blood lymphocytes in the presence of IL-2 for 4 to 7 days.

Return to patient

Lymphocytes

Interleukin 2

Tumor-bearing dog

Incubate 4-7 days

Activated lymphocytes

A vaccine designed to enhance survival in recurrent canine melanoma has been approved by U.S. Department of Agriculture. This vaccine consists of an *Escherichia coli* expression plasmid engineered to express the human tyrosinase gene and administered transdermally by a needle-free device. The plasmid contains a cytomegalovirus promoter and a kanamycin resistance selection marker. Vaccinated dogs mount an immune response against the foreign tyrosinase. Tyrosinase is a melanosomal glycoprotein that is essential for melanin synthesis. The immune response to the tyrosinase induces both antibodies and cytotoxic T cells against the dog's melanoma cells, and this response may prevent tumor recurrence. Mean survival after receiving this vaccine was greater than 500 days, as opposed to 280-day survival in unvaccinated dogs.

Some Specific Tumors

Injection Site–Associated Sarcomas

Most local reactions to injected vaccines in cats resolve rapidly and completely. In some cats, however, tumors develop at these injection sites many months or years after vaccination (Figure 33-7). Injection site–associated sarcoma cells have large irregular nuclei, often pleomorphic with a high mitotic index. Aggregates of lymphocytes and macrophages may surround the tumor. These macrophages may have foamy cytoplasm containing bluish granular material. The tumors are mainly fibrosarcomas, malignant histiocytomas, and osteosarcomas. Less common forms include rhabdomyosarcomas, hemangiosarcomas, chondrosarcomas, liposarcomas, and lymphosarcomas. These tumors are highly invasive, and up to 24% may result in distant metastases. Successful treatment requires a combination of radical surgical excision and adjunctive therapy, including radiation, immunotherapy (such as IL-2 treatment), and chemotherapy, but recurrence is common.

Epidemiological studies have linked the development of these sarcomas to vaccination. Thus these tumors were first noticed following the introduction of potent, inactivated, adjuvanted feline vaccines such as those directed against rabies and feline leukemia. Cats with sarcomas occurring at sites where vaccines are currently administered were compared with cats that developed sarcomas at non–vaccine-injection sites. Cats receiving FeLV vaccine were 5.5 times more likely to develop a sarcoma at the injection site than cats that had not received a vaccine. There was a twofold increase in risk with rabies vaccination. However, the risk was not enormously high. It was calculated that 1 to 3.6 sarcomas developed per 10,000 FeLV and rabies vaccines administered. The risk did increase with the number of doses of vaccine administered—a 50% increase following one dose, a 127% increase following two doses, and a 175% increase following three or four vaccines given simultaneously. Vaccine-associated sarcomas tend to occur in younger animals and tend to be larger and more aggressive than sarcomas arising at other sites. They metastasize in 25% to 70% of cases. In one study, injection site sarcomas

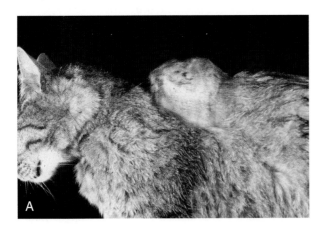

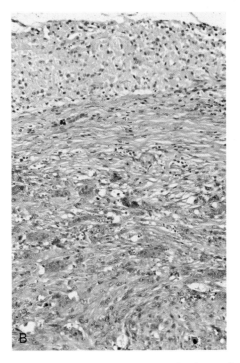

FIGURE 33-7 A, Postvaccinal sarcoma in a cat. Note its characteristic position over the scapulae, where the vaccine has been administered subcutaneously. **B,** A histological section of a postvaccinal sarcoma. This is a fibrosarcoma showing long interwoven bundles of spindle cells (H&E stain).

(Courtesy Dr. M.J. Hendrick.)

developed on average 26 months after rabies vaccination and 11 months after FeLV vaccination. Global, web-based surveys suggest a somewhat lower prevalence of sarcomas (0.63 sarcomas/10,000 cats or 0.32 sarcomas/10,000 doses of all vaccines, or one sarcoma from 31,000 doses administered). It must be pointed out, therefore, that the chances of developing a sarcoma are considerably smaller than the disease risks incurred by unvaccinated cats. Similar vaccination-related injection site sarcomas have been reported in ferrets, dogs, and a horse.

The pathogenesis of these sarcomas is unclear, but it is assumed that carcinogenesis occurs through multiple steps associated with prolonged inflammation or tissue damage. The potent adjuvants found in modern vaccines will result in protection lasting for several years. In addition, these products are administered by the convenient subcutaneous route. As a result, their adjuvants may persist at the injection site for a very long time. Tumor development has also been associated with the use of nonadjuvanted vaccines and even with injection of substances other than vaccines, including long-acting antibiotics or steroids, as well as the presence of persistent suture material, a retained surgical swab, or implanted microchips. There is no evidence that feline sarcoma virus, feline immunodeficiency virus, or feline leukemia viruses cause these tumors.

Prolonged irritation will increase the activation state of the cells involved in inflammation and tissue repair. The repair process involves the production of stem cells that can differentiate to replace damaged ones. These stem cells are long lived and so have plenty of opportunities to accumulate mutations. Signaling pathways may be activated in stem cells, and these pathways will promote cellular self-renewal. Chronic, prolonged irritation could lead to an increase in local stem cells and the possibility that some will mutate. During chronic inflammation, macrophages secrete growth factors and angiogenic factors that enhance cell growth. These factors upregulate NF-κB activity in affected tissues. Oxidants released from activated macrophages may act as carcinogens, especially in rapidly dividing cells. Although the mechanisms are unclear, NF-κB promotes both malignant transformation and metastases and may promote cancer cell formation by inhibiting apoptosis of premalignant cells.

Fibroblasts are stimulated to proliferate at sites of chronic inflammation and wound healing. In some of these fibroblasts, the *sis* oncogene may be activated, whereas in others, there are mutations in the gene coding for the tumor suppressor factor *p53*. The *sis* oncogene codes for the platelet-derived growth factor (PDGF) receptor, and vaccine-associated sarcomas have been shown to express both PDGF and its receptor. In contrast, non–vaccine-associated tumors and normal cat lymphocytes are PDGF negative. It has been suggested, therefore, that lymphocytes within the vaccine-associated sarcomas secrete PDGF, which then serves as a growth factor for the fibroblasts. This combination of abnormalities could result in the loss of growth control in the fibroblasts engaged in the chronic inflammatory process.

The tumor suppressor gene *p53* codes for a nuclear protein that regulates the cell cycle. Wild-type *p53* increases in response to cell damage. This prevents the cell moving through the cell cycle and permits DNA repair before the cell divides. If the cell is severely damaged, *p53* triggers apoptosis and prevents cell damage being transmitted to the next generation. Damaged cells in which *p53* is absent or mutated can continue to divide, giving rise to abnormal and possibly malignant cells. As many as 60% of injection site sarcomas may express mutated *p53*.

Interleukin-23 is a proinflammatory cytokine produced by activated dendritic cells and phagocytic cells. It acts on T cells, promoting Th17 inflammatory responses, upregulating some inflammatory metalloproteases and stimulating angiogenesis. However, it also reduces CD8 T cell infiltration. By reducing T cell infiltration, IL-23 may permit the growth of cancer cells. Animals deficient in IL-23 show increased resistance to chemical carcinogenesis and transplanted tumor growth.

Notwithstanding the above, there is no evidence to prove that injecting less irritating products can reduce the incidence of sarcomas. No specific brands of vaccine, no specific manufacturers, and no other vaccination-associated factors have been associated with an increased prevalence of sarcomas.

To minimize the risks for tumors developing at vaccination sites, it has been recommended that vaccines be administered at standardized sites on cats. For example, current recommendations are to inject rabies vaccine into the right pelvic limb and FeLV vaccine into the left pelvic limb ("rabies, right; leukemia, left"). Vaccines should be administered as distally as possible to permit amputation if required. The site of vaccine administration and the product used should be recorded for each vaccine to help in assessing risk factors.

Transmissible Venereal Sarcoma

Transmissible venereal sarcoma is a tumor transmitted between dogs during copulation. It results from transplantation of tumor cells. (In effect, the tumor cells are infectious agents.) To colonize a new host, these cells must be capable of establishing themselves in allogeneic hosts. This is not always successful, and after an initial growth phase, the tumor eventually regresses and is eliminated. Nevertheless lethal metastases do occur in immunosuppressed dogs. When growing aggressively, these tumor cells fail to express β2-microglobulin, and as a result, MHC class I antigens are not assembled on the cell surface. Exposed dogs, whether or not they develop progressive tumors, develop antibodies to tumor cells, although the serum of dogs with regressive tumors is most effective in inhibiting tumor growth. Thirty to 40% of cells in the regressive phase express MHC classes I and II. Dogs whose tumors regress also develop cytotoxic T cells. If recipient dogs are immunosuppressed, the tendency to malignant growth is enhanced. These tumor cells appear to secrete a cytotoxic factor that kills B cells. Genetic analysis of these cells suggested that they are a clone of cells that originated in a wolf or East Asian breed of dog between 200 and 2300 years ago.

Devil Facial Tumor Disease

The carnivorous marsupial, the Tasmanian Devil (*Sarcophilus harrisii*), is on the brink of extinction as a result of devil facial tumor disease. This is a transmissible tumor spread by direct implantation through bites. The tumors are found primarily on the head and neck and are believed to be of neuroendocrine origin. Animals die within 3 to 6 months of acquiring the tumor and do not appear to mount an immune response to this allograft. The disease has reduced some devil populations by as much as 90%. Although devils have a functioning immune system, they do not reject this tumor because of their limited MHC diversity and so fail to recognize the tumor cells as foreign. The tumor cells express functional MHC class I and II genes, but devil T cells do not respond in mixed lymphocyte cultures (Chapter 32). Thus there is no histocompatibility barrier to tumor growth.

Papillomas

Warts are self-limited tumors of epidermal cells induced by papillomaviruses. The wart virus invades epidermal cells in the basal cell layer of the skin, but these cells do not express viral antigen. Since no viral antigen is expressed in this area where the blood supply is good, the cells are not attacked by lymphocytes. As the infected cells move away from the basal layer toward the skin surface, they also move away from blood vessels, and the chances of immunological attack are minimized. Increasing amounts of virus are shed as the cells move toward the surface into a region devoid of antibodies or lymphocytes. Wart vaccines containing inactivated papillomavirus are available.

Equine Sarcoids

Equine sarcoids are locally aggressive fibroblastic tumors of horse skin associated with infection by bovine papillomavirus. They are remarkably amenable to immunotherapy. If BCG vaccine is infiltrated into the tissues between the tumor and normal skin, regression occurs in about two thirds of cases. The rate of regression depends on the size of the tumor (surgical debulking is required to remove most of the tumor mass), and multiple treatments are usually necessary for a complete cure. Mycobacterial cell walls may also be used to eradicate this tumor. They possess the advantage of not rendering an animal tuberculin positive. Sarcoids are also responsive to other immunostimulants such as killed *P. acnes* and the antiviral drug acyclovir.

Ocular Squamous Cell Carcinoma

Ocular squamous cell carcinoma is a common and economically important tumor of cattle that responds to several forms of immunotherapy. One successful treatment involves inoculation of affected animals with a phenol-saline extract of allogeneic carcinomas. This suggests that these tumors possess characteristic tumor-associated antigens. Indeed sera from affected cattle can react with cancer cells (but not normal cells) obtained from the eyes of other cattle. It is also of interest to note that sera from some cattle with ocular squamous cell carcinoma also react with equine sarcoid and bovine papilloma cells, implying that all three may have a common cause.

Swine Melanoma

The Sinclair melanoma-bearing swine is an inbred line that spontaneously develops melanomas. Most such tumors are benign and regress spontaneously. However, some are malignant and lethal. The tumor regression seen in most of these pigs is immunologically mediated. The tumors are invaded by macrophages, and at the same time the animals generate non-MHC-restricted cytotoxic T cells that are CD4−, CD8−, γ/δ+. Recovering pigs may also generate antibodies against melanoma antigens.

Lymphoid Tumors

Adaptive immunity requires that antigen-sensitive cells stimulated by exposure to antigen respond by division and differentiation. Much of the complexity of the immune system is due to the need for tight control of this cellular response. A failure in this control may result in uncontrolled lymphoid cell proliferation and the development of lymphoid tumors. The surveillance theory was originally proposed when it was observed that immunosuppressed animals and humans had an increased prevalence of tumors. However, an unusually high proportion of these tumors are of lymphoid origin. Therefore it is likely that some of the lymphoid tumors that develop in immunosuppressed individuals result from a failure of immunological control rather than from a failure of surveillance.

Normal immune responses, whether antibody or cell mediated, involve a burst of rapid proliferation in lymphocytes. This burst of proliferation must be carefully controlled (Chapter 20). Although uncontrolled lymphocyte function may induce autoimmunity, uncontrolled lymphocyte proliferation may result in the development of a lymphoma or lymphosarcoma. It is no accident that individuals with autoimmune disease are more likely than normal individuals to develop lymphoid cell tumors.

Several important viruses stimulate nonspecific lymphocyte proliferation. These include the maedi-visna virus, the Aleutian disease parvovirus, and the herpesvirus responsible for malignant catarrhal fever (MCF). MCF is a fatal lymphoproliferative disease of cattle and sheep characterized by lymphadenopathy with widespread tissue accumulations of lymphocytes. Lymphocytes from MCF-infected animals show prolonged growth in tissue culture.

Neoplastic transformation may occur in lymphoid cells of both branches of the immune system at almost any stage in their maturation process. Providing that the tumor cells have not dedifferentiated as a result of very rapid growth (as in acute lymphatic leukemia of calves), it is possible to identify the cells present in a lymphoid tumor by their surface antigens. For example, the presence of cell surface immunoglobulin is characteristic of B cells, whereas the presence of CD3 or CD2 is an identifying feature of T cells.

Bovine Lymphosarcoma

Bovine lymphosarcoma is one of the most common cancers of cattle. It occurs in two main forms: an enzootic form and a sporadic form. The enzootic form of the disease is caused by bovine leukemia virus (BLV), a delta retrovirus. BLV is transmitted by infected lymphocytes. Thus it can be spread by contaminated instruments, by vaccines containing blood, or by biting flies; or calves may be infected in utero. The primary target of the virus is the pre-B cell, although the specific BLV receptor has not been identified. Early in infection the proportion of B cells in peripheral blood increases before there is a significant increase in the number of blood lymphocytes. Eventually some infected animals develop a persistent lymphocytosis (PL) with lymphocyte counts in the range of 20,000 to 80,000/μL. Not all BLV-infected cattle develop PL, although 95% of cattle with this condition are infected with BLV. These lymphocytes may be enlarged, are CD5+, express increased levels of immunoglobulin M (IgM), and show altered glycosylation. Cells in PL are not malignant and can occasionally return to the normal state. BLV becomes stably integrated into these B cells. Some T cells may also contain the BLV provirus. About 1% to 5% of BLV-infected cattle will develop a multicentric lymphosarcoma between 1 and 8 years after infection. Susceptibility to tumor development differs among species. Sheep are very sensitive, cattle have intermediate sensitivity, and goats are the least sensitive. Animals that develop these tumors die within 3 to 6 months. If there is bone marrow involvement, lymphocyte counts can reach 100,000/μL.

BLV is essential for neoplastic transformation but not for the continued growth of tumor cells. The mechanism by which BLV causes tumor development is unclear since there is no rearrangement of any known oncogenes. A viral gene called *Tax* appears to initiate tumorigenesis. Tax is a transactivating protein that can turn on many different cellular genes and that deregulates many different regulatory pathways rather than a single key pathway. Animals with advanced clinical bovine leukosis may be immunosuppressed as a result of the presence in their serum of a suppressor factor (Table 33-1). This suppression is reflected by reduced numbers of T cells and lowered serum IgM levels. Occasionally the neoplastic cells in bovine leukosis may be sufficiently differentiated to secrete immunoglobulin in a manner similar to that seen in myelomas. The cells in the sporadic form of bovine leukosis are predominantly T cells, but some originating from pre-B cells have also been identified.

Lymphomas in Other Species

In sheep, lymphomas are divided fairly evenly between T and B cells, and about 15% are unclassifiable (null cells). Some of these may be due to BLV infection (Box 33-2). A B cell lymphoma inherited as an autosomal recessive condition is recognized in swine. Horses carrying lymphosarcomas are commonly immunosuppressed. This usually involves T cell functions, but B cell function may also be impaired. A case of a horse with a lymphosarcoma with suppressor cell activity has been described. The animal presented with signs of immunodeficiency and was found to be deficient in IgM. The tumor cells grew in the presence of IL-2, possessed many T cell markers, and were noncytotoxic.

In dogs, leukemias may be classified on the basis of the cell type involved (lymphoid or myeloid) and on the basis of the clinical course and cytology (acute or chronic). Chronic

◻ Table 33-1 | Immunosuppressive Effects of Lymphoid Tumors

TUMOR	CELL TYPE	EVIDENCE FOR IMMUNOSUPPRESSION	MECHANISMS
Feline leukemia	T cell	Lymphopenia Prolonged skin grafts Increased susceptibility to infection Lack of response to mitogens	Suppressive viral protein, pI5E Suppressor cells
Marek's disease	T cell	Lack of response to mitogens Depressed cell-mediated cytotoxicity Depressed IgG production	Suppressor macrophages
Avian lymphoid leukosis	B cell	Increased susceptibility to infection	Suppressor lymphocytes
Bovine leukosis	B cell	Depressed serum IgM	Soluble suppressor factor
Myeloma	B cell	Increased susceptibility to infection	Soluble tumor-cell factor Negative feedback
Canine malignant lymphoma	B cell	Predisposition to infection associated with autoimmune disorders	Unknown
Equine lymphosarcoma	T cell	Increased susceptibility to infection	Tumor of suppressor cells

□ Box 33-2 | Lymphomas Differ Greatly Among Dog Breeds

When dog lymphoid tumors are phenotyped, significant differences are seen among breeds. For example, in Irish Wolfhounds, 100% of lymphoid tumors are of T cell origin. In Golden Retrievers, 54% of lymphoid tumors are from T cells, and the other 46% are from B cells. In Cocker Spaniels, only 6.8% are from T cells, whereas 93.2% of are of B cell origin. These different prevalences, however, are shared among related dog breeds. For example, among Toy breeds, 68% of lymphoid tumors are of T cell origin, whereas only 34% of Terrier lymphomas are T cells. Sex and neutering do not influence this distribution. It is likely that these differences in tumor susceptibility result from the major genetic differences among dog breeds.

Modiano JF, Breen M, Burnett RC, et al: Distinct B-cell and T-cell lymphoproliferative disease prevalence among dog breeds indicates heritable risk, *Cancer Res* 65:5654–5661, 2005.

lymphoid leukemia (CLL) is most frequently diagnosed. It is characterized by the presence of large numbers of mature lymphocytes in the blood. Animals may be asymptomatic, and the course of the disease is slow. About 70% of these cases involve T cells (CD3+), and most are large granular lymphocytes (LGLs). Of these LGLs, about 65% are α/β T cells, and the remainder are γ/δ T cells. The non-LGL T cell CLL cases involve α/β T cells. Malignant B cells identified as CD21+, CD79a+ account for about 30% of canine CLL cases. Chronic myeloid leukemias are extremely rare in dogs.

Acute leukemias, which are less common in dogs, may be of lymphoid (B cell) origin (20%) or myeloid origin (70%). The rest of these acute leukemias are difficult to classify and are considered undifferentiated. Many of these tumor cells, both myeloid and lymphoid, express CD34. The prognosis of these acute leukemias is usually very poor.

Lymphosarcomas account for 5% to 7% of canine malignancies. There is no evidence to suggest that these tumors are virus induced. They may be classified according to their apparent site of origin (e.g., multicentric, alimentary, or anterior mediastinal) or, alternatively, by their cell type (e.g., histiocytic, lymphocytic, lymphoblastic, or plasmacytic). The lymphocytic forms are usually of T cell origin. In many cases of canine lymphoma, affected dogs produce antibodies against crude tumor antigens. These antigens are not found on normal lymphoid cells.

Cutaneous T cell lymphomas (mycosis fungoides) are common in old dogs. The lesions consist of CD3+ cells. Eighty percent are CD8+, whereas the remainder are double negative. Most (70%) have γ/δ TCRs, especially if the tumor is confined to the epidermis.

Avian Lymphoid Tumors

Marek's disease is a herpesvirus-induced tumor of T cell origin. Birds with this disease are usually immunosuppressed. Thus their antibody responses, rejection of allografts, and delayed hypersensitivity responses are all depressed. This depression results from several factors, including virus-induced lymphoid destruction and the development of suppressor macrophages. These macrophages restrict the replication of the tumor cells, but in doing so they suppress the resistance of birds to other infections. Lymphoid leukosis is a tumor of B cell origin. Affected birds normally have a depressed antibody response and reduced responses to mitogens. Nevertheless some cases of this disease may present with hypergammaglobulinemia.

For sources of additional information, please visit http://evolve.elsevier.com/tizard/immunology/

Autoimmunity: General Principles

□ Key Points

- Autoimmunity is an inescapable consequence of the way in which the adaptive immune system has evolved.
- Not all autoimmunity is pathological. Autoimmune responses may be mounted against antigens that develop late in life, against antigens hidden within cells, and against antigens that arise as a result of the development of new molecular configurations.
- Most autoimmune diseases result from a failure to ensure that tolerance is maintained against self-antigens.
- There may be a strong genetic predisposition to develop autoimmunity.
- Some autoimmune diseases are triggered by immune stimulants such as virus infections, vaccination, and some drugs.
- The lesions that develop in autoimmune diseases are generated by the mechanisms of hypersensitivity.

Autoimmune diseases are relatively common. They occur in about 5% of humans and probably in a similar proportion of domestic mammals. Most represent the emergence of clones of "rogue" lymphocytes that are directed against normal body components. The fact that they tend to develop late in life suggests that they, like cancer, probably represent the result of multiple random mutations. Thus while one mutation alone may be insufficient to permit an autoimmune response, multiple such mutations may eventually permit self-reactive lymphocytes to develop. Lymphocytes, the key cells of the immune system, are triggered to proliferate by antigens. Given the ubiquity of microorganisms and environmental antigens, lymphocytes are under constant pressure to proliferate. The presence of a constant supply of self-antigens is especially significant. Much of the complexity of the immune system is determined by the need to keep this constant lymphocyte growth in check.

The suppression of lymphocyte growth is managed by multiple mechanisms. These include negative selection within the thymus, the requirement for multiple costimulatory signals, lymphocyte cooperation, and the activities of regulatory cell populations. These regulatory mechanisms often overlap so that the development of self-reactive rogue clones does not occur suddenly. It likely takes multiple accumulated mutations, leading to subtle changes in regulatory pathways, and the loss of control of lymphocyte proliferation. Similar considerations apply to the development of lymphoid tumors. It would be very unusual for autoimmunity to develop as a result of a single mutation in a key molecule.

An inescapable hazard associated with adaptive immunity is the development of autoimmunity. By developing a defense system that can recognize any possible microbial antigenic determinant, vertebrates also developed the potential for self-destruction. The random generation of antigen-binding receptors ensures that many lymphocytes are produced that can bind and respond to self-antigens. It has been estimated that 20% to 50% of T cell receptors (TCRs) and B cell receptors (BCRs) generated in this way will bind to self-antigens with high affinity. These self-reactive cells are usually rigorously suppressed so that only a few animals develop autoimmune disease. However, the reasons why these individuals develop autoimmune diseases are still unclear. Many factors influence susceptibility to autoimmunity. These include sex and age, genetic background, and virus infections. We also know that the development of autoantibodies is a relatively common event that by itself does not inevitably lead to autoimmune disease. Indeed, some autoantibodies serve a physiological function.

Because we do not know precisely what causes autoimmune disease, this chapter reviews some of the many different predisposing factors that have been identified or proposed as well as the mechanisms by which autoimmunity causes tissue damage and disease. As with other immune functions, both B and T cells can mediate autoimmunity. Thus in some autoimmune diseases, the disease is mediated by autoantibodies alone. In others, the damage may be mediated by T cells alone or by some combination of autoantibodies and T cells.

Induction of Autoimmunity

Autoimmune diseases appear to develop spontaneously, and predisposing causes are rarely obvious. Nevertheless they fall into two major categories: they can result from a normal immune response to an unusual or abnormal antigen, or they can result from an abnormal immune response to a normal antigen (Figure 34-1). The second category is probably the most common. In these cases, the mechanisms that normally prevent the development of self-responsive T and B cells fail. Many different environmental factors and genes contribute to this failure, and the failure may not always be complete. Autoimmune diseases may result from an aberrant response to a single specific antigen; alternatively, they may be due to a general defect in the regulation of B or T cell functions.

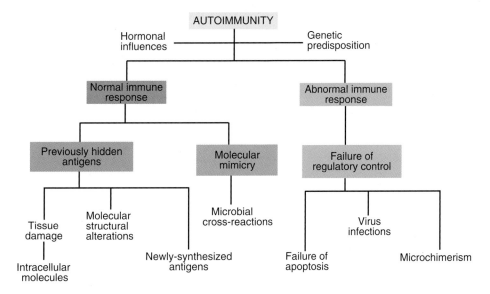

FIGURE 34-1 A simplified scheme for the pathogenesis of autoimmune diseases.

Normal Immune Responses

Many autoimmune responses simply reflect a normal immune response to an antigen that has been previously hidden or are a result of cross-reactivity between an infectious agent and a normal body component. Many naturally occurring autoantibodies play a role in homeostasis and regulation. They are usually low-titer, low-affinity immunoglobulin M (IgM) or IgG antibodies directed against protein fragments, or proteins damaged by oxidation or enzymes.

Antigens Hidden in Cells or Tissues (Cryptic Antigens)

Many autoimmune responses are triggered when nontolerant T cells meet previously hidden autoantigens. After all, T cells can only be made tolerant to autoantigens if the T cells are first exposed to these antigens. There are many autoantigens that do not induce tolerance because they remain hidden within cells or tissues.

Although the control of the immune system requires that most self-reactive cells be eliminated, one should not assume that all autoimmune responses are bad or even cause disease. Indeed, some autoimmune responses have physiological functions. For example, red blood cells must be removed from the blood once they reach the end of their life span. This process is accomplished by autoantibodies. As red cells age, an anion transport protein called CD233 (or band 3 protein) is gradually oxidized, and a new epitope is generated. This new epitope is recognized by IgG autoantibodies. These autoantibodies bind to aged red cells and trigger their phagocytosis by splenic macrophages. CD233 is found on many cell types, and it may be that its exposure on aged cells and their subsequent opsonization is a major elimination pathway.

Many autoantigens are found in places where they never encounter circulating lymphocytes. For example, in the testes, new antigens may appear only at puberty—long after the T cell system has developed and become tolerant to autoantigens. Injury to the testes may permit proteins from damaged tissues to reach the bloodstream, encounter antigen-sensitive cells, and stimulate autoimmunity. Hidden antigens may also be found within cells. For example, after a heart attack, autoantibodies may be produced against the mitochondria of cardiac muscle cells. In chronic hepatitis in dogs, animals develop antibodies to liver membrane proteins. In diseases such as trypanosomiasis or tuberculosis in which widespread tissue damage occurs, autoantibodies to many different tissue antigens may be detected in serum.

Antigens Generated by Molecular Changes

The production of some autoantibodies may be triggered by the development of completely new epitopes on normal proteins. Two examples of autoantibodies generated in this way

are the rheumatoid factors (RFs) and the immunoconglutinins (IKs, after the German spelling).

RFs are autoantibodies directed against other immunoglobulins. When an antibody binds to an antigen, the shape of the immunoglobulin molecule changes in such a way that new epitopes are exposed on its Fc region. These new epitopes may stimulate RF formation. RFs are produced in diseases in which large amounts of immune complexes are generated. These include the autoimmune disease of joints called rheumatoid arthritis and a disease called systemic lupus erythematosus (SLE), in which B cells respond to many different autoantigens.

IKs are autoantibodies directed against the complement components C2, C4, and especially C3. The epitopes that stimulate IK formation are exposed when these complement components are activated. The level of IKs in serum reflects the amount of complement activation; this, in turn, is a measure of the antigenic stimulation to which an animal is subjected. IK levels are thus nonspecific indicators of the prevalence of infectious disease within an animal population. Their physiological role is unclear, but they may enhance complement-mediated opsonization.

Receptor Editing

Both B and T cell antigen receptors are generated by random gene rearrangement. This process inevitably results in the generation of both nonfunctional and autoreactive antigen receptors. Once a complete antigen receptor is formed, however, rearrangement of the receptor gene segments continues. Thus if an immature B cell produces a receptor that binds to a self-antigen, the continuing development of that B cell is blocked while its light chain receptor chains continue to undergo recombination. This is an active process driven by the autoantigen. This replacement of one light chain by another leads to changes in receptor specificity and eventually makes the cells no longer autoreactive. Receptor editing only occurs in immature B cells. Mature B cells that bind autoantigens do not undergo receptor editing but rather are triggered to undergo apoptosis.

Abnormal Immune Responses

Failure of Regulatory Control

Although autoimmunity may be triggered by hidden epitopes, a sustained autoimmune response is necessary for disease to develop. This may result from a failure of the normal control mechanisms of the immune system and can be demonstrated simply by injecting mice with rat red blood cells. Following such an injection, mice not only make antibodies to the rat cells but also develop a self-limited and transient autoimmune response to their own red blood cells. This autoimmune response is rapidly controlled by regulatory cells and lasts for only a few days. If, however, regulatory cell activity in these mice is impaired, as occurs in New Zealand Black (NZB) mice, for example, these autoantibodies will persist to cause red blood cell destruction and anemia.

It is common to find autoimmune diseases associated with lymphoid tumors. For example, myasthenia gravis, an autoimmune disease involving the neuromuscular junction, is commonly associated with the presence of a thymic carcinoma. In humans, there is a fourfold increase in the incidence of rheumatoid arthritis in patients with malignant lymphoid tumors, and there is evidence for a similar association in other mammals. Since many lymphoid tumors result from a failure in immunological control mechanisms, a simultaneous failure in self-tolerance may also occur. Alternatively, some tumors may represent the development of a forbidden clone of cells producing autoantibodies. It is also possible that some lymphoid tumors may develop as a result of prolonged stimulation of the immune system by autoantigens.

Potentially harmful, self-reactive lymphocytes are normally destroyed in the thymus by apoptosis triggered through CD95 (Fas) (Chapter 18). Defects in CD95 or its ligand CD154 (CD95L) cause autoimmunity by permitting abnormal T cells to survive and cause disease. This is well demonstrated in the *lpr* strain of mice. These animals have a mutation that alters the structure of the intracellular domain of CD95 and blocks its functioning. A mutation (called *gld*) in CD95L has a similar effect. Both *lpr* and *gld* mice develop multiple autoimmune lesions accompanied by lymphoproliferation. Some investigators have suggested that mutations in CD95 may contribute to the pathogenesis of lupus in other mammals. The *AIRE* (autoimmune regulator) gene permits multiple self-antigens to be expressed in thymic epithelial cells. T cells that respond to these self-antigens are destroyed. Thus humans with a defective *AIRE* gene develop autoimmunity against multiple endocrine organs, the skin, and other tissues.

Infection-Induced Autoimmunity

Autoimmune diseases are triggered by many environmental factors, and infectious agents are among the most important. Given, however, that infections are very common and autoimmune diseases fairly rare, they clearly cannot account for the entire autoimmune process. For example, mice infected with certain reoviruses develop an autoimmune polyendocrine disease characterized by diabetes mellitus and retarded growth. These reovirus-infected mice make autoantibodies against normal pituitary, pancreas, gastric mucosa, nuclei, glucagon, growth hormone, and insulin. Likewise, in NZB mice, persistent infection with a type C retrovirus leads to the production of autoantibodies against nucleic acids and red blood cells. Bacteria such as *Streptococcus pyogenes, Borrelia burgdorferi,* and *Leptospira interrogans* may trigger autoimmune heart disease, arthritis, and uveitis, respectively. The protozoan parasite *Trypanosoma cruzi* triggers an autoimmune cardiomyopathy.

The situation with spontaneous autoimmune disease is less clear. Many attempts have been made to isolate viruses from patients with autoimmune disease but with mixed results. For example, SLE of dogs and humans has been associated with either a type C retrovirus or paramyxovirus infection. Small quantities of the Epstein-Barr virus genome can be found in the salivary glands of humans with Sjögren's syndrome. Moreover, epidemiological evidence points to some form of a viral trigger for diseases such as multiple sclerosis, rheumatoid arthritis, and insulin-dependent diabetes mellitus in children.

Just how viruses can induce autoimmunity is unclear, but three major mechanisms are recognized; molecular mimicry, epitope spreading, and bystander activation.

Molecular Mimicry Autoimmunity may result from molecular mimicry, a term used to describe the sharing of epitopes between an infectious agent or parasite and an autoantigen (Figure 34-2). B cells may be triggered by a foreign epitope that cross-reacts with an autoantigen. However, they will only respond to this epitope if they receive T cell help. If nearby Th cells also recognize these microbial epitopes as foreign, they may trigger a response that permits the self-reactive B cells to make autoantibodies. Once a B cell response is triggered in this way, the infectious agent may be removed while the autoimmune response continues—a "hit-and-run" process.

Many examples of molecular mimicry are now recognized. For example, the parasite *T. cruzi* contains antigens that cross-react with mammalian neurons and cardiac muscle. Individuals infected with *T. cruzi* make autoantibodies that can cause nervous system and heart disease. Molecular mimicry may also cause the heart lesions of rheumatic fever in children. Antibodies to the cell wall M-protein of group A streptococci cross-react with cardiac myosin. Children infected with certain strains of group A streptococci produce antimyocardial antibodies and develop heart disease. Some strains of streptococci may cause acute glomerulonephritis in children as a result of the production of antibodies cross-reacting with glomerular basement membranes. Other examples of molecular mimicry that may be significant include the Epstein-Barr virus DNA polymerase, which cross-reacts with myelin basic protein and may be involved in the induction of multiple sclerosis, and the poliovirus capsid protein VP2, which cross-reacts with the acetylcholine receptor and may induce myasthenia gravis.

The integrin CD11a/18 (LFA-1) shares an antigenic determinant with the outer surface protein of the Lyme disease bacterium, *B. burgdorferi*. Patients infected with this organism mount an initial immune response that may then develop into an autoimmune response. In about 10% of patients with Lyme arthritis, antibiotics fail to resolve the disease, suggesting that, once triggered, the autoimmune process can proceed in the absence of the bacterium.

Antibodies against microbial heat-shock proteins are found in the serum of humans and rats with rheumatoid arthritis, ankylosing spondylitis, and SLE. Injection of killed *Mycobacterium tuberculosis* in Freund's complete adjuvant can cause arthritis in rats, and T cells from these animals can transfer arthritis to normal syngeneic recipients. These T cells are responding to HSP 60, a mycobacterial heat-shock protein (Chapter 25). Because heat-shock proteins are highly

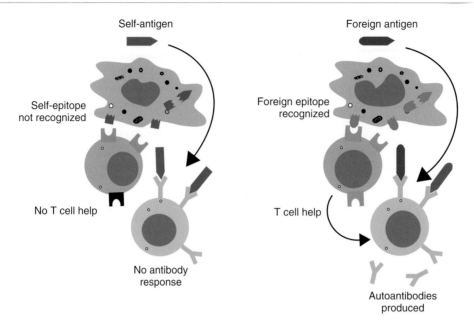

FIGURE 34-2 Cross-reactions with foreign antigens may be sufficient to trigger a helper T cell population that will promote an autoimmune response by B cells. A helper effect triggered by a foreign antigen may inadvertently permit an autoimmune response to occur.

conserved and T cells from rheumatoid arthritis patients are also directed against HSP 60, it has been suggested that molecular mimicry between microbial and mammalian HSP 60 may be important in rheumatoid arthritis.

Ankylosing spondylitis is an autoimmune arthritis of humans that affects the sacroiliac joints, spine, and peripheral joints. Patients also develop acute anterior uveitis (inflammation of the iris and neighboring structures in the eye). More than 95% of humans with ankylosing spondylitis possess the major histocompatibility (MHC) class I allele HLA-B27, whereas in the normal population, the prevalence of this allele is less than 8%. It is believed that the disease results from molecular mimicry between the hypervariable region of HLA-B27 and antigens found in *Klebsiella pneumoniae* and related bacteria. *K. pneumoniae* is found more frequently than normal in the intestine of patients with active ankylosing spondylitis and uveitis, and patients with active disease have elevated levels of IgA against *Klebsiella* in their sera. Cloning of B27 into mice and subsequent infection of these animals with *K. pneumoniae* causes an acute spondylitis.

HLA-B27-like alleles have been cloned from bonobos, gorillas, rhesus, and cynomolgus monkeys, and HLA-B27–associated ankylosing spondylitis has been described in gorillas. Up to 20% of wild gorillas may have spondylitis, and the disease has also been described in a gibbon, in baboons, and in rhesus macaques.

In porcine enzootic pneumonia caused by *Mycoplasma hyopneumoniae,* antibodies to the mycoplasma cross-react with pig lungs, and in contagious bovine pleuropneumonia, there is cross-reactivity between *Mycoplasma mycoides* antigens and normal bovine lung. It is not known to what extent these autoantibodies contribute to the pathogenesis of these diseases. There is a clearer relationship between *Leptospira interrogans*

infection and the development of periodic ophthalmia, the leading cause of blindness in horses (Chapter 35).

Some microbial superantigens may also trigger autoimmunity. The superantigen staphylococcal enterotoxin B activates the same T cells that react with myelin and induces an autoimmune encephalitis. It has been suggested that a bacterial superantigen may trigger rheumatoid arthritis since the T cells in affected joints are enriched in cells bearing certain TCR V domains. The only known agents that can alter V region gene expression in this way are superantigens.

Epitope Spreading In some cases autoimmunity seems to arise from a normal immune response against a foreign antigen that subsequently "spreads" to recognize self-antigens. When an autoimmune response is initiated, the immune response is first directed against a single epitope on the inciting antigen. However, as the process continues, the T and B cell responses diversify, and responses begin to be directed against additional epitopes. At first they will be other epitopes on the same protein. Eventually responses may spread to epitopes on other autoantigens. Epitope spreading has been demonstrated in autoimmune diseases such as thyrotoxicosis and diabetes and may account for some of the difficulties encountered in controlling these diseases.

Bystander Activation When viruses cause tissue damage, previously hidden antigens may be released. These may activate nearby lymphocytes that had not been involved in the antiviral response, Additionally T cells might, in responding to an antigen, produce a mixture of cytokines such as the tumor necrosis factors (TNFs) and nitric oxide, resulting in the death of nearby cells and activation of an autoimmune response. Viruses may induce an inflammatory response that results in the release of multiple cytokines. Pathogens may trigger inappropriate lymphocyte proliferation by acting through pattern-recognition receptors to generate co-stimulatory molecules and proinflammatory mediators. These cytokines may activate previously dormant T cells. As a result the T cells may attack autoantigens that they previously ignored. Evidence suggests that Coxsackie virus–induced diabetes is mediated in large part through bystander activation (Figure 34-3). Prolonged infection with some viruses may induce autoimmunity as a result of chronic activation of the immune responses. Thus a prolonged polyclonal B cell activation may result in the eventual emergence of autoreactive clones.

Microchimerism During pregnancy, mothers and their fetuses may exchange a few cells. Some of these fetal cells may persist in a mother's body for many years after pregnancy. Conversely, a mother's cells may survive for many years in her offspring. These cells are accepted by a tolerant immune system. The process is called fetal microchimerism, and it has been suggested that these persistent cells may be the cause of some autoimmune diseases. In women with the autoimmune disease scleroderma, it is possible to find fetal T, B, and natural killer (NK) cells, as well as fetal monocytes, in the blood. It has been suggested, therefore, that scleroderma is a form of graft-versus-host disease in these patients. Transfer of cells from mother to her fetus may also cause autoimmunity. For example, small numbers of maternal cells can be detected in the blood of most boys with the autoimmune disease dermatomyositis. In all these cases, the number of persistent foreign cells is so small that they cannot be the sole cause of the autoimmune disease.

Predisposing Factors

Genetic Predisposition

Although viruses or other infectious agents may trigger autoimmune responses, it is clear that not all infected individuals develop autoimmune disease. This is because genetic factors are key determinants of disease susceptibility. Genetic analysis of mice has led to the identification of at least 25 gene loci that contribute to autoimmunity if deleted or overexpressed. These include genes that code for cytokines, cytokine receptors, co-stimulators, molecules that regulate apoptosis, molecules that regulate antigen clearance, and members of cytokine or antigen-signaling cascades. Some diseases result from a defect in a single gene such as the *lpr,* or *gld* mutations. Their gene products play a key role in the destruction of self-reactive T cells. In their absence, excessive T cell proliferation and autoimmunity result. Others result from inherited complement deficiencies. More commonly, the role of genes is complex. Thus genes influence the severity of disease, and no specific gene is necessary or sufficient for disease expression. Even if an animal has a complete set of susceptibility alleles at multiple loci, presence of overt disease may depend on the genetic background of the animal. This genetic complexity probably also contributes to differences in disease presentation since these may be determined by different sets of contributing genes. Genetic analysis is also complicated because susceptibility genes may or may not interact with each other. The vulnerability of a target organ to autoimmune damage may also be inherited.

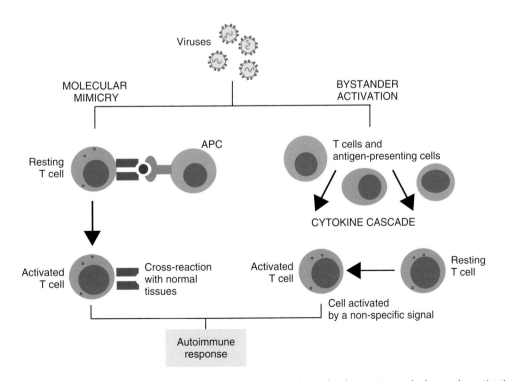

FIGURE 34-3 Viruses may trigger autoimmune responses either by molecular mimicry or by bystander activation.

The genes that are predominantly associated with naturally occurring autoimmune diseases are those in the MHC. MHC molecules regulate the presentation of processed epitopes. In theory, therefore, they determine resistance or susceptibility to many diseases. In practice, there is strong selection against genes that predispose to susceptibility to infectious agents, and MHC genes have been selected for a strong response to most common infectious pathogens. In contrast, autoimmune diseases in old, postreproductive animals do not offer a selective disadvantage, and MHC-linked predispositions have been identified. Studies of humans have shown that almost all autoimmune diseases are linked to multiple MHC loci. Presumably an essential prerequisite for any autoimmune disease is that the autoantigen is appropriately processed and presented on an MHC molecule. Thus the structure of the MHC antigen-binding groove determines whether a specific autoantigen will trigger an immune response. Some MHC alleles appear to protect against autoimmunity, and any predisposition to autoimmunity may be the result of the net effect of both enhancing and protective genes. In addition, most autoimmune diseases are associated with multiple MHC alleles. For example, in humans the combination of HLA-A1, -B8, and -DR3 is associated with increased risk for type 1 diabetes, myasthenia gravis, and SLE.

Breed Predispositions

Dogs have undergone two major population bottlenecks. The first occurred when they were domesticated about 20,000 years ago. The second occurred about 200 years ago when most current dog breeds were created. The development of specific breeds resulted from aggressive selection for behavioral and structural traits. This breed creation, however, also inadvertently selected for mutations in the founder populations. As dog breeds have reduced genetic heterogeneity, so too have they reduced resistance to specific groups of diseases.

The three major classes of immunologically mediated disease (autoimmunity, immunodeficiency, and atopy) tend to be encountered in some dog breeds more commonly than in others. Old English Sheepdogs are unusually prone to develop autoimmune blood diseases. Certain autoimmune diseases, such as polyarteritis nodosa and hypothyroidism, have familial associations. Many domestic dogs, especially those from rare breeds, show restricted MHC polymorphism that can increase autoimmune disease susceptibility. In dogs there are several recognized associations between autoimmunity and MHC alleles. Diabetes mellitus is associated with DLA-A3, -A7, -A10, and -B4; antinuclear antibody production is associated with DLA-12; SLE is associated with DLA-A7; and autoimmune polyarthritis is associated with certain C4 alleles.

Breeds have been developed as a result of aggressive phenotypic selection, in many cases resulting in inbreeding and a lack of genetic diversity. This has had two effects. First, it has permitted deleterious autosomal recessive genes to be expressed, as is seen in the increased prevalence of immunodeficiency syndromes and other immunological disorders. Second, it has

resulted in a loss of MHC polymorphism. For example, DRB1*04 is found in most Boxers, DRB1*2401 may be restricted to Akitas, DRB1*01 predominates in West Highland White Terriers, DQA*0203 is restricted to Dobermans, there is a high incidence of DQA*0102 in Irish Wolfhounds and Chows, and DRB1*0101 is common in Irish Setters. These limited haplotypes ensure that the dogs in these breeds will respond to an unusually narrow range of antigens, thus reducing their resistance to infectious agents. Such dogs will also be more susceptible to autoimmune diseases. The increasing incidence of immunological diseases seen in dogs is largely attributable to careless breeding practices.

Inbred lines of other animals have been produced that are associated with spontaneous development of autoimmune disease. For example, chickens of the OS strain develop autoimmune thyroiditis. Inbred NZB mice spontaneously develop a syndrome that bears a striking resemblance to SLE (Chapter 36). These mice develop immune complex glomerulonephritis. They become hypergammaglobulinemic and hypocomplementemic, and they develop an autoimmune hemolytic anemia. Some also develop lymphoid tumors. NZB mice produce autoantibodies against nuclear antigens, red blood cells, and T cells, and their B cells are polyclonally activated. New Zealand White (NZW) mice are phenotypically normal, but the F1 cross between NZW and NZB mice has an even more severe SLE-like syndrome. In these animals, kidney disease is severe and is associated with high titers of antibodies to nucleic acids. Studies on the inheritance of these traits in mice suggest that they are controlled by a small number of unlinked major genes and a large number of minor genes.

Intestinal Microflora

Because the intestinal microflora influences the development of immunological tolerance (Chapter 22), it may also affect the development of autoimmune disease. For example, mice given oral antibiotics to reduce their intestinal microflora developed less severe experimental allergic encephalomyelitis (EAE) than control animals. In contrast, mice that received antibiotics intraperitoneally developed EAE whose severity was similar to that seen in untreated mice. Protection against EAE was associated with a reduction in the production of proinflammatory cytokines, increased production of interleukin-10 (IL-10) and IL-13 and enhanced Treg activity. A similar result has been observed in experimental autoimmune arthritis where the disease was very much milder in germ-free mice. In this case the mechanism was traced to a reduction in IL-17 production in the intestinal lamina propria. These mice had reduced Th17 activity and thus inflammation. If the intestine of these mice was colonized by a single bacterial species, IL-17 production was restored, autoantibody production began, and arthritis developed rapidly. An opposite effect has been observed on the development of type 1 diabetes in NOD mice. In that case, germ-free mice had a more severe disease than conventional mice.

Mechanisms of Tissue Damage in Autoimmunity

Autoimmune disease results when tissues are damaged by autoreactive T cells or antibodies. This damage is a result of hypersensitivity reactions. However, multiple mechanisms may be involved in any such disease, and these may vary with time.

Type I Hypersensitivity

Milk allergy in cattle is an autoimmune disease in which a milk protein (α casein), normally found only in the udder, gains access to the general circulation and stimulates an immune response. This happens when milking is delayed and intramammary pressure forces the α casein into the circulation. For unknown reasons this triggers a Th2 response and IgE autoantibodies are produced. As a result, affected cows may develop acute anaphylaxis (Chapter 28). A similar condition is seen occasionally in other domestic mammals such as the mare. Although antibodies in milk proteins are commonly found in human serum after rapid weaning, type I hypersensitivity is not a usual sequel.

Type II Hypersensitivity

Autoantibodies may cause cell lysis with the assistance of complement or cytotoxic cells. Thus if autoantibodies are directed against red blood cells, autoimmune hemolytic anemia may result; if directed against platelets, thrombocytopenia will occur; and if against thyroid cells, thyroiditis will result. In one form of this process in humans, autoantibodies against thyroid-stimulating hormone (TSH) receptors on thyroid cells stimulate thyroid activity rather than its destruction. Cell surface receptors are common targets of autoimmune attack. In addition to the TSH receptor, autoantibodies attack the acetylcholine receptor in myasthenia gravis and the insulin receptor in some forms of diabetes. Autoantibodies to β adrenoceptors (Chapter 28) have been detected in some patients with asthma. By blocking β receptors, these antibodies make the airways highly irritable, and affected individuals develop severe asthma.

Type III Hypersensitivity

Autoantibodies form immune complexes with autoantigens, and these complexes may cause inflammation. This is most significant in systemic lupus erythematosus, a disease in which many different autoantibodies are produced. Immune complexes deposited in glomeruli provoke a membranoproliferative glomerulonephritis (Chapter 30). Similarly, in rheumatoid arthritis, immune complexes are deposited in joints and contribute to the local inflammatory response.

Type IV Hypersensitivity

Many autoimmune disease lesions are infiltrated with mononuclear cells, and Th1 responses probably contribute to the pathogenesis of these diseases. Cytotoxic T cells cause demyelination in experimental allergic encephalitis and human multiple sclerosis. Insulin-dependent diabetes mellitus may be due to a cell-mediated response because the diseased pancreatic islets may be infiltrated by lymphocytes, and lymphocytes from diabetics may be cytotoxic for pancreatic islet cells in vitro. Although cytotoxic T cells can kill cells directly, cytokines may also cause tissue damage. For example, TNF-α released by these cells upregulates cell adhesion molecules, including selectins, facilitating migration of neutrophils into the lesions.

For sources of additional information, please visit http://evolve.elsevier.com/tizard/immunology/

Organ-Specific Autoimmune Diseases

□ Key Points

- Domestic mammals suffer from a diverse array of autoimmune diseases. Any organ or tissue is a potential victim of autoimmune attack.
- The most common autoimmune diseases in domestic mammals involve the endocrine system, the skin, and blood cells.
- Treatment of autoimmune diseases usually involves suppression of the destructive inflammatory lesion by corticosteroids. These may be supplemented by the use of other immunosuppressive drugs.

A utoimmune diseases that mainly affect a single organ or tissue presumably result from an abnormal response to a small number of self-antigens and do not necessarily reflect significant loss of control of the immune system as a whole. It is likely that all organs of the body are potentially susceptible to this form of immunological attack. Nevertheless, autoimmune diseases directed against endocrine organs, skin, blood and the nervous system, tend to be most commonly affected. Much depends on the species and breed of an animal as well as its age.

Autoimmune Endocrine Disease

Although domestic animals develop autoimmune endocrine diseases, they differ from humans insofar as these tend to present as single disorders rather than involving multiple endocrine organs. Occasionally a dog may experience two or more autoimmune endocrine disorders simultaneously (autoimmune polyglandular syndrome), but this is very uncommon.

Lymphocytic Thyroiditis

Dogs, humans, and chickens suffer from autoimmune thyroiditis as a result of the production of autoantibodies against thyroglobulin or thyroid peroxidase. These antibodies may also react with triiodothyronine (T_3) or thyroxine (T_4). Affected dogs may also show a delayed skin reaction to intradermally injected thyroid extract, suggesting that cell-mediated immunity contributes to the disease. Several dog breeds are predisposed to thyroiditis, and relatives of affected animals may have antithyroid antibodies although clinically normal. A familial form of hypothyroidism has been demonstrated in Beagles and Great Danes. Dogs from high-risk breeds such as Dobermans tend to develop the disease when young, whereas dogs from low-risk breeds tend to develop it when older. Unfortunately, by the time the disease is diagnosed, the dog may already have been bred. Affected thyroids are infiltrated with plasma cells and lymphocytes, and germinal center formation may occur (Figure 35-1). The invading lymphocytes probably cause epithelial cell destruction through antibody-dependent cell-mediated cytotoxicity (ADCC) and T cell cytotoxicity.

In dogs, clinical signs appear after about 75% of the thyroid is destroyed. These signs are those of hypothyroidism; that is, the animals are fat and inactive and show patchy hair loss. The most common problems are a dry, dull, coarse coat; scaling; hypotrichosis; slow hair regrowth; hyperpigmentation; myxedema; and pyoderma. Other signs include myopathy, hyperlipidemia, hypothermia, anestrus, galactorrhea, diarrhea or constipation, and polyneuropathy. Tests of thyroid function such as a radioimmunoassay for plasma T_4 or T_3 only confirm the existence of hypothyroidism. A thyroid-stimulating hormone (TSH) response test is more useful because it can confirm the inability of the affected thyroid to respond to TSH. (Plasma T_4 levels are measured before and after injection of TSH.) In order to confirm autoimmune thyroiditis, a biopsy must show the characteristic lymphocytic infiltration. Antithyroid antibodies must be detected in serum using an enzyme-linked immunosorbent assay (ELISA), immunoblot, or an indirect fluorescent antibody test (Chapter 41). There is little correlation between antithyroid antibody titers and disease severity. Management of affected animals involves replacement therapy with sodium levothyroxine (synthetic T_4). Improvement should be seen within 4 to 6 weeks. There is no cure for this disease, and the success of treatment depends on effective replacement therapy.

An autoimmune thyroiditis also occurs in the OS (obese) strain of white Leghorn chickens. The thyroids of these birds

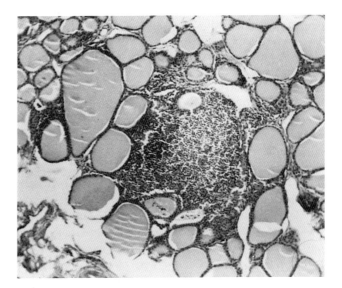

FIGURE 35-1 A lymphocytic nodule in the thyroid of a dog suffering from autoimmune thyroiditis. Original magnification ×100.

(From a specimen provided by Dr. B.N. Wilkie.)

are heavily infiltrated by lymphocytes and plasma cells. Auto-antibodies are directed against thyroglobulin, and affected birds are hypothyroid. These birds also make antibodies against their adrenal gland, exocrine pancreas, and proventricular cells. Neonatal thymectomy prevents the development of lesions.

Hyperthyroidism

Hyperthyroidism is a disease of old cats. Autoantibodies to thyroid peroxidase have been demonstrated in almost one third of cases of feline hyperthyroidism, and about 10% of these animals also have antinuclear antibodies. Lymphocytic infiltration is also observed in about one third of cases, and it is possible that such cases may be immunologically mediated.

Lymphocytic Parathyroiditis

Dogs and cats develop autoimmune hypoparathyroidism. Affected animals usually have a history of neurological or neuromuscular disease, especially seizures. On investigation, affected animals are profoundly hypocalcemic, and serum parathormone levels are severely reduced. Normal parathyroid tissue is replaced by a massive infiltration of lymphocytes and a few plasma cells. Once hypocalcemic tetany is controlled, these animals may be treated by oral vitamin D and calcium administration. It would be logical to administer immunosuppressive therapy.

Insulin-Dependent Diabetes Mellitus

In humans, insulin-dependent diabetes mellitus (IDDM) is an autoimmune disease mediated by autoantibodies against an islet cell enzyme called glutamic acid decarboxylase. Some cases of IDDM in dogs may also be immunologically mediated. The canine disease is associated with pancreatic islet atrophy and a loss of β cells. In some cases, the islets are infiltrated by lymphocytes. Experimentally, circulating mononuclear cells from diabetic dogs have suppressed insulin production by cultured mouse islet cells. Serum from IDDM dogs lysed these islet cells in the presence of complement (Figure 35-2). When dog serum was tested for antibodies against cultured β cells by immunofluorescence, 9 of 23 diabetic dogs showed strongly positive reactions, and an additional 3 showed a weak reaction. Only 1 of 15 normal dogs gave a positive response. Thus cytotoxic cells or antibodies or both may be responsible for β cell destruction in dogs. A familial predisposition to IDDM has been observed in Samoyeds. Genes that may influence the development of canine diabetes mellitus include those for the regulatory cytokines interferon-γ (IFN-γ), interleukin-12 (IL-12), IL-4, and IL-10. These candidate genes were screened for single nucleotide polymorphisms (SNPs) in multiple different dog breeds. Significant associations were observed for IL-4 in Collies, Cairn Terriers, and Schnauzers and for IL-10 in the Cavalier King Charles Spaniel. This suggests that cytokine genes that influence the Th1/Th2 balance may determine susceptibility to diabetes.

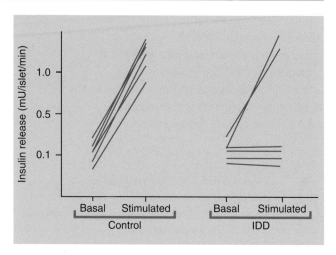

FIGURE 35-2 Insulin release from islets incubated in vitro in the presence of six individual control or insulin-dependent diabetic dog sera, plus complement. Four of the six diabetic dog sera inhibited insulin release from cultured islets.

(From Sai P, Debray-Sachs M, Jondet A, et al: Anti-beta-cell immunity in insulinopenic diabetic dogs, *Diabetes* 33:135–140, 1984.)

Nonobese diabetic (NOD) mice develop spontaneous IDDM associated with infiltration of the pancreatic islets by lymphocytes. Their disease resembles human type 1 diabetes. The development of diabetes in NOD mice is influenced by their microflora. Thus pathogen-free NOD mice that lack MyD88 protein (MyD88 is an adaptor molecule for innate receptors such as the toll-like receptors [TLRs]) do not develop diabetes, whereas totally germ-free MyD88− NOD mice do. If defined commensal microbes are given to these germ-free mice, their diabetes is less severe. Likewise commensal microbes from the intestine of pathogen-free MyD88− NOD mice attenuate the disease when given to germ-free mice. Somehow the interaction of the intestinal microflora with the innate immune system modifies the predisposition of these mice to develop diabetes.

Human patients with type 1 IDDM have circulating antibodies against the 67-kDa isoform of glutamic acid decarboxylase (GAD65) and/or insulinoma antigen-2 (IA-2). Some diabetic dogs also possess such autoantibodies. Thus 4 of 30 diabetic dogs had autoantibodies to GAD65, whereas 3 dogs had autoantibodies to IA-2. Two had autoantibodies to both antigens.

Diabetes mellitus is rare in cattle. Affected animals have atrophied and reduced numbers of pancreatic islets with partial or complete loss of β cells. Lymphocytes commonly infiltrate the remaining islets.

Atrophic Lymphocytic Pancreatitis

The most common cause of an exocrine pancreatic deficiency in dogs is atrophy associated with lymphocyte infiltration. It is seen predominantly in German Shepherds and Rough-Coated Collies. The infiltrating lymphocytes are primarily CD4+ and CD8+ T cells. The CD8+ cells are associated with areas of pancreatic necrosis. Some of these dogs have low levels of antibodies against pancreatic acinar cells, so this may be, in part, an autoimmune disease.

Autoimmune Adrenalitis

Dogs may suffer from lymphocyte-mediated destruction of the adrenal cortex. Affected animals present with depression, weak pulse, bradycardia, abdominal pain, vomiting, diarrhea, dehydration, and hypothermia. As a result of excessive sodium and chloride loss, animals develop hypovolemia and acidosis, leading to circulatory shock, hyperkalemia, and cardiac arrhythmias. Blood corticosteroid levels are low in these animals. This disease has been observed in association with hypothyroidism.

Autoimmune Neurological Disease

An autoimmune brain disease known as experimental allergic encephalomyelitis may be produced by immunizing animals with brain tissue emulsified in Freund's complete adjuvant. After a few weeks, dogs or cats develop focal encephalitis and myelitis, possibly with paralysis. The brain lesions consist of focal vasculitis, mononuclear cell infiltration, perivascular demyelination, and axon damage. Antibodies to brain tissue can be detected in the serum of these animals, although the lesion itself is a result of a cell-mediated response.

A similar encephalitis used to occur following administration of rabies vaccines containing brain tissue to humans. For this reason, the use of adult brain tissue was stopped, and suckling mouse brain tissue obtained prior to myelination is used in the production of rabies vaccines. Postdistemper demyelinating leukoencephalopathy may also be of autoimmune origin, although the production of antimyelin antibodies appears to be common response to central nervous tissue damage, regardless of its cause.

Equine Polyneuritis

Equine polyneuritis (neuritis of the cauda equina) is an uncommon disease of horses affecting the sacral and coccygeal nerves. Affected horses show hyperesthesia followed by progressive paralysis of the tail, rectum, and bladder and localized anesthesia in the same region. The disease may also be associated with facial and trigeminal paralysis. Although sacral and lumbar involvement is usually bilateral, the cranial nerve involvement is often unilateral. A chronic granulomatous inflammation develops in the region of the extradural nerve roots. Affected nerves are thickened and discolored. They show a loss of myelinated axons; infiltration by macrophages, lymphocytes, giant cells, and plasma cells; and deposition of fibrous material in the perineurium. In severe cases the nerve

trunks may be almost totally destroyed. Affected horses have circulating antibodies to a peripheral myelin protein called P2. P2 can induce experimental allergic neuritis in rodents (see later). Although equine polyneuritis may be an autoimmune disease, equine adenovirus-1 has been isolated from its lesions, so the cause is complex. Because of the severe nerve damage, immunosuppressive or antiinflammatory therapy is rarely successful. Neuritis of the cauda equina has also been reported in a dog. The dog presented with a flaccid tail and urinary incompetence. The nerve roots of its cauda equina and lumbar nerves were infiltrated by T and B cells.

Canine Polyneuritis

Canine polyneuritis or coonhound paralysis affects dogs following a bite or scratch from a raccoon. It presents as an ascending symmetrical flaccid paralysis with mild sensory impairment. The bitten limb is usually affected first, but the disease is progressive and will worsen for 10 to 12 days following the bite. In severe cases the dog may develop flaccid quadriplegia and lose the ability to swallow, bark, or breathe. The disease is, however, self-limited, and if respiration is not impaired, the prognosis is good. Dogs usually recover completely. Affected nerves show demyelination and axonal degeneration with macrophage infiltration. An acute polyneuritis similar to coonhound paralysis has also been described following vaccination of dogs with rabies or other vaccines.

Coonhound paralysis and postvaccinal polyneuritis both closely resemble Guillain-Barré syndrome in humans. This syndrome may follow upper respiratory tract infection, gastrointestinal disease, or even vaccination. It is mediated by autoantibodies against peripheral nerve glycolipids. Management of Guillain-Barré syndrome requires plasmapheresis and administration of intravenous immunoglobulins (IVIG). Veterinarians treating canine polyneuritis have traditionally administered corticosteroids, but their effectiveness is unclear.

If sciatic nerve tissue is used to immunize experimental dogs, it provokes experimental allergic neuritis. After a latent period of 6 to 14 days, the animals develop an ascending polyneuritis and gradual paralysis (Figure 35-3). The disease is due to peripheral nerve demyelination resulting from autoimmune attack.

Steroid-Responsive Meningitis-Arteritis

Steroid-responsive meningitis-arteritis (SRMA) is characterized by sterile inflammation of the meningeal arteries and cervical meningitis. Two different forms of the disease are recognized. In the acute form, affected dogs show anorexia, fever, lameness, and listlessness followed by progressive cervical rigidity; hyperesthesia along the vertebral column; generalized, cervical, or spinal pain; ataxia; seizures; and behavioral changes. The typical disease course consists of severe episodes with symptom-free remissions. The less common chronic form may

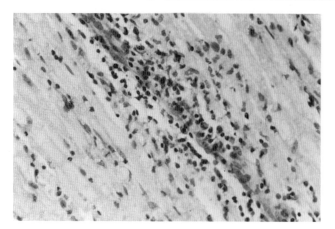

FIGURE 35-3 A section of rat sciatic nerve showing a mononuclear cell infiltration. This is the lesion of experimental allergic neuritis produced by inoculation of rat sciatic nerve in Freund's complete adjuvant. Original magnification ×400.

(Courtesy of Dr. B.N. Wilkie.)

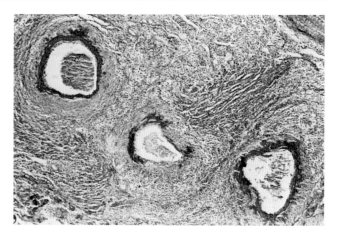

FIGURE 35-4 Meningeal arteries from a dog with meningeal arteritis. Note the periarteritis with fibrinoid necrosis. Original magnification ×125.

(From Harcourt RA: Polyarteritis in a colony of beagles, *Vet Rec* 102:519–522, 1978.)

develop following relapses of acute disease or inadequate treatment. Additional neurological signs consistent with lesions in the brain and spinal cord such as paresis or ataxia may develop. These dogs may have concurrent immune-mediated polyarthritis. The prognosis in young dogs is fair to good since aggressive antiinflammatory and immunosuppressive therapy using prednisolone or prednisone leads to rapid clinical improvement. Once the disease is in remission, the steroid dose should be gradually reduced to the minimum necessary to prevent relapses. Treatment may be stopped 6 months after clinical status, cerebrospinal fluid (CSF) and blood return to normal. It may not be possible to discontinue treatment completely in chronic cases, although azathioprine is effective in such cases. Large dogs, such as Boxers, Weimaraners, and Bernese Mountain Dogs, are commonly affected, although the disease has also been reported in Beagles. Dogs under 2 years of age are most commonly affected.

The CSF in acute cases of SRMA contains high IgA and CXCL8 levels and mature neutrophils. Serum IgA and acute-phase proteins (C-reactive protein and α_2-macroglobulin) are also elevated. Analysis of a patient's T cells indicates that production of IL-2 and IFN-γ are depressed, whereas Th2 production of IL-4 is enhanced and probably accounts for the increased IgA production. About 30% of these dogs have a positive lupus erythematosus (LE) cell test but no detectable antinuclear antibody activity (Chapter 36). In chronic cases the CSF contains predominantly mononuclear cells. On necropsy, the spinal meningeal arteries show fibrinoid degeneration, intimal or medial necrosis, and hyalinization and are infiltrated with lymphocytes, plasma cells, and macrophages, and a few neutrophils (Figure 35-4). Complete obliteration of the blood vessel lumina may occur, whereas rupture and thrombosis of inflamed vessels may lead to hemorrhage, compression, and infarction.

Immune-mediated vasculitis is usually associated with immune complex deposition and neutrophil infiltration in blood vessel walls. In the meningitis described earlier, however, the cellular infiltration may not contain neutrophils. In the Beagle cases, no immunoglobulin deposits were detected in the lesions, although numerous IgG-containing plasma cells were present in the leptomeninges and in the walls of affected vessels.

Necrotizing Meningoencephalitis

Three common inflammatory diseases of the canine central nervous system are recognized. They may be immunological in origin. Canine necrotizing meningoencephalitis (NME) is an inflammatory disease of unknown etiology that has been described in various toy breeds such as Pugs (young females), Maltese Terriers, Pekinese, and Chihuahuas. The necrotic lesions are multifocal and asymmetrical, restricted to the gray and white matter in the cerebra, and are accompanied by a severe meningitis. Macrophages predominate in the lesions, but both scattered T cells and dendritic cells are present in the lesions, whereas B cells are restricted to the meninges. Dogs with NME have autoantibodies to glial fibrillary acidic protein, but the significance of these is unclear. In at least one case, an affected dog had a concomitant glomerulonephritis with smooth linear basement membrane staining for IgG, suggesting the presence of anti–basement membrane antibodies.

A similar disease has been reported in Yorkshire Terriers and French Bulldogs. Called necrotizing leukoencephalitis (NLE), it is characterized by the presence of multiple necrotic foci in the white matter of the forebrain and brainstem. These foci are characterized by cavitation, necrosis, demyelination, and perivascular cuffing. The primary infiltrating cells are T cells. Some investigators consider NLE to be a variant of NME.

A third form of canine nonsuppurative encephalitis is granulomatous meningoencephalitis (GME). This is common and may account for one fourth of canine central nervous system diseases. GME is characterized by the formation of multifocal granulomas in the cerebellum and brainstem. T cells predominate in the lesions. GME may be disseminated, focal or ocular. The prognosis is poor although aggressive immunosuppression with corticosteroids may be beneficial.

Degenerative Myelopathy

Affected dogs show progressive ataxia affecting the hind limbs until they can no longer walk. Forelimb problems eventually develop, and dogs die in 6 to 12 months after disease onset. On necropsy, these dogs have a degenerative myelopathy with widespread demyelination and loss of axons in the thoracolumbar region. The cause of the disease is unknown, but some investigators believe it to be immune mediated. Affected dogs have circulating immune complexes, depressed lymphocyte mitogenic responses, and deposits of IgG and C3 in the lesions and nearby normal tissues. Boxers and Newfoundland dogs affected with inflammatory myopathies have circulating autoantibodies to sarcolemmal autoantigens. It is not clear whether these autoantibodies are a cause or effect of the myopathy. However, detection of these antibodies may be a useful diagnostic test.

Cerebellar Degeneration

Cerebellar degeneration has been observed in Coton de Tulear puppies. It is associated with a depleted granular cell layer and microglial cell activation caused by T cell destruction of granular cells.

Autoimmune Eye Disease

Equine Recurrent Uveitis

The most common cause of blindness in horses is recurrent uveitis (or periodic ophthalmia). Horses suffer recurrent attacks of uveitis, retinitis, and vasculitis. In acute cases, they develop blepharospasm, lacrimation, and photophobia. Each attack gets progressively more severe and gradually spreads to involve other eye tissues until complete blindness results. The eye lesions are infiltrated with Th1 cells and neutrophils with extensive fibrin and C3 deposition. The major autoantigen implicated is the interphotoreceptor retinoid-binding protein with subsequent epitope spreading to the S-protein. Affected horses may also have circulating antibodies to *Leptospira interrogans*. The titer of these antibodies tends to rise during a flare-up of the lesion and drop while in remission. If horses are immunized with either equine cornea or certain serovars of killed *L. interrogans*, they develop corneal opacity 10 days later when antibodies appear in the bloodstream. Partial antigenic identity exists between equine corneas and these *L. interrogans* serovars, and some cases may be due to molecular mimicry with *L. interrogans*. Other cases may be due to infection with *Borrelia burgdorferi* or with the nematode *Onchocerca cervicalis*. Systemic and topical corticosteroid therapy is required to bring the inflammation under control, although the disease usually recurs. Encouraging results have been obtained with slow-release cyclosporine implants.

Uveodermatological Syndrome

Uveodermatological syndrome is a sporadic disease of dogs. A similar disease, Vogt-Koyanagi-Harada syndrome, occurs in humans. Affected dogs develop uveitis and skin depigmentation with whitening of the hair (poliosis) and skin (vitiligo). The eye lesions develop first. Thus most animals present with sudden blindness or chronic uveitis. The early lesions vary from a severe panuveitis to a bilateral anterior uveitis. Some dogs may have retinal detachment, and there may be progressive depigmentation of the retina and iris. Depigmentation of the hair and skin gradually follows the onset of the eye lesions. Some cases may be generalized, involving the eyelids, nasal planum, lips, scrotum, and foot pads (Figure 35-5). These depigmented areas may become ulcerated and crusted.

Histological examination shows a diffuse infiltration of the uveal tract with lymphocytes, plasma cells, and macrophages. Many of the macrophages contain ingested melanin. The skin lesions consist of a mononuclear (macrophages, giant cells, lymphocytes, plasma cells) infiltration of the dermal-epidermal junction (Figure 35-6). The amount of melanin in the epidermis and hair follicles is greatly reduced. In humans, Vogt-Koyanagi-Harada syndrome is believed to be a result of an autoimmune response against melanocytes. In dogs no consistent immunological abnormalities have been observed.

Management of the eye lesions with ocular corticosteroids and of the skin lesions with systemic corticosteroids has been beneficial, although the disease may recur when therapy is

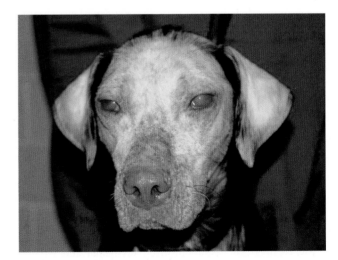

FIGURE 35-5 A case of uveodermatological syndrome. Note ocular clouding, alopecia, and depigmentation of the nasal planum.

(Courtesy of Drs. Robert Kennis, Joan Dziezc, and Larry Wadsworth.)

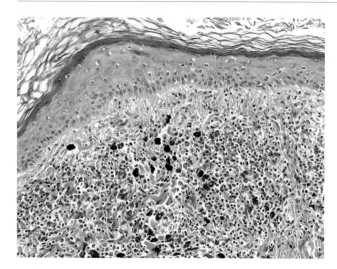

FIGURE 35-6 A histological section of skin from a case of uveodermatological syndrome. Note the major lymphocyte infiltration associated with the skin melanocytes. It is the destruction of these melanocytes that leads to depigmentation.

(Courtesy of Dr. Joanne Mansell.)

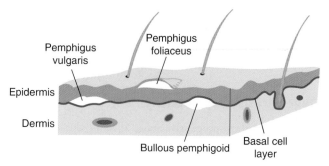

FIGURE 35-7 The differential histology of the autoimmune skin diseases. Note the location of the vesicle in relation to the epidermis.

terminated. Azathioprine may also be given if corticosteroids are insufficient to stop disease progression.

Autoimmune Reproductive Diseases

If the testes are damaged so that hidden antigens are released, an autoimmune response may exacerbate the orchitis. Experimentally, autoimmune orchitis may be produced in male animals by injection of testicular extracts emulsified in Freund's complete adjuvant. Autoantibodies to sperm may also be detected in the serum of some animals following injury to the testes or long-standing obstruction of the seminiferous ducts. For example, dogs infected with *Brucella canis* have chronic epididymitis and become sensitized by sperm antigens carried to the circulation after phagocytosis by macrophages. These sperm antigens stimulate the production of IgG or IgA autoantibodies. The autoantibodies can agglutinate and immobilize sperm, causing infertility.

In stallions and cows, antisperm autoantibodies may be associated with reduced fertility or infertility. In certain lines of black mink, 20% to 30% of older males are infertile as a result of high levels of antisperm antibodies. The animals have a monocytic orchitis, and immune complexes are deposited along the basal lamina of the seminiferous tubules.

Dermatologists recognize an autoimmune dermatitis in which intact female dogs develop a hypersensitivity to endogenous progesterone or estrogen. The disease presents as a bilaterally symmetrical intense pruritus, erythema, and papular eruption. Its development usually coincides with estrus or pseudopregnancy. Corticosteroid treatment may have little effect, but testosterone may help.

Recently there has been an increased interest in production-enhancing vaccines. These vaccines commonly interfere with normal hormone production or reproductive behavior by inducing an autoimmune response. Thus a vaccine designed to neutralize production of gonadotropin-releasing hormone effectively lowers testosterone levels. This results in improved meat quality, faster growth, and reduced aggressive behavior. This vaccine is also used to castrate male pigs and block the production of the steroids associated with boar taint, the offensive odor associated with boar meat. In horses a similar vaccine is used to control estrus and estrus-related misbehavior. Similar vaccines may be used as contraceptives or to treat benign prostatic hyperplasia in dogs. If dogs are immunized with bovine or ovine luteinizing hormone (LH), the autoantibodies produced may neutralize their own LH. Similarly, it is possible to produce autoantibodies that neutralize LH-releasing hormone. As a result, the reproductive cycle is abolished in females, and testicular, epididymal, and prostatic atrophy occurs in male dogs. Other experimental immunocontraceptive vaccines have been directed against prostaglandin $F_{2\alpha}$, reproductive steroids, the LH receptor, and zona pellucida protein.

Sheep immunized with polyandroalbumin (androstenedione-7-carboxyethyl thioester linked to human serum albumin) have about 23% more lambs than untreated sheep. The ewes are given two doses of this vaccine before mating. It is believed that the vaccine induces autoantibodies that reduce serum androstenedione levels.

Autoimmune Skin Diseases

Many different autoimmune skin diseases have been recognized. These diseases may affect hair follicles, basal keratinocytes, or the skin basement membrane. Although hair follicle disease can lead to alopecia, diseases involving basal keratinocytes or basement membranes are often characterized by cell separation within the skin and the consequent development of bullae (blisters or vesicles) (Figure 35-7). As a result, dermatologists use the terms *pemphigus* or *pemphigoid* to describe them, after the Greek word *pemphix* meaning "blister."

Hair Follicle Diseases

Alopecia Areata Alopecia areata is an autoimmune disease characterized by inflammatory hair loss. It has been reported in humans, other primates, dogs, cats, horses, and cattle. In dogs it is a rare disease. The alopecia starts locally, often on the head, but may spread to involve the entire body. It is often symmetrical. The hair follicles are infiltrated with CD4+ and CD8+ T cells and Langerhans cells. IgG antibodies directed against the lower hair follicles can also be detected. C3 or IgM may also be present. The targets of this immunological attack are unclear, but the attack may be directed against a protein called trichohyalin located in the inner root sheath of hair follicles. Alopecia areata responds to corticosteroid treatment, but spontaneous hair regrowth also occurs. Other autoimmune diseases that lead to hair loss include pseudopelade. It differs from alopecia areata in the precise location of the inflammatory infiltrate within the hair follicles. Likewise some cases of pemphigus vulgaris (see later) may also be restricted to hair follicles.

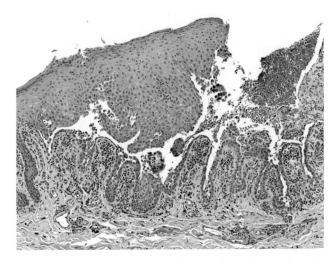

FIGURE 35-8 A section of an oral lesion of pemphigus vulgaris in a dog. Note the cleft formation at the base of the epidermis accompanied by extensive cellular infiltration.

(Courtesy of Dr. Joanne Mansell.)

Blistering Diseases

These are a group of related skin diseases that have been described in humans, dogs, horses, and cats. Known as the pemphigus complex, they are classified according to the location of the lesions within the epidermis. Some lesions develop deep within the epidermis. For example, the most severe form (although very rare) is called pemphigus vulgaris. In this disease, bullae develop around the mucocutaneous junctions, especially the nose, lips, eyes, prepuce, and anus, and on the tongue and the inner surface of the ear. These bullae rupture readily, leaving weeping, denuded areas that may become secondarily infected. Histological examination of intact bullae shows a separation of the skin cells (acantholysis) in the suprabasal region of the lower epidermis (Figures 35-8). The acantholysis results from an autoantibody attack on the structures that bind skin cells together, the desmosomes. In the case of pemphigus vulgaris, the antigen is a desmosome protein called desmoglein-3. The combination of antibodies with desmoglein-3 activates the proto-oncogene *c-myc* and leads to keratinocyte hyperproliferation. As a result, the cells above the lesion proliferate and fail to express adhesion proteins permitting the keratinocytes to separate from each other. Eventually this leads to acantholysis and bulla formation.

Pemphigus foliaceus is a vesicular disease in which the lesions develop superficially in the epidermis. As a result, it is a milder and much more common disease than pemphigus vulgaris. It has been described in humans, dogs, cats, goats, and horses. The bullae are not confined to mucocutaneous junctions or the muzzle. Histology reveals that the bullae formation occurs superficially in the subcorneal region. These bullae are very fragile, rupture easily, and therefore rarely persist. The autoantigen in humans and in some dogs has been identified as desmoglein-1, a cell adhesion protein found in squamous cell desmosomes. In other dogs antibodies of the IgG4 class appear to bind different keratinocyte desmosomal antigens. Some cases of canine pemphigus foliaceus develop after the use of antibiotics such as trimethoprim-sulfadiazine, oxacillin, cephalexin, and ampicillin. They appear to result from the binding of drug thiol groups to cell membranes.

A mild variant of pemphigus foliaceus is pemphigus erythematosus. The lesions in pemphigus erythematosus tend to be confined to the face and ears and are very similar to those of systemic lupus erythematosus (SLE). Indeed, some dogs with pemphigus erythematosus may have antinuclear antibodies in their serum. Panepidermal pustular pemphigus (pemphigus vegetans) is another rare and mild variant of pemphigus foliaceus in which papillomatous proliferation of the base of the bullae occurs on healing.

A fifth form of pemphigus, called paraneoplastic pemphigus, is seen in humans and has been recorded in a dog. It develops in association with lymphoid or solid tumors. It resembles pemphigus vulgaris, but multiple autoantibodies against skin antigens are present.

Direct immunofluorescent examination of pemphigus lesions reveals immunoglobulins deposited on the intercellular cement in a typical "chicken-wire" pattern (Figure 35-9).

It is important to differentiate among the forms of pemphigus for prognostic reasons. Pemphigus vulgaris has a poor prognosis; treatment tends to be unsatisfactory, and the lesions are persistent. In contrast, pemphigus foliaceus is milder, and the results of treatment may be more satisfactory. Treatment of pemphigus primarily involves the use of corticosteroids. In refractory cases, azathioprine, cyclophosphamide, chlorambucil, cyclosporine, or gold salts such as aurothioglucose may be of assistance. As with other autoimmune diseases, the disease often recurs when treatment is stopped.

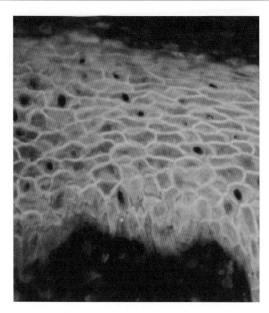

FIGURE 35-9 Direct immunofluorescence of a section of normal dog skin that has been incubated in serum from a dog with pemphigus vulgaris. The intercellular cement is stained.

(Courtesy of Dr. K. Credille.)

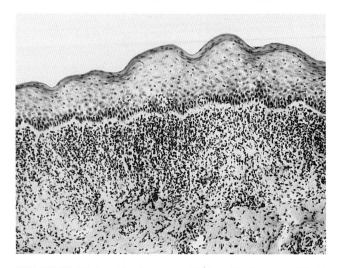

FIGURE 35-10 A section from an oral lesion of bullous pemphigoid in a dog. Note that the cleft is formed below the epidermis. Inflammatory cells are present in the superficial dermis and, to a lesser extent, in the epithelium.

(From Bennett D, Lauder IM, Kirkham D, McQueen A: Bullous autoimmune skin disease in the dog: [1] clinical and pathological assessment, *Vet Rec* 106:497, 1980.)

Skin Basement Membrane Diseases

A second set of blistering diseases is associated with the development of autoantibodies against components of the skin basement membrane. As a result, affected dogs develop subepidermal blisters. Several such diseases have been identified in dogs and other domestic animals. They include bullous pemphigoid, linear IgA dermatosis, and epidermolysis bullosa acquisita.

Bullous Pemphigoid Bullous pemphigoid is a rare skin disease that resembles pemphigus vulgaris. Collies, Shetland Sheepdogs, and Dobermans appear to be predisposed to this disease. It has also been described in humans, pigs, horses, and cats. Multiple bullae develop around mucocutaneous junctions and in the groin and axillae. However, the disease differs from pemphigus vulgaris in that the bullae develop in the subepidermis (and are therefore less likely to rupture). They tend to be filled with fibrin as well as mononuclear cells or eosinophils, and they heal spontaneously (Figure 35-10). Bullous pemphigoid results from the development of autoantibodies against type XVII collagen. This molecule is a component of hemidesmosomes, the structures that attach basal keratinocytes to the basement membrane (Figure 35-11). The presence of IgG on the basement membrane may be demonstrated by immunofluorescence that reveals intense linear staining. The prognosis of bullous pemphigoid is usually poor, but mild cases may recover after treatment with corticosteroids. More commonly, aggressive treatment such as high doses of prednisolone, supplemented if necessary with cyclophosphamide, azathioprine, and chlorambucil, may be required. Some dogs may develop a bullous pemphigoid–like disease in response to

autoantibodies against the basement membrane protein laminin-5.

Linear Immunoglobulin A Dermatosis Another group of skin diseases is characterized by the deposition of IgA in the lamina lucida of the skin basement membrane. One such disease, called dermatitis herpetiformis, has been recorded in a Beagle, whereas a linear IgA dermatosis has been recorded in Dachshunds. Both diseases present with pruritic pustular and papular lesions, resembling pyoderma, with eosinophil-filled subepidermal vesicles. The target autoantigen has been identified as a processed extracellular form of collagen XVII. The drug dapsone has been recommended as the specific treatment for these diseases.

Epidermolysis Bullosa Acquisita A generalized skin disease characterized by severe blistering and ulcerative lesions has been identified in Great Danes. The vesicles originate from erythematous areas on the skin and rapidly progress to ulcers. There is generalized urticaria, oral ulceration, and eventually cutaneous sloughing. A localized variant of the disease has been observed in German Short-Haired Pointers. The dermis and epidermis separate, and neutrophils accumulate within the superficial dermis. The neutrophil infiltration may eventually result in microabscess formation. Secondary changes include ulceration, necrosis, and bacterial infection. Affected animals develop IgA and IgG autoantibodies against the anchoring fibrils of the lower basement membrane (lamina densa). These autoantibodies are specific for type VII collagen and distinctly different from those responsible for bullous pemphigoid. Immunosuppressive therapy may be of benefit, although secondary bacterial infection can cause complications.

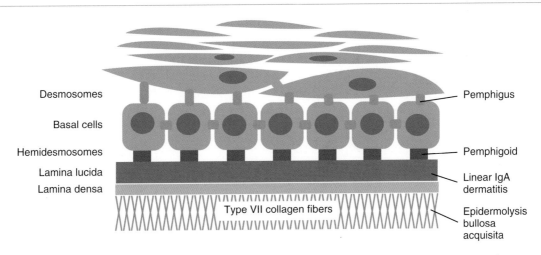

FIGURE 35-11 The structures of the skin showing the major structural features that can act as autoantigens.

An additional subset of canine subepidermal blistering diseases has been shown to result from the production of IgG autoantibodies to another basement membrane component, laminin-332. The skin blistering and ulceration in these cases are associated with microscopic subepidermal vesiculation.

Relapsing Polychondritis

A disease mediated by autoimmunity against type II cartilage has been described in humans and in cats. The animals present with bilateral curling of the ears and ocular changes. The cartilage is infiltrated with plasma cells and lymphocytes. A similar proliferative and necrotizing otitis in kittens is associated with CD3+ T cells found in close approximation to apoptotic keratinocytes, suggesting that some form of T cell–mediated cytotoxicity is occurring. Application of topical tacrolimus cream led to resolution of the lesions within a few weeks.

Autoimmune Nephritis

Horses may develop autoantibodies to glomerular basement membranes that result in glomerulonephritis and renal failure. Immunofluorescence studies of affected kidneys show that the basement membrane is evenly coated with a smooth, linear deposit of immunoglobulin. The autoantibodies may provoke proliferation of the glomerular epithelial cells and epithelial crescent formation. A necrotizing encephalitis associated with an anti–glomerular basement membrane glomerulonephritis has been observed in a West Highland White Terrier.

Immune-Mediated Hemolytic Anemia

Autoantibodies to red blood cell antigens provoke their destruction and cause immune-mediated hemolytic anemia (IMHA). These hemolytic anemias are well recognized in humans and dogs and have been recorded in cattle, horses, cats, mice, rabbits, and raccoons.

Affected dogs are anemic. Thus pallor, weakness, and lethargy are accompanied by fever, icterus, and hepatosplenomegaly. The anemia may be associated with tachycardia, anorexia, vomiting, or diarrhea. Clinical signs are contingent on the speed of development of the disease, its severity, and the mechanism of red cell destruction. This destruction may result from intravascular hemolysis (destruction within the bloodstream) mediated by complement or, much more commonly, by removal of antibody-coated red cells by the macrophages of the spleen and liver (extravascular hemolysis) (Figure 35-12). In dogs the disease occurs more often in females and in spayed dogs. The average age of onset is about 4 to 5 years. There is evidence for a genetic predisposition to IMHA in Cocker Spaniels and Miniature Schnauzers. The causes of IMHA are unknown, although some cases may be attributable to alterations in red cell surface antigens induced by drugs or viruses. In dogs the autoantibodies are primarily directed against red cell glycophorins, the cytoskeletal protein spectrin, and the membrane anion exchange protein CD233 (band 3). About one third of IMHA cases are associated with other immunological abnormalities such as SLE (Chapter 36) or autoimmune thrombocytopenia or with the presence of lymphoid and other tumors. Its onset may be associated with obvious stress such as vaccination (Chapter 24), anaplasmosis, viral disease, or hormonal imbalances as in pregnancy or pyometra.

IMHAs in dogs are classified according to the antibody class involved, the optimal temperature at which the autoantibodies react, and the nature of the hemolytic process (Table 35-1).

Class I: Caused by autoantibodies that agglutinate red cells at body temperature. The agglutination may be seen when a drop of blood is placed on a glass slide. Both IgG and IgM antibodies are involved. Since IgG does not activate complement efficiently, the red cells are mainly destroyed by phagocytosis in the spleen. In very severe cases, a blood

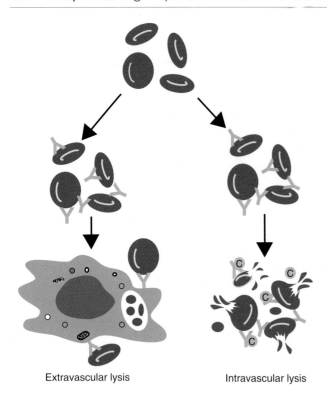

Extravascular lysis   Intravascular lysis

FIGURE 35-12 The basic differences between intravascular and extravascular hemolysis.

smear may show erythrophagocytosis by neutrophils and monocytes.

Class II: IgM antibodies activate complement and destroy red cells by intravascular hemolysis. This results in hemoglobinemia, hemoglobinuria, icterus, and very severe anemia. Affected dogs are anemic, weak, and possibly jaundiced. Kupffer cells in the liver or macrophages in lymph nodes preferentially remove red cells with complement on their surface, so these animals develop hepatomegaly and lymphadenopathy.

Class III: Most cases of IMHA in dogs and cats are mediated by IgG1 and IgG4 antibodies, which bind to red cells at 37° C but do not activate complement or agglutinate the red cells. IgG antibodies can only form short bridges (15 to

25 nm) between cells. As a result, they cannot counteract the zeta potential of the red cells and will not cause direct agglutination. [In contrast, IgM antibodies form long bridges (30 to 50 nm) and can agglutinate cells despite their zeta potential.] Affected red cells are opsonized and removed by splenic macrophages. Splenomegaly is a consistent feature of class III disease.

Class IV: Some IgM antibodies cannot agglutinate red cells at body temperature but can only do so when the blood is chilled. These antibodies are called cold agglutinins. They can be detected by cooling blood to between 10° and 4° C, at which point clumping occurs. The agglutination is reversed on rewarming. As blood circulates through the extremities (tail, toes, ears, and so forth) of affected animals, it may be sufficiently cooled to permit red cell agglutination within capillaries. This can lead to vascular stasis, blockage, tissue ischemia, and, eventually, necrosis. Affected animals may therefore present with necrotic lesions at the extremities, and anemia may not be a significant feature. As might be anticipated, this form of IMHA is most severe in the winter.

Class V: This is mediated by IgM antibodies that bind red cells when chilled to 4° C but do not agglutinate them. These antibodies can only be identified by an antiglobulin test conducted in the cold. They do not induce necrosis of extremities but can activate complement leading to intravascular hemolysis.

Diagnosis

The hematology of affected animals reflects the severe anemia and a regenerative response by the bone marrow. Blood smears commonly show spherocytes, which are small round red cells that lack a central pale area. These spherocytes result from the partial phagocytosis of antibody-coated red cells. The number of spherocytes in blood is a measure of the intensity of red cell destruction.

To diagnose IMHA associated with the presence of nonagglutinating or incomplete antibodies (classes II, III, V), it is necessary to use a direct antiglobulin test (Chapter 41). The red cells of the affected animal are collected in anticoagulant, washed free of serum, and incubated in an antiglobulin serum.

□ Table 35-1 | Classification of Immune-Mediated Hemolytic Anemias

CLASS	PREDOMINANT ANTIBODY	ACTIVITY	OPTIMAL TEMPERATURE (° C)	SITE OF RED CELL REMOVAL	CLINICAL EFFECT
I	G ≫ M	Agglutinin	37	Spleen	Intravascular agglutination
II	M	Hemolysin	37	Liver	Intravascular hemolysin
III	G	Incomplete	37	Spleen	Anemia
IV	M	Agglutinin	4	Liver	Cyanosis and infarction of extremities
V	M	Incomplete	4	Liver	Anemia

The best antiglobulin for this purpose is a polyclonal one with activity against IgM, IgG, and complement. Red cells coated with autoantibody or complement will be cross-linked and agglutinated by the antiglobulin. Occasionally IgM may have a low affinity for the red cells, so it elutes, leaving only complement on their surface.

It is important to emphasize that samples for immunological testing should be collected before immunosuppressive therapy begins. It is also important to note that in the cat, most cases of antiglobulin-positive hemolytic anemia are secondary to feline leukemia virus or *Mycoplasma haemofelis (Haemobartonella felis)* infections. The disease in cats has a more favorable prognosis than in dogs. Monitoring of acute-phase proteins in dogs with IMHA has shown increased concentrations of C-reactive protein and α-1 acid glycoprotein, whereas serum albumin is decreased. The acute-phase response is not predictive of survival, duration of hospitalization, or number of transfusions required, but it normalizes rapidly with disease stabilization.

Treatment of IMHA involves prevention of further hemolysis, treatment of hypoxia, prevention of thromboembolism, and aggressive supportive care. The major cause of death is thromboembolic disease. Administration of high doses of corticosteroids reduces phagocytosis of red cells by mononuclear cells and is the most effective treatment for IgG-mediated disease. Treated animals may respond within 24 to 48 hours. Corticosteroids are of much less benefit in the management of intravascular hemolysis mediated by IgM and complement and do not induce significant immunosuppression in these animals. In such cases, corticosteroid treatment may be supplemented with other immunosuppressive agents such as cyclosporine or cyclophosphamide, but the number of controlled clinical trials of these other drugs are very limited. Low-dose aspirin or heparin may reduce the risk for thromboembolism. Splenectomy should only be considered when more conservative therapy has failed. Although splenectomy may be of assistance in cases of refractory class III disease, no controlled trials have confirmed this.

Acute immunologically mediated anemias occur in horses following infection with *Streptococcus fecalis*, in sheep following leptospirosis, in cats with mycoplasmosis (hemobartonellosis), in dogs with babesiosis, and in pigs with eperythrozoonosis. In these cases IgM cold agglutinins clump red cells from normal animals of the same species when chilled. Antibodies to hemoglobin are found in the serum of cattle severely infected with *Arcanobacterium pyogenes*, perhaps as a result of bacterial hemolysis.

IMHA occurs in horses with lymphosarcomas and melanomas. The animals are depressed and pyrexic and exhibit splenomegaly, jaundice, and hemoglobinuria. Some show red cell autoagglutination. These horses have IgG on their red cells. Dexamethasone treatment can induce remission.

High doses of IVIG have potent antiinflammatory activity and have proved useful in the treatment of some autoimmune diseases in both humans and domestic animals (Chapter 39).

Immune Suppression of Hematopoiesis

In humans, dogs, and cats, autoantibodies to erythroid stem cells may cause red cell aplasia, and autoantibodies to myeloid stem cells may provoke an immune neutropenia. In dogs, red cell aplasia has been associated with the presence of immunoglobulin G (IgG) that inhibits erythroid stem cell differentiation. Severe, persistent, immune-mediated neutropenia does occur in dogs. Diagnosis is based largely on excluding other causes of the neutropenia together with a favorable response to steroid and immunosuppressive therapy. These diseases can only be diagnosed by careful hematological analysis and by demonstration of autoantibodies by immunofluorescence on bone marrow smears. These tests are not easy and have not been validated in domestic species. Affected animals may benefit from high doses of corticosteroids or immunosuppressive therapy. Immune-mediated bone marrow aplasia is rare in cats and usually only affects erythrocyte progenitors. It has been recorded in a ferret.

Autoimmune Thrombocytopenia

Autoimmune thrombocytopenia (AITP) due to an immune attack on platelets has been reported in horses, dogs, and, rarely, cats. Affected animals usually present with multiple petechiae in the skin, gingiva, other mucous membranes, and conjunctiva. Epistaxis, melena, and hematuria may occur. The predominant cause of death in these dogs is severe gastrointestinal hemorrhage. Antibodies against platelet antigens cause extravascular destruction of opsonized platelets in the spleen. As a result, affected animals have unusually low platelet counts and a prolonged bleeding time. The disease is commonly observed in association with IMHA and SLE. The thrombocytopenia seen in animals with multiple myeloma or other lymphoid tumors, with ehrlichiosis and leishmaniasis, or following certain drug treatments may be due to the nonspecific binding of IgG to platelets. (Drug-induced immune-mediated thrombocytopenia in humans is associated with quinine and vancomycin use). In dogs, the average age of onset is 6 years. Predisposed breeds include Airedales, Dobermans, Old English Sheepdogs, Cocker Spaniels, and Poodles. Antibodies to platelets may be measured by direct immunofluorescence on bone marrow aspirates looking for positive staining on megakaryocytes. However, the best test for this purpose is one that measures the release of factor III from platelets after exposure to autoantibodies. This may be performed by incubating platelet-rich plasma with a globulin fraction of the serum under test and estimating the amount of procoagulant activity released. In about 75% of cases the antibodies are of the IgG class. Most cases of AITP in cats are probably secondary to feline leukemia virus infection.

Immunosuppressive doses of corticosteroid are used to treat AITP. Vincristine may also produce a good clinical response since it binds to platelets and kills macrophages when they phagocytose the antibody-coated platelets. There is limited experience with other drugs such as cyclosporine, cyclophosphamide, azathioprine, or leflunomide but some positive results have been reported. Splenectomy may help when other forms of therapy have failed. IVIG therapy may also be beneficial.

Autoimmune Muscle Disease

Myasthenia Gravis

Myasthenia gravis is a disease of skeletal muscle characterized by abnormal fatigue and weakness after mild exercise. It occurs in humans, ferrets, dogs, and cats. Myasthenia gravis results from a failure of transmission of nerve impulses across the

motor endplate of striated muscle as a result of a deficiency of acetylcholine receptors (Figure 35-13). In Jack Russell Terriers, Springer Spaniels, and Fox Terriers, an inherited deficiency of these receptors occurs. This congenital form is therefore a disease of very young dogs.

In adult dogs, however, the acetylcholine receptor deficiency is due to autoantibodies. These IgG antibodies accelerate degradation of the receptors, block their acetylcholine-binding sites, and trigger complement-mediated damage. As a result, the number of available, functional acetylcholine receptors is significantly reduced. Dogs may also make autoantibodies against titin, an intracellular muscle protein, and the ryanodine receptor, a Ca^{2+} release channel in striated muscle.

In normal muscles, the binding of acetylcholine to its receptor opens a sodium channel to produce a localized endplate potential. If the amplitude of the endplate potential is

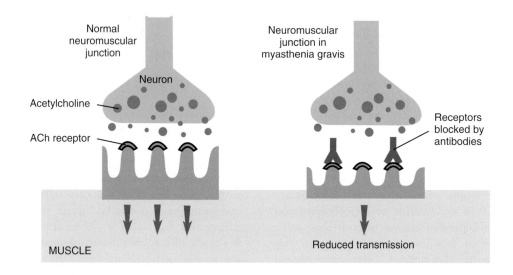

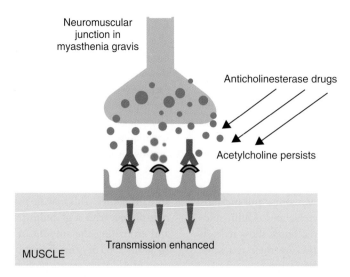

FIGURE 35-13 The pathogenesis of myasthenia gravis. Destruction of acetylcholine receptors prevents effective neuromuscular transmission. Blockage of cholinesterase activity by anticholinesterase drugs permits acetylcholine to accumulate and so enhances neuromuscular transmission.

sufficient, this will generate an action potential and trigger muscle contraction. The endplate potential from a normal neuromuscular junction is more than sufficient to generate a muscle action potential. In myasthenic junctions, however, the endplate potentials fail to trigger action potentials in many muscle fibers. This is manifested as muscle weakness. Repeating the stimulus leads to a progressive increase in weakness as transmission failure occurs at more and more neuromuscular junctions since the amount of acetylcholine released from a nerve terminal usually declines after the first few impulses.

The disease may develop in any breed of dog, but certain breeds are predisposed to it. Breeds such as German Shepherds, Golden Retrievers, Labradors, and Dachshunds appear to develop more severe disease. Rottweilers appear to be at low risk. In cats there appears to be a breed predisposition for Abyssinians and related Somalis.

In some animals the thymus may show medullary hyperplasia, germinal center formation, or even a thymic carcinoma, and surgical thymectomy may result in clinical improvement. About 3% of dog cases and 20% of cat cases are associated with the presence of a thymic tumor.

Animals may present with a history of swallowing difficulty, regurgitation, labored breathing, and generalized muscle weakness. Megaesophagus is common. Clinically different disease forms may be recognized. The disease is classified as focal myasthenia gravis when an animal presents with megaesophagus and various degrees of facial paralysis without limb muscle weakness; generalized myasthenia gravis when limb muscle weakness is associated with facial paralysis and megaesophagus; and acute fulminating myasthenia gravis when the disease rapidly leads to quadriplegia and respiratory difficulty. Almost 60% of cases are generalized or fulminating, whereas the rest are focal. Without treatment, about half of affected animals will die, whereas the others may show spontaneous remissions. Aspiration pneumonia is the main cause of death in myasthenic dogs.

Administration of a short-acting anticholinesterase drug such as edrophonium chloride (Tensilon) leads to a rapid gain in muscle strength. The anticholinesterase, by permitting the acetylcholine to accumulate at the neuromuscular junction, enables the remaining receptors to be stimulated more effectively. Dogs with transient myasthenia gravis may be supported temporarily with long-acting anticholinesterase drugs such as pyridostigmine bromide or neostigmine methyl sulfate. Dogs with progressive disease that show no signs of remission may benefit from immunosuppression. Positive clinical responses have been reported in dogs treated with prednisone or azathioprine or both. However, corticosteroid treatment may result in transient exacerbation of symptoms. Plasmapheresis has been used for short-term therapy to stabilize patients before thymectomy.

Polymyositis

A generalized autoimmune myositis occurs in large dogs such as German Shepherds. The disease may be acute or gradual in onset. The animals show progressive muscle weakness not associated with exercise. Changes in laryngeal muscle function lead to a change in the voice. Megaesophagus may lead to dysphagia and if severe can result in aspiration pneumonia. Affected animals may develop a shifting lameness. Animals may be febrile and develop leukocytosis and eosinophilia. Biopsies show muscle fiber degeneration, necrosis, and vacuolation, and affected muscles may be infiltrated by lymphocytes and plasma cells. About 50% of affected dogs have antinuclear antibodies or antibodies to sarcolemma, or both. Corticosteroids are the treatment of choice. A similar immune-mediated myositis has been recorded in Quarter Horses. It causes rapid atrophy of the gluteal and epaxial muscles. The affected muscles are infiltrated with macrophages and CD4+ lymphocytes with lesser numbers of CD8+ cells and B cells. It too may be treatable with corticosteroids.

Autoimmune Masticatory Myositis

Dogs may develop an autoimmune myositis confined to the muscles of mastication. The major antigen recognized is called masticatory myosin binding protein-C found only in masticatory muscle fibers. Animals present with pain and atrophy or swelling of the masticatory muscles resulting in difficulty in opening (trismus) or closing the jaw. Affected animals may also have conjunctivitis or exophthalmos. Histology of affected muscles shows inflammatory or degenerative lesions affecting the M2 myofibrils. Myositis with lymphocytes and plasma cells predominates, and some lesions may contain many eosinophils. Myofiber atrophy, perimysial or endomysial fibrosis, and muscle fiber necrosis are consistent features. Immunoglobulins may be detected in biopsy specimens of affected muscles, and circulating antibodies to the M2 myofibrils have been demonstrated by an immunoperoxidase assay. Corticosteroids such as prednisone are used for treatment, but the prognosis is guarded. Cavalier King Charles spaniels may be predisposed to this disease.

Canine Cardiomyopathy

English Cocker Spaniels may develop a cardiomyopathy with antinuclear and antimitochondrial autoantibodies and reduced serum IgA levels. It is associated with a specific C4 allotype (C4-4). The autoantigen has not been identified, but in humans similar cardiomyopathies are due to autoantibodies directed against the adenine nucleotide translocator of mitochondria.

Chronic Active Hepatitis

Doberman Pinschers may develop an autoimmune hepatitis. The symptoms are typical of liver disease with anorexia, depression, weight loss, diarrhea, polydipsia, polyuria, icterus, and eventually ascites. The disease commonly presents between 3 and 6 years of age but may have been present subclinically for many years. On necropsy, the liver shows intense inflammation and scar tissue formation around small hepatic vein branches. The lesions contain lymphocytes, plasma cells, and macrophages. The disease eventually causes progressive fibrosis and destruction of hepatocytes. About half of affected dogs develop antibodies to hepatocyte cell membranes. These antibody-positive dogs have more severe disease than dogs without antibodies. In addition, lymphocytes from about 75% of affected dogs respond to liver membrane proteins in vitro. Hepatocytes from affected dogs, but not from normal Dobermans, express major histocompatibility (MHC) class II antigens. This MHC expression correlated with the severity of the disease, whereas corticosteroid treatment reduced both MHC expression and disease severity. It has been suggested therefore that the disease results from a cell-mediated attack on abnormally expressed MHC molecules or an antigen associated with them.

For sources of additional information, please visit http://evolve.elsevier.com/tizard/immunology/

Systemic Immunological Diseases

□ Key Points

- Some autoimmune diseases may result from immunological attack on many different organs at the same time. This probably reflects a major loss of control of the innate and adaptive immune systems.
- Systemic lupus erythematosus (SLE) is a complex autoimmune disease characterized by multiple autoimmune responses together with the presence of autoantibodies to nuclear antigens. Lupus may represent several different disease entities.
- Many different forms of arthritis may also be immunologically mediated. The most significant of these is the erosive arthritis called rheumatoid arthritis. It is associated with the development of autoantibodies to joint components, such as collagens, and of rheumatoid factor (RF), an autoantibody against immunoglobulin G (IgG).
- There is a significant clinical overlap among many of these syndromes, making precise diagnosis difficult.

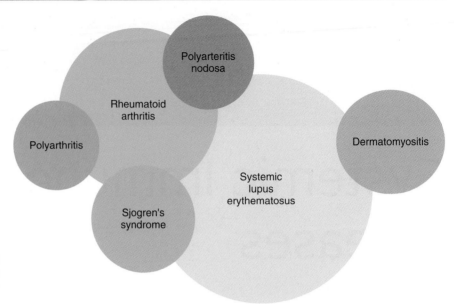

FIGURE 36-1 The interrelationships among the diseases discussed in this chapter. The diagram is somewhat simplified since polyarthritis may be associated with polymyositis.

Animals may suffer from complex inflammatory diseases that involve multiple organ systems. In human medicine, these have been called "rheumatic" diseases, "connective tissue" diseases, or "collagen" diseases based on outdated views on their pathogenesis. These systemic diseases or syndromes are interrelated and have many overlapping clinical features (Figure 36-1). One common feature is extensive and uncontrolled inflammatory responses, and it may be useful to consider them to be forms of innate autoimmunity or "autoinflammatory diseases." Because of their many similarities, it is sometimes difficult to come to a definitive clinical diagnosis.

These innate autoimmune diseases include systemic lupus erythematosus (SLE), rheumatoid arthritis, nonerosive forms of arthritis, vasculitis, dermatomyositis, and Sjögren's syndrome. Although all these diseases have some form of adaptive autoimmune component, they are not simply a result of autoantibodies causing tissue destruction. Most are associated with the presence of immune complexes and complement in tissues leading to chronic inflammation. Many appear to result from uncontrolled inflammatory cytokine production or abnormalities in the complement system. Their initiating factors are unknown, but some may be triggered by infectious agents acting through toll-like receptors (TLRs). All exhibit a significant genetic predisposition, commonly with linkage to the major histocompatibility (MHC).

In humans a large number of inherited inflammatory diseases have been recognized. In many cases these diseases result from defects in the activation of inflammasomes and related molecules. It is predicted that some of these diseases will eventually be recognized in domestic mammal species.

Systemic Lupus Erythematosus

SLE is a complex disease syndrome (or perhaps even multiple diseases) that has been described in humans, other primates,

mice, horses, dogs, and cats. It is characterized by a broad and bewildering diversity of different symptoms and a wide variety of disease courses as symptoms flare and recede over time. The factors that lead to the development of lupus are complex, multifactorial, and poorly defined (Figure 36-2). Its development is affected by environmental factors, including infectious

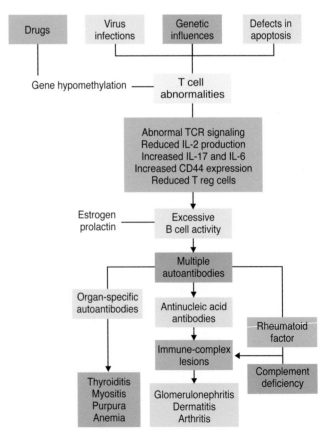

FIGURE 36-2 A diagram showing a possible pathogenesis of systemic lupus erythematosus.

agents, drugs, and food, in association with the combined effects of many different genes. Patients develop a variety of autoantibodies, changes in T cell function, defective phagocytosis, impaired apoptosis, multiorgan inflammation, and oncogene expression.

Pathogenesis

The hallmark of all forms of lupus is the development of autoantibodies against many different nuclear structures, including nucleic acids, ribonucleoproteins, and chromatin. These antinuclear antibodies (ANAs) are found in 97% to 100% of dogs with lupus compared with 16% to 20% of normal control animals. About 16 different nuclear antigens have been described in humans. Dogs differ from humans in that they mainly develop autoantibodies against nuclear proteins such as histones and ribonucleoproteins. These antinuclear antibodies cause tissue injury by several mechanisms. They can combine with free antigens to form immune complexes that are deposited in glomeruli, causing a membranoproliferative glomerulonephritis (Chapter 30). They may be deposited in arteriolar walls, where they cause fibrinoid necrosis and fibrosis, or in synovia, where they provoke arthritis. They may bind to Fc receptors on immune cells, leading to cell activation. The immune responses in SLE are associated with the production of interferon-α (IFN-α) so that the level of this cytokine correlates with disease activity. IFN-α is produced by plasmacytoid dendritic cells. It is believed that in SLE, FcR-, and TLR-mediated uptake of immune complexes and nucleic acids activates plasmacytoid dendritic cells. The IFN promotes inflammatory responses, activating macrophages and autoreactive T cells. ANAs also bind to the nuclei of degenerating cells to produce round or oval structures called hematoxylin bodies in the skin, kidney, lung, lymph nodes, spleen, and heart. Within the bone marrow, opsonized nuclei may be phagocytosed, giving rise to lupus erythematosus (LE) cells (Figure 36-3).

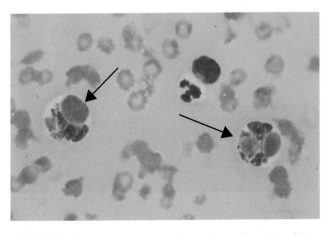

FIGURE 36-3 Two LE cells (*arrows*) from a dog with systemic lupus erythematosus. Original magnification ×1300.

In addition to making antinuclear antibodies, many patients with lupus and related diseases make autoantibodies against two ribonucleoproteins called SSA/Ro and SSB/La. There appear to be significant and consistent clinical differences between patients producing these two types of autoantibody. These antibodies have been detected in dogs.

The production of ANAs in lupus may result from several possible defects. One possibility is that the intracellular TLRs, notably TLR7 and TLR9, lose the ability to discriminate between microbial and self-DNA. If, at the same time, some of their B cells undergo somatic mutation that enables their B cell receptors (BCRs) to bind self-DNA, the ingredients necessary for a profound antibody response to mammalian DNA come together.

Bacterial DNA is a potent antigen and immune stimulant. Since mammalian DNA and bacterial DNA have a conserved backbone structure, it is possible that patients with lupus may respond to bacterial infection by producing cross-reactive antibodies that react with mammalian DNA. For example, the NZB/NZW mouse strain spontaneously develops a lupus-like syndrome when immunized with bacterial DNA. This induces antibodies that bind mammalian double-stranded DNA. These anti-DNA antibodies may form immune complexes and cause arthritis, skin rashes, and vascular disease. Antibody-DNA immune complexes may bind to TLR9 and activate autoreactive B cells by triggering both the TLRs and antigen receptors.

A related defect in some lupus patients appears to be the impaired clearance of apoptotic cells. Normally, apoptotic cells are removed by phagocytosis by macrophages without causing inflammation (Chapter 5). Macrophages from SLE patients, however, show defective phagocytosis of apoptotic cells, which as a result accumulate in tissues. Nuclear fragments from these cells may be trapped and processed by dendritic cells, thereby triggering autoantibody formation. The defect is most obvious in the skin of affected animals, where ultraviolet (UV) radiation leads triggers apoptotic cell death. Nucleic acids from these cells may then act as autoantigens and trigger autoantibody formation. These autoantibodies in turn lead to immune complex deposition and tissue damage. Complement components mediate the efficient clearance of apoptotic cells, so complement deficiencies are associated with the development of lupus-like syndromes. Although a failure of apoptosis leading to activation of autoimmune B cells and multiple autoimmune disorders is a feature of lupus, its initiating cause remains obscure. Although ANAs are characteristic of lupus, many other autoantibodies are produced, suggesting that affected animals may have grossly abnormal B cell function. Affected animals show abnormalities in B cell signaling and migration, overexpression of CD154 (CD40L), and enhanced production of interleukin-6 (IL-6) and IL-10. Some experimental mouse models show overexpression of B cell stimulatory molecules by T cells and dendritic cells. It is therefore possible that the production of multiple autoantibodies in lupus is a combined result of defective apoptosis, overstimulation of B cells, and a failure to eliminate self-reactive B cells.

Autoantibodies to red cells induce a hemolytic anemia. Antibodies to platelets induce a thrombocytopenia. Antilymphocyte antibodies may interfere with immune regulation. About 20% of dogs with lupus produce antibodies to IgG (RFs). Antimuscle antibodies may cause myositis, and antimyocardial antibodies may provoke myocarditis or endocarditis. Antibodies to skin basement membrane cause a dermatitis characterized by changes in the thickness of the epidermis, focal mononuclear cell infiltration, collagen degeneration, and immunoglobulin deposits at the dermoepidermal junction. These deposits form a "lupus band," seen in many other autoimmune skin diseases in addition to lupus (Figure 36-4). In humans, lupus skin lesions are commonly restricted to the bridge of the nose and the area around the eyes since apoptosis is triggered by UV radiation in sunlight. The results of this excessive immune reactivity are also reflected in a polyclonal gammopathy, enlargement of lymph nodes and spleen, and thymic enlargement with germinal center formation. As described in Chapter 7, some lupus patients have a deficiency of the complement receptor CD35. As a result, immune complexes are not bound to red cells or platelets and therefore are not effectively removed from the circulation. These immune complexes may then be deposited in the glomeruli or in joints.

The great variety of autoantibodies produced in lupus can cause an equally great variety of clinical symptoms. Polyarthritis, fever, proteinuria, anemia, and skin diseases are the most common abnormalities, but pericarditis, myocarditis, myositis, lymphadenopathy, and pneumonia have also been reported.

Equine Lupus Equine lupus presents as a generalized skin disease (alopecia, dermal ulceration, and crusting), accompanied by an antiglobulin-positive anemia. The disease is remarkable insofar as affected horses may be almost totally hairless (Figure 36-5). Affected horses are ANA positive, although LE cell tests are equivocal in this species. Skin biopsies show basement membrane degeneration and immunoglobulin deposition typical of lupus. Affected horses may also have glomerulonephritis, synovitis, and lymphadenopathy. Treatment of reported cases has been unsuccessful.

Canine Lupus Lupus affects middle-aged dogs (between 2 and 12 years of age) and affects males more than females. The disease is commonly seen in Collies, German Shepherds, Nova Scotia Duck Tolling Retrievers, and Shetland Sheepdogs, but Beagles, Irish Setters, Poodles, and Afghan Hounds are also affected. Lupus (or positive lupus serology) may occur in related animals, supporting the importance of genetic factors. For example, dogs possessing the MHC class I antigen DLA-A7 are at increased risk and those possessing DLA-A1 and -B5 are at decreased risk for developing disease (Figure 36-6). When dogs affected by lupus are bred, the number of affected offspring is higher than can be accounted for genetically, suggesting that the disease may be vertically transmitted. A type C retrovirus has been suggested as a potential trigger of lupus.

Dogs may present with one or more signs of disease. However, the disease is progressive, so the severity of the lesions and the number of organ systems involved gradually increases in untreated cases. The most characteristic presentation is a fever accompanied by a symmetrical, nonerosive polyarthritis. Indeed, as many as 90% of dogs with lupus may develop arthritis at some stage. Other common presenting signs include renal failure (65%), skin disease (60%), lymphadenopathy or splenomegaly (50%), leukopenia (20%), hemolytic anemia (13%), and thrombocytopenia (4%). Dogs may also show

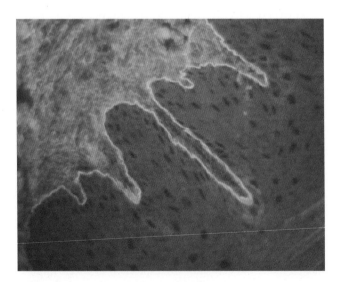

FIGURE 36-4 A lupus band in a section of monkey esophagus. The indirect immunofluorescence assay shows IgG deposition on the skin basement membrane.

(Courtesy Dr. F.C. Heck.)

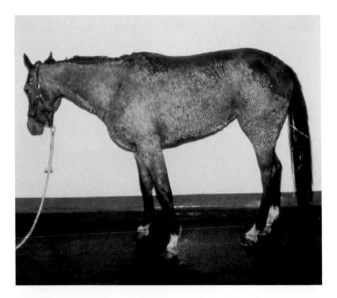

FIGURE 36-5 A filly with systemic lupus erythematosus. Note the generalized alopecia and crusting.

(From Geor RJ, Clark EG, Haines DM, Napier PG: Systemic lupus erythematosus in a filly, *J Am Vet Med Assoc* 197:1489, 1990.)

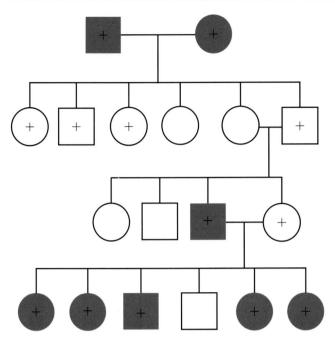

FIGURE 36-6 The inheritance of canine systemic lupus erythematosus. This diagram shows four generations of a single family of dogs. Colored squares (male) or circles (female) denote those animals exhibiting clinical signs of systemic lupus; "+" denotes animals positive for antinuclear antibodies.

(Modified from Teichner M, Krumbacher K, Doxiadis I, et al: Systemic lupus erythematosus in dogs: association to the major histocompatibility complex class I antigen DLA-A7, *Clin Immunol Immunopathol* 55:225, 1990.)

□ Box 36-1 | **Diagnostic Criteria for Systemic Lupus Erythematosus**

Any two of the following must be present:
    Characteristic skin lesions
    Polyarthritis
    Antiglobulin-positive hemolytic anemia
    Thrombocytopenia
    Proteinuria
And either:
    A positive ANA test
Or:
    A positive LE cell test

myositis (8%) or pericarditis (8%) and neurological abnormalities (1.6%). The leukopenia involves a major loss of CD8+ T cells with a somewhat smaller loss of CD4+ T cells so that the CD4/CD8 ratio may climb as high as 6, compared with a normal value of about 1.7. The skin lesions are highly variable but are commonly restricted to areas exposed to sunlight. With this great variety of clinical presentations to choose from, it is not surprising that lupus is so difficult to diagnose.

Several unique variants of lupus have been described in dogs. All are very rare, and many are associated with specific breeds, strongly suggesting a genetic predisposition. For example, vesicular systemic lupus is seen in Shetland Sheepdogs and Rough Collies. It is characterized by vesicular erosive and ulcerative skin lesions, subepidermal vesicles, and immunoglobulin deposition at the dermal-epidermal junction. Affected animals have antibodies against type VII collagen as well as ANAs. It may be treated with aggressive immunosuppressive therapy.

Exfoliative lupus dermatitis has been described in German Short-Haired Pointers. Young adult dogs develop scaling and alopecia on the muzzle, pinnae, and dorsum. Some dogs may exhibit signs of pain and arthritis. Others may develop anemia and thrombocytopenia. Histopathology shows hyperkeratosis with a lymphocytic interface dermatitis similar to that seen in human lupus. IgG is deposited in the epidermal and follicular basement membranes. These dogs have circulating autoantibodies to epidermal basement membranes. Affected animals respond poorly to immunosuppressive therapy. This disease is inherited in an autosomal recessive manner, and the responsible gene is *DFP2* on chromosome 18.

Another lupus-related disease has been described in Gordon Setters. These dogs developed a symmetrical onychodystrophy, malformations, and loss of the claws. As a result, affected animals show lameness, severe discomfort, and acute pain. Some develop ANAs. A related disease of Gordon Setters is possibly black hair follicular dysplasia. In this disease, dogs begin to shed their black hair without normal regrowth. The remaining black hair is either short and stiff or is thin and easily removed. Many affected dogs had positive ANA titers. These two diseases, occurring in the same breed and often in the same individual, may be closely related.

Feline Lupus Lupus is uncommon in cats, in which it usually presents as an antiglobulin-positive anemia. Other clinical manifestations include fever, skin disease, thrombocytopenia, polyarthritis, and renal failure. The ANA test must be interpreted with care in cats since many normal cats are ANA positive.

Diagnosis

A simple diagnostic rule for lupus could be stated as follows: Suspect lupus in an animal with multiple disorders such as those described previously and either a positive test for ANA or a positive test for LE cells (Box 36-1).

ANAs are normally demonstrated by immunofluorescence. Cultured cells or frozen sections of mouse or rat liver on a microscope slide are used as a source of antigen. Dilutions of a patient's serum are applied to this, and the slide is incubated and then washed off. Binding of ANA to the cell nuclei is revealed by incubating the tissue in a fluorescein-labeled antiserum to canine or feline immunoglobulins and then rewashing. Several different nuclear staining patterns have been described for humans and their clinical correlations identified.

In animals, staining patterns have been less thoroughly investigated, and their significance is less clear. Evidence suggests that a homogeneous staining pattern or staining of the nuclear rim is of greatest diagnostic significance but that nucleolar fluorescence is not (Figure 36-7). Dogs whose serum generates a speckled fluorescence pattern tend to have autoimmune diseases other than lupus. Some normal dogs, dogs undergoing treatment with certain drugs (griseofulvin, penicillin, sulfonamides, tetracyclines, phenytoin, procainamide), and some dogs with liver disease or lymphosarcoma may have detectable

ANAs. ANAs are also found in a significant proportion of dogs infected with *Bartonella vinsonii* subsp. *berkhoffii, Ehrlichia canis,* and *Leishmania infantum.* Dogs infected with multiple vector-borne organisms are especially likely to be ANA positive.

Thus nonspecific ANAs may be a result of many different neoplastic, inflammatory, and autoimmune diseases. ANA test results must therefore be used with caution. Administration of propylthiouracil to cats with hyperthyroidism may result in the development of a syndrome resembling lupus. This may include the development of an antiglobulin-positive anemia as well as positive ANA reactions.

LE cells, as previously mentioned, are neutrophils that have phagocytosed nuclear material from apoptotic cells (see Figure 36-3). Their presence may be detected in the bone marrow and occasionally in buffy coat preparations from animals with lupus. It is usually necessary, however, to produce them in vitro. This can be accomplished by allowing the blood of an affected animal to clot and then incubating it at 37° C for 2 hours. During this time, normal neutrophils will phagocytose the nuclei of any apoptotic cells. Pressing it through a fine mesh then disrupts the clot, the resulting cell suspension is centrifuged, and the buffy coat is smeared, stained, and examined. LE cells are not a reliable diagnostic feature of systemic lupus in domestic animals since there is a high incidence of both false-positive and false-negative results.

Treatment

Lupus in animals usually responds well to high doses of corticosteroids (prednisolone or prednisone), accompanied, if necessary, by cyclophosphamide, azathioprine, or chlorambucil. Levamisole (Chapter 39) has also been used with success. However, more drastic measures, such as plasmapheresis, may be needed in refractory cases.

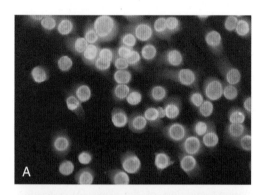
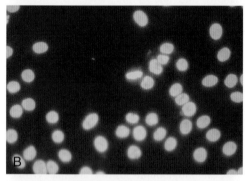
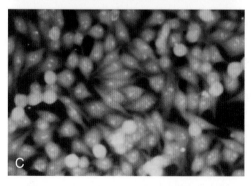

FIGURE 36-7 Three positive ANA reactions. These are indirect fluorescent antibody reactions, in which dog serum under test is layered onto a cell culture. After washing, the bound antibody is detected using a fluorescent antiglobulin. Although "rim" fluorescence **(A)** has traditionally been considered a positive reaction, the staining pattern obtained appears to depend in large part on the way the cells are fixed. These can therefore show diffuse staining **(B)** or nucleolar fluorescence **(C)**.

(Courtesy Dr. F.C. Heck.)

Discoid Lupus Erythematosus

Discoid lupus erythematosus is a mild, uncommon variant of SLE characterized by the occurrence of facial skin lesions alone. There are no other pathological lesions, and ANA and LE tests are negative. It occurs in dogs, cats, horses, and humans. Discoid lupus has been described in Collies and Collie crosses, German Shepherds, Siberian Huskies, and Shetland Sheepdogs. They commonly present with nasal dermatitis with depigmentation, erythema, erosion, ulceration, scaling, and crusting. A vesicular form of the disease has been reported in Shetland Sheepdogs. Occasionally the feet may be affected, and some dogs may have oral ulcers. C3, IgA, IgG, or IgM may be detected in the skin basement membrane in a typical lupus band. The skin lesions may be infiltrated with mononuclear and plasma cells. It is treated with corticosteroids, and the prognosis is good. Since the lesions are exacerbated by sunlight, it is appropriate to use sunscreens and encourage the owner to keep the animal out of intense sunlight.

Discoid lupus in cats is characterized by a nonpruritic scaling and crusting dermatitis almost totally confined to the pinnae of the ear. There may be some ulceration and papule or pustule formation. Skin biopsy shows mononuclear infiltration of the basal cell layer with degeneration of basal cells. Direct immunofluorescence of skin sections shows a lupus band. Affected cats have negative or low ANA titers and negative LE cell tests. Treatment with corticosteroids is effective.

Sjögren's Syndrome

In this syndrome, autoimmune attack on salivary and lacrimal glands leads to conjunctival dryness (keratoconjunctivitis sicca) and mouth dryness (xerostomia). Affected animals subsequently develop gingivitis, dental caries, and excessive thirst. Sjögren's syndrome is often associated with rheumatoid arthritis, systemic lupus, polymyositis, and autoimmune thyroiditis. The first two cases described in dogs were found in a colony maintained for investigations into canine lupus. Affected dogs develop antibodies to nictitating membrane epithelial cells and, less consistently, to lacrimal and salivary glands or to the pancreas, and these organs may be infiltrated with lymphocytes and other mononuclear cells. Most affected animals (90%) are hypergammaglobulinemic and have ANAs (40%) and RFs (34%). Many have other autoimmune lesions such as polyarthritis, hypothyroidism, and glomerulonephritis.

Keratoconjunctivitis Sicca

In keratoconjunctivitis sicca, one of the most common ophthalmic diseases of dogs, tear production is greatly reduced, and animals therefore develop corneal dryness. The resulting abrasion leads to inflammation of the cornea and conjunctiva. A mucoid or mucopurulent ocular discharge, blepharitis, conjunctivitis, and secondary bacterial infections develop. Corneal ulceration may occur and progress to perforation if untreated.

The disease is diagnosed by use of the Schirmer tear test. A 5×30 mm strip of filter paper is placed in the medioventral cul-de-sac for 1 minute. Normal dog tears wet between 14 and 24 mm of paper/minute, but in keratoconjunctivitis sicca cases, the tears usually wet less than 10 mm, and many wet less than 5 mm. The breeds at highest relative risk include English Bulldogs, West Highland White Terriers, Lhasa Apsos, Pugs, Cocker Spaniels, and Pekinese. The disease may be treated by use of artificial tears. It is also logical to use immunosuppressive agents in refractory cases. For example, cyclosporine ophthalmic drops appear to be effective, although it may take 2 to 3 weeks before improved lacrimation is seen.

Keratoconjunctivitis sicca has been reported in a horse. The 3-year-old animal presented with bilateral ulcerative keratoconjunctivitis and improved clinically with ophthalmic cyclosporine therapy. Histological examination of the lacrimal glands showed an eosinophil infiltration with lesser numbers of lymphocytes, plasma cells, and macrophages. Although this suggests an immunological origin for the disease, it must be pointed out that nonimmunological mechanisms such as facial nerve damage can also result in corneal dryness.

Chronic Superficial Keratitis

Chronic superficial keratitis is a common inflammatory ocular disease of dogs in which blood vessels, lymphocytes, plasma cells, and melanocytes invade the superficial corneal stroma. Immunoglobulin deposits may be present. Eventually the pigmented granulation tissue causes corneal opacity. The disease is believed to be immune mediated, although its cause is unknown. It is more prevalent in dogs living at high altitudes, where UV exposure is great. It is also most prevalent in German Shepherds and is associated with specific MHC class II haplotypes.

Autoimmune Polyarthritis

Animals develop immunologically mediated joint diseases, most of which are associated with the deposition of immunoglobulins or immune complexes within joints. Their classification is based on the presence or absence of joint erosion.

Erosive Polyarthritis

Rheumatoid Arthritis The most important immune-mediated erosive polyarthritis in humans is rheumatoid arthritis. Rheumatoid arthritis is a common, crippling disease affecting about 1% of the human population. A very similar disease is seen in domestic animals, especially dogs, in which there is no obvious breed or sex predilection. Dogs with rheumatoid arthritis may present with chronic depression, anorexia, and pyrexia in addition to lameness, which tends to be most severe after rest (e.g., immediately after waking in the morning). The disease mainly affects peripheral joints, which show symmetrical swelling and stiffness. Rheumatoid arthritis tends to be progressive and eventually leads to severe joint erosion and deformities. In advanced cases affected joints may fuse as a result of the formation of bony ankyloses. Radiological findings are variable, but the swelling usually involves soft tissues only, and there may be subchondral rarefaction, cartilage erosion, and narrowing of the joint space.

Pathogenesis Rheumatoid arthritis is a chronic inflammatory disease. It commences as a synovitis with lymphocytes in the synovia and neutrophils in the joint fluid. As the inflammation continues, the synovia swell and proliferate. Outgrowths of the proliferating synovia eventually extend into the joint cavities, where they are called pannus. Pannus consists of fibrous vascular tissue that, as it invades the joint cavity, releases proteases that erode the articular cartilage and, ultimately, the neighboring bony structures. As the arthritis progresses, the infiltrating lymphocytes form lymphoid nodules and germinal centers within the synovia. Amyloidosis, arteritis, glomerulonephritis, and lymphatic hyperplasia are occasional complications of rheumatoid arthritis (Figure 36-8).

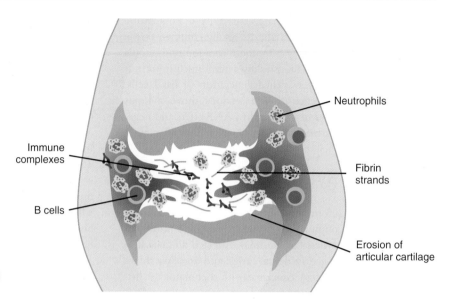

FIGURE 36-8 A schematic diagram showing how joints are damaged in rheumatoid arthritis.

It is probable that many different stimuli, especially infectious agents, trigger rheumatoid arthritis in susceptible animals. Infectious agents implicated in the human disease include Epstein-Barr virus (a herpesvirus), parvoviruses, and mycobacteria. Lyme disease arthritis has many similarities to rheumatoid arthritis. In domestic mammals, *Mycoplasma hyorhinis*, *Erysipelothrix rhusiopathiae,* and *Borrelia burgdorferi* each produce a chronic arthritis that resembles rheumatoid arthritis. Dogs with rheumatoid arthritis have antibodies to canine distemper in their synovial fluids, antibodies that are not present in dogs with osteoarthritis. Immune complexes can be precipitated out of the synovial fluid of dogs with rheumatoid arthritis, and analysis of these complexes by Western blotting shows the presence of canine distemper virus antigens. Thus canine distemper virus may be present in canine rheumatoid joints and may play a role in the pathogenesis of the disease.

Susceptibility to and severity of rheumatoid arthritis in humans are linked to the expression of certain MHC class II molecules (HLA-DR). This susceptibility is associated with the presence of a conserved 5-amino acid sequence located in the HLA-DRB1 antigen-binding groove and known as the "RA shared epitope." Presumably these MHC molecules can bind and present self-peptides. It is interesting to note that this same conserved RA shared epitope is found on canine DLA-DRB1 and is associated with susceptibility to RA in some dog breeds. Some MHC class III genes also affect susceptibility to canine RA. For example, there is an association between possession of the C4 allotype C4-4, low serum C4 levels, and the development of autoimmune polyarthritis. Despite this, it has been estimated that non-MHC genes contribute as much as 75% of the genetic susceptibility to rheumatoid arthritis.

Although rheumatoid arthritis is generally considered an autoimmune disease, the identity of the autoantigens involved is unclear. Three that have been implicated are IgG, collagen, and glycosaminoglycans (Figure 36-9). The development of rheumatoid factors to IgG is characteristic of rheumatoid arthritis. These RFs are directed against epitopes on the C_H2 domains of antigen-bound IgG. They can belong to any immunoglobulin class, including IgE, although IgG RFs are by far the most common. The IgG in rheumatoid arthritis patients is less glycosylated than normal IgG, and it may be that this abnormal IgG can act as an immunogen in a susceptible animal. RFs are found not only in rheumatoid arthritis but also in SLE and other diseases in which extensive immune complex formation occurs. RFs are also present in the serum and synovial fluid of some dogs with osteoarthritis (including cruciate disease) or infective arthritis.

RFs are detected by allowing them to agglutinate antibody-coated particles. In humans, latex beads coated with IgG are used for this purpose. In dogs, it is easier to make a canine antisheep erythrocyte serum and coat sheep erythrocytes with this in a subagglutinating dose. After washing, these coated erythrocytes will agglutinate when mixed with RF-positive dog serum.

Although RFs are of diagnostic importance, their clinical significance is unclear. RFs are found in joint fluid, where their titer tends to correlate with the severity of the lesions, and the lesions themselves may be exacerbated by intraarticular inoculation of autologous immunoglobulins. Nevertheless, some individuals with rheumatoid arthritis may not have detectable RFs, and it is not uncommon to find others who have no arthritis despite the presence of RF in their serum. Thus the measurement of RF in dogs is of doubtful specificity.

Other evidence suggests that autoantibodies to collagen may be important. Type II collagen is the predominant form of collagen in articular cartilage and may act as an autoantigen. Autoantibodies to type II collagen can be detected in the serum and synovial fluid of dogs with rheumatoid arthritis, infective arthritis, and osteoarthritis. Affected humans develop a cell-mediated response to denatured collagen II and III, and horses with chronic, nonsuppurative arthritis, osteoarthritis, or traumatic arthritis develop antibodies to horse collagens I and II.

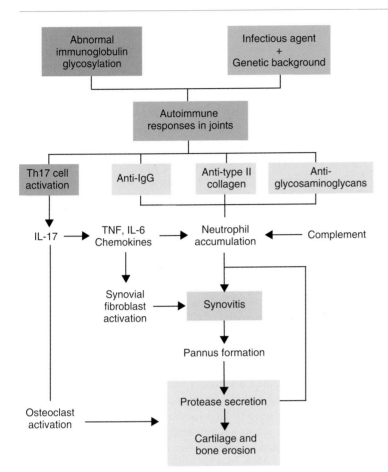

FIGURE 36-9 A schematic diagram showing the possible pathogenesis of rheumatoid arthritis.

These antibodies, as well as immune complexes, can therefore be found in the synovial fluid of horses with many different joint diseases. An autoimmune disease that closely resembles rheumatoid arthritis develops in rats immunized with type II collagen. Evidence from experimental mice and some humans suggests that T cells directed against hyaluronic acid, heparin, and chondroitin sulfates may induce an arthritis resembling rheumatoid arthritis.

Some immunologists believe that rheumatoid arthritis may result from immune responses against citrullinated antigens. Citrulline is an amino acid derived from arginine. It is believed that this conversion plays a role in the preparation of intracellular proteins for apoptosis. Citrullinated antigens are expressed in inflamed joints. Patients develop high levels of autoantibodies to citrullinated antigens before rheumatoid arthritis lesions develop, and these autoantibodies appear to be specific for this disease. They are rarely found in healthy people or in other diseases. It is possible therefore that the key initial lesion in this disease involves autoimmunity to these modified proteins.

Whatever the precise initiating factors, the first stage in the development of rheumatoid arthritis probably involves unregulated activation of Th17 cells within the synovial membrane. The presence of IL-17 produced by these cells activates synovial fibroblasts, cytokines such as IL-1, IL-6, IL-22, granulocyte-macrophage colony-stimulating factor, and tumor necrosis

factor-α (TNF-α) are produced by stromal and endothelial cells. Levels of IFN-γ and IL-2 are very low in synovial fluid, suggesting that Th1 cells are not important in this disease. Inflammatory chemokines such as CCL2 (MCP-1), CCL3 (MIP-1α), and CXCL8 (IL-8) also accumulate. The production of IL-17, together with multiple chemokines, C5a, leukotriene B_4, and platelet-activating factor, results in the accumulation of large numbers of neutrophils in the synovial fluid. Phagocytosis of immune complexes and tissue debris leads to protease escape and the release of oxidants. IL-1, IL-17 and TNF-α stimulate cartilage degradation by activating fibroblast-like cells that line the synovia and by stimulating the release of metalloproteases. Metalloprotease-2 and metalloprotease-9 from chondrocytes and macrophages are raised in canine RA joint fluid. These enzymes degrade the articular cartilage and ligaments. Activated platelets may enter the joint space and aggravate the process by producing more IL-1. More importantly IL-17, TNF-α, and high mobility group box protein-1 (HMGB1) produced by activated T cells activate bone-destroying osteoclasts. These osteoclasts cause the characteristic erosion of periarticular bone. Collectively these reactions lead to bone and cartilage erosion and the characteristic joint pathology.

Macrophage cytokines also trigger synovial angiogenesis. Circulating lymphocytes home to these newly formed capillaries, emigrate into the tissues, and aggregate around the blood vessels. These infiltrating lymphocytes are primarily activated CD4+ T cells. B cell emigration into the tissues eventually leads to local RF production. The RFs form immune complexes and activate complement. Some immune complexes may precipitate out within the superficial layers of the articular cartilage.

The progressive development of inflammation within the joint leads first to morning stiffness. The joints become warm as the blood flow increases, but because the inflammation is restricted to the synovia, the skin rarely becomes red. The animal may show depression and fatigue as a result of the systemic effects of IL-1 and TNF-α. If the joints develop effusions, they will be obviously swollen. As the disease progresses, the grossly inflamed synovia invades the cartilage, ligaments, and bone and destroys the articular cartilage. Synovial lining cells, small blood vessels, and fibroblasts proliferate. Large numbers of macrophages are found in the pannus, as well as MHC class II–positive B cells and dendritic cells.

Diagnosis Diagnosis of rheumatoid arthritis in animals is generally based on the criteria established for human rheumatoid arthritis. They are listed in Box 36-2. Most should have been present for at least 6 weeks. In addition, steps should be taken to exclude SLE (by testing for ANA) and to exclude any infectious cause for the arthritis.

Treatment Treatment of canine rheumatoid arthritis with drugs tends to be unsatisfactory, and the long-term prognosis of the disease is poor. Nonsteroidal antiinflammatory drugs, such as aspirin, carprofen, or etodolac, have been the first choice in treating early, uncomplicated cases of rheumatoid arthritis, although their efficacy is unclear. Corticosteroids such as prednisolone should be reserved for late, severe cases in which salicylates have proved inadequate. Local steroid injections into affected joints will produce rapid relief and clinical remission. However, the joints are still subjected to stress, disease progression is not slowed, and the corticosteroids delay healing and promote articular degeneration. Their use may therefore permit articular damage to proceed unabated. Recently, encouraging results have been obtained in humans by the aggressive use of the immunosuppressive agent methotrexate. Monoclonal antibodies to TNF-α (infliximab), to CD4, to thymocytes, or to IL-2R have also been beneficial in preventing bone erosions in humans, as has administration of recombinant TNF-α receptors (etanercept). The

immunosuppressive drug leflunomide appears to be as effective as methotrexate. Slow-acting immunosuppressive agents, such as the gold salts, sodium aurothiomalate, and aurothioglucose, and antimalarials, such as chloroquine, are also used in humans, but they are expensive, results have been erratic, and experience with these in animals is limited. (Gold salts inhibit the release of HMGB1 from activated macrophages). Appropriate surgery may improve joint stability and reduce pain.

Nonerosive Polyarthritis

The second major group of immune-mediated arthritides includes those in which the joint cartilage is not eroded and the inflammatory lesion is largely confined to the joint capsule and synovia. Many of these clinically resemble rheumatoid arthritis but may be differentiated by their nonerosive character.

Equine Polyarthritis/Polysynovitis Polyarthritis has been reported in foals in association with a lupus-like syndrome. In these cases affected foals (up to 3 months of age) present with multiple swollen joints involving all four limbs and a persistent fever. In some cases other synovial sheaths, including tendon sheaths and bursae, are affected. The synovial effusions are sterile, but synovial biopsies show lymphocyte and plasma cell infiltration with some immunoglobulin deposits. The cells in the joint fluid are mainly neutrophils. These animals are negative for RF, ANA, and LE cells. Many of these animals have a lesion within the thorax, especially *Rhodococcus equi* pneumonia. This is classified as a type II disease (see later). It is possible that immune complexes originating in the lungs may lodge in the synovia and trigger the synovitis. The polyarthritis usually resolves as the primary lesion resolves.

A type I immune-mediated polyarthritis has also been recorded in horses. In these cases animals lose weight, develop an intermittent fever, and have effusions in multiple joints leading to stiffness. They have systemic signs of inflammation, including anemia, leukocytosis, hyperfibrinogenemia, and hyperglobulinemia. The synovial effusion is sterile, and immunoglobulins are present in the synovial membrane. The condition usually resolves with steroid and immunosuppressive therapy.

Canine Polyarthritis Dogs may develop several distinct nonerosive polyarthritides, which can be divided into at least three major categories: arthritis associated with SLE, arthritis associated with a myositis, and idiopathic polyarthritis. Breeds that are predisposed to polyarthritis include German Shepherds, Irish Setters, Shetland Sheepdogs, Cocker Spaniels, and Springer Spaniels. The main clinical features of polyarthritis are stiffness, pyrexia, anorexia, and lethargy. Leflunomide appears to be an effective alternative to oral corticosteroids for the treatment of this disease.

Lupus Polyarthritis Polyarthritis is a common feature of SLE. Diagnosis is contingent on making a firm diagnosis of

---

□ **Box 36-2** | **Diagnostic Criteria for Canine Rheumatoid Arthritis**

• Stiffness or joint pain, especially after periods of inactivity

• Symmetrical joint swelling, especially if multiple joints are involved

• Sterile synovial fluid containing inflammatory cells

• Positive rheumatoid factor test

• Erosive polyarthritis with characteristic histology

lupus. Thus it is necessary to show multiple-system involvement, a significant titer of serum ANAs, and immunopathological features consistent with lupus.

Polyarthritis with Polymyositis A disease characterized by both nonerosive polyarthritis and polymyositis is recognized in young dogs. Most recorded cases have been seen in Spaniels. The animals are stiff and have painful joints, fever, lethargy, weakness, muscle atrophy, and muscle pain. They are negative for both ANA and RF. The arthritis is nonerosive and symmetrical, involving multiple joints. The animals have a symmetrical inflammatory myopathy with myalgia, atrophy, and muscle contracture. The synovial fluid shows high white cell counts, especially neutrophils. Muscle biopsy specimens show a neutrophil or mononuclear cell infiltrate, or both, with muscle fiber atrophy and degeneration. Synovial biopsy specimens show a neutrophil and mononuclear cell infiltration with a fibrinous exudate. IgG, IgM, and complement are deposited in the walls of the synovial vessels. Animals may be treated with corticosteroids and immunosuppressive agents such as cyclophosphamide.

Idiopathic Polyarthritis Most cases of canine polyarthritis fit none of the categories described previously. Although these cases are nonerosive and possess the characteristics of type III hypersensitivity, their precise etiology is unknown. They can be classified into four types (Table 36-1). Type I disease is polyarthritis alone. Type II disease is a reactive arthritis associated with infections in the respiratory or urinary tract, tooth infections, or cellulitis. Type III disease is associated with the presence of gastroenteritis, diarrhea, or ulcerative colitis. It is not clear whether this type of disease is truly distinguishable from type II disease. Type IV disease is associated with the presence of tumors, including seminomas and carcinomas.

An example of type I polyarthritis is the juvenile polyarthritis syndrome seen in Akitas between the ages of 9 weeks and 8 months. These dogs have a cyclical high fever lasting 24 to 48 hours before resolving and evidence of severe, incapacitating joint pain with soft tissue swelling. Radiology shows hepatosplenomegaly and lymphadenopathy. Some animals may have meningitis or meningoencephalitis. Their erythrocytes may be antiglobulin positive. Synovial fluid shows no evidence of infection, although large numbers of neutrophils are present. The dogs are usually negative for RF and ANA. Pedigree analysis suggests that the disease is inherited. Some dogs respond positively to corticosteroid treatment. In refractory cases azathioprine may also be required.

Idiopathic polyarthritis tends to be most common in male dogs, and about half of the cases are seen in young dogs between 1 and 3.5 years of age. Most of the animals show systemic signs such as fever, anorexia, and lethargy. The animals are lame and have a history of stiffness after rest. The most commonly affected joints include the stifle, elbow, and carpus. The onset of lameness is sudden in most cases and is associated with obvious muscle atrophy. There is no significant joint erosion, although periarticular soft tissue swelling and synovial effusions are common. Some cases may have proliferative periosteal changes. All cases are negative for RF and ANA. The joint fluid is sterile. Synovial biopsies show hypertrophy with a neutrophil or a mononuclear cell infiltration, or both. Fibrin deposits are seen in most cases, as is fibrosis. Most lesions contain IgM, IgG, and complement deposits, and some contain IgA-producing plasma cells. Some affected dogs may have a glomerulonephritis. Animals respond well to corticosteroids. The prognosis for idiopathic polyarthropathy is generally better than that for the other forms of immune-mediated arthritis.

Feline Polyarthritis Chronic progressive polyarthritis of male cats is characterized by polyarthritis with either osteopenia or periosteal new bone formation. Periarticular erosions and eventual collapse or subchondral erosions, joint instabilities, and deformities closely resembling those of rheumatoid arthritis are also seen. Affected cats are commonly infected with feline syncytia-forming virus (FSV) or feline leukemia virus (FeLV), or both. (The incidence of FSV in these cats is 2 to 4 times higher, and the incidence of FeLV is 6 to 10 times higher than in normal cats.) It is described here because of suggestions that it is of immunological origin. These suggestions are based on the massive lymphocyte and plasma cell infiltration of affected joints and the presence of an immune complex type of glomerulonephritis. However, affected cats are RF and ANA negative, and their serum immunoglobulin levels tend to be close to normal. Corticosteroids lessen the severity of clinical signs. Combination therapy with corticosteroids and azathioprine or cyclophosphamide can induce temporary remissions.

Cruciate Ligament Rupture Immunological abnormalities are associated with spontaneous rupture of the anterior cruciate ligament in dogs. For example, the synovia of affected dogs contains B cells and IgG-positive plasma cells. In addition, the

---

◻ **Table 36-1 | Classification of Nonerosive Polyarthritis in Dogs**

TYPE	DISEASE ASSOCIATIONS
I	Uncomplicated polyarthritis without other disease associations
II	Polyarthritis associated with infectious lesions remote from the joints (e.g., respiratory or urinary infections)
III	Polyarthritis associated with gastrointestinal disease
IV	Polyarthritis associated with neoplastic disease remote from the joints

From Bennett DJ: Canine idiopathic polyarthritis, *Small Anim Pract* 28:909–928, 1987

synovia contains numerous MHC class II–positive, CD1c+ dendritic cells closely resembling the lesions seen in rheumatoid arthritis. Cruciate ligaments are mainly composed of type I collagen. Autoantibodies to both type I and type II collagen are found in synovial fluid following cruciate ligament rupture (secondary to osteoarthritis). These antibodies are largely bound in immune complexes. They are unlikely to be of major significance and probably represent a secondary response to local damage. CXCL8 (IL-8) levels rise in joints before cruciate ligament rupture, implying that inflammation precedes rupture.

Dermatomyositis

A familial disease of dogs that resembles dermatomyositis in humans has been described in Collies and Shetland Sheepdogs. The disease is inherited as an autosomal dominant condition involving a locus on chromosome 35, although expression is highly variable. Dogs develop dermatitis with a less obvious myositis. Puppies appear normal at birth, but skin lesions develop between 7 and 11 weeks of age, and myositis develops between 12 and 23 weeks. In other studies, the dermatitis developed at 3 to 6 months of age, and myositis was detected after the dermatitis was investigated. The dermatitis first develops on the face; subsequently, lesions may spread to the limbs and trunk, especially over bony prominences. These early lesions are erythematous and eventually lead to vesicle and pustule formation. Once the vesicles rupture, they ulcerate and crust. Lesions may be found on the bridge of the nose and around the eyes and show hair loss and changes in pigmentation. There may be enlargement of the lymph nodes, draining the affected areas. The clinical course and severity are variable, but skin lesions usually resolve by 1 year of age.

Muscle disease follows the onset of skin disease, but there is no correlation between the severity of the two lesions. The most common sign of myositis is masseter and temporal muscle atrophy. Some severely affected puppies may have difficulty eating as a result of the myositis and thus grow poorly. If the muscles of the esophagus are affected, megaesophagus may develop, and secondary aspiration pneumonia results. Generalized lymphoid hyperplasia may also develop in these dogs. Many dogs outgrow the disease and are left with moderate hyperpigmentation, some hypopigmentation and alopecia, and some atrophy of the muscles of mastication. Other dogs develop a progressive disease with severe dermatitis and myositis. Dogs with progressive disease may also develop signs of immunosuppression, especially pyoderma and septicemia, as well as demodicosis. On necropsy, myositis may be seen in the esophagus and arteritis in the skin, muscle, and bladder.

The onset and progression of the disease are correlated with a rise in circulating immune complexes and serum IgG, but the reason for these increases is unclear. Circulating immune complexes and IgG levels return to normal as the disease resolves, suggesting a causative association. Histology shows a nonspecific inflammatory dermatitis. Muscle biopsy, especially

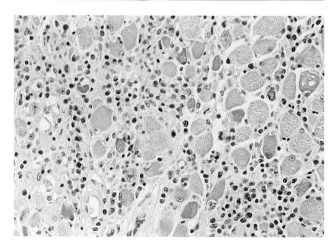

FIGURE 36-10 A section of esophagus from a dog with dermatomyositis. Note the fragmented myofibers as well as the infiltration by lymphocytes, plasma cells, and macrophages. H&E stain; original magnification ×200).

(From Hargis AM, Prieur DJ, Haupt KH, et al: Postmortem findings in four litters of dogs with familial canine dermatomyositis, *Am J Pathol* 123:480–496, 1986.)

of the temporal muscle, shows multifocal accumulations of lymphocytes, plasma cells, and macrophages as well as a few neutrophils and eosinophils. The myofibers are atrophied and may show fragmentation and vacuolation (Figure 36-10). Symptomatic and corticosteroid treatment may be of benefit in severely affected cases.

Immune Vasculitis

Several forms of immune-mediated vasculitis have been described in domestic animals. Their precise relationships are unclear, and as a result, they have been given several different names, including canine juvenile polyarteritis, polyarteritis nodosa, and leukocytoclastic vasculitis.

Canine juvenile polyarteritis primarily affects Beagles less than 2 years of age. The animals show episodes of anorexia, persistent fever of greater than 40° C, and a hunched stance with lowered head and a stiff gait, indicating severe neck pain. The clinical signs may show cyclical remissions and relapses. The animals have a neutrophilia and elevated acute-phase proteins. These dogs have elevated serum IgM and IgA but normal IgG. The proportion of B cells in the blood is increased, but their T cells are decreased, as is their response to mitogens. On necropsy there are few gross lesions. There may be some hemorrhage in lymph nodes. Histologically there is a systemic vasculitis and perivasculitis. In the acute disease there is necrotizing vasculitis with fibrinoid necrosis and a massive inflammatory cell infiltration involving the small and medium-sized arteries of the heart, mediastinum, and cervical spinal cord (Figure 36-11). Immunoglobulins are deposited in the walls of small- and medium-sized arteries. During remissions, the vascular lesions consist of intimal and medial fibrosis and a mild perivasculitis, the residue of previous acute vasculitis.

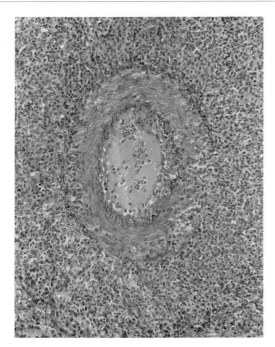

FIGURE 36-11 An extramural coronary artery from a Beagle suffering from juvenile polyarteritis. This medium-sized muscular artery is characterized by medial necrosis, ruptured elastic laminae, and severe perivascular accumulations of neutrophils, lymphocytes, and macrophages. H&E stain.

(From Snyder PW, Kazacos EA, Scott-Moncrieff JC, et al: Pathologic features of naturally occurring juvenile polyarteritis in beagle dogs, *Vet Pathol* 32:337–345, 1995.)

Chronically affected dogs may develop generalized amyloidosis. In many ways, this disease resembles Kawasaki disease of children, the leading cause of acquired heart disease in the United States.

Polyarteritis nodosa occurs in humans, pigs, dogs, and cats. It is characterized by a widespread, focal necrosis of the media of small and medium-sized muscular arteries. The lesions are found in many organs, especially in the kidney. Vessels in the skin are rarely involved.

On occasion, focal vascular lesions characterized by neutrophil infiltration may develop in small blood vessels throughout the body, but especially in skin. Affected dogs have mucocutaneous ulcers, bullae, edema, polyarthropathy, myopathy, anorexia, intermittent fever, and lethargy. Although called hypersensitivity vasculitis, a foreign antigen can be found in only a small proportion of cases. For this reason, a better name for this condition may be leukocytoclastic vasculitis. The cause or causes of polyarteritis nodosa and hypersensitivity vasculitis are unknown. The histology of both diseases suggests that they are a form of type III hypersensitivity reaction, perhaps triggered by an infectious agent. Immunosuppression with corticosteroids, together with cyclophosphamide, has given encouraging results in treating canine hypersensitivity vasculitis. Polyarteritis nodosa is usually detected as an incidental finding on necropsy, although ocular defects may present clinically if the arteries of the eye are involved.

For sources of additional information, please visit http:// evolve.elsevier.com/tizard/immunology/

Primary Immunodeficiencies

□ Chapter Outline

□ Key Points

- As a result of genetic mutations, defects may develop in the developing immune system, resulting in immunodeficiency in newborn animals.
- Many different inherited defects have now been identified in domestic animals, especially in inbred breeds in which heterozygosity is reduced.
- Defects in innate immunity include deficiencies in phagocytosis, leukocyte adherence, and intracellular killing, leading to increased susceptibility to bacterial diseases.
- Defects in T cell function generally predispose an animal to overwhelming virus infections.
- Defects in B cell function and immunoglobulin production predispose animals to overwhelming bacterial disease.
- Combined immunodeficiencies are most severe since affected animals lack resistance to all infectious agents.

Any defect in either the innate or adaptive immune systems usually becomes apparent when affected animals show unusual susceptibility to infectious or parasitic diseases. These diseases may be due to pathogenic organisms or, if the defect is very severe, opportunistic infections by organisms that are not normally able to cause disease. Deficiencies in the immune systems may be a result of inherited defects (primary immunodeficiencies); alternatively, the deficiencies may be a direct result of some other cause (secondary or acquired immunodeficiencies). This chapter describes some of the primary immunodeficiencies recorded in domestic animals.

One feature of primary immunodeficiencies in domestic animals is breed susceptibility. Examples of breed-associated immunodeficiencies include the increased risk for canine parvoviral enteritis in Doberman Pinschers and Rottweilers. German Shepherds may have increased susceptibility to canine distemper, whereas Mexican Hairless Dogs may have defective cell-mediated immune responses. It must also be recognized that the genetic composition of many breeds varies geographically, and problems with a specific breed in one country may not occur in others.

Inherited Defects in Innate Immunity

Inherited deficiencies in innate immunity include defects in the various stages of phagocytosis as well as the complement deficiencies described previously (Chapter 7). Phagocytic defects are well recognized in domestic animals.

Chédiak-Higashi Syndrome

Chédiak-Higashi syndrome is an inherited disease of Hereford, Japanese black, and Brangus cattle, Aleutian mink, blue smoke Persian cats, white tigers, beige (*bg/bg*) mice, Orca whales, and humans. It is an autosomal recessive disease resulting from a mutation in a gene (*LYST*) that encodes a protein that controls lysosomal membrane fusion. The *LYST* gene is found on bovine chromosome 28. In Chédiak-Higashi cattle, there is a missense A:T → G:C mutation that results in replacement of a histidine with an arginine residue. The defect produces abnormally large secretory lysosomes in neutrophils, monocytes, eosinophils, and pigment cells (Figure 37-1). The enlarged neutrophil granules result from the fusion of primary and secondary granules. The leukocyte granules of affected animals are more fragile than those of normal animals, rupturing spontaneously and causing tissue damage, such as cataracts in the eye. These leukocytes have defective chemotactic responsiveness, reduced motility, and reduced intracellular killing. Cytotoxic T cells fail to excrete their granzyme-rich lysosomes.

Clinically, the syndrome is associated with multiple abnormalities. In hair, the melanosomes also fuse together, causing the dilution of coat color (sometimes only obvious in the newborn) and light-colored irises (pseudoalbinism). Other eye abnormalities include photophobia, and animals may develop cataracts. Their eyes have a red fundic light reflection rather than the normal yellow-green. Because of the neutrophil

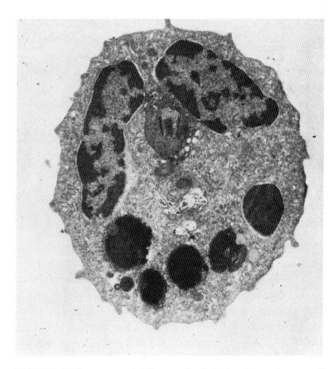

FIGURE 37-1 A neutrophil from a Chédiak-Higashi syndrome calf with enlarged cytoplasmic granules.

(Courtesy Dr. H.W. Leopold.)

defects, affected animals may be more susceptible to respiratory infections and neonatal septicemia. Some affected breeds of cattle, such as Herefords, tend to be more susceptible to infection than others, such as Japanese black cattle. The Chédiak-Higashi gene also impairs the function of natural killer (NK) and cytotoxic T cells. As a result, affected animals may show increased susceptibility to tumors and to viruses such as the Aleutian disease virus in mink. Platelets from affected animals also contain enlarged lysosomes, and their function is abnormal. Affected animals tend to bleed abnormally after surgery and develop hematomas at injection sites. Death from acute hemorrhage is common.

Chédiak-Higashi syndrome may be diagnosed by examining a stained blood smear for the presence of grossly enlarged granules within leukocytes or by examining hair shafts for enlarged melanosomes. Treatment is symptomatic.

Pelger-Huët Anomaly

Pelger-Huët anomaly is an inherited disorder characterized by a failure of granulocyte nuclei to segment into lobes. The neutrophils therefore appear on first sight to be very immature (a left shift). The anomaly is usually detected when an animal is observed to have a persistent left shift that cannot be reconciled with its good health. Although Pelger-Huët neutrophils closely resemble band forms, their nuclear chromatin is condensed, reflecting their maturity. In humans, the anomaly is due to a mutation in the gene coding for lamin B, a nuclear membrane receptor that interacts with chromatin to determine the shape of the nucleus. Pelger-Huët anomaly has been observed in humans, Arabian horses, domestic short-hair cats, and various dog breeds such as Cocker Spaniels, Basenjis, Boston Terriers, Foxhounds, and Coonhounds. In Foxhounds and Australian Shepherds, the anomaly is inherited as an autosomal dominant trait. Pelger-Huët anomaly has a minimal effect on the health of animals. Nevertheless, fewer pups are weaned from affected dogs than from unaffected ones. In addition, Pelger-Huët neutrophils are less able to emigrate from blood vessels in vivo. This reduced mobility may be due to inflexible nuclei. B cell responses may also be impaired since normal canine B cells exposed to serum from affected dogs show depressed responses to antigens.

Canine Leukocyte Adhesion Deficiency

In order for neutrophils to leave inflamed blood vessels, they must first bind to vascular endothelium. This adhesion is mediated by neutrophil integrins. In the absence of these integrins, neutrophils cannot bind to endothelial cells and are unable to emigrate into tissues (Figure 37-2). Thus bacteria in tissues can grow freely without fear of attack by neutrophils. Canine leukocyte adhesion deficiency (CLAD) results from a defect in the integrin CD11b/CD18 (Mac-1). In Mac-1-deficient dogs, neutrophils cannot respond to chemoattractants, trap complement-coated bacteria (Mac-1 is a complement receptor), or bind to endothelial cells. Affected dogs suffer recurrent

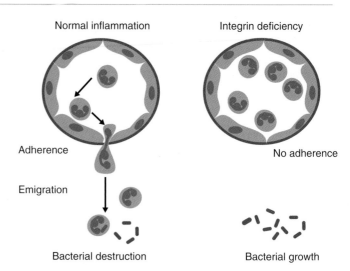

FIGURE 37-2 Integrins are required to bind neutrophils firmly to blood vessel walls. This permits the neutrophils to emigrate to sites of bacterial invasion. In the absence of integrins, neutrophil emigration fails to occur. As a result, invading bacteria can grow unmolested in the tissues.

infections, despite the fact that their blood neutrophils are greatly elevated.

CLAD has been described in Irish Red Setters (as well as in the related Red and White Setter breed), in which it is an autosomal recessive disease. Affected animals die early in life as a result of recurrent severe bacterial infections (osteomyelitis, omphalophlebitis, gingivitis), lymphadenopathy, impaired pus formation, delayed wound healing, weight loss, and fever. Animals have a marked leukocytosis (>200,000/μL), primarily a neutrophilia and eosinophilia. Although these granulocytes look normal, functional tests reveal defects in adhesion-dependent activities, including impaired adhesion to glass or plastic surfaces or to nylon wool fibers. They cannot ingest C3b-opsonized particles. Normal canine granulocytes aggregate after activation with phorbol myristate acetate, but those of CLAD animals do not. Migration in response to chemotactic stimuli is poor. Neither CD11b nor CD18 can be detected by immunofluorescence.

The lesion results from a single missense mutation at position 107 in the β chain of the CD18 gene, which results in the replacement of a highly conserved cysteine residue (Cys36) by a serine. As a result, the mutation disrupts a disulfide bond in CD18, altering its structure and function. CD11b (the α chain) is not expressed because it must be associated with the β chain before the dimer can be expressed on the cell surface. A diagnostic test for the CLAD mutation has been developed. Thus genomic DNA is amplified by polymerase chain reaction (PCR) using primer sets for the mutated region. The PCR products may then be sequenced and the presence of the mutation determined. Matched related bone marrow allografts from normal animals have been given to CLAD dogs and effectively treated the disease.

Canine granulocytopathy syndrome was an autosomal recessive disease observed in Irish Setters. Some investigators have suggested that the disease is identical to CLAD, but because it was described before integrins were discovered, this cannot be confirmed. These animals had suppurative skin lesions, gingivitis, osteomyelitis, pododermatitis, and lymphadenopathy. Affected dogs had a pronounced leukocytosis, and their neutrophils were morphologically normal, although there was a persistent left shift. The affected animals were hypergammaglobulinemic and anemic as a result of the persistent infections. Their lymph nodes showed diffuse, suppurative, nongranulomatous lymphadenitis, which is inconsistent with a diagnosis of CLAD. Examination of the neutrophils of these dogs showed that their respiratory burst was depressed, as reflected by a decrease in glucose oxidation. Nevertheless, they were more effective than normal cells at reducing nitroblue tetrazolium, implying that O_2^- was produced in greater quantities than normal or, perhaps, that it was not effectively removed. Despite this, these cells were unable to kill opsonized *Escherichia coli* or *Staphylococcus aureus,* suggesting that they had a killing defect rather than an adhesion defect.

A form of canine neutrophil dysfunction related to CLAD has been reported resulting from excessive downregulation of β_2-integrin. This occurs in mixed-breed dogs that present with recurrent pyogenic infections. Their neutrophils produce significantly reduced amounts of CD18 and hence β_2-integrin. As a result of this reduced expression, defects occur in several adhesion-dependent neutrophil functions, including superoxide production.

Bovine Leukocyte Adhesion Deficiency

An integrin deficiency has been reported in Holstein calves. Bovine leukocyte adhesion deficiency (BLAD) is an autosomal recessive trait characterized by recurrent bacterial infections, anorexia, oral ulceration, gingivitis, periodontitis, chronic pneumonia, stunted growth, delayed wound healing, peripheral lymphadenopathy, and a persistent extreme neutrophilia. Affected calves usually die between 2 and 7 months of age. The survivors grow slowly and may develop amyloidosis. These calves have large numbers of intravascular neutrophils but very few extravascular neutrophils, even in the presence of invading bacteria.

BLAD results from a point mutation in the gene coding for CD18 (Figure 37-3). As a result, an aspartic acid residue is replaced by a glycine, and functional CD18 is not produced. In the absence of this chain, complete integrins cannot be assembled. Neutrophils fail to attach to vascular endothelial cells and cannot emigrate from blood vessels. Healthy carriers have a single copy of the mutated gene and thus have abnormally low levels of CD18 (Figure 37-4). Through the use of a PCR test, the presence of the altered gene can be demonstrated. In this way it has been shown that one bull, Osborndale Ivanhoe, with thousands of registered sons and daughters, was a carrier of this gene. As a result, the defective gene was widespread and common among Holstein cattle in the United States (14% of bulls, 5.8% of cows). Fortunately, carrier animals can be rapidly detected and removed from breeding programs.

Because CD18 integrins are also expressed by T cells attracted to sites of antigen invasion, BLAD calves show poor delayed hypersensitivity responses. Their neutrophils show reduced responsiveness to chemotactic stimuli and diminished superoxide production and myeloperoxidase activity. They have increased expression of Fc receptors but decreased binding and expression of C3b and IgM on neutrophils, implying an alteration in receptor function. This is reflected by greatly reduced endocytosis and killing of *S. aureus.*

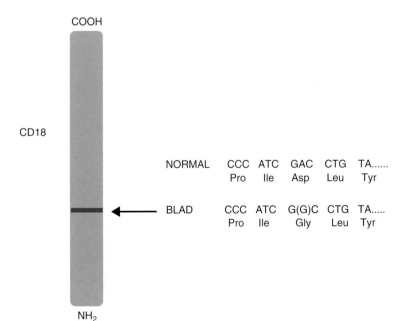

NORMAL	CCC	ATC	GAC	CTG	TA......
	Pro	Ile	Asp	Leu	Tyr

BLAD	CCC	ATC	G(G)C	CTG	TA.....
	Pro	Ile	Gly	Leu	Tyr

FIGURE 37-3 The BLAD mutation. The mutation involves replacement of a cytosine by a guanosine in the CD18 gene. As a result, an aspartic acid residue (A) is replaced by a glycine residue (G). The mutation occurs in a highly conserved region of the CD18 molecule and prevents formation of a biologically active molecule.

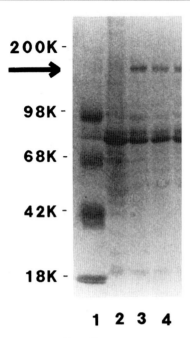

FIGURE 37-4 A Western blot of bovine Mac-1. An extract has been made from the neutrophils of a BLAD calf *(lane 2)* or from clinically normal calves *(lanes 3 and 4)*. The extracts have been electrophoresed and blotted onto nitrocellulose. The bands are stained to show the presence of glycoproteins. Note that CD18 *(arrow)* is absent from the lysate of neutrophils from a BLAD calf. Lane 1 shows molecular weight standards (kDa).

(From Kehrili ME, Schmalstieg FC, Anderson DC, et al: Molecular definition of the bovine granulocytopathy syndrome: identification of deficiency of the Mac-1 [CD11b/CD18] glycoprotein, *Am J Vet Res* 51:1826–1836, 1990.)

Canine Cyclical Neutropenia

Canine cyclical neutropenia (gray collie syndrome) is an autosomal recessive disease of Border Collies. Affected dogs have dilution of skin pigmentation, eye lesions, and regular cyclic fluctuations in leukocyte numbers. Their hair is a characteristic silver-gray color, and their nose is gray—a diagnostic feature. The loss of neutrophils occurs about every 11 to 12 days and lasts for about 3 days. It is followed by normal or elevated neutrophil counts for about 7 days. Severe neutropenia suppresses inflammation and increases susceptibility to bacterial and fungal infections. (Their neutrophils also have reduced myeloperoxidase activity, so the disease is not entirely due to a neutrophil deficiency). In humans, the disease is due to a defect in the gene coding for neutrophil elastase, an enzyme found in azurophil granules. The animals have severe enteric disease, respiratory infections, mouth infections (gingivitis), bone disease (arthralgia), and lymphadenitis and rarely live beyond 3 years. Because platelet numbers also cycle, affected dogs may also have bleeding problems, including gingival hemorrhage and epistaxis. Immunoglobulin levels rise as a result of the recurrent antigenic stimulation, but complement levels cycle in conjunction with the neutropenia. The disease begins to express itself as maternal immunity wanes. Affected puppies

are weak, grow poorly, have wounds that fail to heal, and have a high mortality rate. If they are kept alive by aggressive antibiotic therapy, chronic inflammation may lead to amyloidosis.

Treatment involves the repeated use of antibiotics to control the recurrent infections. If endotoxin is administered repeatedly, it can stimulate the bone marrow and stabilize neutrophil, reticulocyte, and platelet numbers. Lithium carbonate has a similar effect. Unfortunately, both endotoxin and lithium carbonate are toxic, and the disease recurs when the treatment is discontinued.

Other Examples of Defective Neutrophil Function

An inherited defect in neutrophil bactericidal activity has been reported in Dobermans. Dogs had bronchopneumonia and chronic rhinitis that developed soon after birth and persisted despite antimicrobial therapy. Although their chemotaxis and ingestion were apparently normal, their neutrophils were unable to kill *S. aureus*. Since these cells showed reduced reduction of nitroblue tetrazolium and superoxide production, it was suggested that there was a defect in the respiratory burst pathway.

Young Weimaraner dogs have been described as suffering from an immunodeficiency syndrome with a wide range of clinical signs. These include recurrent fevers, diarrhea, pneumonia, pyoderma, osteomyelitis, stomatitis, and osteomyelitis. They may have defective neutrophil function, as shown by a depressed chemiluminescent response to phorbol ester, implying a defect in the respiratory burst mechanism. Their IgG levels may be significantly lower than normal and their IgM and IgA levels somewhat reduced; the other immunological parameters of these animals fall within normal ranges.

A persistent neutropenia attributable to a deficiency of granulocyte colony-stimulating factor (G-CSF) has been reported in a 3-year-old male Rottweiler. The animal had a fever due to multiple recurrent infections, especially a chronic bacterial arthritis in the presence of a persistent neutropenia. A bioassay showed that the animal was not making G-CSF. Its myeloid stem cells responded readily to additional G-CSF, suggesting that they were functionally normal. Bone marrow examination suggested that its neutrophil precursors had failed to mature.

A possible autosomal recessive neutropenia has been described in Border Collies. This disease, called trapped neutrophil syndrome, resulted in recurrent bacterial osteomyelitis and gastroenteritis. Animals presented with persistent fever and lameness due to lytic bone lesions. They had myeloid hyperplasia and dense accumulations of neutrophils in the marrow but few in the blood. The neutropenia apparently resulted from an inability of the neutrophils to escape from the bone marrow into the bloodstream, perhaps as a result of a deficiency of granulocyte-macrophage colony-stimulating factor. In humans this disease has been called myelokathexis.

Inherited Defects in the Adaptive Immune System

The inherited immunological defects have served to confirm the overall arrangement of the immune system, as outlined in Figure 37-5. For example, if both the cell- and antibody-mediated immune responses are defective, it may be assumed that the genetic lesion operates at a point before thymic and bursal cell processing—that is, a stem cell lesion. A defect that occurs only in thymic development is reflected in an inability to mount cell-mediated immune responses, although antibody production may be normal. Similarly, a lesion restricted to B cells is reflected by impaired antibody responses.

Recent advances in molecular genetics have enabled many new primary immunodeficiency disorders to be identified in humans. For example, at least 10 different mutations can result in severe combined immunodeficiency. Likewise mutations in many different genes can disable B cell function and result in immunoglobulin deficiencies.

Immunodeficiencies of Horses

Horses are among the few domestic animals whose economic worth has permitted a thorough analysis of neonatal mortality. As a result, a significant number of primary immunodeficiency syndromes have been identified in this species (Figure 37-6).

Severe Combined Immunodeficiency

The most important congenital equine immunodeficiency is the severe combined immunodeficiency syndrome (SCID). Affected foals fail to produce functional T or B cells and have very few circulating lymphocytes. If they suckle successfully, they will acquire maternal immunoglobulins. Once these have been catabolized, however, these foals cannot produce their own antibodies and eventually become agammaglobulinemic. Affected foals are therefore born healthy but begin to sicken by 2 months of age. The precise time of onset depends on the quantity of colostral antibodies absorbed. All die by 4 to 6 months as a result of overwhelming infection by a variety of low-grade pathogens. Severe bronchopneumonia is the predominant presenting sign. Organisms that have been implicated in this bronchopneumonia include equine adenovirus, *Rhodococcus equi*, and *Pneumocystis* (an opportunistic fungal pathogen). The disease is manifested by a nasal discharge, coughing, dyspnea, weight loss, and fevers. Affected foals may also develop enteritis, omphalophlebitis, and many other infections. *Cryptosporidium parvum* and many different bacteria have been implicated in the enteritis.

On necropsy, the spleens of these foals lack germinal centers and periarteriolar lymphoid sheaths. Their lymph nodes lack lymphoid follicles and germinal centers, and there is cellular depletion in the paracortex. The thymus in these animals may be difficult to find. By using large quantities of blood, it is possible to demonstrate the presence of functional NK cells. Neutrophil and monocyte functions are also normal in these foals.

SCID is an autosomal recessive disease, and its occurrence therefore indicates that both parents carry the mutation. Accurate diagnosis is of great importance since the presence of the mutation reduces significantly the value of the parent animals. Thus all suspected cases must be confirmed by postmortem examination. The clinical diagnosis of SCID requires that at least two of the following three criteria be established: (1) very low (consistently below 1000/ mm^3) circulating lymphocytes; (2) histology typical of SCID—that is, gross hypoplasia of the primary and secondary lymphoid organs; and (3) an absence of IgM from presuckle serum. (The normal equine fetus synthesizes small amounts of IgM. As a result, IgM in normal

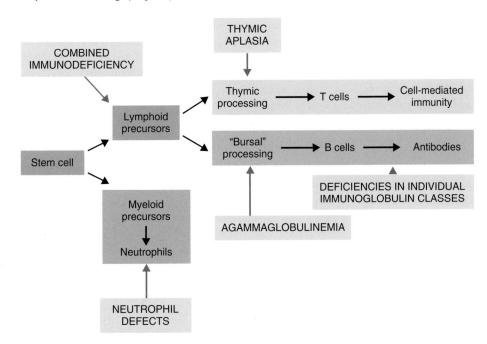

FIGURE 37-5 The points in the immune system where development blocks may lead to immunodeficiencies.

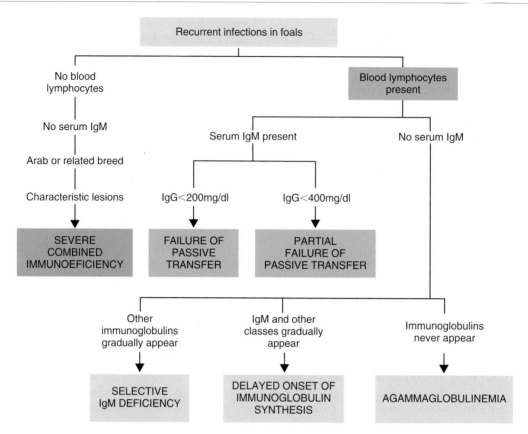

FIGURE 37-6 The differential diagnosis of the equine immune deficiencies.

newborn foals is about 160 μg/mL. If the foal successfully suckles, it will obtain immunoglobulins of all isotypes from the mare's colostrum. However, the half-life of IgM is only about 6 days, so maternal IgM will disappear within a few days of birth. Thus a normal foal will always have some IgM in its serum, but a SCID foal will have none.)

Molecular Basis of Equine Severe Combined Immunodeficiency When the antigen receptors (B cell receptors [BCRs] and T cell receptors [TCRs]) are synthesized, large segments of DNA are excised so that *V, D,* and *J* gene segments can be rejoined (Chapter 17). Several enzymes are involved in this recombination process. Some cut the DNA strands, and others rejoin them. Studies on the cells of SCID foals show that although the enzymes that cut the DNA are normal, there is a defect in the large multicomponent enzyme that rejoins the cut ends. The specific defect lies in the gene coding for the catalytic subunit of an enzyme called DNA-dependent protein kinase *(DNA-PK_{cs})* (Figure 37-7). In the mutant *DNA-PK_{cs}* gene, a loss of five nucleotides results in a frameshift, premature termination of the peptide chain, and a deletion of 967 amino acids from the C-terminus of the molecule, including its entire kinase domain (Figure 37-8). Functional *DNA-PK_{cs}* is totally absent from affected foals. Because of this deficiency, broken DNA strands cannot be rejoined, and neither T cells nor B cells can form functional V regions. In the absence of both TCRs and BCRs, affected foals cannot respond to antigens. Since *DNA-PK_{cs}* is needed to rejoin broken strands of DNA,

it also plays a key role in other DNA repair processes. Thus the cells from SCID foals are unable to repair DNA damaged by radiation (Figure 37-9).

The presence of the mutant *CID* gene in horses can be detected by means of a PCR. A sample of DNA is obtained from horse skin cells. A primer set designed to amplify only DNA containing the 5-base pair deletion and another set designed to amplify only the normal allele are used to determine whether the mutant gene is present. This test has demonstrated that the frequency of the *CID* gene in Arabian horses is 8.4%. Based on this, it would be expected that 0.18% of Arabian foals would be homozygous for the trait and hence clinically affected. Pedigree analysis suggests that the SCID trait was introduced to the United States by a single stallion in the 1920s.

Immunoglobulin Deficiencies

Primary agammaglobulinemia is a rare disease of foals. Affected animals have no identifiable B cells (cells with surface immunoglobulins) and have very low immunoglobulin levels. Their lymphoid tissues contain no primary follicles, germinal centers, or plasma cells. Nevertheless, their blood lymphocytes can respond to mitogens and produce the cytokine migration inhibitory factor (MIF). Intradermal inoculation of phytohemagglutinin induces a typical type IV delayed hypersensitivity reaction. Affected foals experience recurrent bacterial infections but can survive for 17 to 18 months. The disease should be suspected in a foal having a normal lymphocyte count but

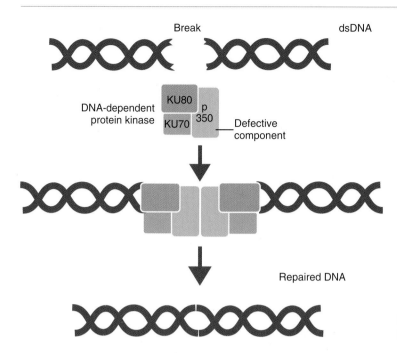

FIGURE 37-7 The defect in DNA dependent protein kinase that prevents DNA repair in SCID foals.

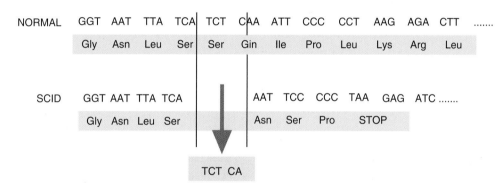

FIGURE 37-8 The gene deletion in the equine *DNA-PK* gene that leads to premature termination of the molecule.

lacking both IgM and IgG. It may be confirmed by showing normal T cell responses to mitogens and an absence of B cells.

Selective IgM deficiencies have been described in foals. Serum IgM levels in these animals are at least two standard deviations below normal, but IgG and IgA levels and B cell numbers are normal. In most cases, foals have septicemia or recurrent respiratory tract infections, often involving *Klebsiella pneumoniae* or *R. equi,* and die by 10 months of age. Some affected foals live longer and respond to therapy but fail to grow, have recurrent respiratory infections, and die by 24 months of age. Most affected foals have been Arabians or quarter horses, suggesting that the disease may have a genetic basis. IgM deficiency has also been described in adult horses over 2 years of age. In many cases such horses have a lymphoreticular neoplasm.

A single case of IgG deficiency has been described in a 3-month-old foal with salmonellosis. The animal had normal IgA and IgM but no germinal centers, lymphoid follicles, splenic follicles, or periarteriolar lymphoid sheaths. Serum IgG was extremely low.

Between 2 and 3 months of age, some foals experience a transient hypogammaglobulinemia as a result of a delayed onset of immunoglobulin synthesis. These animals may have recurrent infections during the period when their immunoglobulin levels are low. Lymphocyte numbers and responsiveness remain normal at this time.

Common Variable Immunodeficiency

Common variable immunodeficiency is the second most common primary immunodeficiency syndrome in humans (after selective IgA deficiency.) It is a heterogeneous group of sporadic diseases all characterized by a failure of B cells to make antibodies. The genetic basis of the disease is therefore variable. In most cases, the B cell deficiency is secondary to defects in CD4+ T cell function. Mutations in genes coding for tumor necrosis factor (TNF) receptors and other co-stimulatory molecules also result in loss of helper T cell function. Unlike the other primary immunodeficiencies, most cases are diagnosed in adults.

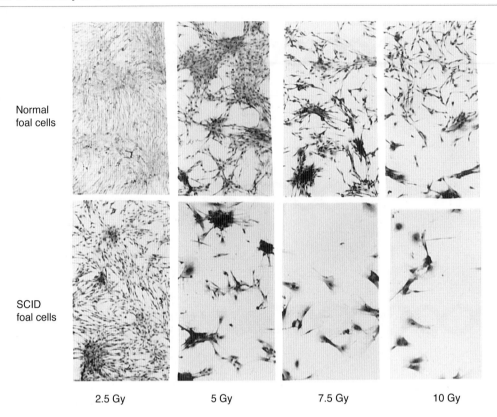

Normal
foal cells

SCID
foal cells

2.5 Gy   5 Gy   7.5 Gy   10 Gy

FIGURE 37-9 The effect of radiation on normal foal fibroblasts and on fibroblasts from a SCID foal. Equivalent numbers of cells were exposed to varying amounts of ionizing radiation as indicated and cultured in chamber slides. Five days later the slides were fixed, stained, and photographed. Note that there are many fewer SCID cells surviving this treatment since they are unable to repair their DNA. (Courtesy Dr. K. Meek.)

Cases of common variable immunodeficiency have been recorded in horses. Although they resemble primary immunodeficiencies in their sporadic nature and severity, they usually occur in animals older than 3 years of age. Typically, the horses present with recurrent infections that are not responsive to medical treatment. Bacterial meningitis may be a consistent feature. Their serum contains only trace levels of IgG and IgM, no detectable IgG3, and very low IgA levels. Sometimes individual IgG subclasses are deficient, whereas IgA levels are normal. T cell numbers are normal, but B cells are undetectable, and there is no response to the B cell mitogen lipopolysaccharide. On necropsy, there are no B cells in lymphoid organs, blood, or bone marrow. Some horses may have severe liver disease, a feature also seen in humans. It is suspected that these individuals have an underlying defect that is only expressed when the immune system is stressed by infection. Other cases have included horses between 2 and 5 years old with a selective IgM deficiency. Many develop a concurrent lymphosarcoma, and limited evidence suggests that they have excessive regulatory T cell function.

Foal Immunodeficiency Syndrome

This primary immunodeficiency syndrome was first described in the highly inbred Fell and Dales pony breeds. It presents as a B cell immunodeficiency accompanied by a profound anemia. Affected foals appear normal at birth but fail to thrive. Their hematocrit and B cell numbers decline over 4-12 weeks until clinical disease develops. Affected animals lack germinal centers and plasma cells. Their B cell numbers decline to less than 10% of normal and serum immunoglobulin levels drop rapidly once maternal antibodies are catabolized. The loss of these immunoglobulins coincides with the development of clinical disease. T cell numbers remain within the normal range. Animals develop severe respiratory disease caused by opportunistic pathogens such as adenoviruses and diarrhea caused by cryptosporidium. At the same time, they develop a profound progressive, non-regenerative anemia which alone may be sufficient to cause death. Foals inevitably die or are euthanized by 1-3 months of age.

The syndrome is inherited as an autosomal recessive condition. It results from a mutation in the gene coding for a protein called sodium/myoinositol co-transporter (*SLC5A3*). (The mutation switches a single amino acid from proline to leucine.) This protein controls cellular osmotic regulation and is required for lymphoid cell survival and erythropoiesis. Because this mutation may occur in any horse breed, the original name, Fell pony Immunodeficiency syndrome, has been changed to Foal Immunodeficiency Syndrome. A PCR-based test is available that can be used to determine whether a foal carries the mutant gene. Heterozygous carriers can be identified and bred in such a way that they have healthy offspring.

Incidence of Immunodeficiencies

The most important immunodeficiency in foals is not inherited but results from a failure to absorb sufficient colostral antibodies from the mare (Chapter 21). This failure of passive transfer may affect up to 10% of all foals. SCID occurs in 2% to 3% of Arab foals and is 10 times more common than selective IgM deficiency. Selective IgM deficiency is, in turn, 10 times more common than agammaglobulinemia.

Immunodeficiencies of Cattle

Severe Combined Immunodeficiency

A combined immunodeficiency has been recorded in an Angus calf. The animal was apparently normal when born and suckled normally. It became ill, however, at 6 weeks of age when it developed pneumonia and diarrhea. The animal was lymphopenic and severely hypogammaglobulinemic. It had undetectable IgM and IgA and a low level of IgG, which was believed to be due to residual maternal antibodies. The animal died within a week with systemic candidiasis. It had a hypoplastic thymus consisting of epithelial cells but no thymocytes. It had no detectable lymph nodes and a hypoplastic spleen that had no lymphocytes within its periarteriolar lymphoid sheaths. The syndrome thus closely resembled equine SCID.

Selective Immunoglobulin G2 Deficiency

IgG2 deficiency has been reported in red Danish cattle. About 1% to 2% of this breed are completely deficient in this immunoglobulin subclass and as a result have an increased susceptibility to pneumonia and gangrenous mastitis. Up to 15% may also have low IgG2 levels, although this does not appear to cause any ill effects.

Hereditary Parakeratosis

Certain Black Pied Danish and Friesian cattle carry an autosomal recessive trait of thymic and lymphocytic hypoplasia (trait A-46). Affected calves are born healthy, but by 4 to 8 weeks they begin to experience severe skin infections. If untreated, they die within a few weeks, and none survive for longer than 4 months. Affected calves have exanthema, hair loss on the legs, and parakeratosis around the mouth and eyes. There is depletion of lymphocytes in the GALT and atrophy of the thymus, spleen, and lymph nodes. These animals are T cell deficient and have depressed cell-mediated immunity but normal antibody responses. Thus they mount a normal antibody response to tetanus toxoid but respond poorly to dinitrochlorobenzene or tuberculin, both of which induce cell-mediated reactions. If these calves are treated by oral zinc oxide

or zinc sulfate, they recover the ability to mount normal cell-mediated responses. If, however, the zinc supplementation is stopped, the animals will relapse within a few weeks. It is probable that these animals have a reduced ability to absorb zinc from the intestine. Zinc is an essential component of the thymic hormone thymulin (Chapter 12) and is therefore required for a normal T cell response.

Other Immunodeficiencies

A transient hypogammaglobulinemia associated with a delayed onset of immunoglobulin synthesis has been recorded in a Simmental heifer, and a case of thymic aplasia with absence of hair has been described in calves. It is probably similar to the "nude" mutation seen in mice and cats (discussed later).

Immunodeficiencies of Dogs

Combined Immunodeficiencies

A severe combined immunodeficiency resulting from a defect in the catalytic subunit of the DNA-dependent protein kinase (DNA-PK$_{cs}$) has been identified in Jack Russell Terriers. From a single breeding pair of terriers, 12 of 32 siblings died from opportunistic infections between 8 and 14 weeks of age. These animals showed a SCID phenotype with lymphopenia, agammaglobulinemia, and thymic and lymphoid aplasia. The disease appeared to be inherited as an autosomal recessive condition. It resulted from a point mutation, leading to stop codon formation and premature termination of the peptide chain 517 amino acids before the normal C-terminus. Affected dogs showed severely diminished expression of DNA-PK$_{cs}$. As in equine SCID, the defect blocks gene splicing during *V(D)J* recombination in TCR and immunoglobulin variable regions. The carrier frequency of this gene is 1.1%.

An X-linked SCID has been recorded in Basset Hounds and Cardigan Welsh Corgis. The disease is characterized by stunted growth, increased susceptibility to infections, and absence of lymph nodes. Clinically, animals are healthy during the immediate neonatal period as a result of maternal antibodies. However by 6 to 8 weeks, as the levels of maternal antibodies decline, the animals begin to develop infections. At first these are relatively mild infections, such as superficial pyoderma and otitis media. Eventually, they become more severe, and untreated animals die of severe pneumonia, enteritis, or sepsis by 4 months of age. Common infections include canine distemper, generalized staphylococcal infections, adenoviral and parvoviral infections, and cryptosporidiosis. It is interesting to note that *Pneumocystis* pneumonia has not been recorded in these dogs. This immunodeficiency is an X-linked disorder since breeding of a carrier female to a normal sire results in approximately half the males in each litter being affected and all the females being phenotypically normal.

On examination these dogs are lymphopenic (~1000/µL). Their CD4/CD8 ratio is, however, approximately 15:1, compared with normal dogs that have a ratio of 1.7:1. This indicates a major drop in CD8+ cell numbers. The absolute number of T cells is less than 20% of normal. The dogs have normal numbers of B cells. The few lymphocytes in the blood are unresponsive to mitogens. The puppies have normal IgM levels but very low, or no, IgG and IgA. These dogs do not make antibodies against antigens such as tetanus toxoid.

On necropsy the thymus of affected dogs is approximately 10% of the normal weight and lacks a defined cortex (Figure 37-10). Their lymph nodes and tonsils are very small and dysplastic and may be very difficult to find. When present, the nodes are disorganized and contain very few small lymphocytes. Their spleens contain large periarteriolar lymphoid nodules with occasional small lymphocytes and few plasma cells. The bone marrow in these dogs appears normal. Approximately 40% of the thymocytes of these dogs are CD4−, CD8−, compared with 16% in normal dogs.

The disease results from a mutation in the gene coding for the γ chain of the IL-2R *(IL-2Rγ)*. The same chain is also a component of the IL-4, IL-7, IL-9, and IL-15 receptors and has been designated the common γ chain, γc. In affected Basset Hounds, a loss of four bases in the γc gene causes a frameshift. As a result of this frameshift, a stop codon is generated. Thus, instead of the complete protein, only a small peptide is produced, and no functional protein is made. A second SCID mutation has been described in Cardigan Welsh Corgis. In these animals a single cytosine residue is inserted into the γc gene so that a stop codon is generated before the transmembrane domain, resulting in a failure to synthesize the complete chain (Figure 37-11). As a result this peptide is not expressed on the cell surface. In both cases, the mutation does not interfere with IL-2 production, but the lymphocytes of these

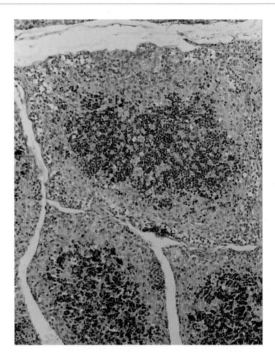

FIGURE 37-10 Photomicrograph of the thymus of a basset hound with X-linked immunodeficiency. Note the lack of a defined cortex and the scattered foci of dark-staining lymphocytes. (H&E stain.)

(From Snyder PW, Kazacos EA, Felsburg PJ: Histologic characterization of the thymus in canine X-linked severe combined immunodeficiency, *Clin Immunol Immunopathol* 67:55–67, 1993.)

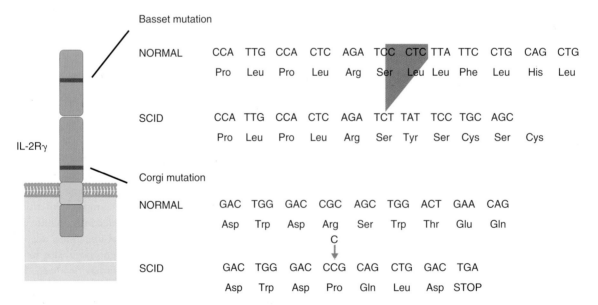

FIGURE 37-11 The two defined canine X-linked SCIF mutations in the *IL-2Rγ* gene. In the Corgi mutation, the insertion of a single cytosine residue into the gene leads to the generation of a stop codon and premature termination of peptide synthesis. In the Basset mutation, deletion of four bases causes a frameshift mutation and also leads to the generation of a stop codon (not shown).

(Data from Henthorn PS, Somberg RL, Fimiani VM, et al: IL-2R gamma gene microdeletion demonstrates that canine X-linked severe combined immunodeficiency is a homologue of the human disease, *Genomics* 23:69–74, 1994; and from Somberg RL, Pullen RP, Casal ML, et al: A single nucleotide insertion in the canine interleukin-2 receptor gamma chain results in X-linked severe combined immunodeficiency disease, *Vet Immunol Immunopathol* 47:203–214, 1995.)

animals are unresponsive to IL-2. In the absence of a γc chain, mature T cells will not develop.

Experimentally, affected dogs may be "cured" by bone marrow allografts. Reconstitution with normal bone marrow results in the appearance of normal donor T cells and a mixed chimerism ranging from 30% to 50% donor B cells. It is interesting to note, however, that SCID dogs kept alive by stem cell allografts begin to age prematurely at 2 to 3 years. They develop intestinal malabsorption and neural cell tumors. Presumably the absence of *DNA-PK$_{cs}$* prevents the repair of other cells, leading to premature aging.

Immunoglobulin Deficiencies

A selective IgM deficiency has been reported in two related Doberman pinschers. One animal was asymptomatic, whereas the other had a chronic mucopurulent nasal discharge and bronchopneumonia. Both these animals had high IgA, low IgG, and very low IgM. They experienced only a chronic nasal discharge, so the clinical significance of this deficiency is in doubt.

Selective deficiencies of IgA have been observed in several breeds of dogs, but German Shepherds are especially predisposed to a range of infectious disorders, including mycoses, anal furunculosis, deep pyoderma, and small intestinal bacterial overgrowth. This suggests that they may have deficiencies in mucosal immunity. Consistent with this is the observation that German shepherds in the United Kingdom have normal IgM and IgG levels but significantly reduced levels of IgA (~80 mg/dL, as opposed to 170 mg/dL in control dogs.) Likewise, dogs of this breed have significantly lower concentrations of IgA in their tears compared with other breeds. They have normal numbers of IgA-producing plasma cells, implying that the deficiency may be due to defective synthesis or secretion of IgA. German Shepherds have significantly reduced median IgA levels in feces compared with control dogs of other breeds. Many have IgA concentrations below the 95% confidence limit of the control population, and some lack detectable fecal IgA. Their fecal IgG and albumin levels tend to be higher than controls.

Shar-pei puppies with recurrent cough, nasal discharge, conjunctivitis, and pneumonia, as well as demodicosis and *Microsporum canis* infections, have been identified as having a selective IgA deficiency (<15 mg/dL). Likewise, abnormally low IgA concentrations have been found in a high percentage of clinically normal Shar-pei dogs. A high prevalence of atopic disease is observed in these dogs, a feature also seen in IgA-deficient humans.

A primary IgA deficiency has been described in an inbred Beagle colony. The colony had a history of parainfluenza and endemic kennel cough due to *Bordetella bronchiseptica*. Despite vaccination, these animals continued to experience recurrent respiratory tract infections and otitis. Immunoelectrophoresis and radial immunodiffusion showed that affected dogs had normal serum IgG and IgM levels but very little IgA (<5 mg/dL). Phenotypically normal parent dogs had very low IgA levels. Four affected dogs had circulating anti-IgA antibodies. Their T and B lymphocyte numbers and lymphocyte responses

to mitogens were normal, as was their response to tetanus toxoid. They had a normal number of plasma cells secreting IgG and IgM but no plasma cells secreting IgA. When two affected animals were mated, four out of five pups in a litter were IgA deficient. The disease was not sex linked.

A transient hypogammaglobulinemia has been seen in two animals from a litter of Spitz puppies that experienced recurrent upper respiratory tract infections between 8 and 16 weeks of age. These dogs had normal T cell numbers and mitogen responses. They had low immunoglobulin levels and low antibody titers to vaccine antigens at 16 weeks. These puppies responded very weakly to tetanus toxoid when it was administered at 4 months. By 6 months, however, immunoglobulins had risen to normal levels, and the puppies regained their health. It is believed that these puppies experienced a delayed onset of immunoglobulin synthesis. Symptomatic treatment is sufficient to support these animals until their immune system becomes functional.

Cavalier King Charles Spaniels with *Pneumocystis* pneumonia had IgG concentrations that were significantly lower in infected dogs (median, 3.2 mg/mL) than in breed- and age-matched control dogs (median, 8.5 mg/mL). IgM levels, in contrast, were significantly higher in the affected dogs. IgA levels were within the normal range. Lymphocyte counts in affected dogs were normal or high. This may well be an IgG-deficiency syndrome.

Pneumocystis pneumonia has been observed repeatedly in young miniature dachshunds. The affected animals are usually less than 1 year old and appear to be immunodeficient. Serum electrophoresis shows a marked reduction in IgM, IgG, and IgA. In addition, lymphocyte responses to both phytohemagglutinin and pokeweed mitogens are severely depressed. There is a reduction in B cell numbers. Although the *Pneumocystis* pneumonia responds to aggressive therapy, these animals rarely do well and die young.

T Cell Deficiencies

A family of inbred Weimaraners has been reported as having immunodeficiency and dwarfism. The animals appeared normal at birth, but at 6 to 7 weeks they developed a wasting syndrome characterized by emaciation and lethargy. The puppies began to experience recurrent infections that eventually killed them. On necropsy their thymuses were atrophied and lacked a cortex. These animals had normal immunoglobulin levels, their helper cell activity was unimpaired, and their secondary lymphoid organs appeared normal. Their lymphocytes were unresponsive to mitogens. Growth hormone treatment caused thymic cortical regeneration and a dramatic clinical improvement. However, growth hormone did not restore lymphocyte responsiveness to mitogens. The disease is almost certainly due to a deficiency of growth hormone as a result of a lesion in the hypothalamus and confirms that the thymus requires growth hormone to function.

Lethal acrodermatitis has been identified in Bull Terriers. This is a complex immunodeficiency syndrome associated with growth retardation, skin lesions (acrodermatitis, chronic pyoderma, paronychia), diarrhea, recurrent pneumonia, and abnormal behavior. The puppies were weak at birth and did not nurse well. Some showed a lighter pigmentation than their littermates. When weaned, they had difficulty eating and failed to grow. Small, crusted lesions developed between the digits, and a pustular dermatitis developed around the eyes and mouth at 6 to 10 weeks. The lesions developed into a severe pyoderma. Fungi such as *Malassezia* and *Candida* were readily isolated from the lesions. Diarrhea developed early in the disease, and respiratory tract infections were common. The puppies became depressed and sluggish and died by 15 months of age, with a median survival of 7 months. They had a neutrophilia, normal IgG and IgM levels but significantly lower IgA levels, and hypercholesterolemia. Plasma zinc levels were unusually low. They showed depressed lymphocyte mitogen responses. On necropsy there was a severe loss of T cells so that the puppies lacked a thymus, and the lymph nodes and spleen were very small. The disease is inherited as an autosomal recessive disease, and the parents of affected puppies could be traced to one common ancestor. Because of its similarities to trait A-46 of cattle, these dogs were treated with oral zinc (discussed earlier). Very high doses resulted in some clinical improvement, but this could not be sustained.

German Shepherd pyoderma is, as its name implies, a chronic skin disease that occurs in middle-aged German Shepherds and is associated with infection with coagulase-positive staphylococci. These cases do not respond well to antibiotic therapy, and it is believed to reflect some form of underlying genetic or immunological defect. Although affected dogs appeared to mount normal humoral responses, limited studies have shown reduced lymphocyte responses to mitogens, an imbalance of lymphocyte subsets (CD4 cells are depressed, CD8 cells are increased), and a decline in the level of CD21+ B cells. (The complement receptor CD21 plays a role in B cell activation). When the number of CD3+ T cells and B cells were examined in normal dog skin and in the skin of dogs with pyoderma, it was found that the B cell numbers were similar but that the number of T cells infiltrating the lesions in German Shepherds was significantly reduced. Studies of T cell function in these animals have also demonstrated a functional defect. This suggests that T cell dysfunction may play a role in the pathogenesis of pyoderma in this breed.

Uncharacterized Immunodeficiencies

The veterinary literature contains several reports of dogs with severe recurrent infections caused by organisms that are not normally considered to be highly pathogenic. Protothecosis has been recorded in dogs. One third of the cases have been in Collies, suggesting an inherited predisposition. Weimaraners are unusually susceptible to some systemic bacterial infections; German Shepherds are susceptible to generalized systemic *Aspergillus* infections, whereas some Rottweiler and Doberman families are unusually susceptible to parvovirus infection. None of these have been shown to be due to primary immunodeficiencies, and all require further investigation.

Immunodeficiencies of Cats

Hypotrichosis with Thymic Aplasia

The nude mouse has long been accepted as an important mouse model of immunodeficiency. Nude mice are a strain of hairless mice that fail to develop a functional thymus. This disease has been described in rats, guinea pigs, and calves. A similar mutation has been described in Birman kittens. These kittens were born without any body hair (Figure 37-12). On necropsy they also had no thymus and had depletion of lymphocytes in the paracortex of lymph nodes, spleen, and Peyer's patches. Thus they were effectively T cell deficient. Analysis of the pedigree suggested that the disease was inherited as an autosomal recessive disease.

Immunodeficiencies of Mice

Nude Mice

The best-known mouse model of immunodeficiency is the nude mouse. Nude mice are a strain of hairless mice whose thymic epithelial cells are nonfunctional as a result of a defect in the gene for a transcription factor called FoxN1. (Similar mutations have been observed in rats, guinea pigs, calves, and cats.) Because their thymic epithelial cells fail to function, the primitive thymus in nude mice develops into cysts with walls of immature epithelial cells that do not produce mature T cells. They do possess a limited number of immature T cells and B cells so that a few lymphocytes may be found in peripheral blood. Normal thymus grafts, by restoring epithelial cell function, permit the T cells of nude mice to mature and develop immune competence. Nude mice are deficient in conventional

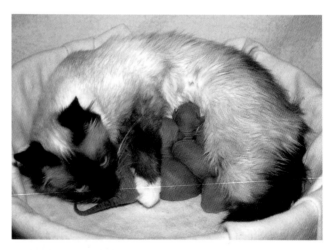

FIGURE 37-12 Kittens born with an autosomal recessive form of congenital hypotrichosis with thymic aplasia-nude kittens.

(From Casal ML, Straumann U, Sigg C, et al: Congenital hypotrichosis with thymic aplasia in nine Birman kittens, *J Am Anim Hosp Assoc* 30:600–602, 1994. Courtesy Dr. M.J. Casal.)

cell-mediated immune responses, as reflected by prolonged allograft survival and lack of responses to T cell mitogens. Their IgG and IgA levels also are depressed, presumably as a result of a loss of helper T cells.

Although nude mice show enhanced susceptibility to virus-induced tumors, they fail to develop more than the normal level of spontaneous tumors. This observation was, for many years, a major objection to the immunological surveillance theory because if T cells destroy tumors, T cell–deficient animals should have an increased incidence of tumors. However, nude mice possess normal numbers of NK cells, which may protect them in the absence of T cells.

Severe Combined Immunodeficiency Mice

SCID mice have very low numbers of B cells and T cells. Development of B cells is halted before expression of cytoplasmic or cell membrane immunoglobulins. T cell development is also arrested at a very early stage, and those lymphocytes that do reach the bloodstream are CD4−, CD8−. They have no immunoglobulins and are unable to mount cell-mediated immune responses. *Scid* mice survive relatively well for about a year in specific-pathogen-free facilities but eventually die of *Pneumocystis* pneumonia. The defects in *scid* mice result from an inability to rearrange their BCR or TCR V region genes correctly. Several different mutations in the DNA joining enzymes have been identified. As a result the cells cannot produce functional receptors, and no functional T or B cells are produced. As in SCID horses, the mouse *scid* mutations also increase sensitivity to ionizing radiation since these animals are unable to repair DNA damage. About 15% of *scid* mice are "leaky"; they have low levels of immunoglobulins of limited heterogeneity and can reject allografts. Antigen-presenting cells, myeloid and erythroid cells, and NK cells are normal in *scid* mice.

Moth-Eaten Mice

Moth-eaten mice have a defective T cell system but produce excessive quantities of immunoglobulins and develop autoimmune disease. Their name comes from their appearance. Within a few days of birth, neutrophils invade their hair follicles and cause patchy loss of pigment. These animals lack cytotoxic T cells and NK cells. Mice that are *me/me* have a short life span and usually die as a result of lung damage. The thymus of these animals involutes unusually early, and the emigration of prethymocytes into the thymus is impaired. The B cell hyperactivity may be due to excessive production of some B cell–stimulating cytokines.

X-Linked Immunodeficiency

Xid mice have a recessive, X-linked B cell defect so that they are unable to respond to certain T-independent carbohydrate antigens. They lack certain B cell subsets. Mice that are *bg/nu/xid* are severely immunosuppressed since they lack T, B,

and NK cells. Lightly irradiated *bg/nu/xid* mice can accept human bone marrow xenografts.

Immunodeficiencies of Humans

Many different immunodeficiency syndromes have been reported in humans. It is anticipated that investigators will succeed eventually in identifying most of these syndromes in domestic animals as well.

The most important phagocytic deficiency syndrome of humans is chronic granulomatous disease. This has not yet been reported as occurring in domestic animals, although it undoubtedly does. Children affected with chronic granulomatous disease have recurrent infections characterized by the development of septic granulomas in lymph nodes, lungs, bones, and skin. The neutrophils of these children are less capable than normal cells of destroying organisms such as staphylococci and coliforms. Their specific lesion is a defect in one of the subcomponents of the NADPH oxidase (NOX) complex.

Infants suffer from several different forms of combined immunodeficiency. The most severe is reticular dysgenesis, which results from a defect in the development of both myeloid and lymphoid stem cells. Other combined immunodeficiencies result from defects in the development of both T and B lymphoid stem cells. Some of these CID cases are due to a deficiency of the enzyme adenosine deaminase. In other cases there is a defect in the genes coding for interleukin-2 (IL-2) or IL-7 receptors, for recombinase-activating gene proteins, for CD25, for the CD3γ chain, or for MHC class I or class II molecules. The standard treatment for all these diseases is a stem cell allograft.

T Cell Deficiencies

The DiGeorge anomaly results from a failure of the third and fourth thymic pouches to develop. In consequence, no thymic epithelial tissue develops, and few cells populate the T-dependent areas of the secondary lymphoid tissues. Since these infants have no functional T cells, they can neither mount a delayed hypersensitivity reaction nor reject allografts. The importance of T cells in protection against viruses is emphasized by the observation that infants with the DiGeorge anomaly generally die of virus infections but remain resistant to bacteria.

B Cell Deficiencies

The most severe of the B cell deficiencies, called Bruton-type agammaglobulinemia, is an X-linked recessive disease that affects early B cell development. Affected infants are devoid of all immunoglobulin classes. They experience recurrent infections due to bacteria such as pneumococci, staphylococci, and streptococci but are usually resistant to viral, fungal, and protozoan infections. The disease results from a mutation in a receptor tyrosine kinase. Inherited deficiencies of individual immunoglobulin classes have also been recorded in humans. As might be anticipated, there are many possible combinations of deficiencies in IgG, IgM, IgA, and IgE, and a tendency to give each a specific name leads to confusion. One of the most important of these is Wiskott-Aldrich syndrome. In this disease, a selective IgM deficiency is associated with multiple infections, eczema, and thrombocytopenia. Another such syndrome is ataxia-telangiectasia, in which serum IgA and IgE levels are extremely low or absent and cerebellar and cutaneous abnormalities exist. Affected children, lacking an effective surface immune system, have recurrent bacterial respiratory tract infections. Ataxia-telangiectasia results from a defect in DNA repair mechanisms. In another disease called hyper-IgM syndrome, a defect in the CD40 ligand leads to a defect in late B cell development and a failure in the IgM class switch so that affected individuals have high levels of IgM but very low (or absent) IgG and IgA. Patients suffer from recurrent respiratory tract infections. The most common human primary immunodeficiency is an IgA deficiency that affects 1 in 600 Caucasians. Some of these individuals are asymptomatic; others suffer from an increased frequency of respiratory and gastrointestinal infections. The genetic defect appears to lie within the MHC complex.

Immunodeficiencies of Chickens

Birds of the hypothyroid OS strain have a selective IgA deficiency. Birds of the UCD 140 line have a selective IgG deficiency called hereditary dysgammaglobulinemia. These birds have normal immunoglobulin levels for about 50 days after hatching; then their IgG drops, and their IgM and IgA rise. In addition to hypogammaglobulinemia, UCD 140 strain birds develop immune complex lesions, and it has been suggested that a vertically transmitted virus mediates this disease.

For sources of additional information, please visit http:// evolve.elsevier.com/tizard/immunology/

Secondary Immunological Defects

□ **Key Points**

- Immunodeficiencies caused by damage to the immune system (secondary immunodeficiencies) are not uncommon in domestic animals.
- The most important causes of immunosuppression are viral infections. To survive within a host, viruses may cause profound immunodeficiency either by infecting and killing lymphocytes or by causing them to become cancerous.
- Other important causes of immunodeficiencies include stress, both physical and mental, some environmental toxins, malnutrition (both starvation and obesity), and old age.

The immune system, like any body system, is subject to destruction and dysfunction as a result of attacks by pathogenic and environmental agents. Among the most important of these agents are microorganisms, especially viruses, toxins, stress of various types, old age, and malnutrition.

Virus-Induced Immunosuppression

Viruses that affect the immune system may be divided into those that affect primary lymphoid tissues and those that affect secondary lymphoid tissues. Both types of virus can cause profound immunodeficiencies. For example, in chickens, the infectious bursal disease virus (IBDV) destroys lymphocytes in the bursa of Fabricius. IBDV is not completely specific for bursal cells; it also destroys cells in the spleen and thymus. These tissues usually recover, whereas the bursa atrophies. The resulting immunosuppression, as might be predicted, is most evident in young birds infected soon after hatching, at a time when the bursa is actively engaged in generating B cells.

One of the most important animal viruses that destroys secondary lymphoid organs is canine distemper. Canine distemper virus, although it can multiply in many different cell types, has a predilection for lymphocytes, epithelia, and nervous tissue. Its primary cellular receptor is CD150, expressed on activated B and T cells. The distemper virus spreads from its initial invasion sites in the tonsils and bronchial lymph nodes to the bloodstream, where it kills both T and B cells and causes a lymphopenia. Subsequently it invades secondary lymphoid organs such as the spleen, lymph nodes, mucosal lymphoid tissues, and bone marrow, where it destroys more cells. The virus also invades and destroys the thymus. The shedding of infected cells from these lymphoid organs enables the virus to reach epithelial tissues and the brain. Canine distemper virus triggers lymphocyte and macrophage apoptosis and produces profound immunosuppression. It also suppresses production of interleukin-1 (IL-1) and IL-2 while stimulating prostaglandin release by macrophages. As a result, lymphocyte responses to mitogens are depressed, immunoglobulin levels fall, and skin allograft rejection is suppressed. This immunosuppression accounts, in large part, for the clinical signs of canine distemper. For example, many dogs with distemper develop *Pneumocystis* pneumonia. (*Pneumocystis* is a fungus that occurs in the lungs. It does not cause disease in immunocompetent animals but produces a severe pneumonia in animals with suppressed immune function. Indeed, the development of *Pneumocystis* pneumonia is evidence of a significant immunodeficiency.) If germ-free dogs are infected by virulent distemper virus, they develop a relatively mild disease, presumably because secondary infection cannot occur.

Loss of lymphocytes is common in virus infections since viral survival and persistence may require immunosuppression (Figure 38-1). Thus a lymphopenia occurs in feline panleukopenia, canine parvovirus-2 infection, feline leukemia, and African swine fever. Bovine virus diarrhea virus (BVDV) causes destruction of both B and T cells in the lymph nodes, spleen, thymus, and Peyer's patches. As in canine distemper, surviving B cells fail to make immunoglobulins and respond poorly to mitogens. Viral destruction of Peyer's patches causes intestinal ulceration and leads to secondary bacterial invasion. Both persistently infected cattle and normal cattle infected with cytopathic BVDV have depressed neutrophil functions, and

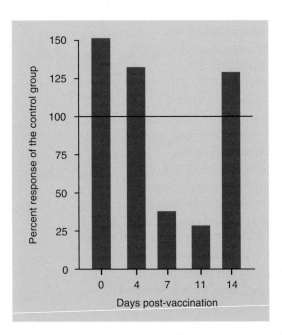

FIGURE 38-1 The immunosuppressive effect of viruses. The effect of administering a mixed vaccine (containing canine distemper, canine adenovirus, canine parainfluenza, canine parvovirus-2, and leptospira) on the response of a puppy's lymphocytes to the mitogen phytohemagglutinin. Control levels were 100%.

(Redrawn from Phillips TR, Jensen JL, Rubino MJ, et al: Effects of vaccines on the canine immune system, *Can J Vet Res* 53:154–160, 1989.)

bacterial clearance from the blood is impaired. A related virus, border disease virus, preferentially infects CD8+ T cells and interferes with their cytotoxic and immunoregulatory functions.

Herpesviruses are also immunosuppressive. For example, equine herpesvirus-1 causes a drop in T cell numbers and depresses cell-mediated responses in foals. Bovine herpesvirus-1 (BHV-1) also causes a drop in T cells and in the responses to T cell mitogens. Although BHV-1 stimulates bovine alveolar macrophages to express increased amounts of MHC class II and promotes antibody-mediated phagocytosis, it also depresses macrophage-mediated cytotoxicity and IL-1 synthesis. Parainfluenzavirus-3 and infectious bovine rhinotracheitis viruses have long been known to interfere with alveolar macrophage function. They inhibit phagosome-lysosome fusion, paving the way for secondary infections with *Mannheimia hemolytica* in stressed calves. Porcine reproductive and respiratory syndrome (PRRS) virus in pigs causes destruction of alveolar macrophages and predisposes affected animals to severe enzootic pneumonia. It also kills dendritic cells, a feature that may account for the ability of PRRS virus to persist in pigs for up to 6 months.

The effect of some viruses on the immune system may be relatively complex or anomalous. In maedi-visna, a neurological disease of sheep caused by a retrovirus, cell-mediated immune responses such as graft rejection are suppressed, whereas B cell responses are enhanced (Chapter 26). Some leukemia viruses may be selectively immunosuppressive, so that depression of the IgG response is greater than that of the IgM response. In equine infectious anemia, the IgG3 response is variably depressed, whereas synthesis of the other immunoglobulin classes remains unaffected.

The results of virus-induced lymphoid tissue destruction are readily seen. Animals are lymphopenic and have reduced lymphocyte responses to mitogens. For example, responses to phytohemagglutinin are depressed in influenza, measles, canine distemper, Marek's disease, Newcastle disease, feline leukemia, bovine virus diarrhea, and lymphocytic choriomeningitis. Destruction of lymphoid tissues may also result in hypogammaglobulinemia or a reduced response to antigens. Thymic atrophy and lymphopenia are common manifestations of many virus infections, and before any primary immunodeficiency syndrome is diagnosed, rigorous steps must be taken to exclude the possibility that it is, in fact, secondary to a virus infection.

Retrovirus Infections in Primates

More than 40 lentiviruses have been isolated from nonhuman primates, especially African species. These simian immunodeficiency viruses include SIV_{mac} isolated from a rhesus macaque (*Macaca mulatta*) in a laboratory; SIV_{agm} from an African green monkey (*Chlorocebus sabaeus*); SIV_{sm} from a sooty mangabey (*Cercocebus atys*); SIV_{mnd} from a mandrill (*Mandrillus sphinx*); and most important, SIV_{cpz} from a chimpanzee (*Pan troglodytes*). SIV_{cpz} is the ancestor of HIV-1, whereas SIV_{sm} is the ancestor of HIV-2. All these isolates selectively invade CD4+ T cells. When SIV_{mac} infects rhesus macaques and other Asian species, it stimulates a strong but ineffective immune response. Viral replication continues and eventually causes an immunodeficiency syndrome similar to human AIDS. The infection is believed to be transmitted sexually. Clinical disease progression is slow, but the animals eventually develop lymphadenopathy, severe weight loss, chronic diarrhea, lymphomas, neurological lesions, and opportunistic infections by organisms such as *Pneumocystis*, *Mycobacterium avium-intracellulare*, *Candida albicans*, and *Cryptosporidium parvum*. The macaques are immunosuppressed as a result of depletion of CD4+ T cells, macrophages, and dendritic cells. The virus invades both T cells and macrophages using two cellular receptors, CD4 and either the receptor for the chemokine CCR5 or for CXCR4. About 25% of infected animals do not mount a significant response to SIV and die within 3 to 5 months as a result of a severe SIV encephalitis. Macaques that mount an immune response usually die 1 to 3 years after infection. Spontaneous recovery does not occur. The other SIVs cause persistent viremia but rarely result in disease in African primates. This is because they rapidly develop an antiinflammatory response that prevents chronic T cell activation and apoptosis.

Type D Simian Retroviruses

An acquired immunodeficiency syndrome (AIDS) develops in primates infected with one of several endogenous type D simian retroviruses (SRVs). These viruses, much more common than the lentiviruses, are transmitted by biting; vertical transmission rarely occurs. SRVs have a much broader tissue tropism than the SIVs and, in addition to lymphocytes and macrophages, can also infect fibroblasts, epithelial cells, and the central nervous system. The SRVs destroy both B and T cells, leading to death from opportunistic infections. The syndrome is associated with a profound drop in serum IgG and IgM levels and a severe lymphopenia. Monocyte function is unimpaired, but surviving lymphocytes do not respond to mitogens. Affected monkeys are also profoundly neutropenic. On necropsy, the monkeys have a generalized lymphadenopathy, hepatomegaly, and splenomegaly. There is a loss of lymphocytes from the T-dependent areas of the secondary lymphoid organs. B cell areas show an initial hyperplasia of the secondary follicles followed by the loss of these follicles and an absence of plasma cells. These histological changes are very similar to those seen in AIDS in humans. In many cases, normally innocuous agents such as *Pneumocystis*, cytomegalovirus, *C. parvum*, and *C. albicans* cause infection. Some affected monkeys develop tumors such as fibrosarcomas. About half of the infected animals develop neutralizing antibodies and survive the disease. The others die from septicemia or diarrhea with wasting.

Retrovirus Infections in Cats

Feline Leukemia

Feline leukemia virus (FeLV) is an oncogenic retrovirus that can cause both proliferative and degenerative diseases in cats (Figure 38-2). Three naturally occurring viral variants are recognized based on the structure of their gp70 protein. FeLV-A is the predominant, naturally transmitted variant. It is present in all FeLV-infected cats. The other variants are only found in association with FeLV-A. When FeLV-A combines with endogenous retroviral sequences (sequences that are stably integrated into the cat genome and are normally never expressed but are genetically transmitted), FeLV-B is formed. FeLV-B is found in about 50% of viremic cats and has a greater propensity than FeLV-A to cause tumors. FeLV-C is found in about 1% to 2% of infected cats and arises from FeLV-A through a mutation in the envelope gene. It is much more suppressive for bone marrow than FeLV-A.

FOCMA A unique surface protein, called feline oncornavirus cell membrane antigen (FOCMA), is expressed on FeLV-infected cells. It is coded for by endogenous retroviral genes within the cat genome. It is not expressed on normal cells but rather on cells infected with FeLV. It was originally believed that the presence of FOCMA on a cell membrane identified the cell as an FeLV-induced tumor cell. Of those cats that fail to make neutralizing antibodies to FeLV and remain viremic, about 80% develop antitumor activity by making antibodies against FOCMA. A cat that makes antibodies to FOCMA can usually destroy virus-induced tumor cells. Unfortunately, antibodies to FOCMA do not confer protection against the FeLV-induced degenerative diseases, and viremic cats that fail to

produce anti-FOCMA antibodies are fully susceptible to all the FeLV syndromes, including lymphosarcoma. Some feline lymphosarcoma cells may express FOCMA in the absence of evidence of FeLV infection.

Transmission FeLV is shed in saliva and nasal secretions and is thus transmitted between cats by grooming. On natural exposure to FeLV, about 70% of cats become infected, but the remaining 30% do not. Of the infected cats, about 60% become immune, and 40% become viremic. Of the viremic cats, 10% cure spontaneously, whereas the remaining 90% remain infected for life. Of these persistently viremic animals, about 15% live normal healthy lives, but the remaining animals die within 3 to 5 years from FeLV disease. Lymphoid tumors develop in 15% to 20% of FeLV-infected cats. Persistently viremic cats have a half-life of 1 year.

Pathogenesis Once FeLV infects a cat, the virus first grows in the lymphoid tissues of the pharynx and tonsils. This is followed by a transient viremia as it spreads throughout the body and infects the other lymphoid organs. A mild lymphopenia occurs 1 to 2 weeks after infection. This is of variable duration but lasts longer in young cats than in adults. There is also a variable neutropenia. Antibodies develop between 7 and 42 days after the onset of infection, and the virus is cleared between 28 and 42 days. Virus can be found in the thymus at day 1, in blood between 2 and 145 days, and in lymphoid organs between 3 and 28 days. The presence of both antibodies and virus results in the production of immune complexes and the development of a membranoproliferative glomerulonephritis. Some cats may lose their viremia but remain latently infected. In latently infected animals, the virus persists in the bone marrow, but there is no virus in the blood, and virus-neutralizing antibodies are present. Treatment with steroids or culturing bone marrow cells in vitro allows productive re-expression of the virus. Stress (e.g., crowding, shipping) may cause a recurrence of viremia in 5% to 10% of cats. The presence of neutralizing antibodies does not correlate well with the disease state, and challenging recovered cats may not provoke a secondary antibody response. Prenatal or early infection of kittens with FeLV can also result in a persistent viremia.

Tumors Cats probably have the highest prevalence of lymphoid tumors of any domestic mammal. Most of these lymphoid tumors are caused by FeLV. They include lymphosarcoma, reticulum cell sarcoma, erythroleukemia, and granulocytic leukemias. The lymphosarcoma caused by FeLV is usually of T cell origin, although FeLV grows in cells of many types and is not restricted to lymphoid tissues. Some FeLV lymphomas in the intestine may be of B cell origin. When tumors develop in FeLV-infected cats, not all can be shown to contain the virus. The proportion of virus-positive tumors ranges from 100% of myeloid leukemias to 30% of alimentary lymphomas. In young cats FeLV-induced tumors are mainly of T cell origin. In older cats, they tend to originate from both T and B cells.

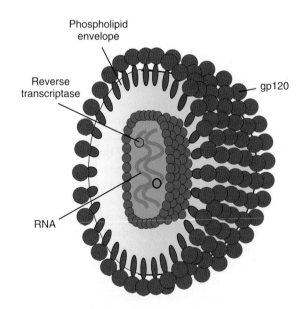

FIGURE 38-2 The structure of a typical retrovirus such as feline leukemia virus or feline lentivirus.

Phospholipid envelope

Reverse transcriptase

gp120

RNA

Immunosuppression

T Cell Defects FeLV develops T cell tropic variants as a result of mutations in their envelope genes. These immunodeficiency-inducing variants replicate to high numbers in T cells. They enter T cells by binding to two receptors. One receptor is a phosphate transporter protein (Pit1). The second is a novel cell surface protein called FeLIX ("FeLV infectivity X-essory protein"). The lymphopenia in FeLV-infected cats is due to a loss of CD4+ T cells. CD8+ T cells may also drop in the early stages of the disease so that the CD4/CD8 ratio may remain within normal limits. (The CD4/CD8 ratio in normal cats ranges from about 0.4 to 3.5, with a median value of about 1.9.) CD8+ T cell numbers eventually recover, and the CD4/CD8 ratio then drops. B cell numbers may also be depressed, but this depends on the severity of secondary infections. Kittens infected with FeLV develop a wasting syndrome associated with thymic atrophy and recurrent infections. Depending on the severity of the secondary infections, this may be associated with either lymphoid atrophy or lymphoid hyperplasia. In cats without secondary infection, lymphoid atrophy is associated with loss of cells from the paracortical areas of lymph nodes. Changes in the spleen are less marked but may result in a reduction in the entire white pulp. As a result of T cell loss, FeLV infected cats have depressed cell-mediated immunity. This depression is probably due to the effects of p15e, the immunosuppressive envelope protein of the FeLV virus, which is produced in very large quantities by dying cells. The p15e suppresses the responses of cats to FOCMA, suppresses lymphocyte mitogen responses, and blocks the responses of T cells to IL-2. As a result, FeLV-infected cats may carry skin allografts for about twice as long as normal cats (24 days compared with 12). Leukocytes of infected cats produce significantly less IL-2 than leukocytes from normal cats. This decline is especially marked in cats with leukemia or lymphosarcoma arising in the thymus. This immunosuppression also predisposes viremic cats to secondary diseases such as feline infectious peritonitis, mycoplasmosis, toxoplasmosis, septicemia, and fungal infections. Bone marrow stem cells are also inhibited by p15e, preventing production of erythroid cells and causing a nonregenerative anemia.

B Cell Defects In contrast to the severe T cell dysfunction, B cell activities in FeLV-infected cats are only mildly impaired. There may be poor responses to low doses of antigen as well as reduced IgM production, but serum IgG levels remain normal. Because B cell function and antibody production are relatively normal in chronically infected cats, antibodies to the virus are produced in large quantities. These antibodies combine with circulating virions or soluble proteins to form immune complexes. The immune complexes are deposited in the renal glomeruli and cause severe mesangioproliferative glomerulonephritis, leading to hypoproteinemia, edema, uremia, and death. Viral antigens binding to erythrocytes can also cause an antiglobulin-positive hemolytic anemia. Immune complexes also activate the classical complement pathway. As a result, complement will be consumed, and FeLV cats may have very low levels of complement. This loss may reduce resistance to tumors since normal cat serum infused into leukemic cats can cause tumor regression.

FeLV-AIDS During natural FeLV infection, a highly immunosuppressive form of the virus may develop. Called FeLV-AIDS, this causes fatal immunodeficiency in nearly 100% of infected cats. The isolate consists of two virus populations. One, designated 61E, is replication competent but does not induce immunodeficiency disease by itself. The other, 61C, is replication defective, but when inoculated together with 61E, it induces a fatal immunodeficiency syndrome.

The immunodeficiency syndrome is characterized by progressive weight loss and lymphoid hyperplasia followed by severe lymphoid depletion, chronic diarrhea, and opportunistic infections. The onset of disease is preceded by an inability to respond to T-independent antigens. As early as 9 weeks after infection, the CD4+ T cells produce lower levels of B cell stimulatory cytokines. This is followed by a drastic drop in CD4+ T cells, whereas CD8+ T cell and B cell numbers remain normal. The clinical defect in FeLV-AIDS is an inability to mount antibody responses, although in vitro B cell function appears to be normal. The immunodeficiency is associated with mutations in a 34-amino acid sequence at the C-terminus of viral gp70. The mutation changes the conformation of the surface glycoprotein and prevents the virus from blocking infection by additional virions, leading to subsequent cell killing.

Immunity About 40% of cats infected with FeLV do not mount an adequate immune response against the virus and become persistently infected. Persistently infected cats remain viremic. The remaining 60% of infected cats mount a strong immune response. These cats develop virus-neutralizing antibodies to the major envelope glycoprotein, gp70. Immune cats also develop virus-specific cytotoxic T cells to viral gag/pro antigens. These prevent the virus from invading cells, and these cats become strongly immune. Antibodies against antigens other than gp70 may also play a role in immunity.

Three types of effective vaccines are currently available against FeLV. One type contains supernatant fluid from a cell line persistently infected with FeLV. This fluid contains several of the major protein antigens of FeLV. The second type of FeLV vaccine consists of inactivated whole virions from tissue culture, which are usually administered with a powerful adjuvant. The third type of FeLV vaccine is a canarypox vectored recombinant product that can be administered without an adjuvant. Widespread vaccination has significantly reduced the prevalence of this disease in the United States. These vaccines do appear to differ in their ability to prevent latent infections, although they are effective in preventing the development of clinical disease.

Diagnosis The introduction of sensitive molecular diagnostic techniques to replace serologic assays has changed our views on persistent FeLV infections. Real-time and reverse-transcriptase polymerase chain reaction (PCR) assays are much more

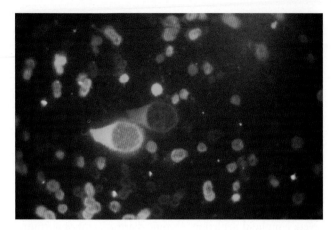

FIGURE 38-3 A positive indirect immunofluorescence assay for FeLV in a peripheral blood smear.
(Courtesy Dr. F.C. Heck.)

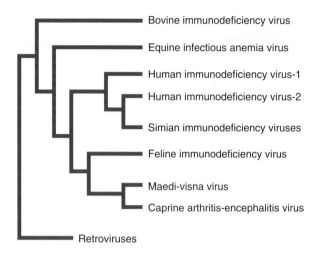

FIGURE 38-4 A dendrogram showing the relationships of the major lentiviruses.

sensitive and specific than virus isolation, antigen detection, or immunofluorescence. These tests have shown that many cats may have FeLV DNA integrated into their cells but never develop an antigenemia. Vaccines may be able to prevent the development of clinical disease but not proviral integration. These latent infections may persist for years, and viremia or disease develops occasionally. On the other hand, this integrated viral DNA may also be required for long-term protection. Other cats may have both detectable viral nucleic acids and antigenemia (i.e., active infections). FeLV antigenemia may be detected by an antigen-capture ELISA, by the membrane filter technique, or by rapid immunochromatography of blood or serum. A direct immunofluorescent test on a buffy coat smear using antibodies to group-specific antigen can detect cell-associated antigen and hence intracellular viremia (Figure 38-3). Alternative testing methods include testing saliva or tears using material collected on a swab or filter paper strips.

Feline Immunodeficiency Virus

Feline immunodeficiency virus (FIV) was originally isolated from cats with clinical immunodeficiency. The virus is an enveloped, single-stranded RNA virus belonging to the lentivirus subgroup of retroviruses. It is differentiated from FeLV (a γ-retrovirus) by the biochemical requirements of its reverse transcriptase. (FIV reverse transcriptase requires magnesium, whereas FeLV requires manganese.) FIV is related to HIV, the cause of AIDS (Figure 38-4). FeLV and FIV are distinctly different viruses, and antibodies made against one do not react with the other. Nevertheless, approximately 12% to 33% of FIV-infected cats may also be infected with FeLV, an especially potent immunosuppressive mixture. At least five different genetic clades (or subtypes) of FIV have been identified. Subtype variations may account for differences in pathogenicity, tissue tropism, and clinical disease.

Transmission FIV is spread by territorial free-roaming male cats through aggressive biting. As a result, it occurs predominantly in old male cats that spend a lot of time outdoors. Oral exposure is a potential route of infection in suckling kittens, and chronically infected queens transmit the virus to more than half their kittens in utero. Noninfected kittens from chronically infected queens show reduced neonatal viability. FIV can also be sexually transmitted. In households where cats live together nonaggressively, sharing food or water bowls and undergoing mutual grooming, the infection is poorly spread. In the United States, 1% to 3% of normal healthy cats and 10% to 15% of chronically ill cats are infected with FIV. In other countries, such as Japan, the infection rate may be as high as 44%.

Pathogenesis Experimental FIV infection is characterized by four distinct clinical stages. The acute stage lasts for several weeks. Infected cats develop a fever about 3 to 10 weeks after exposure to FIV. The virus is carried to local lymph nodes, where it replicates in T cells. It then spreads to other lymph nodes throughout the body. FIV can be isolated from infected cats as early as 10 to 14 days after infection. Viremia increases until day 21, peaks again at 7 to 8 weeks, and then declines. Disease severity varies from no clinical signs to generalized lymphadenopathy and lymphoid hyperplasia. Cats can develop fever, anorexia, dehydration, and diarrhea with mild pneumonitis, conjunctivitis, and nephritis. They may develop a mild lymphopenia and a severe neutropenia at this time. The lymphopenia is due to a loss of CD4+ T cells. Cats rarely die at this stage unless they are also infected with FeLV, in which case they die of a panleukopenia. Antibodies to FIV develop 2 to 6 weeks after infection and persist throughout infection. Most cats recover from the acute stage and appear clinically healthy.

The asymptomatic, or latent, stage may last as long as 10 years and is longer in young than in older cats. Cats appear healthy during this stage, but their CD4+ T cell numbers drop progressively. Their lymph nodes show gradual hypoplasia, leading to aplasia. Cats may also develop bone marrow suppression, including leukopenia and anemia. Thus this stage is marked by progressive impairment of immune function, but it may be many years before severe immunodeficiency and AIDS-like signs develop.

The gradual onset of progressive generalized lymphadenopathy marks the third stage of the disease. This lasts for months to years and is associated with vague signs of ill health, such as recurrent fever, inappetence, weight loss, chronic stomatitis, arthritis, and behavioral abnormalities. Lymph nodes develop follicular hyperplasia. As a result of the growing immunodeficiency, cats may develop secondary but not opportunistic infections. These are mainly bacterial infections affecting the oral cavity, skin, and digestive tract. Cats show some weight loss (<20%), anemia, lymphopenia, and neutropenia.

The final stage is a severe AIDS-like disease that lasts for a few months until the cat dies. Cats show a weight loss of greater than 20%. Secondary lymphoid tissues show follicular involution. Because of their severe immunodeficiency, opportunistic infections develop. These can include feline herpesvirus type 1, rodent poxviruses, vaccine-induced rabies, FeLV, staphylococcal infections, anaerobic infections, tuberculosis (*M. avium-intracellulare*), *Cryptococcus,* toxoplasmosis, mange, lungworms, and heartworms. The animals have anemia, lymphopenia, and neutropenia. Malignancies and ocular and neurological disease also occur. In naturally infected cats, clinical findings are highly variable because of the great variety of potential secondary infections. They can include chronic fever, oral cavity disease (periodontitis, gingivitis, stomatitis) leading to inappetence or pain on eating, chronic upper respiratory tract disease, chronic enteritis leading to persistent diarrhea, and conjunctivitis. Some cats may experience cystitis, chronic skin disease, fever, anorexia, lethargy, abortion or reproductive problems, vomiting, anemia, leukopenia, lymphosarcoma, and myeloproliferative disorders. Neurological signs have been described in FIV-infected cats, and the virus has been shown to infect the central nervous system. Half of FIV-infected cats have neurological dysfunction, as demonstrated by abnormal behavior, convulsions, ataxia, paralysis, and nystagmus. FIV is associated with demyelination in the dorsal columns of the spinal cord, vacuolization of the myelin sheaths in the spinal nerve roots, and perivascular and perineuronal mononuclear cell infiltration. Ocular lesions, especially anterior uveitis, conjunctivitis, and glaucoma, have also been noted.

Immunosuppression FIV can replicate in CD4+ and CD8+ T cells, B cells, megakaryocytes, neuronal cells, and macrophages. Some strains only replicate well in lymphocytes, whereas other strains replicate well in both lymphocytes and macrophages. Some FIV strains can also grow in fibroblasts in vitro. Primary targets of FIV infection are the lymphocytes. However, as infection persists, the virus increasingly affects macrophages. In clinically ill cats with a high viral load, macrophages are the major sites of viral replication. FIV-infected cats have fewer neutrophils, a lower proportion of T cells, and a higher proportion of B cells compared with uninfected animals.

FIV binds specifically to CD134 expressed on a subset of CD4+ T cells. This binding, in conjunction with binding to the α-chemokine receptor CXCR4 (CD184), is required for FIV to infect a cell. CD134 glycoprotein is upregulated on activated CD4+ T cells but not on activated CD8+ T cells.

Most naturally infected cats have a critical loss of CD4+ T cells (Figure 38-5). This loss is a result of destruction of infected cells, decreased production, and premature apoptosis. The surviving CD4 cells may show reduced responses to mitogens. FIV cats may show a shift away from a Th1 cytokine production pattern. They may also show an increase in CD8+ T cells. As a result, the CD4/CD8 ratio of FIV-infected cats may drop from a normal value of about two to less than one. FIV chronically activates CD4+, CD25+ regulatory T (Treg) cells, which further contributes to the immunosuppressive effect by downregulating IL-2 production and inhibiting CD4+ T cells proliferation. Affected cats show decreased IL-2 and Il-12

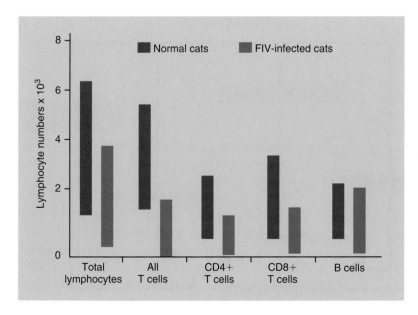

FIGURE 38-5 The numbers of cells in different lymphocyte populations (pan T, CD4, CD8, B cells) for 11 normal cats and 11 cats infected with feline immunodeficiency virus.

(From Novotney C, English RV, Housman J, et al: Lymphocyte population changes in cats naturally infected with feline immunodeficiency virus, *AIDS* 4:1213–1218, 1990.)

production as well as increased IL-10. Thus the rise in the IL-10/IL-12 ratio is especially immunosuppressive.

The lymphopenia that develops in both FeLV and FIV infections is due to a loss of T cells (Figure 38-6). CD4+ T cells are depressed in both, but the depression is much greater in FIV-infected animals. FIV-infected cats show a rapid drop in T cell numbers, whereas their B cells are unaffected. Their CD8+ T cells recover, but their CD4+ T cells fail to do so. Within 6 months of FIV infection, there is a measurable drop in CD4+ T cells. The response to thymus-dependent and -independent antigens initially remains unchanged. By 2 to 3 years after the onset of infection, however, the drop in CD4+ T cells continues, and the response to thymus-dependent antigens is profoundly depressed, while the response to thymus-independent antigens is unchanged. Other changes include reduced responses to T cell mitogens and IL-2, and reduced production of IL-2. Affected cats may upregulate IL-10 transcription, further contributing to their immunodeficiency. FIV-infected cats may have normal numbers of CD8+ T cells and B cells and normal levels of IgM and IgA. Indeed more than 25% of FIV-infected cats may be hypergammaglobulinemic as a result of polyclonal B cell activation Affected cats may also have immune complexes in their blood and deposited in renal glomeruli.

FIV infects T cells by first binding to CD134. But when the serum of FIV-infected cats is analyzed, 63% express autoantibodies to CD134! These anti-CD134 antibodies effectively block FIV infection ex vivo. These autoantibodies bind to a cryptic epitope on CD134 that is only exposed when FIV binds to CD134. The autoantibodies displace the viral glycoprotein and prevent infection. The presence of antibodies to CD134 correlates with lower viral loads and better health status of FIV-infected cats.

Immunity and Diagnosis Clinical symptoms are not sufficient to reliably diagnose FIV infection. The infection is

therefore diagnosed by testing for antibodies in serum by ELISA or immunochromatography and should be confirmed by Western blotting or PCR. Antibodies appear as early as 2 weeks after infection, and most cats are positive by 60 days. These antibodies persist for the life of the animal, although they may become undetectable in terminal disease. Maternal antibodies persist in most kittens born to FIV-positive queens for the first 8 to 12 weeks of life regardless of whether the kitten is infected. Some may remain seropositive for up to 16 weeks. These antibodies afford protection and kittens that receive high levels of antibodies from vaccinated or infected queens are protected.

Once infected with FIV, a cat will remain infected for life. However, viral regression may occur in kittens vertically infected by their mothers. At 3 to 4 months of age, these kittens may lose detectable antibody and virus in their blood, although the virus persists at low levels in bone marrow and lymph nodes and can be detected by PCR.

Envelope glycoproteins stimulate strong cell-mediated and humoral immunity in cats. Good results have been obtained using inactivated whole FIV and certain DNA vaccines. An adjuvanted, inactivated vaccine against FIV clades A and D is commercially available.

Treatment Treatment of FIV infection is symptomatic and involves the use of antibiotics to control bacterial infections, fluid therapy, and possibly dietary supplements. AZT (zidovudine, azidothymidine) is the only drug known to have an antiviral effect in clinically affected cats. It appears to improve the health of affected cats and increases both their quality of life and survival. Unfortunately, AZT-resistant strains of FIV may develop, and the drug seems to be of limited benefit in clinically ill cats. Encouraging results have also been obtained by the use of bone marrow allografts in association with antiviral therapy.

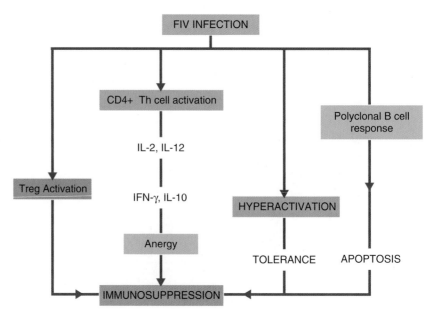

FIGURE 38-6 The major immunosuppressive pathways activated in FIV infections.

Retrovirus Infections in Cattle

Bovine Immunodeficiency Virus

Bovine immunodeficiency virus (BIV) is a lentivirus originally isolated from a cow with lymphosarcoma. The BIV-infected animal showed lymph node hyperplasia, lymphocytosis, central nervous system lesions, loss of weight, and weakness. When used to infect calves, BIV shows limited pathogenicity. The animals develop transient lymphocytosis, lymphadenopathy, and a nonsuppurative meningoencephalitis. BIV infection may also cause minor changes in the response of lymphocytes to mitogens and may suppress some neutrophil functions such as antibody-dependent cell-mediated cytotoxicity several months after infection. BIV can also infect sheep. In this species, experimental infection is associated with an increase in CD2+ and CD4+ T cells, as well as in the CD4/CD8 ratio, between 6 and 8 months after inoculation. The sheep showed no signs of illness by 1 year after inoculation and appeared to have normal immune function. BIV can also cause a chronic infection of rabbits, leading to splenomegaly and lymphadenopathy.

Jembrana disease is a lentivirus infection that occurs in Balinese cattle (*Bos javanensis*). It causes intense lymphoproliferation in the lymph nodes and spleen in these cattle. Animals that recover are completely immune.

Retrovirus Infections in Dogs

Several different retroviruses have been isolated from dogs. Some have been claimed to be lentiviruses, although the existence of a "canine immunodeficiency virus" has not been established. For example, a lentivirus has been isolated from the mononuclear cells of a leukemic German Shepherd in Israel. This virus does not appear to be closely related to the other major lentiviruses. On inoculation into newborn Beagles, it caused pronounced lymphadenopathy.

Another retrovirus has been isolated from a dog in the United States. This animal had anemia, neutropenia, lymphopenia, and thrombocytopenia, as well as depressed humoral and T cell–mediated immune responses. On necropsy the dog showed depletion of lymphoid organs and bone marrow hypoplasia. Yet it also had plasma cell infiltrates in many organs as well as multiple secondary infections. This retrovirus was of the C-type, and it possessed a gene related to the polymerase gene of bovine leukemia virus. It is also interesting to note that this animal had received multiple blood transfusions, a route of infection well recognized for HIV.

A lentivirus has also been isolated from a dog with hemorrhagic gastroenteritis. This animal showed a lymphopenia and agammaglobulinemia with lymphoid and bone marrow hypoplasia. The virus could grow in canine lymphocytes and thymocytes; it had a magnesium-dependent reverse transcriptase. The virus was present in bone marrow, intestine, and lymph nodes. It caused reduced synthesis of IL-2 and reduced responsiveness to IL-2, and it was cytotoxic for lymphocytes.

Circovirus Infections

Circoviruses are small, nonenveloped DNA viruses that tend to damage lymphoid tissues. They include the chicken anemia agent, which infects hemocytoblasts in the bone marrow and precursor T cells in the thymus, beak-and-feather disease virus, which can cause lymphoid atrophy in psittacine birds, and porcine circovirus-2 (PCV2), which is associated with postweaning multisystemic wasting syndrome (PMWS). PMWS is an acquired immunodeficiency syndrome of piglets characterized by wasting, lymphadenopathy, and respiratory disease with occasional pallor, jaundice, and diarrhea. Some affected piglets have a profound lymphocyte depletion, initially involving CD4+, CD8+, and double-positive T cells. T cell areas in tonsils and lymph nodes are depleted, and there is an absence of follicles in the cortex. Some pigs develop a necrotizing lymphadenitis as a result of hypertrophy and hyperplasia of their high endothelial venules, leading to thrombosis and necrosis. IgM-positive B cells are also reduced in more chronic cases. PCV2 also interferes with endocytosis by dendritic cells. Lymphoid depletion is directly related to viral load in lymphoid organs. Infected piglets suffer from a variety of secondary and opportunistic infections. Although PCV2 is the most likely causative agent, it has proved difficult to reproduce the disease consistently, and other factors including environmental factors, other infectious agents, and possibly immune stimulation are also involved.

Juvenile Llama Immunodeficiency Syndrome

A severe immunodeficiency syndrome has been recognized in young llamas. It has not been reported in other South American camelids. The disease is not due to failure of passive transfer since the median age of onset ranges from 2 to 30 months. Most affected animals are clinically normal and grow well until weaning. Initial signs include failure to grow, weight loss, and repeated multiple opportunistic infections with a variety of bacterial, fungal, and protozoan organisms. Respiratory tract infections are common. *Pneumocystis* infection has been recorded in some animals. The animals have low to low-normal lymphocyte numbers. They have depressed lymphocyte responses to mitogens such as phytohemagglutinin, concanavalin A, and streptococcal protein A. Lymph node biopsy specimens show marked depletion of T cells in the paracortical areas, and the primary follicles in the B cell areas are small and lack germinal centers. The animals also have low serum IgG levels and respond very poorly to *Clostridium perfringens* vaccines. Thus both T and B cell responses are depressed. The cause of this syndrome is unknown. Some investigators have detected reverse-transcriptase activity in tissues and have seen particles on electron microscopy that are compatible with a retrovirus infection. Nevertheless, the consistent occurrence of this disease in young llamas suggests that it may be inherited. Although treatment is supportive, the long-term prognosis for these animals is poor.

Other Causes of Secondary Immunodeficiency

Microbial and Parasite Infections

Immunosuppression generally accompanies infestation with *Toxoplasma* or trypanosomes, helminths such as *Trichinella spiralis*, arthropods such as *Demodex*, and bacteria such as *M. hemolytica*, the actinobacilli, and some streptococci (Chapters 25 to 27).

Toxin-Induced Immunosuppression

Many environmental toxins such as polychlorinated biphenyls, polybrominated biphenyls, dieldrin, iodine, lead, cadmium, methyl mercury, and DDT are immunosuppressive. $CdCl_2$ and $HgCl_2$ both inhibit phagocytosis by bovine leukocytes at very low concentrations. Higher concentrations are required to inhibit NK cell function and cell proliferation.

Mycotoxins are important immunosuppressants in cattle or poultry fed moldy grain. The most prevalent of these are derived from *Fusarium* species. These include the trichothecenes (T-2 toxin and deoxynivalenol) and the fumonisins. Deoxynivalenol administered to pregnant sows resulted is a low level of IgA in their colostrum and reduced IgA and IgG in their piglets 12 to 48 hours after first suckling. In dairy cattle deoxynivalenol causes immunosuppression, greater susceptibility to mastitis, and high somatic cell counts in milk. T-2 toxin depresses the response of calf lymphocytes to mitogens and decreases the chemotactic migration of neutrophils. T-2 toxin also reduces IgM, IgA, and C3 levels in cattle. Trichothecenes are also immunosuppressive in pigs and birds. Fumonisin B1 inhibits division of both T and B cells in piglets, increases interferon-γ (IFN-γ) production while suppressing IL-4 production, and increases susceptibility to *Escherichia coli* infections. Aflatoxins from *Aspergillus* species increase the susceptibility of chickens to *Salmonella* as a result of depressed phagocytosis. They increase the susceptibility of dairy cattle to mastitis. They depress piglet growth and reduced immune responses to *Mycoplasma*. Toxin-induced immunosuppression may be especially important in wild carnivores situated at the top of the food chain. A good example of this is seen in seals feeding on environmentally contaminated fish. These animals show depressed responses to vaccines, impaired mitogenic responses, lowered delayed hypersensitivity responses, and reduced NK cell numbers. This immunosuppression may decrease their resistance to phocine morbillivirus.

Malnutrition and Immunity

It has long been recognized that famine and disease are closely associated, and we tend to assume that malnutrition leads to increased susceptibility to infection. The effects of malnutrition on immune functions are however complex. Especially since malnutrition includes not only deficiencies but also excesses or imbalances of individual nutrients (Box 38-1).

In general, severe nutritional deficiencies reduce T cell function and therefore impair cell-mediated responses, at the same time sparing B cell function and humoral immunity. Thus starvation rapidly induces thymic atrophy as well as the level of thymic hormones. The number of circulating T cells drops, and cells are lost from the T cell areas of secondary lymphoid organs. Delayed hypersensitivity reactions are reduced, allograft rejection is delayed, and IFN-γ production is impaired. Some studies have suggested that protein starvation selectively suppresses Th2 responses such as IL-4 and IgE production, leading to increased susceptibility to parasite invasion.

Adipose Tissue Adipose tissue was long considered a resting tissue where fat reserves were stored until needed. It is increasingly clear, however, that adipose tissue plays a key role in both innate and adaptive immunity. The two key cell types found in adipose tissue are adipocytes and macrophages. Both produce multiple cytokines. For example, adipocytes produce two major cytokines (also called adipokines): leptin and adiponectin.

Leptin is a 16-kDa protein that binds to receptors in the hypothalamus and suppresses the appetite. The amount of leptin in blood is proportional to the amount of fat in the

---

◻ Box 38-1 | Intestinal Microflora and Obesity

The intestinal microflora exerts a profound influence on many metabolic processes throughout the body, and it has been suggested that it also influences obesity. For example, mice that lack TLR5 become obese. If these mice are treated with antibiotics to eliminate their intestinal microflora, obesity does not develop. When intestinal bacteria were transferred to microflora-depleted mice, the obesity syndrome developed. Other studies have shown that the diversity of the intestinal microflora and its metabolic pathways are consistently different in obese and lean humans and mice. Although it was originally believed that the intestinal microflora was "more efficient" in obese individuals, it is now believed that products from the microflora influence the immune system through the pattern-recognition receptors on innate immune cells to promote inflammation and adipose tissue deposition. This also explains why antibiotics in animal feed act as growth promoters. Perhaps obesity is contagious!

Sandoval DA, Seeley RJ: The microbes made me eat it, *Science* 328:178–179, 2010.

body. The fatter an animal, therefore, the more leptin is produced, and appetite is correspondingly suppressed. Conversely, caloric restriction and weight loss lead to a loss of adipocytes, a drop in leptin levels, and an increase in appetite (Figure 38-7). Breed-specific differences in leptin levels occur in dogs. The significance of this is unknown. In cats, leptin levels rise after spaying, which probably accounts for the weight gain commonly observed in these animals. In horses, leptin levels in colostrum are two to three times those in blood, and it has been suggested, therefore, that this leptin may be is required for intestinal development. Leptin is a potent macrophage activator. It enhances NK cell development and activation. Leptin also enhances Th1 cell production of IFN-γ, tumor necrosis factor-α (TNF-α), and leptin itself, thus generating an autocrine feedback loop.

Adiponectin is an adipokine that counteracts the activities of leptin. Its concentration is inversely related to body weight, and it has strong antiinflammatory activity. In lean animals, it decreases production of IL-8, IFN-γ, IL-6, and TNF-α while increasing the production of IL-1RA and IL-10. Adiponectin also regulates glucose and fatty acid metabolism. In obesity, adiponectin production drops, and adipose tissue macrophages

then produce a cytokine called resistin that increases insulin resistance leading to diabetes.

Adipose tissue in lean humans contains about 10% macrophages, whereas in obese humans, it may contain 50% macrophages. Leptin activates macrophages and dendritic cells. It increases their TNF-α, IL-6, and IL-1 production and upregulates expression of MHC class II. The increased IL-6 production by adipose tissue–associated macrophages promotes Th17-mediated responses. The abundant adipose tissue macrophages in obese individuals are classically activated M1 macrophages that release multiple proinflammatory cytokines. These cytokines decrease the sensitivity of other cells to insulin. Conversely, lean individuals with little fat have small numbers of alternatively activated M2 macrophages. These cells are activated by IL-4 and IL-13. The major source of these cytokines is eosinophils. (Since eosinophils are activated by parasitic worms, it is of interest to speculate that the weight loss observed in parasitized animals may be mediated by eosinophils.)

In lean animals, where leptin levels are low, macrophage activation is suppressed, inflammatory responses are reduced, and there is a shift from Th1 to Th2 responses while increasing Treg cells. In obese animals, however, widespread classic

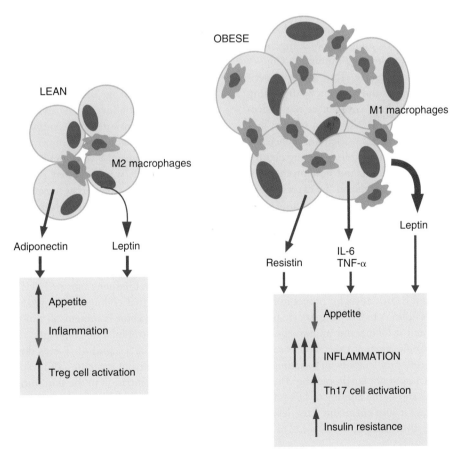

FIGURE 38-7 Obese adipose tissue is rich in classically activated (M1) macrophages that, in association with large quantities of leptin, generate proinflammatory cytokines, resulting in enhanced inflammation throughout the body. Lean adipose tissue, in contrast, contains small numbers of alternatively activated (M2) macrophages and produces little leptin, tending to suppress inflammatory reactions. Adiponectin contributes to this antiinflammatory effect, whereas resistin is proinflammatory.

macrophage activation predisposes to inflammatory diseases such as atherosclerosis, arthritis, and autoimmunity as well as to cancer. There is a clear link between obesity and inflammation. Given the increasing obesity of pets as well as some of the effects of rapid growth in food animals, veterinarians would be well advised to take this link into account.

Severe starvation has little effect on B cell functions. The B cell areas in lymphoid tissues and the number of circulating B cells remain unchanged. Serum immunoglobulins of all classes may remain normal or even rise. Secretory IgA levels commonly drop, but secretory IgE may rise, suggesting abnormal immunoregulation. Starvation, however, results in depressed complement levels and impairment of neutrophil and macrophage chemotaxis, the respiratory burst, release of lysosomal enzymes, and microbicidal activity.

Several trace elements are required for optimal functioning of the immune system. The most important are zinc, copper, selenium, and iron. Deficiencies of any of these are immunosuppressive. Zinc is especially critical to the proper functioning of the immune system since it acts as an ionic signaling messenger to promote T cell activation. Zinc-deficient pigs have reduced thymus weight, depressed cytotoxic T cell activity, depressed B cell activity, and depressed NK cell activity. They show decreased antibody production to T-dependent antigens. If pregnant animals are deprived of zinc, their offspring are immunosuppressed. Phagocytic cells from zinc-deficient animals show reduced chemotaxis and microbial ingestion. Mild zinc supplementation may promote immunity. Copper deficiencies are also immunosuppressive. Thus a copper deficiency reduces neutrophil numbers and function by depressing superoxide production. It also reduces lymphocyte responsiveness to mitogens; reduces T, B, and NK cell numbers; and enhances mast cell histamine release. Selenium deficiency depresses the function of most immune cells, reducing neutrophil activity, T and NK cell responses, and IgM production. Supplementation with selenium upregulates the expression of the IL-2R and prevents oxidative damage to immune cells. Iron deficiency is immunosuppressive for cell-mediated responses. However, the effects of this on resistance to infection may be complex since many pathogens require iron to replicate. A magnesium deficiency suppresses immunoglobulin levels.

Three vitamins, A, D, and E, are critical for proper immune function. Deficiencies of vitamin A reduce lymphocyte proliferation, NK cell activity, and cytokine and immunoglobulin production (Figure 38-8). Some vitamin A metabolites such as retinoic acid enhance T cell proliferation and cytotoxicity. Retinoic acid is especially important in promoting Th2 differentiation in the intestine and in the homing of IgA-positive B cells to mucosal surfaces. It also maintains Treg levels in the intestinal mucosa and thus maintains tolerance to food antigens (Chapter 22).

Vitamin E is a major antioxidant in cell membranes and is important in regulating the oxidants produced by phagocytic cells. Vitamin E deficiency depresses immunoglobulin levels through its effects on Treg cells and decreases lymphocyte

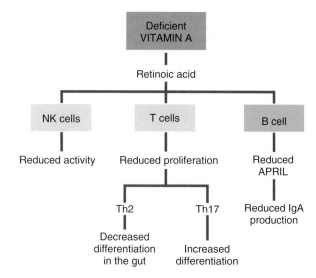

FIGURE 38-8 The functions of vitamin A and its metabolite, retinoic acid in immunity.

responses to mitogens. Animals deficient in vitamin E also show reduced IL-2 and transferrin receptor expression and depressed phagocytic function. Vitamin E is one of the few vitamins for which supplementation has been shown to enhance immune responses and disease resistance. The importance of vitamin E for proper functioning of the immune system has been seen in an inbred population of donkeys whose foals were dying from overwhelming bacterial infections at 3 to 5 months of age. Investigations revealed that these foals were agammaglobulinemic but also lacked detectable vitamin E in their serum. Vitamin E supplementation by injection caused an immediate clinical improvement in an affected foal, and within 2 months immunoglobulin levels were within normal limits. It was suggested that affected foals lacked a vitamin E transfer protein that prevented them from absorbing the vitamin. All subsequent foals in this herd received supplemental vitamin E and remained healthy.

When a bacterium such as *Mycobacterium tuberculosis* interacts with toll-like receptor 1 (TLR1) or TLR2 on macrophages, it upregulates many different genes and enhances their antimicrobial activity. One gene activated by TLR1 or TLR2 signaling in humans is that coding for the vitamin D receptor (Figure 38-9). This receptor is present on most immune system cells, including neutrophils, macrophages, and T cells. Binding of vitamin D to its receptor on T cells downregulates IFN-γ and IL-2 expression and promotes Th2 responses. It also promotes Treg cell differentiation in the skin. Binding to the receptor on macrophages, in contrast, promotes their activation and the production of cathelicidin and β-defensin-2. It is no coincidence that resistance to tuberculosis is directly related to serum vitamin D levels and that humans with a deficiency of vitamin D have significantly decreased resistance to this infection. It has been suggested that mice use nitric oxide rather than vitamin D as an intermediate in innate signaling because they are nocturnal, whereas humans acquire vitamin D from

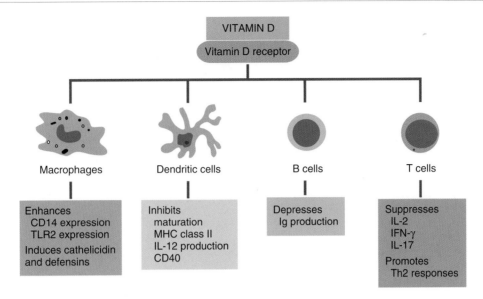

FIGURE 38-9 The importance of vitamin D in immunity. Note that vitamin D is a potent stimulator of innate immunity by enhancing production of antimicrobial peptides. It is, however, somewhat suppressive of adaptive immune responses.

sunshine on exposed skin. It is unclear whether similar mechanisms operate in domestic mammals.

Taurine deficiencies in cats can result in a neutropenia, although mononuclear cell numbers may rise. The neutrophils of taurine-deficient cats show decreased respiratory burst activity and phagocytosis. Although these cats may show a hypergammaglobulinemia, there is regression of germinal centers, suggesting a loss of B cell activity.

The effects of malnutrition may be reflected in altered resistance to infectious diseases. Because bacteria can readily survive and multiply in body tissues despite malnutrition of the host, starvation commonly increases the severity of bacterial infections such as pneumonia. Viruses, in contrast, require healthy host cells in which to grow. Malnutrition, by rendering host cells unhealthy, may therefore increase resistance to viruses. Overnutrition can also influence susceptibility to viruses. For example, overfed dogs show an increased susceptibility to canine distemper and canine adenovirus-1.

Exercise and Immunity

Regular moderate exercise boosts immune function. For example, increased antibody responses are seen in mice that get moderate exercise, compared with unexercised control mice. Exercise also raises blood neutrophil counts, enhances NK cell activity, promotes lymphocyte responses to mitogens, and increases blood levels of IL-1, IL-6, and TNF-α. Although mild exercise is good for immune function, high-intensity exercise, prolonged exhaustive exercise, or overtraining may induce a functional immunodeficiency. In horses, blood lymphocytes show a decreased proliferative response for up to 16 hours after a race. Acute exercise in the unfit animal can be especially stressful. Unfit horses subjected to strenuous exercise

showed significantly raised steroid levels, resulting in reduced proliferation of their lymphocytes to mitogens and influenza virus antigens and reduced neutrophil chemotactic responsiveness and chemiluminescence (a measure of respiratory burst activity) (Figure 38-10). These animals show a decline in their CD4/CD8 ratio as well as in both the number and activity of their NK cells. The age of an animal may moderate the effect of exercise on immune responses. For example, strenuous exercise significantly reduces lymphocyte proliferative responses in young horses yet has much less effect on older animals. This resistance of older horses to exercise-induced immunosuppression may result from their reduced steroid production.

The complex effects of extreme exercise on the immune system are well seen in dogs undergoing long endurance sled races. The proportion of dogs with low total globulin immediately after racing was significantly greater than before racing. In some of these dogs it remained low 4 months after the race. IgG was also lower after racing than before racing. Likewise serum IgM and IgE were higher before racing, although IgA was higher after racing. These changes in immunoglobulins might well affect resistance to infectious diseases.

Transportation stress is well recognized as predisposing to the development of respiratory disease in horses. A major reason for the impairment of respiratory defenses in transported horses is prolonged head elevation. With the head held high, mucociliary clearance is significantly reduced. Over time, this elevation permits the accumulation of bacteria, particulates, and inflammatory exudates in the trachea. After 24 hours of head elevation, significant pulmonary inflammation develops. It takes about 12 hours of free head movement for this inflammation to decline to normal levels. Transportation stress in calves has been reported to increase leukocyte and neutrophil counts and NK cell activity and to reduce T cell numbers.

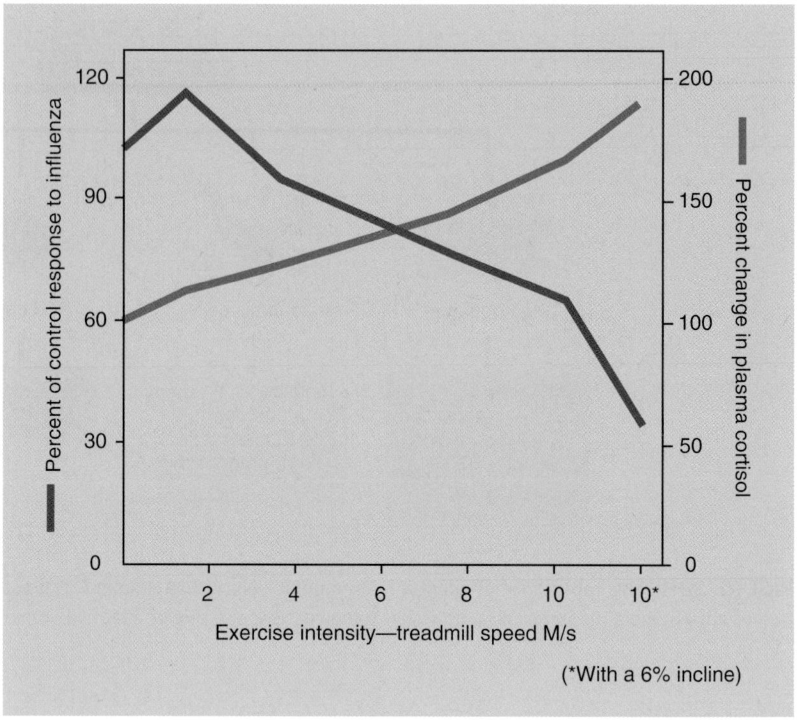

FIGURE 38-10 Although a moderate amount of exercise is good for the immune system, excessive exercise causes severe stress that can be immunosuppressive. In this example, six thoroughbred horses were subjected to a treadmill-based exercise challenge of various intensities (speed and incline). Blood samples were assayed for plasma cortisol levels by radioimmunoassay, and influenza virus–specific lymphocyte proliferation was assayed by thymidine incorporation. A clear relationship exists among exercise intensity, the stress response, and immune responsiveness.

(From data kindly provided by Drs. S.G. Kamerling, P.A. Melrose, D.D. French, and D.W. Horohov.)

Posttraumatic Immune Deficiency

Severely traumatized or burned animals commonly die of sepsis as a result of immunodeficiency. This is largely due to the production of large amounts of IL-10 and other immunosuppressive cytokines by macrophages. Corticosteroids, prostaglandins from damaged tissues, and a small protein called suppressive active peptide, which appears in serum following a burn, all have immunosuppressive properties. The deficiency develops within minutes or hours and recovers as wounds heal. It affects T cell, macrophage, and neutrophil function, but B cell function appears to be normal. As a result, delayed hypersensitivity reactions, allograft rejection, and T-dependent antibody responses are all impaired. IL-2 and IL-2R production are reduced. CD8+ cells are increased in injured individuals, suggesting that regulatory cell function may be enhanced. Macrophages lose antigen-presenting ability as they express decreased levels of MHC class II. Neutrophil and macrophage phagocytosis and respiratory burst activities are both impaired. Although surgery may result in some suppression of lymphocyte responses to mitogens, evidence suggests that routine surgery has no significant effect on the response of healthy animals to vaccination.

Age and Immunity

Innate Immunity Innate, cell-mediated, and humoral immune responses all decline with advancing age, a phenomenon called immunosenescence (Figure 38-11). For example, neutrophils and macrophages from the aged have an impaired ability to produce a respiratory burst and to produce nitrogen

oxidants. As a result, they are less able than cells from the young to kill ingested bacteria. Macrophage numbers decline in aged animals and express lower levels of TLRs. When stimulated with known TLR ligands, they secrete reduced amounts of IL-6 and TNF-α. Aged macrophages show reduced responses to activating agents such as IFN-γ. Aged Beagles (>8 years of age) show decreased neutrophil phagocytosis (a decline of 39% in their ability to kill *Lactococcus lactis*). Young dogs (<1 year of age) had significantly higher levels of messenger RNA for IL-8R, L-selectin, and IL-1β–converting enzyme compared with older dogs.

Dendritic cells from aged individuals are less effective at antigen presentation. Their reduced ability to present antigen to T cells results from changes in surface antigen expression and cytokine production. Their reduced ability to stimulate B cells is due to reduced immune complex binding. NK cells from elderly individuals are less effective at killing tumor cells. These defects in innate immunity may be more profound than defects in adaptive immunity in elderly individuals. Thus there may be a link between low-grade inflammation in the aged and geriatric syndromes such as the frailty of old age, a phenomenon called inflammaging. This low-grade inflammatory state has been identified in aged horses, where it may be due to pituitary pars intermedia dysfunction (PPID) secondary to neurodegeneration in the hypothalamus. Aged horses with PPID have increased blood levels of IL-8. The peripheral blood mononuclear cells from old horses produce more inflammatory cytokines than those from young horses. Likewise the cells from fat old horses produce more cytokines than cells from thin old horses. Reducing body weight and fat in old horses significantly reduces the percentage of IFN-γ– and

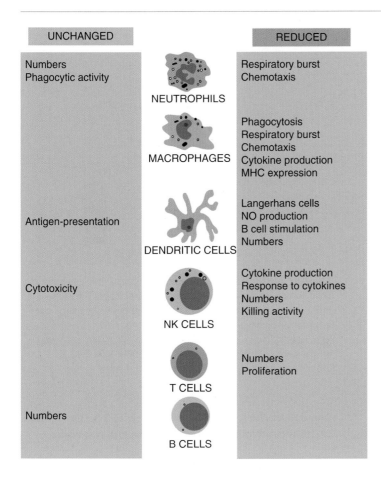

UNCHANGED		REDUCED
Numbers Phagocytic activity	**NEUTROPHILS**	Respiratory burst Chemotaxis
	MACROPHAGES	Phagocytosis Respiratory burst Chemotaxis Cytokine production MHC expression
Antigen-presentation	**DENDRITIC CELLS**	Langerhans cells NO production B cell stimulation Numbers
Cytotoxicity	**NK CELLS**	Cytokine production Response to cytokines Numbers Killing activity
	T CELLS	Numbers Proliferation
Numbers	**B CELLS**	

FIGURE 38-11 The changes in the immune system that occur with aging.

TNF-α-positive lymphocytes and monocytes and serum levels of TNF-α. The reverse was the case when weight and fat increased. Thus age-related obesity plays a role in the changes in the inflammatory response seen in older animals.

Lymphoid Organs Aging is associated with progressive dysregulation and structural changes in primary and secondary lymphoid organs. Thymic involution is the most obvious of these changes. Ileal Peyer's patches involute after sexual maturity in dogs. Old dogs have a decreased white pulp in the spleen. Lymph node changes vary depending on their location but include cortical atrophy and medullary fibrosis. Cats between 10 and 14 years of age had lower white cell, lymphocyte, and eosinophil counts than cats between 2 and 5 years of age. Absolute numbers of T cells, B cells, and NK cells were also lower in aged animals. Serum IgA and IgM, however, were higher in the aged group. There were no differences in their complement activity or their acute-phase responses. In Labradors, absolute numbers of leukocytes, lymphocytes, monocytes, granulocytes and CD3+, CD4+, CD8+, and CD21+ lymphocytes decreased significantly with increasing age.

B Cell Responses The bone marrow is relatively unaffected by old age, and an aged bone marrow can reconstitute the body as well as a young one. If aged B cells are mixed with young T cells, the response is relatively normal. If the reverse is attempted (i.e., mixing young B cells with aged T cells), the B cells respond poorly. Somatic mutation in immunoglobulin V region genes ceases in old animals so that antibody affinity tends to be lower than in young animals. Nevertheless, immunoglobulin concentrations do not decline in old age. Old dogs show little decline in antibody responses, although old horses have reduced antibody responses to influenza vaccination.

T Cell Responses The greatest impact aging has on the immune system is the decline of cell-mediated responses with age. The relative percentages of lymphocytes and CD4+ cells decrease, whereas the percentage of granulocytes and CD8+ cells increases. As a result, there is a decline in the CD4/CD8 ratio. There is significant thymic involution, leading to a decline in the numbers of CD4+ T cells and in the export of cells from the thymus. In addition, the lymphocyte population of the aged changes from a naïve population to a memory cell population. T cells from aged animals lose their ability to progress through the cell cycle. As a result, early events in the T cell response to antigens, such as activation of protein kinase C and the rise in intracellular calcium, are impaired. Even after expressing IL-2 receptors and being exposed to IL-2, aged T cells may not respond effectively to antigens. T cells from old dogs and horses show a decline in responses to mitogens. Analysis shows that some aged T cells continue to produce normal amounts of IL-2, but many do not. Thus aged T cell populations are mixtures of fully functional and impaired cells. In old horses (>20 years), there is a significant decrease in the proportion of CD8+ T cells and a rise in the CD4/CD8 ratio compared with young animals. Horses more than 20 years of age have reduced lymphocyte responses to mitogens, and this deficiency cannot be overcome by exposure to additional IL-2.

Aging causes increased susceptibility to certain viral infections, including herpesviruses. This increased susceptibility of aged mice results from excessive production of IL-17 by NK cells. This in turn leads to increased neutrophil recruitment and enhanced tissue damage. These mice also show a coincident decrease in IFN-γ production leading to a failure to control viral replication. Both of these changes are necessary to account for the increased lethality of herpesviruses in aged mice. A similar imbalance could well occur in other aged mammals.

Although aged animals may mount poorer primary responses to vaccines, their memory responses tend to remain unaffected. Elderly animals generally have persistent protective antibody levels and do respond by elevations in titer upon boosting. There is a difference with novel antigens. A recent study of dogs receiving rabies vaccine for the first time showed that a significant decrease in antibody titers and a corresponding increase in vaccine failures occurred in older dogs (Chapter 24).

Feeding a low-calorie diet has been shown to extend the life span of dogs significantly. One possible reason for this lengthened life span is the prevention of immunosenescence. Prolonged calorie restriction in dogs retarded age-related declines in lymphoproliferative responses, in absolute numbers of lymphocytes and in the T, CD4, and CD8 subsets. This may result from low circulating leptin levels. Calorie restriction appears to have no effect on neutrophil phagocytic activity, antibody production, or NK activity.

Despite the previous comments, young animals may show poorer resistance to some invaders than mature animals. This appears to be especially important in sheep. Lambs are more susceptible than mature sheep to parasitic and infectious diseases during the first year of life. Older sheep tend to show greater resistance to internal parasites such as *Haemonchus*, *Trichostrongylus*, and *Ostertagia*. Sheep younger than 1 year of age are more susceptible than mature sheep to virus diseases such as bluetongue and contagious ecthyma. Young sheep, 4 to 8 months of age, have a lower proportion of CD4+ T cells in their blood than mature sheep. Lymphocytes from young sheep produce less IFN-γ than those from adult sheep. Older sheep produce more antibodies to *Brucella abortus* lipopolysaccharide and responded more intensely to the contact sensitizer dinitrochlorobenzene. However, the two age groups did not differ in B cell or WC1+ T cell numbers and mounted comparable responses to diphtheria toxoid and tetanus. This mild

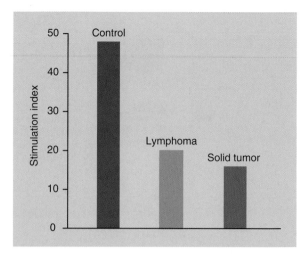

FIGURE 38-12 Immunosuppression in dogs with lymphomas or solid tumors compared with normal control dogs. The stimulation index is a measure of the response of lymphocytes to the mitogenic lectin phytohemagglutinin.

(Data taken from Weiden PL, Storb R, Kolb HJ, et al: Immune reactivity in dogs with spontaneous malignancy, *J Natl Cancer Inst* 53:1049–1056, 1974.)

immunodeficiency in lambs presumably reflects the immaturity of their immune system during the first year of life.

Other Secondary Immunodeficiencies

Immunodeficiencies may result from a wide variety of insults to the body. For example, immunoglobulin synthesis is generally reduced in individuals with absolute protein loss (patients with the nephrotic syndrome, heavily parasitized or tumor-bearing individuals, and patients who have experienced severe burns or trauma). Stress may result in immunodeficiencies. For example, it is possible to provoke a combined immunodeficiency syndrome by chilling newborn puppies for 5 to 10 days. Diverse stressors such as rapid weaning, sleep deprivation, general anesthesia, prolonged transportation, and overcrowding are all effective immunosuppressants. Physical destruction of lymphoid tissues can result in immunodeficiencies. For example, loss of lymphoid tissue leading to immunosuppression may occur in tumor-bearing animals, especially if the tumors themselves are lymphoid in origin (Figure 38-12). Adult horses with chronic diarrhea are immunosuppressed, as reflected by reduced IgA and reduced lymphocyte responses to mitogens. Some endocrine diseases such as thyrotoxicosis and diabetes mellitus may also result in immunosuppression.

For sources of additional information, please visit http:// evolve.elsevier.com/tizard/immunology/

Drugs and Other Agents That Affect the Immune System

□ Key Points

- There are many drugs that can suppress immune responses. The most widely used are corticosteroids. These prevent the activation of NF-κB and block many immune functions.
- Immunosuppressive drugs used to prevent allograft rejection or to treat autoimmune disease may either be nonspecific inhibitors of cell division or specifically block the activation of T cells by interfering with signal transduction.
- Drugs employed to stimulate the immune system commonly include microbial molecules that activate toll-like receptors (TLRs) in a nonspecific fashion.
- Cytokine therapy may eventually be useful in veterinary medicine, but the toxicity and cost of these molecules have so far prevented widespread clinical use.

Many clinical situations exist in which it is desirable to either stimulate or suppress the adaptive immune system, and many different drugs and techniques are available to do this. Indeed, this area of immunology is a discipline in its own right, called immunopharmacology.

Suppression of the Immune System

The methods available for inhibiting adaptive immune responses may be classified into two main groups. Older techniques generally involved administering treatment that, by inhibiting all cell division, reduced the response of T and B cells to antigens. This approach is crude and dangerous since other rapidly proliferating cell populations, such as intestinal epithelium and bone marrow stem cells, may also be severely damaged with potentially disastrous consequences. Recently, it has proved possible to selectively eliminate responding T cells by the use of specific antisera or monoclonal antibodies or by the use of highly selective immunosuppressive drugs.

Nonspecific Immunosuppression

Radiation

Radiation is immunosuppressive because it prevents cell division. It affects cells by several different mechanisms. The simplest of these is through ionizing rays hitting an essential, unique molecule, such as DNA, within the cell. A loss of even one nucleotide results in a permanent mutation of a gene, with potentially lethal effects on the progeny of the affected cell. Radiation also causes ionization of water and the formation of highly reactive free oxygen and hydroxyl radicals within the cell. The hydroxyl radicals react with dissolved oxygen to form toxic peroxides that destroy DNA and inhibit cell division. Although radiation is of some use in prolonging graft survival in experimental animals, especially laboratory rodents, the amount of radiation required for effective prolongation of graft survival in dogs is so high that it is lethal.

Corticosteroids

Corticosteroids are among the most commonly used immunosuppressive and antiinflammatory agents. Their effects, however, differ among species. Mammals may be classified as corticosteroid sensitive or resistant depending on the ease by which they can be depleted of lymphocytes. Laboratory rodents and humans are much more sensitive to the immunosuppressive effects of corticosteroids than are the major domestic mammals, and care should be taken not to extrapolate laboratory animal results directly to other species.

The effects of corticosteroids on cell function have a common pathway (Figure 39-1). Corticosteroids are absorbed directly into cells, where they bind to receptors in the cytosol. The corticosteroid-receptor complexes are then transported to the nucleus, where they stimulate the synthesis of IκBα, the inhibitor of NF-κB. In a resting cell, NF-κB is inactive since its nuclear binding site is masked by IκBα. When a lymphocyte is stimulated, the two molecules dissociate, the IκBα is degraded by proteasomes, and the released NF-κB moves to the nucleus and activates genes involved in inflammation and immunity. Corticosteroids, however, stimulate the production of excess IκBα. This excess continues to block NF-κB-mediated processes, including cytokine synthesis and T cell responses. As a result, corticosteroids suppress both immunological and inflammatory processes.

Corticosteroids influence immunity in four areas (Box 39-1): they affect leukocyte production and circulation; they influence the effector mechanisms of lymphocytes; they modulate the activities of inflammatory mediators; and they modify protein, carbohydrate, and fat metabolism.

The effects of corticosteroids on leukocytes vary among species. In horses and cattle, the number of circulating eosinophils, basophils, and lymphocytes declines within a few hours

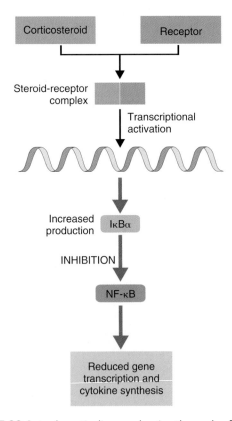

FIGURE 39-1 A schematic diagram showing the mode of action of corticosteroids. Normally, signal transduction and cytokine synthesis occur when the transcription factor NF-κB dissociates from its inhibitor IκBα. The released IκBα is rapidly degraded. Corticosteroids stimulate the synthesis of excessive amounts of IκBα, which binds to NF-κB and continues to prevent its activation.

☐ Box 39-1 | **Effects of Corticosteroids on the Immune System**

Neutrophils

Neutrophilia
Depressed chemotaxis
Depressed margination
Depressed phagocytosis
Depressed ADCC
Depressed bactericidal activity
Stabilization of membranes
Inhibition of phospholipase A_2

Macrophages

Depressed chemotaxis
Depressed phagocytosis
Depressed bactericidal activity
Depressed IL-1 and IL-6 production
Depressed antigen processing

Lymphocytes

Depressed proliferation
Depressed T cell responses
Impaired T cell–mediated cytotoxicity
Depressed IL-2 production
Depressed lymphokine production

Immunoglobulins

Minimal decrease

Complement

No effect

corticosteroid treatment, although in cattle corticosteroids may increase serum interferon (IFN) levels. The effects of corticosteroids on antibody responses are variable and depend on timing and dose. In general, B cells tend to be corticosteroid resistant, and enormous doses are usually required to suppress antibody synthesis. It is interesting to note, however, that in horses, moderate doses of dexamethasone suppress IgG1 and IgG4 responses while having no apparent effect on IgG3 responses. Corticosteroids also upregulate the expression of CD121b. This is a decoy receptor that can bind active IL-1 but will not transduce a signal, effectively blocking IL-1 activity.

Synthetic corticosteroids suppress acute inflammation. They inhibit increases in vascular permeability and vasodilation. As a result they prevent edema formation and fibrin deposition. At the same time, they block the emigration of leukocytes from capillaries. They inhibit the release of lysosomal enzymes and impair antigen processing by macrophages. Corticosteroids can also inhibit phospholipases and so prevent the production of leukotrienes and prostaglandins. In the later stages of inflammation, they inhibit capillary and fibroblast proliferation (perhaps by blocking IL-1 production) and enhance collagen breakdown. As a result, corticosteroids delay wound and fracture healing.

When systemic corticosteroid therapy is initiated, prednisolone or methylprednisolone are usually the agents selected for small animal treatment, and betamethasone and dexamethasone are commonly employed in large animal practice. Cats may require significantly higher doses than dogs to achieve a significant clinical response. Once a response has been induced, the dose of corticosteroids should be gradually reduced by lengthening the dose interval and then decreasing the amount given. This treatment is not without risks since it has the potential to suppress the pituitary-adrenal axis and induce Cushing's syndrome. By suppressing inflammation and phagocytosis, corticosteroids may render animals highly susceptible to infection.

Cytotoxic Drugs

Cytotoxic drugs inhibit cell division by blocking nucleic acid synthesis and activity. The major cytotoxic drugs currently in use are alkylating agents, folic acid antagonists, and DNA synthesis inhibitors.

Alkylating Agents Alkylating agents cross-link DNA helices, preventing their separation, and thus block cell division. The most important of these is cyclophosphamide (Figure 39-2). Cyclophosphamide is toxic for resting and dividing cells, especially for dividing immunocompetent cells. It impairs both B and T cell responses, especially the primary immune response. It blocks mitogen and antigen-induced cell division and the production of IFN-γ. It prevents B cells from renewing their antigen receptors. Early in therapy, cyclophosphamide tends to destroy more B cells than T cells. In long-term therapy it affects both cell populations. It also suppresses macrophage function. Cyclophosphamide may be administered

of corticosteroid administration as a result of sequestration in the bone marrow. The numbers of neutrophils, on the other hand, increase as a result of decreased adherence to vascular endothelium and reduced emigration into inflamed tissues. Neutrophil, monocyte, and eosinophil chemotaxis are suppressed by corticosteroids, but neutrophil random migration is enhanced. Corticosteroids suppress the cytotoxic and phagocytic abilities of neutrophils in some species, but in others, such as the horse and goat, they have no effect on phagocytosis. Macrophage production of prostaglandins and cytokines such as interleukin-1 (IL-1), as well as antigen processing, is reduced in some species.

Corticosteroids cause apoptosis of thymocytes and thus induce thymic atrophy. They also suppress the ability of T cells to produce cytokines. The most important exception to this is IL-2, which is not regulated by NF-κB (Chapter 8). Lymphocyte proliferation in response to foreign cells is suppressed, suggesting that there is interference with the recognition of MHC class II molecules. Corticosteroids also block production of lymphotoxin. NK and some antibody-dependent cellular cytotoxicity (ADCC) reactions may be refractory to

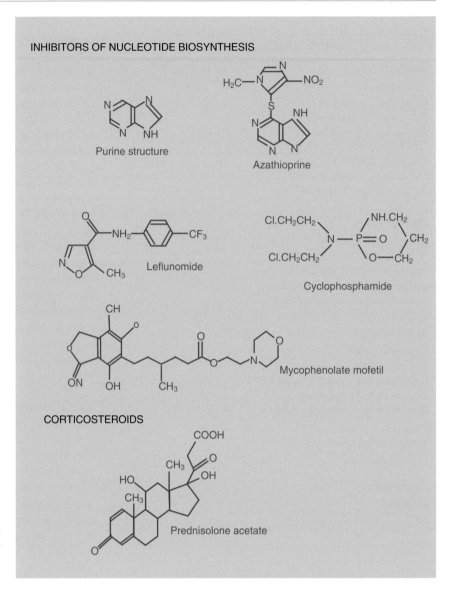

INHIBITORS OF NUCLEOTIDE BIOSYNTHESIS

Purine structure

Azathioprine

Leflunomide

Cyclophosphamide

Mycophenolate mofetil

CORTICOSTEROIDS

Prednisolone acetate

FIGURE 39-2 The structure of some commonly employed immunosuppressive drugs and the normal compounds with which they compete. Cyclophosphamide acts by cross-linking DNA chains.

parenterally or orally and is inactive until biotransformed in the liver. It has a half-life of about 6 hours and is largely excreted through the kidney. It is of interest to note that corticosteroids enhance the metabolism of cyclophosphamide and so reduce its potency. The main toxic effect of cyclophosphamide is bone marrow suppression, leading to leukopenia with a predisposition to infection. Other adverse effects may include thrombocytopenia, anemia, and bladder damage. Cyclophosphamide may be of benefit in the treatment of lymphoid neoplasia and in the treatment of immune-mediated skin diseases, although its potential toxicity suggests that other, less-toxic alternatives be considered first.

Folic Acid Antagonists Methotrexate is a folic acid antagonist that binds to dihydrofolate reductase and blocks the synthesis of tetrahydrofolate, inhibiting the synthesis of thymidine and purine nucleotides. As a result, it can suppress antibody formation. Its side effects are similar to those caused by cyclophosphamide. It is widely used for the treatment of rheumatoid arthritis in humans.

DNA Synthesis Inhibitors Azathioprine is a nucleoside analog that suppresses lymphocyte activation and mitosis. It is metabolized in the liver to 6-mercaptopurine, which inhibits DNA and RNA synthesis. T and B cells are especially susceptible to this effect. It can suppress both primary and secondary antibody responses if given after antigen exposure. Azathioprine has significant antiinflammatory activity since it inhibits the production of macrophages. It has no effect on the production of cytokines or immunoglobulins by lymphocytes but tends to suppress T cell–mediated responses to a greater extent than B cell responses. Its major toxic effects include bone marrow depression affecting leukocytes rather than platelets or red cells, acute pancreatitis, and gastroenteritis. Azathioprine is useful in the control of allograft rejection. It is favored by many clinicians for the treatment of immune-mediated skin diseases because of its combination of antiinflammatory and immunosuppressive activity. It is commonly used in association with corticosteroids. If azathioprine is used in dogs, marrow function should be monitored and the dose reduced if necessary. There are breed-related variations in azathioprine metabolism in dogs that may affect its effectiveness and toxicity.

Selective Immunosuppression

Calcineurin Inhibitors

Perhaps the single most important step in the development of routine, successful organ allografting has been the development of very potent but selective immunosuppressive agents. Of these, cyclosporine has been by far the most successful. Cyclosporine (also called ciclosporin) is an immunosuppressive polypeptide derived from a soil fungus, *Tolypocladium inflatum*. This fungus yields several natural forms of cyclosporine,

of which the most important is cyclosporin A, a circular peptide of 11 amino acids (Figure 39-3). As a result, cyclosporine has two distinct surfaces that allow it to bind two proteins simultaneously. When it enters the T cell cytosol, one surface binds to an intracellular receptor called cytophilin, whereas the other binds and blocks the intracellular transmitter calcineurin, a serine-threonine phosphatase (Figure 39-4). Cyclosporine therefore inhibits signal transduction and blocks production of IL-2 and IFN-γ by T cells. The primary effect of cyclosporine treatment is therefore the blocking of Th1 responses. It has indirect suppressive effects on macrophages, B cells, natural killer (NK) cells, neutrophils, eosinophils, and mast cells.

Because cyclosporine inhibits IFN-γ production by activated T cells, it prevents the induction of MHC class I

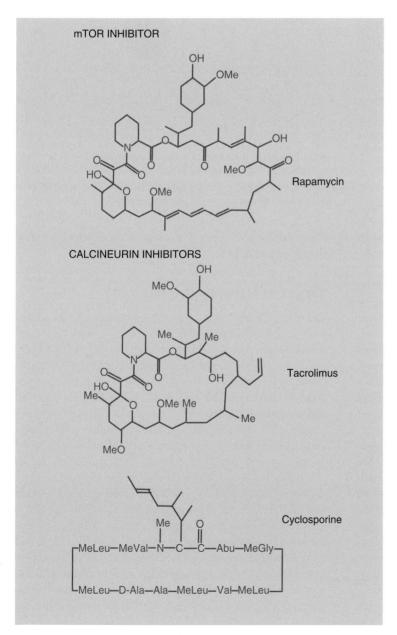

FIGURE 39-3 The structure of the immunosuppressive drugs rapamycin, tacrolimus, and cyclosporine. abu, aminobutyric acid.

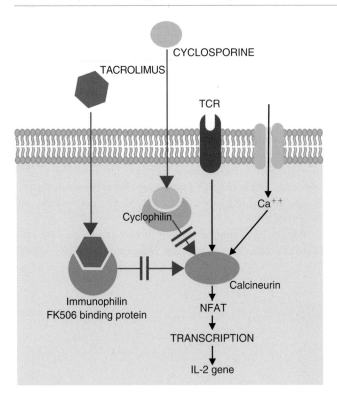

CYCLOSPORINE

TACROLIMUS

TCR

Ca⁺⁺

Cyclophilin

Calcineurin

Immunophilin
FK506 binding protein

NFAT

TRANSCRIPTION

IL-2 gene

FIGURE 39-4 The mode of action of cyclosporine and tacrolimus. Both prevent activation of the signaling molecule calcineurin. As a result the transcription factor NF-AT is inhibited, and activation of genes such as those for IL-2 production are prevented.

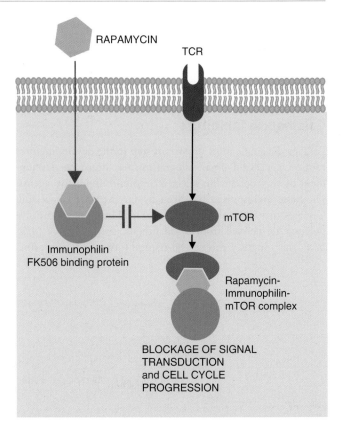

RAPAMYCIN

TCR

mTOR

Immunophilin
FK506 binding protein

Rapamycin-
Immunophilin-
mTOR complex

BLOCKAGE OF SIGNAL
TRANSDUCTION
and CELL CYCLE
PROGRESSION

FIGURE 39-5 The mode of action of rapamycin. This drug blocks activation of the aptly named mTOR (mammalian target of rapamycin). As a result numerous cell functions are blocked, including gene activation pathways and cell cycle progression.

expression on allografts. Since corticosteroids have a similar effect, the combination of corticosteroids and cyclosporine is especially potent and can enhance survival of allografts while leaving other immune functions intact. It therefore has a significant advantage over other older immunosuppressants. The use of cyclosporine has made tissue transplantation a routinely successful and safe procedure. In cats that received renal allografts from unrelated blood group–compatible donors and were treated with cyclosporine and prednisolone, mean survival was greater than 12 months. Cyclosporine also inhibits several hypersensitivity reactions. It is as effective as corticosteroids in treating canine atopic dermatitis. It is useful in a variety of immunologically mediated dermatologic diseases and appears to have a wide safety margin in dogs. The major adverse effect reported is gastroenteritis.

Tacrolimus is a macrolide antibiotic that acts as a calcineurin blocking agent in a manner similar to cyclosporine (see Figure 39-4). It inhibits the production of several key cytokines, including IL-2, IL-3, IL-4, IL-5, IFN-γ. and TNF-α. Tacrolimus is much more potent than cyclosporine in inhibiting T and B cell responses. It is also superior to cyclosporine in preventing or reversing allograft and xenograft rejection in humans and can prevent graft vascular disease (Chapter 32). Unfortunately, it causes severe intestinal toxicity in dogs, resulting in ulceration, vasculitis, anorexia, and vomiting. Topical tacrolimus has been used successfully to treat atopic

dermatitis, discoid lupus erythematosus, and pemphigus erythematosus in dogs.

Target of Rapamycin Inhibitors

The macrolide antibiotic rapamycin (sirolimus) and the related molecule everolimus specifically inhibit a multifunctional serine kinase known as mammalian target of rapamycin (mTOR). mTOR plays a critical role in regulating T cell activation by integrating the signals received from specific antigen, co-stimulatory receptors, and cytokines and directing the T cell differentiation into effector, regulatory, or memory pathways (Figure 39-5). mTOR also acts on nondividing macrophages and dendritic cells to orchestrate many of their activities by associating with MyD88, activating IFN regulatory factors, and inhibiting caspase-1. Rapamycin acts on macrophages and dendritic cells, enhancing IL-12 and nitric oxide production but inhibiting IL-10. This in turn promotes Th1- or Th17-mediated inflammation. Rapamycin inhibits B and T cell proliferation by blocking stimulatory signals from IL-2, IL-4, and IL-6. It enhances regulatory T (Treg) cell production and promotes tolerance. It acts synergistically with calcineurin inhibitors and is much superior to cyclosporine in preventing or reversing allograft and xenograft rejection in humans. Because it blocks endothelial cell and fibroblast proliferation, rapamycin can prevent graft vascular disease (Chapter 32), although it also inhibits wound healing. When given to aged mice, rapamycin significantly increases their life span. It is believed to act as a dietary restriction mimetic. Unfortunately, it also induces severe intestinal toxicity in dogs, causing ulceration, vasculitis, anorexia, and vomiting.

Inosine Monophosphate Dehydrogenase Inhibitors

Mycophenolate mofetil significantly prolongs canine allograft survival but is severely toxic to the canine gastrointestinal tract. It acts selectively on activated lymphocytes since it preferentially inhibits the purine pathway enzyme inositol monophosphate dehydrogenase found in activated but not resting lymphocytes. This leads to reduced production of guanosine monophosphate and prevents synthesis of DNA. It therefore blocks both B and T cell proliferation, T cell differentiation, antibody formation, and dendritic cell maturation. When given with cyclosporine, mycophenolate mofetil prevents renal allograft rejection between unrelated mongrel dogs. It has been reported to be effective in controlling canine autoimmune diseases such as immune-mediated thrombocytopenia and hemolytic anemia, meningoencephalitis, polymyositis, and pemphigus foliaceus, as well as systemic histiocytosis (Chapter 10).

Leflunomide

Leflunomide is an antiinflammatory agent that inhibits pyrimidine synthesis. It may induce production of Treg cells. It has been used for the prevention of allograft rejection in dogs. It has also been applied to several canine autoimmune and inflammatory diseases, especially in cases refractory to corticosteroid treatment or in which corticosteroids are contraindicated.

Depletion of Lymphocytes

Because of the many adverse side effects of the nonspecific cytotoxic drugs (not the least important of which is an increased predisposition to infection), a considerable effort has been made to find more specific alternative immunosuppressive procedures. One relatively simple technique that largely depletes T cells is to administer an antiserum specific for T lymphocytes. Antilymphocytic serum (ALS) suppresses the cell-mediated immune response and leaves the humoral immune response relatively intact. In practice, ALS is of variable efficiency and causes severe side effects. ALS-treated mice have been shown to accept rat xenografts, whereas clinical use of ALS in humans has not been universally accepted as useful. A much more specific antiserum with precise targeting is monoclonal anti-CD3. Anti-CD3 is directed only against T cells and is effective in reversing allograft rejection in humans. An even more specific monoclonal antibody is anti-CD25. This binds to the α chain of the IL-2 receptor and prevents lymphocyte activation. Anti-CD25 helps prevent renal allograft rejection and, since it does not cause T cell depletion, has fewer side effects and leads to fewer opportunistic infections than ALS.

Monoclonal antibodies against canine CD4 and CD8 have been used to control rejection of canine renal allografts. They are very effective, even with highly mismatched mongrel dogs. Both anti-CD4 and anti-CD8 must be used together, and their immunosuppressive effect lasts for about 10 days. (The dogs develop neutralizing antibodies against these monoclonal antibodies.) These are especially effective in combination with cyclosporine.

In some diseases, especially those due to excessive immune function, it may be beneficial to neutralize excessive cytokine activity using monoclonal antibodies. Thus it is possible to use neutralizing antibodies against a cytokine or against its receptor. The most successful anticytokine antibody employed in humans is that directed against TNF-α (infliximab) and is used to suppress inflammation in rheumatoid arthritis and Crohn's disease.

Intravenous Immunoglobulin Therapy

Although immunoglobulin replacement is appropriate for animals with antibody deficiencies, intravenous immunoglobulin (IVIG) therapy is immunosuppressive. Human IVIG is used to treat autoimmune and inflammatory disease in domestic animals. This is a pooled IgG preparation derived from a large number of healthy donors. Administered intravenously, its beneficial effects are mediated by IgG immunoglobulins with sialic acid on their Fc region. Removal of the sialic acid reduces its antiinflammatory effect. It appears to bind and block either a sialic acid–specific receptor on regulatory macrophages or some form of Fc receptor on effector macrophages and dendritic cells. This then inhibits the activities of autoantibodies. It may also function in part by blockading FcRn and accelerating autoantibody degradation (Chapter 35). Administration of IVIG has been shown to increase production of transforming growth factor-β (TGF-β) and IL-10 by Treg cells. In dogs it may act by saturating Fc receptors on monocytes. IVIG may also interfere with Fas-mediated apoptosis.

When administered to dogs, IVIG causes a mild thrombocytopenia, leucopenia, increased total plasma protein, increases in fibrin degradation products, thrombin-antithrombin complexes, and C-reactive protein. In effect it enhances blood coagulation and some inflammatory responses. It also binds to canine monocytes and lymphocytes (CD4, CD8, and B) and appears to inhibit antibody-mediated phagocytosis by monocytes. IVIG has been used to treat successfully autoimmune diseases such as immune-mediated hemolytic anemia and thrombocytopenia, and pemphigus, as well as severe cutaneous drug reactions such as erythema multiforme and

□ Box 39-2 | **Immunosuppressive Fatty Acids**

Inflammation is mediated by many different molecules, including lipids such as the leukotrienes and prostaglandins. Certain dietary polyunsaturated fatty acids omega-3 and omega-6 acids especially, are the precursors of these prostanoids and can regulate their production. Omega-6 fatty acids such as arachidonic acid tend to be proinflammatory, whereas the omega-3 fatty acids such as eicosapentaenoic acid and docosahexaenoic acid tend to have antiinflammatory effects since they suppress eicosanoid production. The omega-3 fatty acids also promote production of resolvins and protectins. These molecules suppress NF-κB signaling and inhibit the production of inflammatory cytokines such as IL-1 and TNF-β. They tend to be immunosuppressive as well, suppressing B, total T, and Th cells in cat skin. They do not appear to influence Tc or NK cell populations, IL-2 responses, delayed hypersensitivity, or immunoglobulin levels. The feeding of oils containing omega-3 fatty acids such as fish oil, evening primrose oil, and flaxseed oil may therefore reduce skin inflammatory responses and be of significant clinical benefit in the treatment of allergic skin diseases.

Stevens-Johnson syndrome. Most authors report positive clinical responses with minimal adverse reactions (Box 39-2).

Stimulation of the Immune System

There are many situations in veterinary medicine in which it is desirable to enhance innate or adaptive immunity, for example, the enhancement of resistance to infection and the treatment of immunosuppressive diseases. Immunostimulants vary according to their origin, their mode of action, and the way in which they are used. In contrast to adjuvants, immunostimulants need not be administered together with an antigen to enhance an immune response.

Bacteria and Bacterial Products

A wide variety of bacteria have been employed as immunostimulants. These usually act as sources of pathogen-associated molecular patterns and stimulate one or more TLRs. As a result, they activate macrophages and dendritic cells and stimulate cytokine synthesis. The most potent of these cytokine synthesis enhancers is bacille Calmette-Guérin (BCG), the live attenuated vaccine strain of *Mycobacterium bovis*. BCG generally enhances B and T cell–mediated responses, phagocytosis, allograft rejection, and resistance to infection. Unfortunately, whole BCG induces tuberculin hypersensitivity in treated

animals and is therefore unacceptable for use in farm animals. To prevent sensitization, purified cell wall fractions of BCG have therefore been developed. These have been used to treat equine sarcoids and ocular squamous cell carcinoma. They are also of benefit in the treatment of upper respiratory tract infections in horses. Several active constituents have been identified. One of these is trehalose dimycolate, which promotes nonspecific immunity against several bacterial infections and may provoke regression of some experimental tumors. Another is muramyl dipeptide (MDP), a simple mycobacterial glycopeptide that enhances antibody production, stimulates polyclonal activation of lymphocytes, and activates macrophages. Because MDP is rapidly excreted in the urine, its biological activity is enhanced by incorporation into liposomes. Polymerization and conjugation with glycopeptides or synthetic antigens can also enhance the immunostimulating effects of MDP. MDP prolongs survival time and decreases metastases in dogs with osteosarcoma.

Killed anaerobic corynebacteria, such as *Propionibacterium acnes*, also promote antibody formation. These bacteria are phagocytosed by macrophages and presumably stimulate cytokine synthesis through TLRs. *P. acnes* has a complex activity since it stimulates macrophages and the antibody response to thymus-dependent antigens, but it has a variable effect on the response to thymus-independent antigens. Killed *P. acnes* has been of benefit in the treatment of staphylococcal pyoderma, malignant oral melanoma in dogs, feline leukemia in cats, and respiratory disease in horses. Other bacterial components, such as staphylococcal cell walls (especially staphylococcal phage lysate), some streptococcal components, and components of *Bordetella pertussis*, *Brucella abortus*, *Bacillus subtilis*, and *Klebsiella pneumoniae*, all have immunostimulating activity.

Unmethylated CpG nucleotides can bind to the dendritic cell and macrophage receptor TLR9, activate antigen-presenting cells, and trigger a potent Th1 cytokine response. When administered with antigens, these nucleotides act as potent adjuvants. When administered alone, they can act as immunostimulants and greatly enhance innate immunity.

Complex Carbohydrates

Certain complex carbohydrates derived from yeasts—namely, zymosan, glucans, aminated polyglucose, and lentinans—can also activate macrophages. These may function as adjuvants and potentiate resistance to infectious agents. Fish such as trout, salmon, and catfish appear to respond especially well to these immunostimulants when incorporated in the diet. As a result, immunostimulation by complex carbohydrates, especially glucans, is routine in aquaculture.

Immunoenhancing Drugs

A broad-spectrum anthelmintic, levamisole, functions in a manner similar to the thymic hormone thymopoietin (Chapter 12); that is, it stimulates T cell differentiation and T cell response to antigens. Levamisole enhances bovine lymphocyte blastogenesis at suboptimal mitogen concentrations, enhances interferon production, and increases FcR activity in bovine macrophages. It probably also enhances cell-mediated cytotoxicity, lymphokine production, and suppressor cell function. Levamisole stimulates the phagocytic activities of macrophages and neutrophils. It promotes the activation and maturation of dendritic cells. Its effects are greatest in animals with depressed T cell function; it has little or no effect on the immune system of healthy animals. Levamisole may therefore be of assistance in the treatment of chronic infections and neoplastic diseases but may exacerbate disease caused by excessive T cell function.

Vitamins

Some vitamins, most notably A, D, and E, play a key role in regulating immunity.

Vitamin A metabolites, especially retinoic acid, enhance cytotoxicity and T cell proliferation by stimulating IL-2 production. Conversely vitamin A–deficient mice have defective helper T cell activity. Retinoic acid can inhibit B cell proliferation and inhibit B cell apoptosis. Retinoic acid also enhances dendritic cell antigen presentation and maturation. Vitamin A metabolites can modulate the Th1-Th2 balance as well as the differentiation of Treg and Th17 cells. Retinoic acid also regulates the gut-homing abilities of T and B cells, and a vitamin A deficiency is associated with impaired gastrointestinal immune responses and increased susceptibility to gastrointestinal and respiratory diseases. Vitamin A supplementation reduces diarrhea in malnourished children.

Vitamin D, as described previously (Chapter 25), also plays a key role in immunity. The most important form, vitamin D_3, is synthesized within the skin or the liver, kidneys, and lymphoid tissues. Macrophages and dendritic cells require vitamin D for the production of the antimicrobial peptide cathelicidin. The vitamin D receptor is upregulated by IL-15 triggered by T cell receptor (TCR) activation.

Vitamin E and selenium affect immune responses and disease resistance in poultry, pigs, and laboratory animals. A deficiency of vitamin E ([dl]-α-tocopheryl-acetate) results in immunosuppression and reduced resistance to disease. On the other hand, supplementation of diets with vitamin E can enhance certain immune responses and lead to increased resistance to disease. Lymphocyte responses to pokeweed mitogen are higher in pigs with high vitamin E levels. Vitamin E supplementation given to cows for several weeks before calving prevents the decline in neutrophil function and macrophage function that normally occurs in the immediate postparturient period. Vitamin E promotes B cell proliferation; the effect is most marked in the primary immune response. It can act as an adjuvant when administered with *Brucella ovis* vaccine, clostridial toxoid, and *Escherichia coli* J5 vaccine. In some cases this increased antibody production may lead to increased disease resistance. Vitamin E can reduce the age-related decline in immune function by a direct action on T cells

and by suppressing macrophage prostaglandin E_2 production. Supplemental vitamin E may enhance immunity in some animals and elderly humans.

Cytokines

Since purified cytokines produced by recombinant DNA techniques are now readily available, many investigators have investigated their use in the treatment of disease. By administering additional cytokines, it has been assumed that the amount of these molecules in the normal animal is rate limiting and that administering additional material in pure form will somehow promote disease resistance or healing. also It has also been assumed that by administering a single new cytokine, one will not trigger mechanisms that will regulate its activity or even neutralize its effects. None of these assumptions may be valid. The major cytokines (IL-1, IL-2, IL-12, colony-stimulating factors, and the IFNs) have all been tested on animals in vivo. Unfortunately, the administration of purified cytokines has usually had minimal effects on disease processes and has been accompanied by significant adverse effects.

Theoretically, administration of interferons should inhibit virus replication as well as stimulate some cellular functions such as neutrophil activity, thereby promoting disease resistance. This has proved to be an oversimplification. High doses of interferons are very toxic and cause severe fever, malaise, and appetite loss. They inhibit hematopoiesis and cause thrombocytopenia and granulocytopenia. They can also cause liver, kidney, and neural toxicity. In addition, IFNs seem to be relatively poor antiviral agents.

Recombinant human IFN-α (rHuIFN-α) has been used to treat rhinopneumonitis caused by bovine herpesvirus-1 (BHV-1) and rotavirus-induced diarrhea in calves. Recombinant bovine interferons (rBoIFN-α or rBoIFN-γ) have also been used to treat BHV-1, *Mannheimia hemolytica, Histophilus somni,* vesicular stomatitis, coliform mastitis, brucellosis, and salmonellosis in calves and transmissible gastroenteritis in piglets. Recombinant porcine IFN-γ has been used on *Actinobacillus pleuropneumoniae* infections in pigs. Porcine IFN-α (PoIFN-α) is a powerful adjuvant for foot-and-mouth disease vaccine in swine. Both human and bovine IFN-α have been used for the treatment of feline leukemia. Recombinant feline IFN-ω has also been tested in feline leukemia virus and feline immunodeficiency virus infections. In almost all cases, high-dose IFN treatment of infectious diseases has produced some positive responses. These are not impressive, however, and the treatment may have toxic side effects, such as fever, inappetence, and malaise.

Recombinant IL-2 has been administered to pigs at the same time that they were vaccinated against *A. pleuropneumoniae* or pseudorabies and to calves vaccinated against BHV-1. Although it enhances immunity, IL-2 is very toxic. It causes severe side effects, including malaise, a capillary leak syndrome, diarrhea, and fever (Chapter 33). It is interesting to note, however, that relatively low doses of rHuIL-2, when injected directly into papillomas or carcinomas of the vulva in cattle, induced a positive response in more than 80% of cases, and some complete regressions were observed.

In addition to the trials described previously, studies have been conducted using IL-1 and granulocyte-macrophage colony-stimulating factor (GM-CSF). rBoIL-1β is an effective adjuvant in some experimental vaccines. rBoGM-CSF enhances neutrophil functions. Encouraging results have been obtained using IL-12 to promote Th1 cell function. Despite this, clinical trials employing purified cytokines have generally produced disappointing results.

For sources of additional information, please visit http:// evolve.elsevier.com/tizard/immunology/

Evolution of the Immune System

Key Points

- Invertebrates rely exclusively on the use of innate immune mechanisms to protect themselves against infectious agents.
- The jawless fish mainly rely on innate immunity, although they also possess a remarkably complex and diverse antigen-binding receptor system.
- Cartilaginous fish are the first vertebrates to utilize an adaptive immune system.
- It is suggested that the appearance of adaptive immunity occurred relatively suddenly during the evolutionary process with the incorporation into the fish genome of a microbial transposon containing recombinase genes.
- Jawed fish and all the more developed vertebrates possess both antibody and cell-mediated immune systems, although the details differ between species.
- The major chicken immunoglobulin is called IgY because it is structurally different from mammalian IgG.

All animals, regardless of their complexity or evolutionary history, must be able to defend themselves against invading microorganisms that might cause disease or death. Both invertebrates and vertebrates possess innate immune defenses triggered by "danger signals" such as tissue damage or microbial invasion. The mammalian type of adaptive immune system, however, evolved only after the emergence of the jawless fishes or cyclostomes. Thus, adaptive immune mechanisms such as antibody production or antigen-responsive lymphocytes are found only in the advanced vertebrates.

The diverse subsystems of the innate immune system evolved at different stages of phylogeny in response to the threats imposed by various pathogens. Different subsystems may have changed in relative importance based on specific needs or changes in anatomy and physiology. The relative contribution of these subsystems in any individual species probably reflects the optimal mixture that evolved to ensure maximal protection for that species. Specific components of the innate immune system may therefore vary greatly among species, or even within the same class of organism.

Changes in innate subsystem use clearly occurred at different stages of phylogeny. Natural killer (NK) cells, the use of type I interferons (IFNs), and certain specialized leukocytes such as eosinophils and basophils occur only in vertebrates. Likewise subsystems that depend on an intact vasculature do not work in invertebrates that have an open circulatory system.

Immunity in Invertebrates

Invertebrates are classified based on the presence of a body cavity or coelom (Figure 40-1). The acoelomates include the sponges and coelenterates (jellyfish and sea anemones). The coelomates evolved further into two major lines. One line includes the annelids, mollusks, and arthropods, collectively called the protostomes. The other line, including the echinoderms, protochordates, and chordates, is called the deuterostomes. It is from deuterostome-like ancestors that the vertebrates evolved. Invertebrates rely exclusively on physical barriers and innate immune defenses to exclude microbial invaders.

Physical Barriers

Physical barriers are most obvious in the arthropods. Tough chitinous exoskeletons can protect arthropods against all types of attackers. The horseshoe crab (*Limulus polyphemus*) not only has a hard exoskeleton but also can protect itself against bacteria in polluted water by secreting a specialized glycoprotein through pores in the carapace. On contact with endotoxins, this glycoprotein coagulates, sealing the pores and immobilizing any invading bacteria. Likewise, if bacteria enter horseshoe crab hemolymph, clotting factors are activated by lipopolysaccharides (LPSs) and result in local clot formation that traps invaders. Other invertebrates such as the coelenterates,

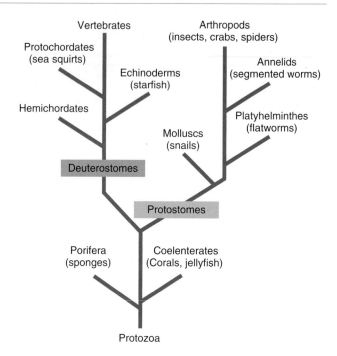

FIGURE 40-1 A phylogenetic tree showing the major divisions of the invertebrates.

annelids, mollusks, and echinoderms secrete masses of sticky mucus when attacked, thus immobilizing potential invaders. This mucus may contain antimicrobial peptides.

Innate Immunity

Invertebrates use three major innate defense subsystems: phagocytosis by blood or body cavity cells; protease cascades that lead to fluid clotting, melanin formation, and opsonization; and the production of a wide variety of antimicrobial peptides. Their initial defensive response is to use rapidly attacking phagocytic cells. This can be highly efficient, killing more than 99% of the invading bacteria. The few surviving bacteria, however, are somewhat more resistant to phagocytic cells than normal. These survivors induce the second stage of the response, the production of potent antibacterial peptides that wipe out any surviving bacteria and ensure that none survive to permit the development of resistance.

Phagocytosis In 1884, the Russian biologist Elie Mechnikov discovered phagocytosis when examining starfish larvae. He showed that mobile cells attacked rose thorns introduced into the coelom of these larvae. Since then, phagocytosis has been shown to be a universal defense mechanism within the animal kingdom. Several different types of phagocytic cells are recognized in coelomate invertebrates. They occur in blood (hemocytes) and in the body cavity (coelomocytes). These cells behave like mammalian phagocytes and undertake chemotaxis, adherence, ingestion, and digestion. They contain proteases, and in some invertebrates, such as mollusks, they produce potent oxidants. Some phagocytes can aggregate and plug wounds to prevent bleeding. Where phagocytic cells cannot control the invaders, they may be walled off in cellular nodules somewhat similar to vertebrate granulomas.

Invertebrates can produce cytokine-like molecules. One of these, an interleukin-1 (IL-1)-like molecule, may activate phagocytic cells and stimulate phagocytosis. LPS stimulation of mollusk hemocytes may stimulate the release of TNF-like, IL-6-like, or IL-1-like proteins. Cell surface adhesive proteins such as integrins are found in arthropods such as *Drosophila* or freshwater crayfish. These may promote hemocyte degranulation and activation of the prophenoloxidase system.

Prophenoloxidase (proPO)-Activating System

This system, found in arthropod hemolymph, consists of multiple enzymes that, when activated, generate a cascade of proteases leading to the production of the inert polymeric pigment melanin (Figure 40-2). The system is activated by the interaction of bacterial and fungal LPSs, peptidoglycans, and glucans with hemocytes. Activation also occurs through cuticular and hemolymph proteases. The proPO system generates phenoloxidase, a sticky enzyme that binds to foreign surfaces. This enzyme acts on tyrosine and dopamine to generate melanin and deposit it around inflammatory sites. Melanin polymer is deposited in the tissues surrounding invaders to form an impermeable barrier that blocks their nutrient uptake. Oxidizing agents and other antimicrobial molecules are also generated during melanin synthesis.

Antimicrobial Peptides

When bacteria infect insects, their pathogen-associated molecular patterns (PAMPs) are recognized by toll-like receptors (TLRs) and other receptors. Because of their dependence on innate immunity, invertebrates have evolved many different pattern-recognition receptors. In the sea urchin (*Strongylocentrotus purpuratus*), for example, there are 222 different *TLR* genes and more than 200 *NOD*-like genes. TLRs have been identified in even the least developed invertebrates such as the sponges. In contrast to mammals, in which TLRs directly recognize pathogens, drosophila Toll is

activated by a protein ligand (called spätzle) that is generated after pathogen recognition.

As a result of activation of these pathways, arthropod cells produce diverse antimicrobial peptides. These peptides are mainly produced in the fat body (the functional equivalent of the mammalian liver), although some may be produced locally on body surfaces. The peptides appear about 2 hours after bacterial invasion and reach peak levels at 24 hours. In some insects, the activity is short lived and disappears in a few days; in others, it may last for several months. About 400 different antimicrobial peptides, including defensins, have been identified in invertebrates. Invertebrates also generate lectins that can bind microbial carbohydrates such as LPSs, glucans, mannans, and sialic acid. These include C-type lectins and pentraxins and are thus analogous to mammalian acute-phase proteins. These invertebrate lectins act as opsonins and enhance activation of the prophenoloxidase system. Insects also produce the antibacterial enzyme lysozyme.

The complement system is ancient, with some components originating long before the emergence of vertebrates. Two complement-like proteins, C3 and Bf, have been traced back as far as the coelenterates. It is likely that the ancestral C3 was proteolytically activated by Bf and then formed a covalent thioester bond with foreign molecules. When the chordates emerged around 900 Mya, molecules such as MBL and the MASPS were recruited to the complement system to establish the lectin pathway. Proteins homologous to mammalian MBL, ficolins, MASPs, C3, C2/factor B, and a C3 receptor have been identified in ascidians (sea squirts). Thus invertebrates have both alternative and lectin pathways. Once activated through these pathways, invertebrate complement can opsonize microbial invaders.

RNA Interference

The intracellular RNA interference pathway (RNAi) is a gene-silencing system that appears to have evolved to prevent viruses from replicating within infected cells. It is especially important as a defense system in invertebrates (Figure 40-3). RNA normally occurs only in a single-stranded (ss) form. Long segments of double-stranded RNA (dsRNA) are not present in healthy eukaryotic cells, but they do occur if a cell is infected by RNA viruses. When a virus-infected cell produces dsRNA, it is rapidly degraded into many short fragments by an enzyme called dicer. These fragments, or small-interfering RNAs (siRNAs) are then stabilized by a protein complex called the RNA-induced silencing complex (RISC). Half of these siRNAs will be complementary to the viral messenger RNAs (mRNAs) and as a result can serve as templates and bind them. Once these viral mRNAs have been captured by binding to the RISC complex, they are degraded rapidly, and viral replication effectively blocked.

Adaptive Immunity

Invertebrates do not make antibodies. The ability to mount adaptive immune responses arose with the jawed vertebrates. Nevertheless, proteins belonging to the immunoglobulin

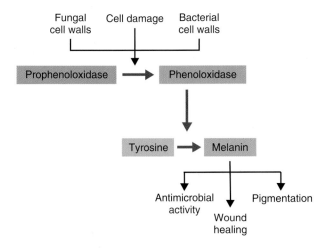

FIGURE 40-2 The prophenoloxidase pathway is an enzyme cascade system found in many invertebrates, in which it serves a key defensive role.

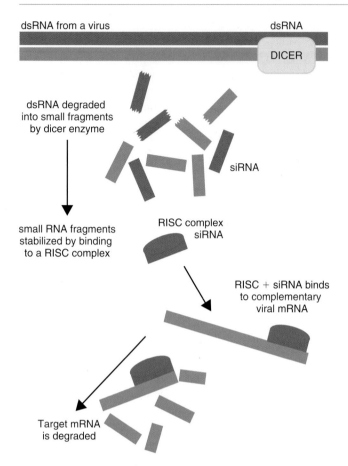

dsRNA from a virus

dsRNA

DICER

dsRNA degraded
into small fragments
by dicer enzyme

siRNA

small RNA fragments
stabilized by binding
to a RISC complex

RISC complex
siRNA

RISC + siRNA binds
to complementary
viral mRNA

Target mRNA
is degraded

FIGURE 40-3 The mechanism of RNA interference, an important defensive mechanism in invertebrates (and plants). Double-stranded RNA should not be present in the cytoplasm of normal healthy cells. Its presence indicates that an RNA virus is infecting a cell. This dsRNA is degraded by an enzyme called dicer into short fragments (short-interfering RNA). The short fragments are then stabilized by a set of proteins called the RISC complex. Half of these siRNA fragments will be complementary to viral messenger RNAs within the cell. As a result, they will bind specifically to the mRNA. Once this happens the mRNA will be degraded.

superfamily have been detected in arthropods, echinoderms, and mollusks as well as in protochordates. Some of these proteins can bind specifically to foreign molecules. In insects, there is a protein member of the immunoglobulin superfamily called Dscam that can be extensively diversified by alternate splicing. Isoforms of Dscam are expressed in immune tissues and secreted as soluble proteins into the hemolymph. *Drosophila* species have the potential to express more than 18,000 isoforms of this molecule. Individual hemocytes may express 14 to 50 forms of Dscam that can bind to bacteria and enhance their phagocytosis. It is not known how self-recognition by Dscam is prevented.

Graft Rejection

Invertebrates can reject allografts and xenografts. For example, cell-mediated allograft rejection occurs in sponges, coelenterates, annelids, and echinoderms. When two identical sponge colonies are placed side by side and made to grow in contact with each other, no reaction occurs. If, however, sponges from two different colonies are made to grow in contact, local destruction of tissue occurs along the area of contact as each sponge attempts to destroy the other.

Annelids such as earthworms can reject both allografts and xenografts. The rejection of xenografts (from other species of earthworms) takes about 20 days. Cells invade the graft, and the grafted tissue turns white, swells, becomes edematous, and eventually dies. If the recipient worms are grafted with a second piece of skin from the same donor, the second graft is rejected faster than the first. This ability to reject second grafts rapidly may be adoptively transferred by coelomocytes from sensitized animals.

Immunity in Vertebrates

There are seven classes of living vertebrates: jawless fish, cartilaginous fish, bony fish, amphibians, reptiles, birds, and mammals (Figure 40-4).

The fish emerged about 450 Mya, long before the appearance of the mammals. The least developed living fish belong to the class Agnatha, the jawless fish, or cyclostomes such as the lampreys and the hagfish. Considerably more complex than the cyclostomes are the Chondrichthyes. These are the fish with cartilaginous skeletons and include the rays and sharks (the elasmobranchs). The most complex fish are the bony fish of the class Osteichthyes, which include the overwhelming majority of modern fish, the teleosts. Because they emerged so long ago, fish are much more diverse than mammals, and major differences exist between the immune systems of each class.

There are two major orders of amphibians: the less evolved Urodela, which includes long-bodied, tailed amphibians such as the salamanders and newts; and the Anura, an advanced, tailless order that includes the frogs and toads. These too differ significantly in their immune capabilities.

Three subclasses of reptiles currently exist: the Anapsida, which includes the turtles; the Lepidosaura, which consists of the lizards and snakes; and the Archosauria, which includes the crocodiles and alligators.

The dinosaurs were sufficiently different from true reptiles to be put in a class of their own, the Dinosaura. Although most dinosaurs disappeared 65 Mya at the end of the cretaceous period, their modern descendants are the birds, the members of the class Aves. Unlike the reptiles, birds are (and dinosaurs were) endothermic, or warm blooded. As a result of this, birds share with mammals all the benefits that come from greatly increased physiological and biochemical efficiency.

The mammals consist of three orders: the prototherians, composed of the monotremes, or egg-laying mammals such as the platypus and the echidna; the metatherians, composed of the marsupials or pouched mammals, such as the opossum and the kangaroos; and the eutherians, or placental mammals. The marsupials and eutherians are each other's closest relatives. The

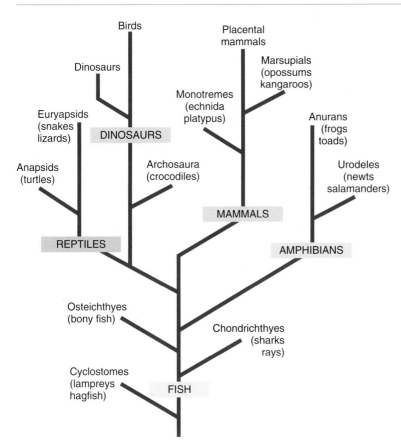

FIGURE 40-4 A simplified phylogenic tree showing the major relationships among the vertebrates.

two groups diverged about 172 Mya. The bulk of this book is devoted to the immunology of eutherian mammals.

Immunity in Cyclostomes

The most primitive of living vertebrates are the cyclostomes, the fish without jaws, including the lampreys and the hagfish. These fish make several different types of proteins that can bind to bacteria and enhance phagocytosis by leukocytes. Some of these proteins resemble complement. Their amino acid sequences resemble C3, C4, and C5, and they contain a hidden thioester bond. Lampreys have an ortholog of mammalian C1q that acts as a lectin. Cyclostomes possess both the alternate and lectin pathways but lack the lytic components of complement. The lamprey complement system thus promotes phagocytosis rather than lysis. Lamprey C3 has features of the common ancestor of mammalian C3 and C4, and lamprey factor B resembles the common ancestor of factor B and C2.

Cyclostomes have two types of blood leukocytes. One population resembles monocytes. The other population looks like lymphocytes. Lacking the appropriate recombinases, cyclostomes cannot make antibodies or T cell receptors (TCRs). Instead, they mount a different form of adaptive humoral response through the use of a population of variable lymphocyte receptors (VLRs) unrelated to immunoglobulins. There are major two types of VLR: VLRA is only found on cell surfaces, and VLRB is both secreted and cell bound.

Cyclostomes generate enormous diversity in their VLRs by rearranging their DNA through a process related to gene conversion. This involves inserting variable numbers of leucine-rich modules into an incomplete VLR germline gene. These modules are obtained from a large library of such modules located at each end of the *VLR* gene and are inserted into the middle of the VLR to generate a functional gene. As a result, the binding site of these VLRs is lined by hypervariable positively selected amino acids. It is calculated that they may be able to assemble as many as 10^{14} unique receptors in this way. It also appears that each lamprey lymphocyte expresses a specific VLR, suggesting that clonal selection operates in this system. Both types of VLR are probably anchored to the lymphocyte membrane, but VLRB may be released after antigenic stimulation. T cell stimulants enhance VLRA production rather than VLRB.

The production of VLRs therefore represents a very different mechanism from that involving immunoglobulin or TLR diversity, which emerged around the same time (about 450 Mya). This serves to emphasize yet again the benefits of a lymphocyte-based adaptive immune system capable of combating both extracellular and intracellular pathogens. Most advanced vertebrates developed T and B cells. The jawless fish developed VLRA and VLRB.

Hagfish kept under good conditions in a warm environment can reject skin allografts. First grafts take about 72 days at 18° C to be rejected; second grafts are rejected in about 28 days. This rejection is presumably due to innate mechanisms.

Immunological "Big Bang"

The adaptive immune system depends on possession of two key antigen receptor systems, the TCR and the B cell receptor (BCR). Both require the rearrangement of *V, D,* and *J* gene segments to form functional, antigen-binding receptors. Invertebrates and cyclostomes cannot rearrange these genes, but cartilaginous and bony fish can. Sometime during the 100 million years between the divergence of jawless and jawed vertebrates and the emergence of cartilaginous and bony fish, about 450 Mya, the enzymatic machinery needed for the recombination of *V* gene segments emerged. The mechanism of this sudden appearance is unknown. It has been suggested, however, that a transposon carrying the precursors of the recombinase-activating genes *RAG1* and *RAG2* (most likely a bacterial integrase) was successfully inserted into an immunoglobulin superfamily *V*-like gene within the germline of the early jawed vertebrates (Figure 40-5). As a result, the immunoglobulin gene could be expressed only after splicing mediated by the RAG enzymes. Thus emerged, in a major evolutionary leap, the ability to generate antigen-binding sites and functional immunoglobulins. This, for the first time, permitted animals to respond specifically to previously encountered antigens. The advantages of this new "improved" system were such that it is now a feature of all jawed vertebrates. This did not, of course, result in discarding of the innate immune defenses. Lectins, the complement system, and the NK cell system remain essential components of vertebrate immunity. It is also important to point out that adaptive immunity did not confer invincibility to infectious agents. It simply made life more difficult for them and conferred an incremental selective advantage on animals with such defenses. The selective advantage of adaptive immunity came with an attendant cost—the potential for autoimmune disease.

Immunity in Jawed Fish

Innate Immunity

Fish employ innate subsystems such as TLRs that are similar to those found in mammals. There are six major families of vertebrate TLRs, and within each family, the TLRs recognize a general class of PAMP. The functions and binding specificities of each TLR family have largely remained unchanged as the vertebrates evolved. (The microbes have not changed, so neither have the TLRs). Orthologs of fish TLR 14, 21, 22, and 23 have not been found in mammals. Fish are resistant to the toxic effects of LPS since fish TLR4 does not recognize LPS. Fish are, of course constantly exposed to aquatic viruses and must defend themselves accordingly. Triggering of the type I IFN system through TLRs is important for fish innate immunity.

In fish inflammatory responses, granulocytes arrive first, and their numbers peak after 12 to 24 hours. This is followed by a wave of macrophages and possibly lymphocytes. The granulocytes are attracted by microbial products and soluble tissue mediators. The response tends to be prolonged, and macrophage numbers peak after 2 to 7 days. In fish, granulocytes originate from the anterior kidney, whereas the macrophages develop from blood monocytes. Fish macrophages are found in many sites, especially the mesentery, splenic ellipsoids, kidney, and atrium of the heart.

Teleost neutrophils are similar in morphology and probably function to mammalian neutrophils and are frequently seen in inflammatory lesions. These neutrophils are phagocytic, and their numbers increase in response to infections. They possess most of the enzymes of mammalian neutrophils. It has been suggested that in some species, neutrophils may carry out their bactericidal function extracellularly rather than intracellularly. The release of oxidants from neutrophils at inflammatory sites may cause severe tissue damage. The fat of fish is highly unsaturated as an adaptation to low temperatures. Polyunsaturated fats are prone to oxidation, and free radicals may therefore oxidize tissue lipids. Fish, therefore, require a powerful means of modulating this response. The brown pigment melanin can quench free radicals, and melanin-containing cells are common in the lymphoid tissues of most bony fish as well as in inflammatory lesions. It probably protects tissues against oxidants produced by phagocytic cells.

Both bony and cartilaginous fish can produce lysozyme, lectins, defensins, complement, and acute-phase proteins. Lysozyme is present in fish eggs and may protect the developing embryo. This fish lysozyme is much more broadly reactive than the mammalian enzyme and is active against both Gram-positive and Gram-negative bacteria. Fish acute-phase proteins include C-reactive protein, serum amyloid A, and serum amyloid P. However, their rise is much less pronounced than

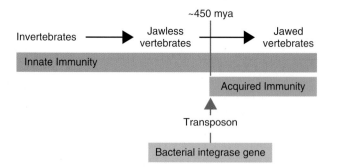

FIGURE 40-5 Innate immunity is a feature of all animals, both vertebrates and invertebrates. Adaptive immunity, in contrast, is found only in the jawed vertebrates, that is, animals more evolved than the jawless fish. It has been suggested that the ability to mount an adaptive immune response depends on the transfer of a bacterial integrase gene to a vertebrate germ cell through a transposon.

in mammals. A mannose-binding lectin has been identified in species such as the Atlantic salmon. Natural cytotoxic cells similar to mammalian NK cells have been described in bony fish. They are produced in the anterior kidney. Antimicrobial peptides called piscidins are found in the mast cells and phagocytic cells of bony fish. Electron microscopy suggests that these peptides can enter phagosomes and probably play a role in killing both extracellular and intracellular invaders.

Cartilaginous and bony fish possess all three complement pathways, namely, the classical, alternate, and lectin activator pathways. The gene duplications required for the development of the classical pathway appeared before the appearance of cartilaginous fish. The fish lytic pathway generates a terminal complement complex similar to that formed in mammals, although it works at a lower optimal temperature (~25° C). Unlike other vertebrates, in which C3 is coded for by a single copy gene, in bony fish, C3 is produced in multiple functional isoforms. For example, rainbow trout have four C3 isoforms, carp have eight, and sea bream have five. They differ in their structure and in their ability to bind to different activating surfaces. It has been suggested that this complement polymorphism may permit the most effective destruction of different invading microorganisms. As in mammals, C3 is the complement component at highest concentration in fish serum. Regulatory proteins similar to C4-binding protein and factor H have been identified in sand bass.

Adaptive Immunity

Both cartilaginous and bony fish can mount adaptive immune responses and have a complete set of lymphoid organs except for a bone marrow (Figure 40-6). They have a thymus located just above the pharynx that arises from the first gill arches. In immature fish, small pores lead from the pharynx to the thymus, suggesting that it may be stimulated directly by antigens in the surrounding water. Thymectomy in fish can lead to prolongation of allograft survival and reduced antibody responses. Antibodies or antigen-binding cells may be detected in the thymus during an immune response, suggesting that it contains both T-like and B-like cells. Although the thymus may involute in response to hormones or season, age involution is inconsistent, and the thymus may be found in many older fish.

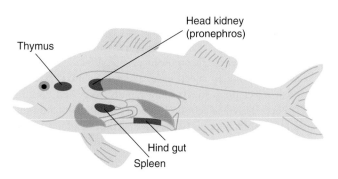

FIGURE 40-6 The lymphoid organs of a bony fish.

The kidneys of fish differentiate into two sections. The opisthonephros or posterior kidney is an excretory organ that serves the same function as the mammalian kidney. In contrast, the pronephros or anterior kidney is a lymphoid organ containing antibody-forming cells and phagocytes. It performs a function analogous to mammalian bone marrow and lymph nodes. Fish have a spleen whose structure and location are similar to those in mammals.

Aggregates of lymphocytes are prominent in the fish intestinal tract. In addition, lymphomyeloid structures that appear to produce granulocytes are found in the submucosa of the esophagus (Leydig organ) and in the gonads (epigonal organ) of sharks. Some species possess both, but others may have only one of these organs. The epigonal organ and the Leydig organ in cartilaginous fish express RAG proteins as well as TdT and other B cell–specific transcription factors and appear to be primary lymphoid organs. The epigonal organ appears to function like mammalian bone marrow as a source of B cells throughout life.

Fish possess aggregations of macrophages that contain pigments such as melanin and hemosiderin. These melanomacrophage centers are found in the spleen, liver, and kidney. Antigens may persist in these centers for long periods, and they appear to be precursors of the germinal centers found in more evolved vertebrates.

Fish possess true lymphocytes that resemble those of mammals. B cells can be found in the thymus, anterior kidney, spleen, Leydig organ, and blood, and their surface immunoglobulins act as antigen receptors. These B cells can mature into plasma cells. Unlike mammalian B cells, however, teleost B cells can phagocytose particles, generate phagolysosomes, and kill ingested microbes. These findings support the idea that B cells may have evolved from an ancestral phagocytic cell and may account for the apparent similarities between macrophages and mammalian B-1 cells. Both helper and cytotoxic T cells can be detected in fish.

Immunoglobulins The cartilaginous fish such as the sharks are the least developed vertebrates known to possess an adaptive immune system. Like other species, they produce a diversity of immunoglobulin isotypes.

Vertebrate light chains can be classified into one of four ancestral "clans" that originated before the emergence of cartilaginous fish. One restricted to elasmobranchs called σ-cart; one in all groups except bony fish called σ, one in all groups except birds (κ); and one in all groups except bony fish (λ). All four have maintained separate identities since their emergence 450 Mya, suggesting that there must be a functional basis for their differences.

Immunoglobulins are present in cartilaginous fish because they possess the recombinant activator genes *RAG1* and *RAG2*. The manner in which these immunoglobulin molecules are coded for by light and heavy chain genes and the structures of the *V*, *J*, and *C* gene segments are similar to those seen in mammals. Nevertheless, they differ from mammals in the organization of immunoglobulin gene segments within the genome.

For example, sharks and other elasmobranch fish have clustered immunoglobulin genes, where V, D, J, and C segments form clusters that are duplicated many times; thus:

$$-VDJC—VDJC—VDJC—VDJC—VDJC—$$

There are 200 to 500 of these VDJC clusters in sharks; each cluster is about 16 kilobases (kb) in size. About half of these clusters appear to be functional. (This arrangement is somewhat similar to that seen in the *TRA* and *TRB* genes in mammals.) Teleost fish, in contrast, have an immunoglobulin heavy chain gene arrangement similar to that of mammals (the translocon pattern), with multiple *VH* genes arranged thus:

$$-V-V-V-V-V-V-V-D-D-J-J-J-J-C—$$

Teleost light chain genes, however, are arranged in the clustered pattern so that, for example, in catfish, heavy chains are arranged in the translocon pattern, and light chain genes are in the clustered pattern. Shark immunoglobulins show evidence of somatic hypermutation.

IgM is the most ancient of the immunoglobulin classes and is found in both bony and cartilaginous fish (Figure 40-7). Cartilaginous fish usually have both pentameric and monomeric serum IgM. Bony fish have tetrameric and monomeric IgM. These different forms may compensate for a lack of IgG. Recently, several additional immunoglobulin isotypes have been identified in elasmobranchs. These include IgNAR (new antigen receptor) in the nurse shark, IgW in the sandbar shark, IgR in the skate, and IgT in the trout. Other species-specific immunoglobulin isotypes include IgZ in zebrafish, IgH in pufferfish, and a chimeric IgM-IgZ in common carp.

IgNAR consists only of heavy chains with no associated light chains. As a result, antigens bind to its single heavy chain variable domain in a manner similar to camel immunoglobulins. The heavy chain of IgW is orthologous to IgD. It occurs in two forms: a conventional form and a short, truncated form similar to the truncated form of avian IgY. IgT gene segments are located upstream of the *IgM* genes, a very unusual arrangement. As might be expected, IgT is produced very early in the life of the developing trout. IgD has been identified in catfish, halibut, salmon, and cod. It has some similarities to mammalian IgD, including coexpression with IgM on the B cell surface as a result of alternative splicing.

An unusual feature of elasmobranch immunity is the existence of immunoglobulin genes rearranged in the germline. These appear to play a role early in development but tend to be silenced in later life when they are replaced by rearranging genes. In the nurse shark, the predominant immunoglobulin in neonates is coded for by a germline-rearranged gene.

Fish antibody responses are characterized by the predominance of IgM and by their relatively poor secondary responses. Fish antibodies in the presence of normal serum as a source of complement can lyse target cells and they are effective at agglutination. There is no evidence that fish antibodies can function as opsonins, nor have Fc receptors been detected on fish phagocytic cells. The blood vessel walls of fish are permeable to IgM. As a result, antibodies are found in most tissue fluids (plasma, lymph, skin mucus). Transfer of antibodies from immunized females to their eggs has been described in the plaice.

Not all antigens are effective immunogens in fish. Soluble protein antigens are poorly immunogenic, in contrast to particulate antigens such as bacteria or foreign erythrocytes that are highly immunogenic. Many cartilaginous fish show seasonal effects on antibody production; that is, under constant conditions of light and temperature, immune responses are poorer in winter than in summer. Social interactions can also influence their immune response—fish kept at high population density are immunosuppressed (Box 40-1).

Cell-Mediated Immunity The acquisition of recombinase activity-enabled fish to generate rearranged TCRs and TCR homologs. Their overall structure is similar to that in mammals. The germline *TCR* genes are not rearranged and are organized in the cluster pattern. Fish have both major histocompatability (MHC) class I and II genes, but these have never been found in agnathans or invertebrates. (MHC class III genes, in contrast, have been found in primitive chordates.) The basic structure of each MHC molecule is conserved, as is the organization of the class I and class II loci, although in teleosts, class I and II loci are on different chromosomes. (Box 40-2).

Cartilaginous fish reject scale allografts slowly, whereas bony fish reject them much more rapidly. Repeated grafting leads to accelerated rejection. The rejected allografts are infiltrated by lymphocytes and show destruction of blood vessels and pigment cells. As in all ectotherms, graft rejection is slower at lower temperatures. Many different cytokines have been identified in fish, including IL-1, IL-2, IL-3, IL-6, TNF-α, TGF-β, IFN-β, and IFN-γ.

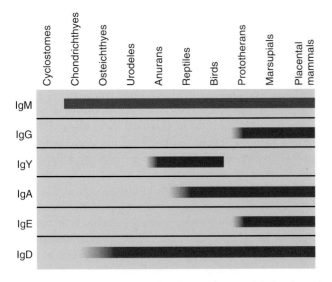

FIGURE 40-7 The evolution of the major immunoglobulin classes.

□ Box 40-1 | **Vaccine-Induced Autoimmunity in Fish**

Oil-adjuvanted vaccines are widely employed in aquaculture for the prevention of infections. Under some circumstances administration of these vaccines to farmed Atlantic salmon can result in polyclonal B cell activation, the production of multiple autoantibodies, and the development of a membranoproliferative glomerulopathy and spondylitis. The autoantibodies are directed against nuclear and cytoplasmic antigens, immunoglobulins (rheumatoid factors), ssDNA, chromatin, thyroglobulin, erythrocytes, and ferritin. These are not nonspecific reactions; rather, each fish develops its own pattern of autoreactivity with different levels of response against each autoantigen. The kidney lesions that develop are consistent with immune complex–mediated reactions. These vaccine-induced reactions may well have an impact on the continuing use of oil-based adjuvants in salmon vaccines.

Koppang EO, Bjerkås I, Haugarvoll E, et al: Vaccination-induced systemic autoimmunity in farmed Atlantic salmon, *J Immunol* 181:4807–4814, 2008.

□ Box 40-2 | **The Curious Case of the Cod!**

The Atlantic cod, (*Gadus morhua*) has a very unusual immune system. It totally lacks MHC class II molecules as well as the chaperone invariant chain (Ii)! In addition, the gene for CD4, the MHC II binding protein on T cells is a truncated pseudogene. As a result, the cod is unable to process and present processed bacterial and parasitic antigens to its T cells in the conventional manner. Despite this, the cod does not appear to be unusually susceptible to infectious diseases in its natural cold water habitat. It must therefore compensate somehow for the lack of an MHC class II pathway. It has accomplished this by greatly expanding the number and complexity of its MHC class I genes. It has, in addition, a uniquely large population of TLR families. The cod thus relies heavily on TLRs, especially on TLR9 to detect bacterial DNA. Atlantic cod also have unusually high levels of serum IgM and abundant neutrophils in their bloodstream.

Star B et al. The genome sequence of Atlantic cod reveals a unique immune system. Nature, 2011, 407:277–210.

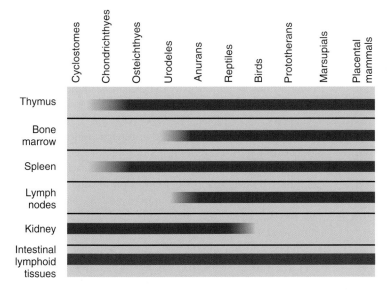

FIGURE 40-8 The evolution of the major lymphoid organs in vertebrates.

Immunity in Amphibians

As vertebrates have evolved, they have shown a progressive increase in the complexity of their immune systems (Figure 40-8). This is well seen in amphibians, in which there are marked differences between the less complex urodeles (tailed amphibians such as the newts and salamanders) and the much more developed anurans such as the frogs and toads. In addition, amphibians go through a complex metamorphosis as they change from the tadpole into an adult form. This has significant effects on the development of the immune system. A notable feature of amphibian innate immunity is the presence of very potent antimicrobial peptides in their skin. Amphibians also possess a complement system that, although similar to that of mammals, is more effective at 16° C.

Urodele Amphibians

Urodeles generally lack a bone marrow, although some salamanders may have a small amount of lymphoid tissue within their long bones. They have a thymus that develops slowly, only appearing at the seventh week of life. Thymectomy delays or blocks rejection of skin allografts. The kidney retains its lymphoid function, as in fish. Stem cells arise from the intertubular areas of the kidney in both urodeles and anurans. In the spleen, the red and white pulps are not separate.

Urodeles produce a monomeric IgM and can mount a good but slow antibody response against bacterial antigens. They do not respond to soluble protein antigens such as serum albumin or ferritin. Other urodele immunoglobulin isotypes are IgY and IgP.

It takes about 28 to 42 days for a skin allograft to be rejected in urodele amphibians. The allograft looks healthy for about 3 weeks, and it is then slowly rejected. Destruction of the pigment cells makes rejection of the graft readily visible because it turns white. Second-set rejection takes about 8 to 20 days in the newt, and the alloimmune memory lasts at least 90 days.

Anuran Amphibians

In contrast to urodeles, a fully functional bone marrow is present in anurans (frogs and toads). Their thymus arises from the second pharyngeal pouches and involutes by about 1 year of age. It also involutes during metamorphosis from the tadpole to the adult stage and then rapidly regenerates. The thymus lies just below the skin posterior to the middle ear. It shows a distinct separation between the outer cortex and central medulla. The thymic cortex is full of proliferating lymphocytes. The medulla contains fewer lymphocytes, but thymic corpuscles are present. Immunoglobulins can be found on about 80% of these thymocytes. Larval thymectomy in the toad reduces their response to foreign red blood cells, but the response to bacterial LPS is unaffected, suggesting this is a T-independent response. Thymectomy slows but does not completely prevent allograft rejection in toads. In frogs and toads, for the first time, boundary layer cells separate the red pulp and the periarteriolar white pulp of the spleen. Structures that resemble lymph nodes are seen in some anuran amphibians. These protolymph nodes consist of a mass of lymphocytes surrounding blood sinusoids. As a result, they filter blood rather than lymph. Nodular lymphoid aggregates do not seem to be present in the intestine of urodeles but are seen in anurans.

Larval anurans such as the bullfrog tadpole have lymphomyeloid organs in their branchial region called ventral cavity bodies. Sinusoids in these organs are lined with macrophages that effectively remove injected particulate antigens from the blood. Removal of these organs renders tadpoles incapable of making antibodies to soluble antigens. They disappear at metamorphosis. Lymphocytes are found in large numbers in the subcapsular region of the liver in fish, amphibians, and reptiles. These lymphocyte accumulations occur close to blood sinuses and may have a stem cell function.

Both adult and larval amphibians have circulating B and T cells. They probably originate in the ventral cavity bodies or the liver. About 80% of circulating lymphocytes carry surface IgM. Frogs possess NK-like and T cytotoxic–like killer cells.

Anuran amphibians have up to five immunoglobulin isotypes and are the least developed vertebrates to show isotype switching. Their IgM consists of either pentamers or hexamers (in *Xenopus*) and one or two low-molecular-weight molecules: IgY with a 66-kDa υ heavy chain and IgX with a 64-kDa χ heavy chain. (IgX is a distinctly different immunoglobulin class not found in other vertebrates [Figure 40-9].) *Xenopus* immunoglobulins also contain two types of light chain (perhaps homologous to mammalian κ and λ chains). Anuran amphibians possess secretory immunoglobulins in bile and the intestine (but not in skin mucus). These consist of IgM and IgX but not IgY. In the axolotl (*Ambystoma mexicanum*), IgY is a secretory immunoglobulin found in close association with secretory component–like molecules. This is different from *Xenopus*, in which IgY behaves like avian IgY or mammalian IgG. Amphibian antibody diversity is generated in a fashion similar to that in mammals.

The gene for the IgD heavy chain (δ) has been identified in the toad *Xenopus tropicalis,* where it is expressed on the surface of mature B cells. The location of the Cδ heavy chain is the same as that found in mammals, immediately 3′ to the *IgM* gene. Sequence analysis, however, shows that xenopus IgD is orthologous to IgW found only in cartilaginous fish and lungfish. This implies that IgD/W was present in these ancestors of all living jawed vertebrates. In contrast to IgM, IgD is structurally highly variable. Thus in different species it shows many duplications, deletions of domains, the presence of multiple splice forms, or even the loss of the entire gene, as in birds. As a result, it probably plays different roles in different vertebrate taxa. An additional isotype, IgF with a φ heavy chain, has also been identified in *Xenopus*. It is unique in having a hinge region. This is the earliest example of such a structure. The IgH locus of *X. tropicalis,* therefore, has the following order: $5'-V_H-D_H-J_H-C_\mu-C_\delta-C_\chi-C_\upsilon-C_\phi-3'$.

Frogs immunized with bacteria or foreign erythrocytes will produce only IgM. Bacteriophages or soluble foreign proteins induce both IgM and IgY. Soluble antigens and bacteriophages can induce both IgM and IgY production in adult toads. The IgY takes up to 1 month to appear, and its level is very low. Anuran larvae will make only IgM antibodies unless immunized several times when low levels of IgY are produced. Amphibians do not mount a secondary response to erythrocytes and bacteria, but memory develops in response to the antigens that stimulate an IgY response. Studies of immunological memory are complicated by the fact that antigens may persist in the circulation for several months after injection. Anaphylaxis-like reactions have been described in amphibians and reptiles.

Amphibians have T cells with functional TCRs, and anurans such as bullfrogs and toads can reject allografts. A first-set reaction takes about 14 days at 25° C. The graft shows capillary dilation, lymphocyte infiltration, and disintegration of pigment cells. Second allografts do not even become vascularized and are destroyed within a few days. If these amphibians are kept in the cold, a skin allograft may take as long as 200 days to be rejected. Delayed hypersensitivity reactions have been described in the axolotl (*Ambystoma*) and *Xenopus* in response to mycobacterial sensitization.

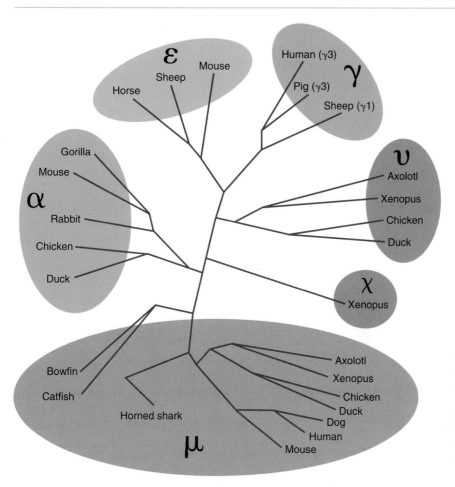

FIGURE 40-9 The evolutionary relationships among the major vertebrate immunoglobulin heavy chains. This is a distance tree constructed by aligning the amino acid sequences of representative vertebrate Ig H-chain constant regions.

(Redrawn from Warr GW, Magor KE, Higgins DA: IgY: clues to the origins of modern antibodies, *Immunol Today* 16:392–398, 1995.)

During amphibian metamorphosis from larval stage to adult, there is a temporary immunosuppression as shown by slowing of allograft rejection. Some allografts may even be tolerated at this time. As tadpoles change into frogs or toads, the thymus shrinks, and there is a drop in the numbers of B cells and antibody levels.

Xenopus has a well-characterized MHC with class I, II, and III regions called XLA. The class II region contains genes for both α and β chains that code for 30- to 35-kDa transmembrane glycoproteins. About 20 class I and 30 class II alleles are believed to exist. The class III region contains a gene for C4. It is interesting to note that although MHC class II molecules are expressed early in larval development on B cells and tadpole epithelia, MHC class I molecules are not expressed before larval metamorphosis.

Immunity in Reptiles

The reptilian thymus develops from the pharyngeal pouches and is structurally similar to that seen in other classes of vertebrates. Both age and seasonal involution of the reptile thymus have been reported. The thymus shrinks in winter and enlarges in summer. The reptilian spleen usually shows a clear separation between red and white pulps.

Lymphomyeloid nodes that resemble lymph nodes are seen in reptiles. They have a simple structure consisting of a lymphoid parenchyma with phagocytes and intervening sinusoids. Primitive lymph nodules surrounding the aorta, vena cava, and jugular veins are also found. Lymphocytes and plasma cells are found in nodules in the intestinal wall of all the more evolved vertebrates. Some turtles and snakes have lymphoid aggregations that project into the cloacal lumen, called the cloacal complex. These aggregates are larger in adults than in young turtles and are therefore not primary lymphoid organs and cannot be regarded as a primitive bursa. A few lymphocytes are found in the kidney of reptiles.

The reptiles that have been studied possess IgM, IgD, and IgY. The IgM of turtles is comparable to mammalian IgM in size, chain structure, and carbohydrate content. The IgY is found in both the full-sized and truncated isoforms (although some turtles may have only the truncated isoform). Geckos (*Eublepharis* species) produce a form of IgA. Sequence analysis shows that while its C_H1 and C_H2 domains are homologous to *Xenopus* IgY, its C_H3 and C_H4 domains are homologous to *Xenopus* IgM! It appears therefore that recombination between *IgY* and *IgM* genes gave rise to this IgA. Alligators possess two different forms of immunoglobulin light chain, perhaps homologs of mammalian κ and λ.

Green anole lizards express three immunoglobulin heavy chain isotypes: IgM, IgD, and IgY. The IgM chain lacks a cysteine in C_H1, suggesting that the heavy and light chains in IgM may not be covalently associated. As in some birds, two forms of IgY are produced: a full-length form and a truncated form. These lizards completely lack an *IgA* gene in their IgH locus.

Three C3 genes are present in the cobra. One codes for functional C3 in serum. The other two are expressed only in the venom gland and encode a C3c-like molecule present in venom that forms a stable C3-convertase in the presence of factor B.

Turtles and lizards immunized with bovine serum albumin, pig serum, or red blood cells can mount both primary and secondary antibody responses. The antibody produced in the primary response is IgM; the antibody produced in the secondary response is IgY. All reptile antibody responses appear to be T-dependent responses. Secondary responses and IgY antibody production do not occur in response to certain bacterial antigens such as *Salmonella adelaide*, *Brucella abortus*, or *Salmonella typhimurium*. The reader may recollect that a similar situation occurs in mammals, in that thymus-independent antigens such as *Escherichia coli* LPS induce a prolonged IgM response that is distinctly different from that induced by soluble protein antigens (Chapter 15).

As in other ectotherms, the rate of allograft rejection is temperature dependent. Turtles, snakes, and lizards reject allogeneic skin grafts in about 40 days at 25° C. Graft-versus-host disease can be induced by injection of cells from their parents into newborn turtles and can lead to death. The severity of the disease depends on the genetic disparity between the turtles. Mortality, however, is greater at 30° C than at 20° C. Other evidence of cell-mediated immune responses such as mixed lymphocyte reactions and delayed hypersensitivity reactions has been demonstrated in reptiles.

Immunity in Birds

Most studies on the avian immune system have focused on chickens. Thus the statements to follow, although generally true of chickens, may not necessarily apply to the other approximately 10,000 bird species. The birds diverged from the mammalian line about 300 Mya, which has provided ample opportunity for the immune systems of mammals and birds to evolve major differences.

Analysis of the complete chicken genome provides some interesting insights into the evolution of the immune system in this species. For example, it has proved possible to identify chicken orthologs of several immune-related genes that were previously believed to be confined to mammals. These include cathelicidin, colony-stimulating factors, and IL-3, IL-4, IL-7, IL-9, IL-13, and IL-26. Chickens have TLR1, TLR2, TLR3, TLR4, TLR5, and TLR7 but not TLR8, TLR9, or TLR10. It is also of interest to note that some gene families are found in chickens to a much greater extent than humans. Many of these have roles in immunity and host defense. They include some immunoglobulin receptors, MHC class I molecules, NK cell receptors, and T cell antigens. The significance of this expansion is unclear, but it may simply reflect the different histories of exposure to infectious agents encountered by birds and primates.

Avian Major Histocompatibility Complex Molecules

Based on the results obtained in chickens, it has been widely assumed that the avian MHC is small and simple. For example, the chicken MHC occupies only 92 kb and contains only 19 genes. It is divided into two independent regions designated MHC-B and MHC-Y. Both are located on microchromosome 16, but they are separated by the nucleolar organizer region (Figure 40-10). The B region contains three gene clusters. Cluster 1, or the B-F/B-L region, contains a two class I α chain genes (*B-F*), a *C4* gene, and two class II β chain genes (*B-L*). There is a single class II α chain gene located about 5 centimorgans from the β chain gene. Two clusters (V and VI) form the *B-G* or class IV region. The *B-G* gene products are membrane proteins ranging from 40 to 48 kDa. These molecules can form monomers, homodimers, and heterodimers and are mainly found on red cells and thrombocytes. Related *B-G* molecules are found at low levels on lymphocytes. Their function is unknown. The Y region consists of two clusters containing two MHC class I and two MHC class II loci. They differ from the B region loci in that their products are not expressed

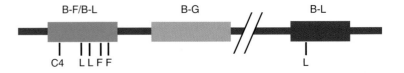

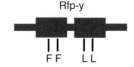

FIGURE 40-10 Structure of the chicken B region (*top*) and the Y region (*bottom*). *F* genes are class II genes, and *L* genes are class I genes.

on red cells. Genes within the Y region also regulate NK cell recognition. The B locus of the turkey is very similar to that of the chicken. It is a small, constricted locus with 34 genes in near-perfect synteny with that of the chicken MHC-B.

In the common chicken haplotypes, only one class I and one class II molecule are dominantly expressed. Since viruses contain relatively few proteins, MHC-dependent disease susceptibility depends on virus antigens binding to the dominant MHC class I molecule. As a result, possession of specific haplotypes determines viral disease susceptibility. For example, the haplotype B^{21} is associated with resistance to Marek's disease, whereas the B^{19} haplotype is associated with susceptibility. Chickens homozygous for B^1 generally have high adult mortality, are highly susceptible to Marek's disease, and respond poorly to *Salmonella pullorum* or to human serum albumin. Birds homozygous for B^5 are able to mount a better antibody response and develop less severe lesions in response to infection with *Eimeria tenella* than B^2 homozygous birds. Certain MHC genotypes (B$^{A4/A4}$ and B$^{A12/A12}$) are significantly over-represented in birds suffering from bacterial arthritis and osteomyelitis caused by *Staphylococcus aureus*.

Neither chickens nor turkeys are typical of birds as a whole. Passerine birds, for example, have a complex MHC structure with multiple duplicated copies of each class of gene, pseudogenes, and longer introns and intergenic regions. Even the kiwi, a very primitive bird, has at least five MHC class II genes.

The thymus in birds and in primitive mammals is similar to that seen in eutherian mammals. Germinal centers are not seen in fish, amphibian, or reptile spleens. In contrast, the germinal centers of bird lymphoid organs are large and well defined. Although birds are commonly considered not to possess lymph nodes, they do possess structures that can be considered to be their functional equivalent. These avian lymph nodes consist of a central sinus that is the main lumen of a lymphatic vessel. The sinus is surrounded by a sheath of lymphoid tissue that contains germinal centers (Figure 40-11). Avian lymph nodes have no external capsule.

The bursa of Fabricius has been described in Chapter 12. Bursectomy results in a loss of antibody production, although bursectomized birds can still reject skin allografts. These results have been interpreted to suggest that the bursa is a primary lymphoid organ whose function is to serve as a maturation and differentiation site for the cells of the antibody-forming system. The bursa, however, contains some T cells; it can trap antigens and undertake some antibody synthesis. Birds also have large numbers of lymphocytes in the cecal tonsils and in the skin.

Bird lymphocytes originate in the yoke sac and migrate either to the bursa or to the thymus. Immature lymphocytes that enter the thymus mature under the influence of molecules produced by thymic epithelial cells, and cells with recognizable T cell markers emigrate from the thymus. T cells constitute between 60% and 70% of blood lymphocytes.

Chicken NK cells are asialo-GM$_1$ positive and may share surface antigens with T cells. They are probably large granular lymphocytes. NK activity is found in the thymus, bursa, spleen, and intestinal epithelium. They attack human cancer

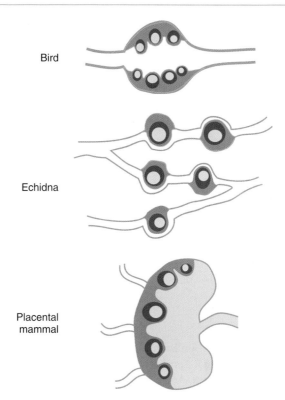

FIGURE 40-11 The structure of lymph nodes in birds, echidna, and placental mammals.

cells, lymphoid leukosis, leukemia virus, and Marek disease virus-infected cells.

Immunoglobulin Classes

There are three principal immunoglobulin classes in birds (chickens): IgY, IgM, and IgA. Avian IgD genes have not yet been identified.

Immunoglobulin Y The principal immunoglobulin in chicken serum is called IgY. Although somewhat similar to mammalian IgG, it has sufficient molecular differences to warrant a different designation. Like the immunoglobulins of mammals, IgY consists of two heavy and two light chains (Figure 40-12). The heavy chains, called upsilon (υ) chains, usually consist of one variable and four constant domains, and the complete molecule is about 180 kDa. However, some birds have a truncated isoform that has only two constant domains (it lacks the third and fourth constant domains). This isoform is about 120 kDa. Some birds such as ducks and geese have both full-sized and truncated IgY. Others, such as chickens, have only full-sized molecules.

The truncated isoform of IgY is produced as a result of alternative splicing of heavy chain mRNA. Its correct name is therefore IgY(ΔFc). Because the molecule lacks an Fc region, it cannot activate complement nor bind to Fc receptors. Its function is unclear. There has, however, been a tendency during evolution to make low-molecular-weight

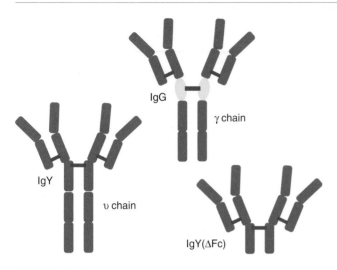

FIGURE 40-12 The structure of IgY and IgY(ΔFc) compared with mammalian IgG.

immunoglobulins. Similar truncated immunoglobulins have also been described in some fish (IgM[ΔFc]), some turtles, and the quokka (*Setonix brachyurus*), a marsupial. These low-molecular-weight molecules may offer some selective advantage. For example, it has been suggested that they will not trigger potentially lethal hypersensitivity reactions. Evidence from mallards (*Anas platyrhynchos*) suggests that the ratio of IgY(ΔFc) to intact IgY affects the efficiency of phagocytosis and determines whether immune complexes are phagocytosed in the spleen or liver.

Both isoforms of IgY lack a hinge region. Although bivalent, these molecules are somewhat inflexible and only cause precipitation or agglutination in the presence of high salt concentrations. They tend to show somewhat restricted diversity and limited affinity maturation. Studies on the interrelationships of the vertebrate immunoglobulins clearly show that IgY is related to both IgG and IgE in mammals (see Figure 40-8). In fact, it may have arisen from an evolutionary precursor of these two classes.

It is of interest to note that chickens can develop anaphylaxis. The signs of acute anaphylaxis in chickens and other birds are similar to those in mammals, although it is likely mediated by IgY. They show increased salivation, defecation, ruffling of feathers, dyspnea, convulsions, cyanosis, collapse, and death. The major target organ is probably the lung, and death is due to pulmonary arterial hypotension, right-sided heart dilation, and cardiac arrest. The pharmacological agents involved include histamine, serotonin, the kinins, and leukotrienes.

Immunoglobulin M Birds produce primary and secondary responses in a manner similar to mammals. The predominance of IgM production in the primary immune response and of IgY in the secondary response is less marked than in mammals. A monomeric IgM can be detected in chicken eggs and in 1-day-old chicks. It is thought to be derived from oviduct secretions in the hen.

Immunoglobulin A The structure of chicken IgA is similar to IgA in mammals. The only significant difference is that chicken IgA has four heavy chain C domains, whereas mammalian IgA has only three. Chicken serum IgA exists in both dimeric (340 kDa) and monomeric (170 kDa) forms. Intestinal IgA is associated with secretory component.

Generation of Antibody Diversity

Chickens generate antibody diversity in a manner that is quite unlike that seen in mammals. Chickens have only one functional *V* gene and one *J* gene for both light and heavy chains, although they do have 16 different *D* genes. Chicken immunoglobulin diversity is therefore generated by gene conversion. Although they have only one functional *V* gene, chickens have available a large number of *V* pseudogenes that serve as sequence donors. They therefore diversify their *V* genes by gene conversion. During recombination of the *V* and *J* genes, single bases are also added to each gene (N region addition), and joining occurs at random. Chicken immunoglobulins are further diversified by somatic hypermutation and imprecise V-J joining.

A second major difference involves the timing of the process. In mammals, rearrangement of immunoglobulin genes occurs throughout life. Chickens, in contrast, rearrange their immunoglobulin genes as a single wave between 10 and 15 days of embryogenesis, at a period when there is clonal expansion of B cells in the bursa of Fabricius. During that 5-day period, birds generate all the antibody specificities they will need for the rest of their lives. After the bursa degenerates at puberty, the chicken must largely make do with the B cell diversity generated in early life. However, once a mature chicken B cell is stimulated by exposure to an antigen, it can generate additional V region diversity by further gene conversion. If gene conversion is blocked, somatic mutation can occur. Indeed, species that undertake gene conversion also show limited somatic mutation, although the reverse is not true. The chicken can generate about 10^6 different immunoglobulin molecules. This is approximately one order of magnitude less than the mouse.

Chicken T cells can participate in delayed hypersensitivity reactions, graft-versus-host disease, and allograft rejection. Avian homologs of mammalian γ/δ TCR (TCR-1) and α/β TCR (TCR-2 and TCR-3) have been identified. TCR-2 and TCR-3 are subsets of α/β TCRs that use distinctly different V_β gene segments. TCR-2 cells undergo V-DJ joining by gene deletion, whereas TCR-3 cells undergo V-DJ joining by chromosome inversion. The structure of the avian CD3 signaling complex is different from that in mammals insofar as it contains only two dimers, δ/γ-ε and ζ-ζ, rather than three. There is evidence that chickens possess both Th1 and Th2 cells. For example, chicken IL-18 stimulates IFN-γ release from CD4+ T cells.

Birds reject skin allografts in about 7 to 14 days. Histological examination shows massive infiltration of the grafted tissue with lymphocytes. These cells are believed to be T cells since neonatal thymectomy results in a failure to reject grafts. If chicken T cells are dropped onto the chorioallantoic membrane of 13- to 14-day-old chick embryos, the cells will attack the chick tissues. This will result in pock formation on the membrane and splenic enlargement. The grafted cells attack the hematopoietic cells of the recipient. A few days after hatching, chicks become resistant to this form of graft-versus-host attack.

Chickens have at least 12 different blood group systems with multiple alleles. The red cell B system is also the major histocompatibility system in the chicken. A hemolytic disease may be artificially produced in chicken embryos by vaccinating the hen with cock red cells.

Immunity in Monotremes and Marsupials

The least developed mammals, the monotremes, such as the duck-billed platypus (*Ornithorhynchus anatinus*) and the echidna (*Tachyglossus aculeatus*), have a spleen, thymus, and gut-associated lymphoid tissues that are as well developed as those in marsupials and eutherian mammals. However, instead of typical mammalian lymph nodes, they have lymphoid structures consisting of several lymphoid nodules, each containing a germinal center suspended by its blood vessels within the lumen of a lymphatic plexus. Thus, each nodule is bathed in lymph. There is usually just one germinal center per nodule. The evolution of the predominant blood immunoglobulin from IgY to IgG probably occurred very early in mammalian evolution since monotremes possess not IgY but IgG. They have eight different heavy chain isotypes, including two IgG isotypes, two IgA isotypes, IgD, IgE, IgM, and a unique isotype called IgO. IgO is structurally intermediate between IgY and IgG. Although distinctly different from marsupial and eutherian immunoglobulins, they also show overall structural similarity. All the major structural changes that gave rise to the immunoglobulin classes expressed in modern mammals evolved before the separation of the monotremes from the marsupials and placental mammals and probably soon after the split from reptile lineages 300 Mya. Monotremes, like other mammals, produce predominantly IgM in the primary immune response and IgG in secondary immune responses.

The recent complete sequencing of the genome of the marsupial opossum *Monodelphis domestica* has allowed investigators to look at its immune system genes (its immunome) in detail. It contains genes for all the key immune gene families. There has been substantial duplication or gene conversion involving leukocyte receptors, NK complexes, immunoglobulins, type I interferons, and defensins. The opossum genome also contains a new TCR chain expressed early in development before conventional TCRs and may provide protection during the first few days of life before the opossum immune system is functional. This receptor chain, called TCRμ, consists of V, D, and J genes either recombined as in eutherian mammals or prejoined in the germline DNA. It resembles a TCR isoform from sharks and may represent the remains of a very ancient receptor system.

Marsupials produce immunoglobulins in a manner similar to eutherian mammals. They possess four immunoglobulin isotypes: IgM, IgG, IgE, and IgA. The marsupial opossum (*Didelphis*) resembles more primitive vertebrates in that it responds well to particulate antigens, such as bacteria, but responds poorly to soluble antigens. When opossums were inoculated with sheep red blood cells, the primary immune response was long lived and reasonably strong. The secondary response was weaker than the first and lasted for a much shorter period.

Mammals collectively possess a very large number of *VH* genes. When the sequences of their conserved framework regions are analyzed, they can be shown to cluster into three major "clans" (I, II, and III). Comparative studies have shown that these three clans have probably existed for more than 400 million years. Fish *VH* genes are most closely related to mammalian clan III, although they also possess two additional clans not found in mammals. The *VH* genes of birds (chickens), monotremes, marsupials, and some eutherians (rabbits, and pigs) also belong to clan III. This has led to the suggestion that clan III is the most ancient of the mammalian clans. However, cattle and sheep also express only a single *VH* gene family, and this belongs to clan II. Humans and mice possess *VH* genes belonging to all three families.

Mammalian Phylogeny

This book has focused on immunity in a small group of domestic mammals. These mammals have been selected not as representatives of mammalian diversity but for the behavioral traits that lend them to domestication or for the ease with which they are maintained in captivity. If we examine their place in mammalian phylogeny, we can see that most domestic animal species are relatively closely related (Figure 40-13). Even domestic pets such as dogs and cats are closer to farm animal species than to primates. Likewise, laboratory animals tend to cluster in a separate group. It is unsurprising, therefore, that significant differences exist among the immune systems of species of interest to veterinarians. It is also clear that if we are to understand the significance of these differences and how they evolved, we must examine the immune systems of other, unrelated mammals. Even within the major domestic herbivores, their phylogeny demonstrates why there are significant differences between their immune systems (Figure 40-14).

Fever

Vertebrates generally respond to antigens faster and more intensely at higher temperatures. Conversely, low temperatures in ectotherms may be significantly immunosuppressive. In

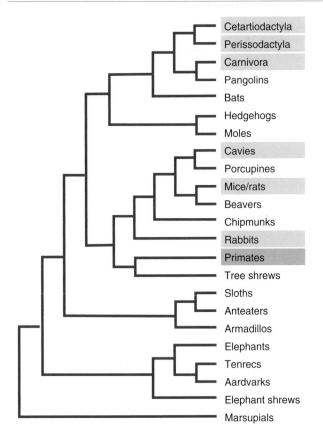

FIGURE 40-13 The currently accepted phylogeny of mammals as based on analysis of gene sequences. Note that none of the domestic animal species can be considered representative of mammals as a whole.

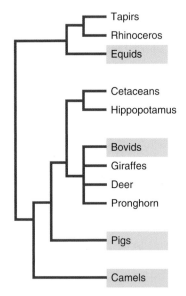

FIGURE 40-14 The molecular phylogeny of the domestic herbivores. Many gaps remain in our knowledge of the immunology of these species.

chilled fish, the lag period following vaccination may be long, or there may be a complete absence of a detectable antibody response. Only certain phases of the antibody response are temperature dependent. For example, secondary immune responses can be elicited at low temperatures provided primary immunization is carried out at a high temperature. The cells that are sensitive to low temperature in fish are helper T cells, and the effect is due to a loss of T cell membrane fluidity and reactivity to interleukins. Acclimatization to low temperatures can also occur. For example, goldfish that are acclimatized at a low temperature may be able to produce a similar number of antibody-forming cells to those that have remained at a warmer temperature. The nature of the antigen is also critical in that certain T cell–dependent mitogens are ineffective at low temperatures, again implying that the target cell is a helper T cell. The environmental temperature influences the rejection of allografts in all ectotherms.

Although it is well recognized that most endotherms such as mammals develop a fever when infected, it is less apparent that ectotherms such as fish or reptiles and even arthropods also develop fever in response to infection. Ectotherms are unable to change their body temperature by physiological mechanisms. As a result, they cannot develop a fever if maintained in a constant temperature environment. If, however, they are maintained in an environment with cool and warm areas, they will cycle between these areas and maintain their body temperature within well-defined limits. For example, it has been observed that normal iguanas (*Dipsosaurus dorsalis*) maintain their temperature between 37° and 41° C. However, iguanas infected with the bacterium *Aeromonas hydrophila* modify their behavior so that they spend more time in the warm environment (Figure 40-15). As a result, their temperatures cycle between 40° and 43° C. Once the bacterial infection is cured, the iguanas resume their normal behavior. Thus the iguanas effectively induce a fever by their behavior. A similar behavioral fever is seen in goldfish kept in two interconnected tanks maintained at different temperatures. In response to microbial infection, the fish will choose to spend more time in the warmer water, effectively raising their body temperature. The benefits of this to ectotherms are obvious because, as pointed out earlier, their immune systems function much more efficiently at higher temperatures. Many insects also respond to fungal or bacterial infections by developing a behavioral fever. That is, they raise their mean body temperature by spending more time in a warmer environment. It is interesting to note, however, that not all insect pathogens can stimulate such a response and that not all insects respond in the same way. For example, the bacterium *Serratia marcescens* can elicit a fever in the desert locust but not in the domestic cricket.

Some mammals hibernate, most notably bears, bats, and some rodents. During hibernation, periods of metabolic depression known as torpor are interspersed by transient activity called arousal. During torpor, the body temperature may fall to less than 10° C. This affects both the innate and adaptive immune systems. Torpor drastically reduces blood leukocyte

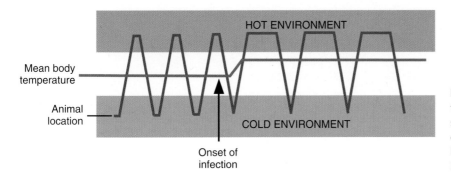

Mean body
temperature

Animal
location

Onset of
infection

FIGURE 40-15 A fever can be induced in ecto-therms by modifications in behavior. Simply spending more time in a warm environment will effectively raise average body temperature. This behavioral response occurs in response to micro-bial infection.

numbers, complement levels, phagocytosis, TNF-α and IFN-γ production, T cell proliferation, and antibody synthesis. For example, if bats are cooled to about 8° C, they cease antibody production, but rewarming permits rapid resumption of anti-body synthesis. This cessation of the antibody response in hibernating bats may allow them to act as persistent carriers of viruses such as rabies and increases their infection risk, as shown by the development of white-nose syndrome, a fungal infection in hibernating bats. Hibernating animals also fast, and this too may have significant effects on immune function.

For sources of additional information, please visit http:// evolve.elsevier.com/tizard/immunology/

Immunodiagnostic Techniques

Key Points

- The detection of antibodies in serum may be of assistance in the diagnosis of an infectious disease. Specific antibodies may also be used to identify the presence of an antigen.
- The most sensitive and specific tests are those that directly detect the antigen or antibody of interest. These are called primary binding tests. An example of a primary binding test is an enzyme-linked immunosorbent assay (ELISA).
- Secondary binding tests tend to be the easiest to perform but are less sensitive than primary binding tests. Examples include precipitation and agglutination tests.
- Tertiary tests directly measure protection. They are usually complex and so may not lend themselves to rapid testing. An example is a virus neutralization test.
- Serological tests are judged by the number of false-positive results they generate (their *specificity*) and by the number of false-negative test results they generate (their *sensitivity*).
- In general highly sensitive tests tend to have low specificity, and vice versa.

Immune responses are used in two ways to diagnose disease. First, specific antibodies may be used to detect or identify an antigen of interest. These antigens can be associated with an infectious agent, or can simply be molecules that need to be located or measured. Second, by detecting specific antibodies in serum, it is possible to determine whether an animal has been previously exposed to an infectious agent. This may establish a diagnosis or determine the degree of exposure of the population to that agent. The measurement of antigen-antibody interactions for diagnostic purposes is called serology.

Serological techniques can be classified into three broad categories. Primary binding tests directly measure the binding of antigen to antibody (Table 41-1). Secondary binding tests measure the results of antigen-antibody interaction in vitro. These tests are usually less sensitive than the primary binding tests but may be simpler to perform or require less complex technology. The third category, in vivo tests, measure the actual protective effect of antibodies in an animal.

Reagents Used in Serological Tests

Serum

The most common source of antibodies is serum obtained from clotted blood. Serum may be stored frozen and tested when convenient. If necessary, the serum can be depleted of complement activity by heating to 56° C for 30 minutes.

Antiglobulins

Immunoglobulins are antigenic when injected into an animal of a different species. For example, purified dog immunoglobulins can be injected into rabbits. The rabbits respond by making specific antibodies called antiglobulins. Depending on the purity of the injected immunoglobulin, it is possible to make nonspecific antiglobulins against immunoglobulins of all classes, or very specific antiglobulins directed against single classes. Antiglobulins are essential reagents in many immunological tests.

Monoclonal Antibodies

Hybridoma-derived monoclonal antibodies are pure and specific, can be used as standard chemical reagents, and can be obtained in almost unlimited amounts (Chapter 15). As a result, monoclonal antibodies frequently replace conventional antiserum as reagents in immunodiagnostic tests.

Specific Antibodies

When detecting antigens in tissues or body fluids, the first steps may involve the use of a specific antibody against the antigen of interest. Although these antibodies are often made by immunizing mammals, there is a growing interest in using chicken IgY antibodies. Birds may react very strongly against mammalian antigens. Chickens produce large amounts of IgY antibodies that become concentrated in the egg yolk. It may be much more convenient to harvest large amounts

□ Table 41-1 | **Smallest Amount of Antibody Protein Detectable by Selected Immunological Tests**

TESTS	PROTEIN (μg/mL)
Primary Binding Tests	
ELISA	0.0005
Competitive radioimmunoassay	0.00005
Secondary Binding Tests	
Gel precipitation	30
Ring precipitation	18
Bacterial agglutination	0.05
Passive hemagglutination	0.01
Hemagglutination inhibition	0.005
Complement fixation	0.05
Virus neutralization	0.00005
Bactericidal activity	0.00005
Antitoxin neutralization	0.06
In Vivo Test	
Passive cutaneous anaphylaxis	0.02

LIVERPOOL JOHN MOORES UNIVERSITY
LEARNING SERVICES

of antibody from egg yolks than have to bleed animals repeatedly. Antiglobulins may then be used to detect the bound IgY.

Primary Binding Tests

Primary binding tests are performed by allowing antigen and antibody to combine and then measuring the immune complexes formed. In order to measure these reactions, one of the reactants must be chemically labeled. Radioisotopes, fluorescent dyes, colloidal metals, and enzymes have all been used as labels in these tests.

Radioimmunoassays

Assays that use radioisotopes as labels have the advantage of being exquisitely sensitive. On the other hand, isotope detection systems are expensive. This expense, combined with the hazards of radioactivity and the need to dispose of radioactive material in a safe manner, has ensured that radioimmunoassays are only used when highly sensitive assays are required.

Radioimmunoassays for Antibody

The radioallergosorbent test (RAST) measures specific IgE in the serum of allergic animals. In this technique, antigen-impregnated cellulose disks are immersed in test serum so that any antibody binds to the antigen. After washing to remove unbound antibody, the disk is immersed in a solution containing radiolabeled antiglobulin (e.g., anti-IgE). The antiglobulin binds only if IgE has bound to the antigen. The amount of radioactivity bound to the disk is therefore a measure of the level of specific IgE antibody activity in the serum.

Radioimmunoassays for Antigen

Competitive immunoassays are based on the principle that unlabeled antigen will displace radiolabeled antigen from immune complexes (Figure 41-1). These tests are exquisitely sensitive and are commonly used to detect trace amounts of drugs. The antigen (or drug) is labeled with a radioactive isotope such as tritium (H^3), carbon-14, or iodine-125. When radiolabeled antigen is mixed with its specific antibody, the two combine to form immune complexes that can be precipitated out of solution. Any radioactivity remaining in the supernatant fluid is due to the presence of unbound antigen. If unlabeled antigen is added to the mixture, before adding the antibody, it will compete with the radioactive antigen for antibody-binding sites. As a result, some labeled antigen will be unable to bind, and the amount of radioactivity in the supernatant will increase. If a standard curve is first constructed based on the use of known amounts of unlabeled antigen, the amount of antigen in a test sample may be measured by reference to this standard curve.

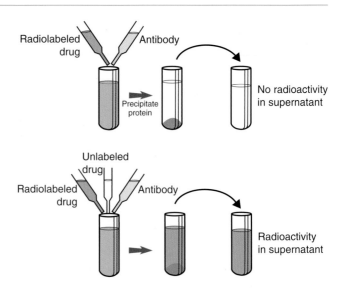

FIGURE 41-1 The principle of competitive radioimmunoassay. Unlabeled antigen in the test solution displaces labeled antigen from immune complexes. The amount of labeled antigen released will be proportional to the amount of unlabeled antigen added.

Immunofluorescence Assays

Fluorescent dyes are commonly employed as labels in primary binding tests, the most important being fluorescein isothiocyanate (FITC). FITC is a yellow compound that can be chemically linked to antibodies without affecting their reactivity. When radiated with invisible ultraviolet or blue light at 290 and 145 nm, FITC re-emits visible green light at 525 nm. This fluorescence can be readily seen under a fluorescent microscope. FITC-labeled antibodies are used in the direct and indirect fluorescent antibody tests.

Direct Fluorescent Antibody Tests

Direct fluorescent antibody tests are used to identify the presence of antigen in a tissue sample. Antibody directed against a specific antigen such as a bacterium or virus is first labeled with FITC. A tissue section or smear containing the organism is fixed to a glass slide, incubated with the labeled antiserum, and then washed to remove any unbound antibody (Figure 41-2). When examined by darkfield illumination under a microscope with an ultraviolet light source, the organisms that bind the labeled antibody will fluoresce brightly. This test can identify the presence of small numbers of bacteria in a sample. For example, it can be used to detect *M. avium* subspecies *paratuberculosis* in feces, or to detect bacteria such as *Dichelobacter nodosus*, *Listeria monocytogenes*, or clostridia in diseased tissues (Figure 41-3). It may also be employed to detect viruses in tissue culture or in tissues from infected animals. Examples include the detection of rabies virus in the brains of infected animals or feline leukemia virus in infected cat leukocytes (Figure 38-3).

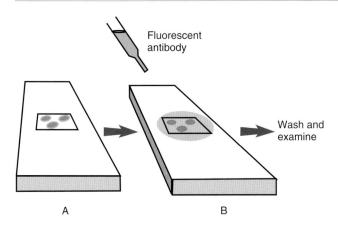

FIGURE 41-2 The direct fluorescent antibody assay. This technique is used to detect antigen by means of FITC-labeled antibody.

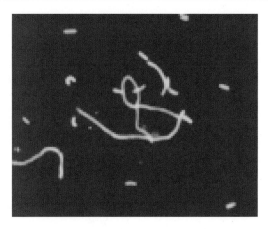

FIGURE 41-3 Direct immunofluorescence of a smear of *Clostridium septicum*. (See also Figs. 22-9 and 38-3.)

(Courtesy Dr. John Huff.)

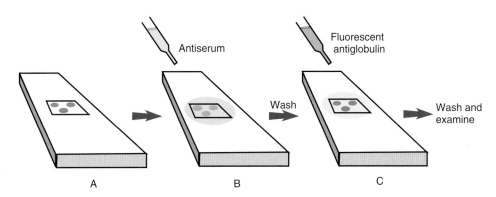

FIGURE 41-4 The indirect fluorescent antibody test may be used to detect either antigen or antibody. The antigen, in a section smear or culture, will bind antibody from serum. After washing, this antibody may be detected by binding to FITC-labeled antiglobulin.

Indirect Fluorescent Antibody Tests

Indirect fluorescent antibody tests can be used to measure antibodies in serum or to identify specific antigens in tissues or cell cultures. When measuring antibody levels, antigen is employed as a tissue smear, section, or cell culture on a slide or coverslip. This is incubated in serum suspected of containing antibodies to that antigen. The serum is then washed off, leaving only specific antibodies bound to the antigen (Figure 41-4). These bound antibodies may then be visualized by incubating the smear in FITC-labeled antiglobulin. When the unbound labeled antiglobulin is removed by washing and the slide examined, the presence of fluorescence indicates that antibody was present in the test serum. The quantity of antibody in the test serum may be estimated by examining increasing dilutions of serum on different antigen preparations.

The indirect fluorescent antibody test has two advantages over the direct technique. Since several labeled antiglobulin molecules will bind to each antibody molecule, the fluorescence will be considerably brighter than in the direct test. Similarly, by using antiglobulins specific for each immuno-

globulin class, the class of the specific antibody may also be determined.

Particle Concentration Fluorescence Immunoassays

Immunofluorescence assays can be automated and quantitated by means of particle immunoassays (Figure 41-5). For example, antigen-coated, submicrometer polystyrene particles can be mixed with test serum. After incubation, the particles are recovered by vacuum filtration, washed to remove unbound antibody, and exposed to a fluorescent antiglobulin. After filtering the suspension again and washing to remove unbound antiglobulin, the particle suspension can be placed in a spectrofluorometer and the intensity of particle-bound fluorescence measured. This provides a measure of the level of antibodies in the test serum. A very useful variation on this is the competitive assay used as a rapid test for antibodies to *Brucella abortus* in cattle. In this case, *Brucella* antigen-coated polystyrene particles are mixed with a standard amount of fluorescent anti-*Brucella* serum and the serum under test. If positive, the unlabeled test serum blocks the binding of

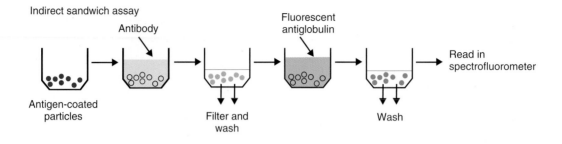

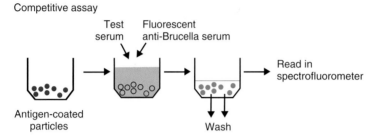

FIGURE 41-5 The principle of the particle concentration fluorescence immunoassay.

fluorescent antibodies to the particles. The more antibody in the test serum, the greater is the inhibition of fluorescent antibody binding.

Immunoenzyme Assays

Among the most important immunoassays employed in veterinary medicine is the ELISA. As with other primary binding tests, ELISAs may be used to detect and measure either antibody or antigen.

Microwell Enzyme-Linked Immunosorbent Assay Tests

The most common form of ELISA is used to detect and measure specific antibodies. In order to perform this assay, microwells in polystyrene plates are first filled with an antigen solution (Figure 41-6). Proteins bind firmly to polystyrene surfaces, so that after unbound antigen is removed by vigorous washing, the wells remain coated with a layer of antigen. These coated plates can be stored until required. The serum under test is added to the wells. Any antibodies in the serum will bind to the antigen layer. After incubation and washing to remove unbound antibody, the presence of any bound antibodies can be detected by adding a solution containing an antiglobulin chemically linked to an enzyme. This labeled antiglobulin binds to the antibody and, following incubation and washing, can be detected and measured by adding a solution containing the enzyme substrate. The enzyme and substrate have been selected to ensure that a colored product develops in the tube. The intensity of the color that develops is therefore proportional to the amount of enzyme-linked antiglobulin that is bound, which in turn is proportional to the amount of antibody present in the serum under test. The color intensity may be estimated visually or, preferably, by spectrophotometry.

One modification of this technique is the antibody sandwich ELISA, which can be used to detect and measure a specific antigen (Figure 41-7). The wells in polystyrene plates are coated with specific antibody (capture antibody) before testing. To conduct the test, the antigen solution to be tested is added to each well. The capture antibody will bind any antigen present in the test solution. This step is followed, after washing, by specific antibody, which also binds the antigen (the detection antibody). After washing to remove unbound antibody, enzyme-labeled antiglobulin, and substrate, as described for the indirect technique, are added. (It is important that the capture antibody and the detection antibody are from a different species and that a species-specific antiglobulin is used for visualization of the detection antibody. This will avoid false-positive results caused by binding of the antiglobulin to the capture antibody in the absence of antigen.) In this assay, the intensity of the color reaction is related directly to the amount of bound antigen. Because these tests involve the formation of antibody-antigen-antibody layers, they are called sandwich ELISAs. Sandwich ELISAs are used to detect circulating virus in blood from cats with feline leukemia.

Another common modification of this technique is the labeled-antigen ELISA used to detect antibodies. This is favored in manufactured diagnostic kits. The antigen is bound to the microwells before testing (Figure 41-8). The serum to be tested is added, followed, after washing, by labeled antigen. Any serum antibodies present will bind the labeled antigen to the microwell where it can be measured.

A competitive ELISA can be used to measure hapten molecules or viral antigens (Figure 41-9). In this technique, the microwell is coated with specific antibody before testing. In a

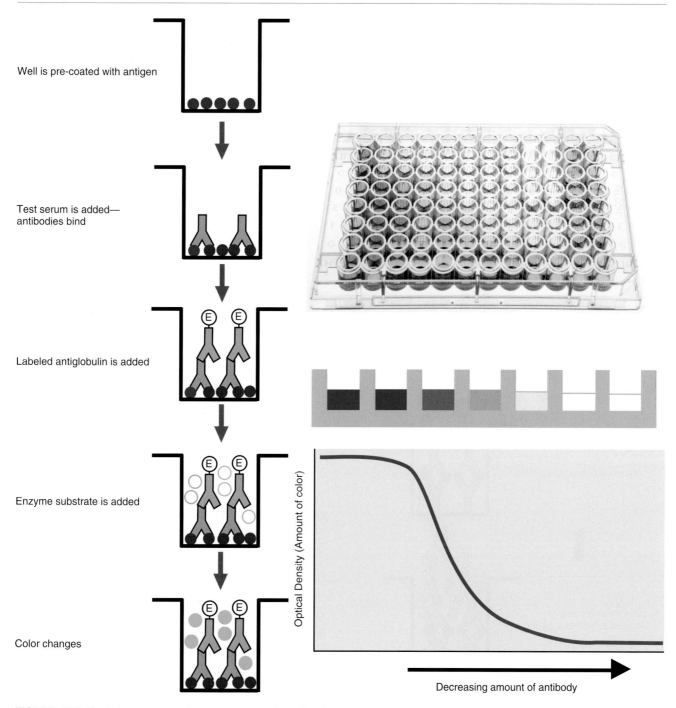

Well is pre-coated with antigen

Test serum is added—antibodies bind

Labeled antiglobulin is added

Enzyme substrate is added

Color changes

Optical Density (Amount of color)

Decreasing amount of antibody

FIGURE 41-6 The indirect ELISA technique. Antigen is bound to the wells in a styrene plate. The presence of bound antibody is detected by means of an enzyme-labeled antiglobulin. Addition of the enzyme substrate leads to a color change proportional to the amount of bound antibody. This color change can be estimated visually or read in an ELISA reader (a specially adapted spectrophotometer).

single reaction, the test sample and enzyme-labeled antigen are placed in the well where the antigens compete for the antibody-binding sites. The amount of labeled antigen bound to the microwell is inversely related to the concentration of antigen in the test sample. This technique is faster than other ELISA techniques. It can be made very sensitive if the sample antigen is permitted to react with the antibody before the labeled antigen is added.

Western Blotting

One solution to the problem of identifying protein antigens in a complex mixture is by use of a technique called Western blotting. This is a three-stage primary binding test (Figure 41-10). Stage 1 involves electrophoresis of a protein mixture on gels so that each component is resolved into a single band. Stage 2 involves blotting or transfer of these protein bands to

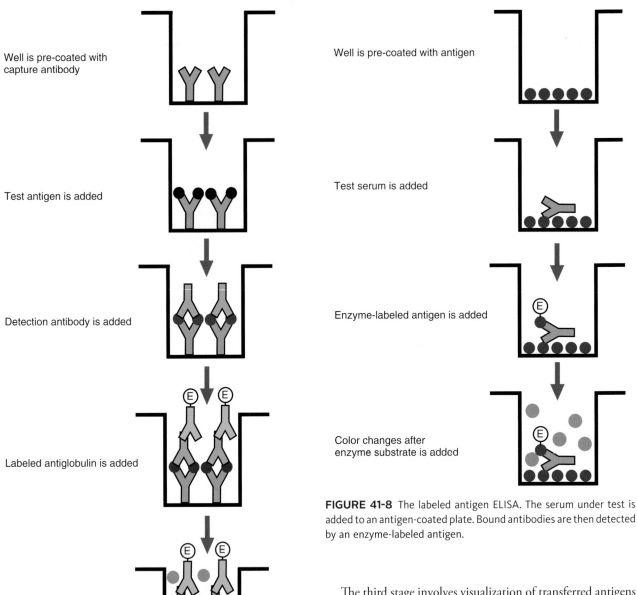

Well is pre-coated with capture antibody

Test antigen is added

Detection antibody is added

Labeled antiglobulin is added

Color changes after enzyme substrate is added

Well is pre-coated with antigen

Test serum is added

Enzyme-labeled antigen is added

Color changes after enzyme substrate is added

FIGURE 41-7 The antibody sandwich ELISA. Antigen is bound to the plate by means of an antibody. The presence of that bound antigen is detected by sequential addition of a second antibody and an enzyme-labeled antiglobulin. Addition of the enzyme substrate leads to a color change proportional to the amount of bound antigen.

FIGURE 41-8 The labeled antigen ELISA. The serum under test is added to an antigen-coated plate. Bound antibodies are then detected by an enzyme-labeled antigen.

an immobilizing nitrocellulose membrane. This is accomplished by placing the membrane on top of the gel and sandwiching the two between sponges saturated with buffer. The membrane-gel sandwich is supported between rigid plastic sheets and placed in a buffer reservoir, and an electrical current is passed between the sponges. The protein bands are transferred from the gel to the membrane without loss of resolution.

The third stage involves visualization of transferred antigens by means of an enzyme immunoassay or radioimmunoassay. When an enzyme immunoassay is employed, the membrane is first incubated in specific antiserum. After the membrane has been washed, an enzyme-labeled antiglobulin solution is added. When this is removed by washing, substrate is added, and a color develops in the bands where the antibody has bound to antigen. When isotope-labeled antiglobulin is used, an autoradiograph must be made and the labeled band identified by darkening of a photographic emulsion. Western blotting is used to identify the important antigens in complex microorganisms or parasites (Figure 41-11). A variant form of the Western blot is the dot blot. Antigen solution is drawn through a nitrocellulose membrane so that any protein binds to the membrane. The presence of the antigen can be determined using specific antiserum and enzyme-labeled antiglobulin in sequence. After exposure to enzyme substrate, the presence of a stained dot is a positive reaction. (Use of nasal washings as a source of the antigen, such as when trying to detect respiratory viruses, is called a snot-blot!).

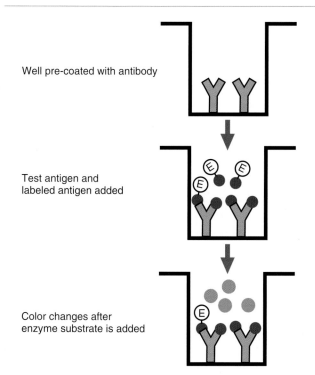

FIGURE 41-9 The competitive ELISA. Labeled and unlabeled antigen compete for binding to antibody. Addition of the enzyme substrate leads to a color change inversely proportional to the amount of test antigen bound.

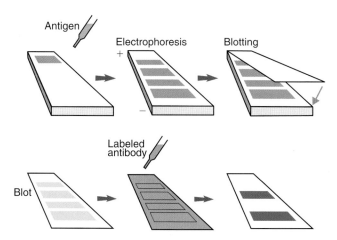

FIGURE 41-10 The Western blotting technique. Serum is separated by electrophoresis and blotted onto nitrocellulose paper; the antigen bands are revealed by use of specific antibody and an enzyme- or isotope-labeled antiglobulin. The blotting stage may be a passive transfer or an electric potential may be used to accelerate the blotting process.

It is possible to put "dots" of many different monoclonal antibodies on a single sheet of nitrocellulose. They may then be exposed to a complex labeled antigen mixture such as a cell protein extract, and after washing and developing, the relative concentrations of many different antigens can be visualized. This is known as an antibody microarray.

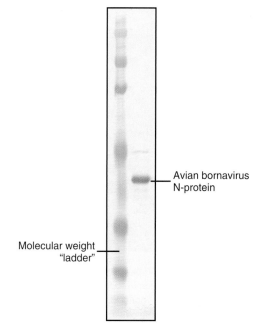

FIGURE 41-11 A Western blot assay. In this example, the serum of a bird was tested for the presence of antibodies to avian bornavirus N-protein. Proteins from a culture of avian bornavirus were first separated by electrophoresis. The electrophoresed material was then blotted onto nitrocellulose paper. Serum from the bird to be tested was allowed to react with the viral proteins and unbound antibodies removed by washing. Finally, the presence of bound antibodies was revealed using an enzyme-labeled antiglobulin followed by enzyme substrate. The N-protein is revealed as a colored band of the correct size. The stained bands on the left are markers of defined molecular weights.

(Courtesy Dr. I. Villanueva.)

ELISAs can be used to test fluids other than blood. For example, saliva or tears can be tested for the presence of feline leukemia virus. In most cases these are simply modified versions of the serum ELISA tests. However, in one such test, a hard plastic swab with antibody to feline leukemia virus bound to the tip is rubbed throughout the cat's mouth. The antibodies on the swab are protected by a sugar coating that is removed by soaking before the test. The antibody on the swab will bind any viral antigen in the saliva. The swab is then inserted into a tube containing enzyme-labeled monoclonal antibodies against feline leukemia virus antigens. After washing, the swab is placed in a solution of the enzyme substrate and the color change noted. This technique is much less sensitive than testing blood directly but is very convenient.

Immunohistochemistry

Enzymes conjugated to immunoglobulins or antiglobulins can be used to locate specific antigens in tissue sections. Horseradish peroxidase is the most widely employed label. The tests are performed in a manner similar to the immunofluorescence tests. In the direct immunoperoxidase test, the tissue section

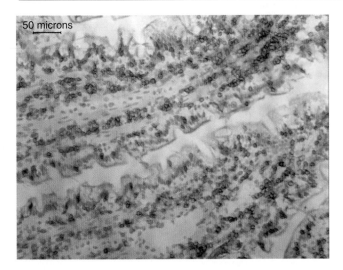

FIGURE 41-12 The immunoperoxidase technique showing the presence of α/β T cells in the lamina propria and epithelium of canine duodenum. Cells binding the monoclonal antibody are exposed to peroxidase-labeled specific antiglobulin. The presence of the peroxidase is revealed as a brown deposit.

(From German AJ, Hall EJ, Moore PF, et al: The distribution of lymphocytes expressing alphabeta and gammadelta T-cell receptors, and the expression of mucosal addressin cell adhesion molecule-1 in the canine intestine, *J Comp Pathol* 121:249–263, 1999.)

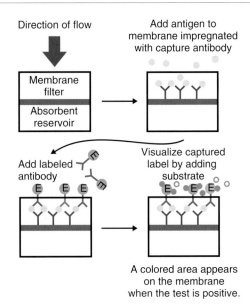

FIGURE 41-13 An immunofiltration technique. Captured antibody is immobilized on a membrane, and reagent samples are allowed to flow through sequentially. The final labeled product is seen as a colored bar or dot. In practice this method is used in the form of a plastic-mounted kit.

(Courtesy IDEXX Laboratories, Inc.)

is treated with the enzyme-labeled antibody. After washing, the tissue is incubated in a solution of the appropriate enzyme substrate. Bound antibody is detected by the development of a brown stain at the site of antibody binding (Figure 41-12). In the indirect test, bound antibody is detected by means of a labeled antiglobulin. This technique has a significant advantage over immunofluorescence techniques in that the tissue can be examined by conventional light microscopy and can be stained so that structural relationships are easier to see.

Disposable Immunoassay Devices

Recent years have seen the development of simple immunoassays that can be employed in the clinic and will give useful information in a very short time. These assays simply provide all necessary reagents in excess, and the sample to be tested becomes the limiting feature. Most disposable devices use this form of assay because the use of excess reagents makes the accurate metering of the sample unnecessary. Examples include immunofiltration and immunochromatography assays.

Immunofiltration

Membrane filter or flow-through devices use a capture antibody immobilized on a membrane filter (Figure 41-13). One simple method uses a nylon membrane coated with antibody. It is set on a support base connected to an absorbent bed. A

test sample, such as blood containing antigen, flows through the antibody-coated membrane, followed at specific intervals by defined volumes of labeled antibody conjugate, wash solution, and enzyme substrate. A positive result, where antigen has bound, may be visualized as a colored dot or the creation of a plus sign. In this test, the negative sign area is formed by material that binds the enzyme conjugate (or by enzyme coupled to the matrix), and the other vertical bar that forms the plus sign is formed by capture antibody bound to the matrix. A modification, which allows the use of whole blood, includes either a blood-solubilizing dilution system or a prefilter to remove cells. Because of the high surface area within these membranes, assay times can be relatively short. This form of test is commonly employed for the diagnosis of feline leukemia, feline immunodeficiency virus, and heartworm infections.

Immunochromatography

To make assays even faster and easier to read, immunochromatography assays are being increasingly employed. In their simplest form, these involve allowing an antigen solution (such as infected blood) to flow laterally through a porous strip. As the solution passes through the strip, it first passes through a zone where it meets and solubilizes dried labeled antibody and forms immune complexes. This antibody may be labeled with either colloidal gold (pink color) or colloidal selenium (blue color). The fluid then flows through a detection zone containing immobilized antibody against the antigen. This captures any immune complexes. As a result, a pink or blue line

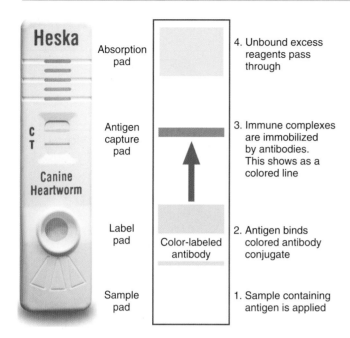

Heska

Absorption pad — 4. Unbound excess reagents pass through

Antigen capture pad — 3. Immune complexes are immobilized by antibodies. This shows as a colored line

Label pad — Color-labeled antibody — 2. Antigen binds colored antibody conjugate

Sample pad — 1. Sample containing antigen is applied

C
T

Canine Heartworm

FIGURE 41-14 Immunochromatography. A sample containing antigen flows through a porous strip, and positive reactions are shown by the appearance of a colored band.

(Courtesy Heska Inc.)

develops in the detection zone in a positive test (Figure 41-14). This simple procedure permits multiple samples to be analyzed in a simple one-step procedure. A positive control band can be developed as well, and the use of an effective prefilter can permit the use of whole blood. This assay is used for the detection of heartworm or feline leukemia antigens. Similar assays may be used to detect viruses such as rota or parvoviruses and bacteria such as salmonella.

Immunochromatography systems are made in several different formats. For example, the sample containing the antigen of interest can be applied to a porous membrane at one end of the strip. Then capillary action can draw the solution through a conjugate pad, a solid-phase detection zone, and into an absorption pad. Buffer may be added to speed the flow of antigen solution. In another form of this assay, the antigen solution is dropped onto a pad containing antibody. This is followed by wash buffer that drives the immune complexes through the pad to an area containing labeled antiglobulin. The immune complexes are captured at this point. Then buffer can be applied at the other end of the pad and used to flush labeled complexes back to the detection zone where they form a colored band. These tests can also be employed for antibody detection using cocktails of recombinant antigens bound to the substrate. Such a test is available for the diagnosis of tuberculosis in animals.

Antibody Labels

Although radioisotopes and enzymes are commonly used as labels for primary binding tests, both have disadvantages. For example, radioactive isotopes may have a short half-life, are

potentially hazardous, and may require expensive detection devices. Enzymes, though stable and relatively cheap, are large molecules that may inhibit antibody activity or lose enzymatic activity in the process of being bound to antiglobulin. One alternative is to use the small molecule biotin and its specific binding protein avidin. Biotin can bind to proteins without affecting their biological activity. Avidin binds very strongly and specifically to biotin and may be conjugated with enzymes.

The most popular enzymes used in ELISAs include alkaline phosphatase, horseradish peroxidase, and β-galactosidase. Enzyme assays involving the production of luminescent products, such as luciferase, may be many times more sensitive than conventional enzyme assays but require sophisticated instruments to measure the luminescence produced. Colored dyes linked to antibodies have been used in dipstick assays. Reagents linked to ferritin or colloidal gold may be used to identify the location of antigens in cells examined by electron microscopy because such labels are electron dense. As described previously, colloidal gold and colloidal selenium are colored and may be used as labels in simple immunochromatography tests.

The Flow Cytometer

Because of the importance of identifying cell immunophenotypes, considerable effort has gone into developing rapid identification methods for cell surface antigens. Immunophenotypes can now be automatically analyzed in great detail and with high efficiency using a flow cytometer (Figure 41-15). In this instrument a suspension of cells is pumped through a very narrow tube so that the cells pass through in single file. A laser beam is directed through the cell stream, and the effects of each cell on the light beam are measured. The scatter of the light beam in a forward direction can be used to give a measure of a cell's size. The light scattered to the side by a cell gives a measure of a cell's surface roughness and internal complexity. A combination of these two parameters can be used to identify all the leukocytes in a blood sample.

The flow cytometer can, however, be used to measure much more than this. If a cell suspension is mixed with a fluorescent monoclonal antibody, the labeled antibody will bind to cells carrying the appropriate antigen on its surface. This subpopulation can be characterized and counted (Figures 41-16 and 41-17). By using antibodies labeled with different colors of fluorescent dyes, the expression of multiple cell surface antigens can be analyzed simultaneously. It is possible to use the flow cytometer to follow sequential changes in the immunophenotype of mixed-cell populations (Figure 41-18).

Secondary Binding Tests

The reactions between antigens and antibodies are commonly followed by a secondary reaction. If antibodies combine with soluble antigens in solution, the resulting complexes may precipitate. Antibodies binding to particulate antigens (e.g.,

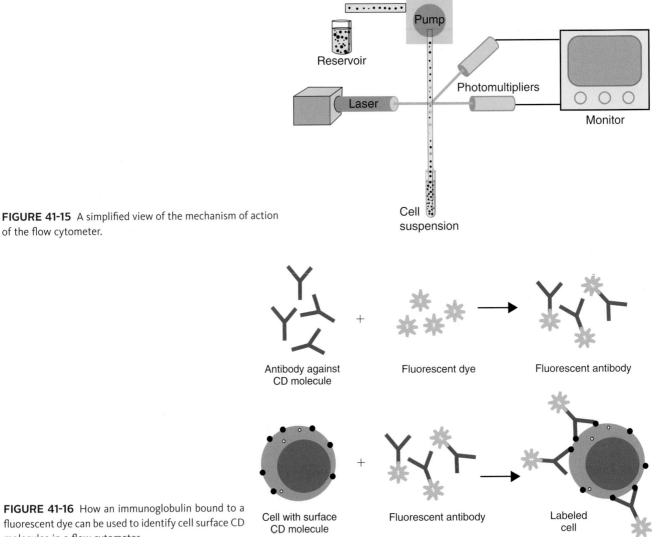

FIGURE 41-15 A simplified view of the mechanism of action of the flow cytometer.

FIGURE 41-16 How an immunoglobulin bound to a fluorescent dye can be used to identify cell surface CD molecules in a flow cytometer.

bacteria or red blood cells) may make them clump or agglutinate. If an antibody can activate the classical complement pathway and the antigen is on a cell surface, cell lysis may result. These reactions can be employed in many different serological assays.

Precipitation Tests

If a solution of soluble antigen is mixed with a strong antiserum, the mixture becomes cloudy within a few minutes, and then flocculent; finally a precipitate settles to the bottom of the tube within an hour. The precipitate consists of antigen-antibody complexes. If increasing amounts of soluble antigen are mixed with a constant amount of antibody, the amount of precipitate that develops is determined by the relative proportions of the reactants. No obvious precipitate is formed at low antigen concentrations. As the amount of antigen increases, larger quantities of precipitate form until the amount is maximal. However, with the addition of yet more antigen, the amount of precipitate gradually diminishes, until none is present in tubes containing a large excess of antigen (Figure 41-19). Equine IgG3 antibodies behave in a somewhat different fashion, producing a distinct flocculation over a very narrow range of antigen concentrations (Figure 41-20).

In the first stage of these reactions, only a little antigen is complexed to antibody, so little precipitate is deposited. In the tubes where most precipitation occurs, both antigen and antibody are completely complexed, and neither can be detected in the supernatant fluid. This is called the equivalence zone, and the ratio of antibody to antigen is optimal. When antigen is added to excess, a precipitate does not form, although soluble immune complexes are present, and free antigen may be detected in the supernatant fluid.

This pattern results from the fact that antibodies are bivalent and therefore can cross-link only two epitopes at a time, but complex antigens are generally multivalent, possessing many epitopes (Figure 41-21). Where there is excess antibody, each antigen molecule is covered with antibody molecules, preventing cross-linkage and thus precipitation. When the

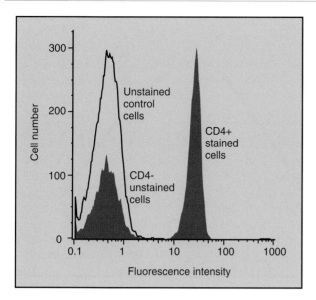

FIGURE 41-17 A typical flow cytometer readout from labeling a cell population with antiequine CD4. The intensity of fluorescent labeling increases from left to right. Thus unlabeled control cells form the unshaded left peak. When a mixture of CD4$^+$ and CD4$^-$ cells is examined it forms two distinct peaks (*shaded area*). The left peak consists of unlabeled (CD4$^-$) cells. The right peak consists of labeled (CD4$^+$) cells. The area under each peak is a measure of the size of each cell subpopulation.

(Courtesy Dr. R.R. Smith III.)

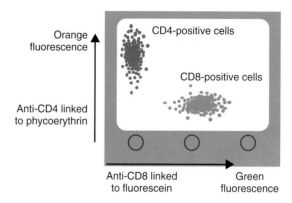

FIGURE 41-18 The pattern seen on a flow cytometer screen when analyzing lymphocyte populations stained with two different fluorescence-conjugated antibodies. It is usual to label one population with a green dye and the second population with a red or orange dye.

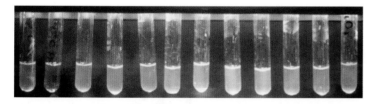

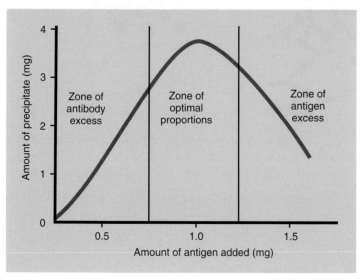

FIGURE 41-19 The effect of mixing increasing amounts of antigen (bovine serum) with a constant amount of antibody (rabbit antiserum). The tube with the greatest amount of precipitate is the one in which the ratio of antigen to antibody is optimal. A quantitative precipitation curve of this test shows this effect graphically.

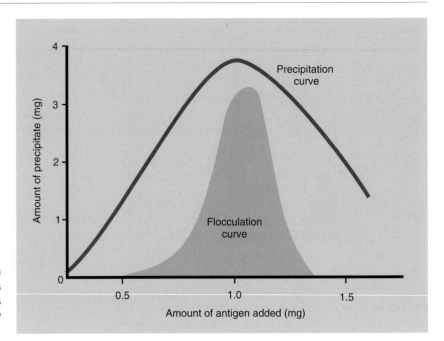

FIGURE 41-20 A quantitative precipitation curve of the type obtained when horse serum is used as a source of antibody. Flocculation occurs only over a narrow range of antigen-antibody mixtures.

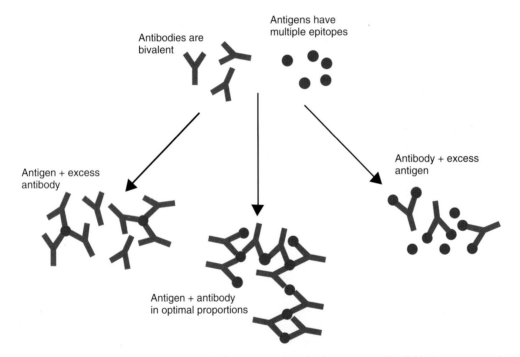

FIGURE 41-21 The mechanism of immunoprecipitation. In both antigen and antibody excess, small, soluble, immune complexes are produced. However, at optimal proportions, large insoluble complexes are generated.

reactants are in optimal proportions, the ratio of antigen to antibody is such that cross-linking and lattice formation are extensive. As this lattice grows it becomes insoluble and eventually precipitates. In mixtures in which antigen is in excess, each antibody molecule binds two antigen molecules. Further cross-linkage is impossible, and since these complexes are small and soluble, no precipitation occurs. Mononuclear phagocytes are most efficient at binding and removing complexes formed at optimal proportions and in antibody excess. Small immune

complexes formed in antigen excess are poorly removed by phagocytic cells but are deposited in vessel walls and in glomeruli, where they cause type III hypersensitivity (Chapter 30).

Immunodiffusion

One simple method of demonstrating immune precipitation is immunodiffusion or gel diffusion. Round wells, about 5 mm in diameter and about 1 cm apart, are cut in a layer of clear

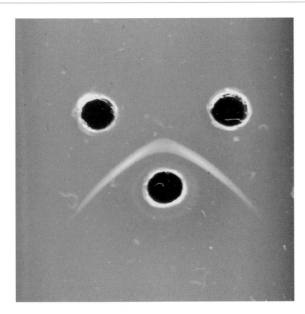

FIGURE 41-22 Precipitation in agar gel. Antigen and antibody diffusing from their respective wells precipitate in a region where optimal proportions are achieved. In this example, the antigen is identical in both top wells. As a result, the precipitation lines fuse to show complete identity.

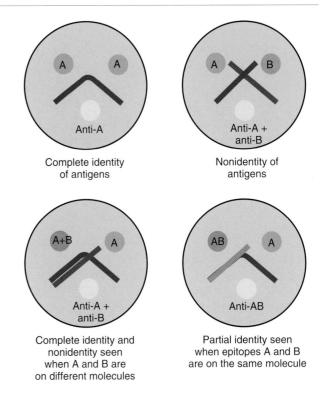

FIGURE 41-23 The gel diffusion technique to determine the relationship of two antigens.

agar. One well is then filled with soluble antigen and the other with antiserum; the reactants diffuse out radially. Where the reactants meet in optimal proportions, an opaque white line of precipitate appears (Figure 41-22).

If the solutions used contain several different antigens and antibodies, the components are unlikely to reach optimal proportions in exactly the same position. Consequently, a separate line of precipitate is produced for each interacting set of antigens and antibodies. This test can be used to determine the relationship between antigens. If two antigen wells and one antibody well are set up as in Figures 41-22 and 41-23, lines will form between each antigen well and the antibody well. If these two lines join, the two antigens are probably identical. If the lines cross, the two antigens are completely different. If the lines merge with spur formation, a partial identity exists, indicating that one antigen possesses epitopes not present in the other. The Coggins test is a gel diffusion method used to detect antibodies against equine infectious anemia virus in horse serum. In this test an extract of infected horse spleen or a cell culture antigen reacts with the serum of the horse under test in agar gel, and the development of a line of precipitate constitutes a positive reaction. A similar test is used to identify cattle infected with bovine leukemia virus.

Radial Immunodiffusion If an antigen solution diffuses into agar in which specific antiserum has been incorporated, a ring of precipitate will form around the antigen well. The area of this ring is proportional to the amount of antigen in the well. A standard curve may therefore be constructed using known amounts of antigen (Figure 41-24). Unknown solutions

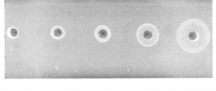

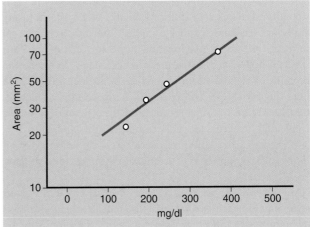

FIGURE 41-24 A radial immunodiffusion assay. The area of precipitation is proportional to the concentration of antigen. In this case antiserum to bovine IgA is incorporated in the agar and is used to measure bovine serum IgA levels.

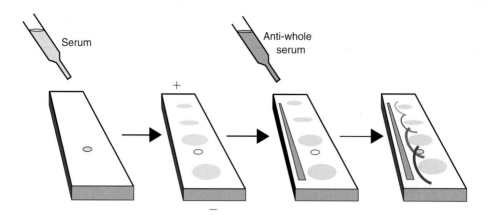

FIGURE 41-25 The technique of immunoelectrophoresis (see text for details).

of antigen can then be accurately assayed by comparing the ring diameters from unknowns with the standard curve. This test is used to measure serum immunoglobulin levels in newborn foals (Chapter 21).

Immunoelectrophoresis and Related Techniques

Although conventional gel-diffusion techniques give a separate precipitation line for each antigen-antibody system in a mixture, it is often difficult to resolve all the components in a complex mixture. One way to improve the resolution of the system is to first separate the antigen mixture by electrophoresis before undertaking immunodiffusion. This technique is called immunoelectrophoresis and is used to identify proteins in body fluids (Figure 41-25).

Immunoelectrophoresis involves the electrophoresis of the antigen mixture in agar gel in one direction. A trough is then cut in the agar parallel to this line of separated proteins. Antiserum against the whole serum is placed in this trough and allowed to diffuse laterally. When the diffusing antibodies encounter antigen, curved lines of precipitate are formed. One arc of precipitation forms for each of the constituents in the antigen mixture. This technique can resolve the proteins of normal serum into 25 to 40 distinct precipitation lines (Figure 41-26). This technique has been used to identify the absence of a normal serum protein, as in animals with a congenital deficiency of some complement components. It is also used to detect the presence of excessive amounts of an individual component, as in animals with myeloma (Figure 15-22).

If, instead of being permitted to passively diffuse into agar-containing antiserum as in the radial immunodiffusion technique, the antigen is driven into the antiserum agar by electrophoresis, the ring of precipitation around each well becomes deformed into a rocket shape. The length of the rocket is proportional to the amount of antigen placed in each well. This technique is called rocket electrophoresis.

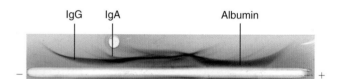

FIGURE 41-26 Immunoelectrophoresis of pig serum showing the lines of precipitation produced by some of the major serum proteins. (See also Figure 15-22.)

Titration of Antibodies

Although the simple detection of antibodies or antigen is sufficient for many purposes, it is usually desirable to quantitate the reaction. One way of measuring specific antibody levels is by titration. The serum under test is diluted in a series of decreasing concentrations (Figure 41-27). Each dilution is then tested for activity. The reciprocal of the highest dilution giving a positive reaction, called the titer, provides an estimate of the amount of antibody in that serum.

Agglutination

Because antibodies are bivalent, they can cross-link particulate antigens such as bacteria or foreign red cells, resulting in their clumping or agglutination. Antibodies differ in their ability to cause agglutination; for example, IgM antibodies are more efficient than IgG antibodies (Table 41-2). If excess antibody is added to a suspension of antigenic particles, then, just as in the precipitation reaction, each particle may be so coated by antibody that agglutination is inhibited. This lack of reactivity at high concentrations of antibody is termed a prozone. Another cause of prozone formation is the presence of antibodies that cannot cause agglutination. These nonagglutinating antibodies are also called incomplete antibodies. The reason for their lack of agglutinating activity is not completely understood; one possibility is that the epitopes with which they react

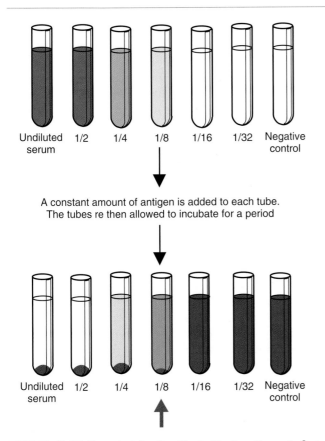

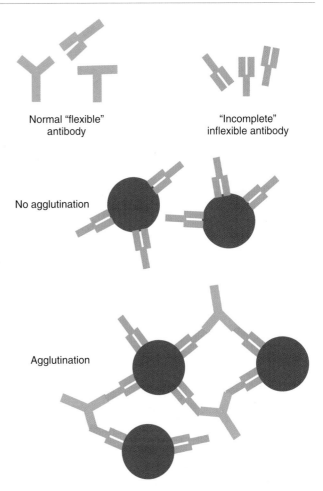

FIGURE 41-28 The direct antiglobulin test. The presence of the antiglobulin is required to agglutinate particles coated with nonagglutinating antibody.

FIGURE 41-27 The principle of antibody titration. Serum is first diluted in a series of tubes. A constant amount of antigen is then added to each tube, and the tubes are incubated. At the end of the incubation period, the last tube in which a reaction has occurred is identified. In this example, agglutination has occurred in all tubes up to a serum dilution of 1:8. The agglutination titer of the serum is said to be 8.

lie deep within the surface coat of the particle, so deep that cross-linking cannot occur. An alternative suggestion is that they are capable of only restricted movement in their hinge region, causing them to be functionally monovalent (Chapter 29).

Antiglobulin Tests

If it is necessary to test for the presence of nonagglutinating antibodies on the surface of particles such as bacteria or erythrocytes, a direct antiglobulin test may be used. The washed particles may be mixed with an antiglobulin, and if antibodies are present on their surface, agglutination will occur (Figure 41-28).

Passive Agglutination

Since agglutination is a much more sensitive technique than precipitation, it is sometimes useful to convert a precipitating system to an agglutinating one (Figure 41-29). This may be done by chemically linking soluble antigen to inert particles such as erythrocytes, bacteria, or latex beads.

□ Table 41-2 | Role of Specific Immunoglobulin Classes in Serological Assays

PROPERTY	IgG	IgM	IgA	EQUINE IgG3
Agglutination	+	+++	+	−
Complement activation	+	+++	−	−
Precipitation	+++	+	±	±
Time of appearance (days)	3-7	2-5	3-7	3-7
Time to peak titer (days)	7-21	5-14	7-21	7-21

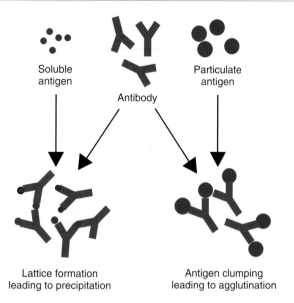

FIGURE 41-29 The relationship between precipitation and agglutination. This is essentially a consequence of the size of the antigenic particle. Large particles agglutinate. Small particles and soluble molecules precipitate.

Erythrocytes are among the best particles for this purpose, and tests that employ coated erythrocytes are called passive hemagglutination tests.

Viral Hemagglutination and Its Inhibition

Some viruses can bind and agglutinate mammalian and avian red cells. This virus-induced hemagglutination may assist in characterizing an unknown virus. Inhibition of viral hemagglutination by antibody can be used either as a method of identifying a specific virus or to measure antibody levels in serum. Hemagglutinating organisms include orthomyxoviruses and paramyxoviruses, alphaviruses, flaviviruses, and bunyaviruses as well as some adenoviruses, reoviruses, parvoviruses, and coronaviruses. They also include some mycoplasma such as *Mycoplasma gallisepticum*.

Complement Fixation

The activation of the classical complement pathway by antibody bound to antigen results in the generation of terminal complement complexes that can disrupt cell membranes. If the antibody binds red cells, these will be ruptured, and hemolysis occurs. This phenomenon can be used to measure serum antibody levels in a test called the complement fixation test.

Complement is a normal constituent of all fresh serum, but the complement in fresh, unheated guinea pig serum is the most efficient in hemolytic tests. Serum used as a source of complement for serological applications should be stored frozen in small volumes. Once thawed, it should be used promptly. It should not be repeatedly frozen and thawed.

The complement fixation test is performed in two parts. First, antigen and antibodies (the serum under test deprived of its complement by heating at 56° C) are mixed and incubated in the presence of normal guinea pig serum as a source of complement. After the antigen-antibody-complement mixture reacts, the amount of free complement remaining in the mixture is measured by adding an indicator system consisting of antibody-coated sheep red cells. Lysis of these cells (seen as the development of a transparent red solution) is a negative result because it indicates that complement was not activated and that antibody was absent from the serum under test (Figure 41-30). Absence of lysis (seen as a cloudy red cell suspension), indicating that complement was consumed (or fixed), is a positive result. It is usual to titrate the serum being tested so that, if antibodies are present in that serum, as it is diluted the reaction in each tube will change from no lysis (positive) to lysis (negative). The titer is the highest dilution of serum in which no more than 50% of the red cells are lysed.

Cytotoxicity Tests

Complement may cause membrane damage, not only to erythrocytes but also to nucleated cells and to protozoa. Antibodies against cell surface antigens thus may be measured by reacting target cells with antibody and complement and estimating the resulting cell death. This form of assay has been employed to tissue type cells by determining which major histocompatibility complex (MHC) class I molecules they are expressing.

Assays in Living Systems

If an organism or antigen possesses biological activity, antibodies can be measured by their ability to neutralize this activity. The activities that may be neutralized include hemolysis of erythrocytes, lysis of nucleated cells, and disease or death in animals. Reactions such as these are subject to a high degree of variability because they tend to change gradually over a wide range of doses of organism or antigen. For this reason, results obtained from a single positive or negative neutralization test are usually of little use. For example, 0.003 mg of tetanus toxin may kill some mice in a test group, but about five times that dose is required to kill all mice in the same group. In addition, if an attempt is made to assess the lowest dose of tetanus toxin that will kill all the animals in a group (the minimal lethal dose), it is found to be highly variable. It is equally difficult to estimate with precision the highest dose of toxin that will just fail to kill all test animals. The most exact method of measuring the lethal effects of a toxin has been to estimate the dose that will just kill 50% of a group of test animals (Figure 41-31). In practice, it is usually not possible to arrive at this 50% end point by direct experimentation. For this reason it is usually necessary to calculate it by plotting the results against the

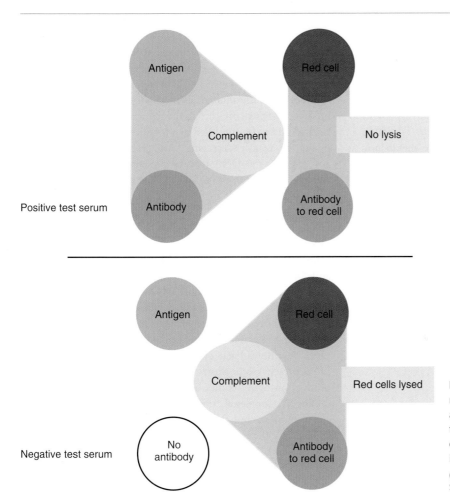

FIGURE 41-30 The principle of the complement fixation test. Complement, if fixed by antigen and antibody, is unavailable to lyse the target cells in the indicator system. In the absence of antibody the complement remains unfixed and is available to lyse the indicator system.

(Modified from Roitt I: *Essential immunology*. Blackwell Science, 1971, Oxford.)

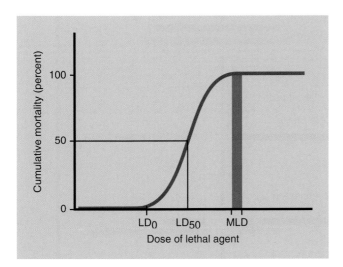

FIGURE 41-31 A cumulative mortality curve showing how the LD_{50} provides a more accurate estimate of the lethal effects of a toxin than either the LD_0 or the MLD.

dose of toxin given and arriving at the 50% end point by calculation.

In the example cited in the previous paragraph, the lethality of the toxin can be estimated by measuring the dose required to kill 50% of a group of experimental animals. This lethal dose is called the LD_{50}. Similarly, the dose of complement that just hemolyses 50% of a red cell suspension is called the CH_{50}. The dose of organisms that infects 50% of animals is the ID_{50}, the dose that just infects 50% of tissue cultures is the $TCID_{50}$, and the dose of antiserum or vaccine that protects 50% of challenged animals is the PD_{50}.

Neutralization Tests

Neutralization tests estimate the ability of antibody to neutralize the biological activity of antigen when mixed with it in vitro. These tests may be used to identify bacterial toxins such as *Clostridium perfringens* α-toxin or staphylococcal α-toxin.

Viruses may be prevented from infecting cells after specific antibody has combined with and blocked their critical attachment sites. This reaction is the basis of the neutralization tests that are employed either for the identification of unknown viruses or for the measurement of specific antiviral antibody. Neutralization tests are highly specific and extremely sensitive. Thus, antiserum to coliphage T4 will neutralize phage-induced lysis of *Escherichia coli* because antibodies can block the receptor on the phage tail, thus preventing its attachment to a bacterium. A single antibody molecule is sufficient to cause this blockage, and a phage neutralization test may therefore detect as little as 0.00005 mg of antibody.

Protection Tests

A protection test is a form of neutralization test carried out entirely in vivo. The protective properties of a specific antiserum are measured by administering it in increasing dilutions to a group of test animals, which may then be challenged with a standard dose of pathogenic organisms or toxin. Although protection tests provide a direct measure of the therapeutic efficacy of an antiserum, they are also subject to great experimental variation because of differences among animals. Animals differ in their susceptibility to infection and in a number of other factors, such as the rate of absorption of antiserum, the level of activity of the mononuclear phagocyte system, and the half-life of the passively administered immunoglobulin. As in neutralization tests, meaningful results can be obtained only if large numbers of animals are employed and if the challenge dose is carefully standardized. It is usual to use a dose of organisms or toxin containing a known number of LD_{50} or ID_{50}. Similarly, the protective effect of an antiserum may be expressed in PD_{50}, the dose required to protect 50% of a group of animals.

Molecular Methods

Although immunological assays have historically provided the most sensitive assays for diagnostic purposes, modern molecular techniques have proved to be even more sensitive and specific. The detection of the nucleic acid of an infectious agent through polymerase chain reactions (PCRs) is often superior to immunological methods (Figure 41-32). This method is based on the ability of very small quantities of nucleic acid to be amplified in a highly specific manner so that it can be readily detected. Thus, for example, very small amounts of viral DNA may be present in a tissue sample. If the tissue is heated, the paired DNA strands will separate into two single strands. If the nucleotide sequence of this DNA is known, specific primers (oligonucleotides of single-stranded DNA) can be added to the tissue, where they bind the viral DNA and act as a template for new DNA synthesis. These primers are selected so that they are complementary to the 3′ ends of the sequence to be amplified. Thus these primers will bind to the ends of the sample DNA—a process called annealing. By adding an enzyme called DNA polymerase, new complementary strands of DNA are then assembled on the primers. The cycle is now repeated: heating → primer annealing → new DNA assembly. Each cycle doubles the amount of specific DNA present, so in theory, 30 such cycles should result in the production of 2^{30} copies of the original DNA sample. Once cycling is completed, the products can be examined by gel electrophoresis and the characteristic DNA bands identified. If necessary the bands may be sequenced to provide assurance that the correct DNA has been amplified.

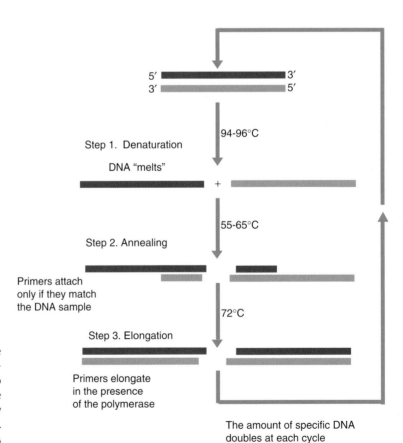

FIGURE 41-32 The principle of the polymerase chain reaction (PCR) test. Essentially by performing a cycle of reactions repeatedly, it is possible to produce large amounts of DNA coding for the gene of interest. Thus the cycle can be driven by repeatedly changing the reaction temperature. Once produced in sufficient amounts, this DNA can be detected by electrophoresis.

As might be anticipated, many different variations of the basic PCR process have been developed. For example, if the nucleic acid of interest is RNA rather than DNA (e.g., detecting an RNA virus), a reverse-transcriptase PCR may be performed. This simply involves the initial conversion of the viral RNA to DNA using a reverse transcriptase, before beginning the PCR cycle.

Real-time PCR uses fluorescence-resonance energy transfer to quantitate the amplification of a specific DNA of interest. As the cycles proceed, the amount of fluorescence increases and can be plotted. With this test, it is possible to measure the initial copy number, and it is less susceptible to contamination errors.

PCR assays are not only useful in detecting the presence of trace amounts of viral nucleic acid in tissues. They can also be used to amplify specific genes from within an animal's own DNA. For example, if the primers are correctly selected, they can be used to amplify normal or abnormal genes. Thus PCR can identify SCID foals or cattle with leukocyte adherence deficiency (Chapter 37).

Diagnostic Applications of Immunological Tests

Obviously, the presence of antibodies to a specific organism in an animal's serum indicates previous exposure to an epitope present on that organism. It does not, however, prove that infection exists or that any concurrent disease is actually caused by the organism in question. For example, the fact that the sera of most healthy horses contain antibodies to *Salmonella typhimurium* does not prove that most horses are suffering from salmonellosis. The presence of antibodies to an organism in a single serum sample is rarely of diagnostic significance. Only if at least two samples are taken 1 to 3 weeks apart and show at least a fourfold rise in titer can a diagnosis be made. This should be done only in conjunction with careful clinical assessment.

A second feature that must be considered in the interpretation of serological tests is the possibility of errors. Technical errors are usually prevented by incorporation of appropriate controls into the test system. Other errors, however, are largely unavoidable. For example, if test results are obtained from a known diseased population and from a known disease-free population, it will be rare to find that the results obtained separate perfectly. Much more commonly, the test results overlap, and the test cannot distinguish normal from diseased with 100% accuracy (Figure 41-33). As a result, irrespective of the selected cut-off point, there will be some correct results and some incorrect ones. There will be four types of result: true-positive and true-negative results and false-positive and false-negative results. A test in which a large proportion of the positive results are true is considered specific, whereas one that correctly identifies the true-negative responses is sensitive. In general, the level of such errors is set by the point used to

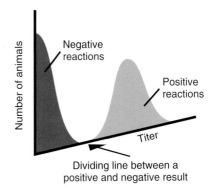

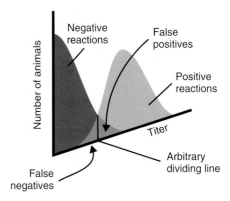

FIGURE 41-33 Schematic diagrams depicting the errors associated with immunological tests. The top diagram depicts an ideal test in which there is no ambiguity in interpreting test results. The bottom diagram depicts a more typical test in which an arbitrary line must be used to separate positive from negative results. By moving this dividing line, the relative proportions of false-positive and false-negative results may be changed.

differentiate positive from negative reactions. If the cut-off point is adjusted downward so that the criterion for a positive test is made less strict, the number of false-positive results will increase, but there will also be a decrease in the number of false-negative results. Thus, highly sensitive tests tend to be relatively nonspecific, and highly specific tests are generally insensitive. The establishment of the cut-off point in reading tests and, from this, the sensitivity and specificity of a test are determined both by the requirements of the test procedure and by the importance of false-positive and false-negative reactions. In ideal tests, it would be desirable for the criteria used in interpreting the test results to be so obvious and absolute that each test would be absolutely sensitive and specific. Unfortunately, such ideal tests are uncommon.

The sensitivity and specificity of any test can be calculated using the number of true-positive (a), false-positive (c), true-negative (d), and false-negative (b) results. The sensitivity of a test is the probability that a test result will be positive when the disease is present (true-positive rate) will be $a/(a + b)$. The specificity of a test is the probability that a test will be negative when the disease is absent (the negative rate will be d/(c + d). Because of the reciprocal nature of sensitivity and specificity (one goes up as the other goes down), it is possible to plot this graphically using a receiver operating characteristic (ROC) curve (Figure 41-34). In this technique, the sensitivity is plotted as a function of 100 minus the specificity for different cut-off points. Each point on the ROC curve thus represents sensitivity/specificity for a given cut-off point. A test with perfect discrimination will thus have an ROC plot that passes through the upper left corner (100% sensitivity and 100% specificity). An investigator can determine the optimal cut-off point by selecting the point on the curve closest to the upper left corner. The area under the curve also provides a measure of how well the test separates the two populations being tested. An area of 1 represents a perfect test, whereas an area of 0.5 represents a test whose results do not differ from random and hence is useless. ROC curve analysis is very useful in determining the best way to interpret a serological test, especially assays such as ELISAs, in which quantitative data is obtained, but their significance is not immediately apparent.

As has been evident from the discussions earlier in this chapter, the advantages and disadvantages of each immunodiagnostic test vary according to the specific requirements of the investigator, the nature of the antigen employed, and the complexity, sensitivity, and specificity of each method. In general, the selection of a diagnostic test represents a compromise among its sensitivity, its specificity, and its complexity. The latter includes the number of steps involved, the time involved, the degree of technical expertise required, its cost, and the nature of the equipment needed to conduct the test. Although precise guidelines cannot be drawn, it is usually most appropriate to use the most sensitive and specific test that can be satisfactorily performed with the available technical

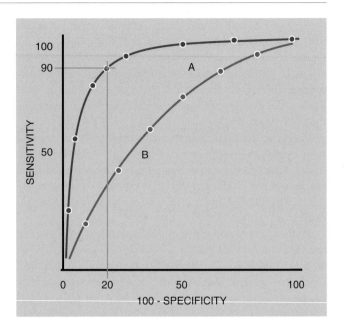

FIGURE 41-34 An ROC curve plots a test sensitivity against 100-specificity for an entire range of cut-off points (e.g., different optical density values in an ELISA test). In a good test, specificity and sensitivity approach 100%, and the appropriate cut-off value may be very obvious. Thus in test A, the best cut-off point would give a sensitivity of 90% and a specificity of 80%. Unfortunately, this is not always the case (B).

assistance and equipment at the lowest cost in the shortest possible time.

For sources of additional information, please visit http:// evolve.elsevier.com/tizard/immunology/

Appendix 1

Annotated List of Selected CD Molecules

Note: Of the 363 officially recognized CD molecules, many have no known function at this time, whereas others do not play a significant role in the immune system. Most are glycoproteins. This list summarizes the key features of only those CD molecules described in the text.

CD1 A family of class Id MHC-like molecules that are antigen-presenting molecules for lipids and glycolipids. Found on thymocytes, macrophages, dendritic cells, NKT cells, and some B cells.

CD2 Also called LFA-2, this is a cell adherence molecule whose ligands are CD58 (nonrodents) and CD48 (rodents only). It is found on T cells and some B cells.

CD3 A collective designation for the signal transducing molecules of the TCR. They are found only on T cells.

CD4 A receptor for MHC class II molecules that plays a key role in the recognition of processed antigen by helper T cells. It is expressed on helper T cells, thymocytes, and monocytes.

CD5 A receptor for CD72. It is found on T cells and a subpopulation of B cells (B-1a cells) in most species, including mice and humans, but not on B cells in rats or dogs.

CD8 This dimeric glycoprotein is a receptor for MHC class I molecules that plays a key role in the recognition of endogenous antigen. It is expressed on cytotoxic T cells

CD9 A glycoprotein expressed on platelets, immature B cells, eosinophils, basophils, and activated T cells.

CD10 An endopeptidase expressed on T and B cell precursors.

CD11 Also called LFA-1, this is an integrin α chain found on leukocytes. Three forms are known, 11a, 11b, and 11c. They bind leukocytes to vascular endothelium.

CD14 This is the receptor for lipopolysaccharide-binding protein and therefore regulates the biological activities of this molecule. It is found on macrophages and granulocytes.

CD15 A complex carbohydrate called Lewis-X. Its sialylated form, sialyl Lewis^x is expressed on NK cells. Its ligand is the selectin CD62. It is found on many cells, especially granulocytes.

CD16 Also called FcγRIII, this is a low-affinity receptor for IgG and for CD4. It is found on NK cells, granulocytes, and macrophages.

CD18 This is the integrin β1 chain found on all leukocytes. It associates with the various forms of CD11. A mutation in the *CD18* gene is responsible for leukocyte adherence deficiency in calves.

CD19 A protein that associates with CD21 and plays a key role in regulating the B cell response to antigen. It is expressed on B cells and their precursors but not on plasma cells. It is also expressed on dendritic cells.

CD21 A complement receptor also called CR2. Its several ligands include CD23 and C3d. It regulates B cell responses in association with CD19. CD21 is found on B cells, some T cells, and dendritic cells

CD22 Also called siglec-2; a B cell inhibitory receptor.

CD23 A receptor for IgE also called FcϵRII. In its soluble form it regulates the production of IgE. It can also regulate B cell responses by binding to CD21. It is found mainly on mature B cells.

CD25 The α chain of the IL-2 receptor. CD25 associates with the IL-2Rβchain (CD122). It is expressed on activated T cells, B cells, and monocytes. CD25 expression is a feature of regulatory T cells.

CD28 The ligand for both CD80 and CD86 that plays a key role in T cell co-stimulation. It is expressed on activated B cells and other antigen-presenting cells. It delivers a stimulatory signal to T cells as opposed to CD152, which delivers a suppressive signal.

CD29 A β_1 integrin expressed on leukocytes and platelets. In conjunction with its α chain (one of the forms of CD49), it binds these cells to extracellular matrix proteins.

CD31 Mediates adhesion between cells that express CD31 (e.g., leukocytes to endothelial cells) in a homophilic manner (CD31 binds CD31 on the apposing cell). It regulates the phagocytosis of dead and dying cells.

CD32 A medium-affinity IgG receptor also called FcγRII, different forms of which are expressed on macrophages, granulocytes, and B cells.

CD33 Siglec-3, a lectin expressed on immature hematopoietic stem cells.

CD34 Also called sialomucin, this glycoprotein is a ligand for certain integrins. It is expressed on endothelial cells and some dendritic cells.

CD35 This is the receptor for the complement components C3b and C4b, so it is also called CR1. It is expressed on granulocytes, monocytes, B cells, NK cells, and primate erythrocytes.

CD36 A pattern-recognition receptor that binds many different ligands, especially lipids. CD36 on intestinal γ/δ T cells binds bacterial lipoteichoic acids and helps trigger innate responses. Found on many different cell types.

CD40 A member of the tumor necrosis factor receptor superfamily. Binding to its ligand CD40L (CD154) on activated helper T cells is essential for a successful antibody response and class switching. It is expressed on all antigen-presenting cells.

CD41 An integrin α chain expressed on platelets and macrophages. It associates with its β chain (CD61) and binds fibrinogen.

CD43 Also called sialophorin or leukosialin, this glycoprotein serves as an antiadhesive molecule on leukocytes. It is expressed on T cells as well as granulocytes, macrophages, NK cells, platelets, and activated B cells.

CD44 A receptor for hyaluronic acid that mediates binding of cells to high endothelial venules. It is expressed in large amounts on T and B cells, monocytes and granulocytes, and many other cells.

CD45 A family of tyrosine phosphatases, some of which are required for signaling through the TCR. Multiple isoforms of CD45 are generated by alternative splicing of three exons. They are found on all cells of hematopoietic origin except red cells.

CD46 Also called membrane cofactor protein. CD46 is a receptor for C3b and C4b. Once bound, these complement components are destroyed by factor I. It is expressed on T cells, B cells, monocytes, granulocytes, NK cells, platelets, fibroblasts, endothelial cells, and epithelial cells, but not on red cells.

CD48 A GPI-linked glycoprotein that is a ligand for CD2 and CD247 in rodents. It is expressed on all blood lymphocytes.

CD49 A family of integrin α chains associated with the CD29 β chain. They are expressed in various forms on leukocytes, platelets, and epithelial cells. Also called very-late antigens (VLAs), their ligands are extracellular matrix proteins.

CD50 ICAM-3, the ligand for DC-SIGN (CD209) on dendritic cells. It is expressed on T cells.

CD51 An integrin α chain found on platelets and endothelial cells. Its β chain is CD61, and its ligand is vitronectin.

CD54 Also called ICAM-1, this glycoprotein is the ligand for the CD11a/CD18 and CD11b/CD18 integrins. It is expressed on a wide variety of cells, most notably vascular endothelial cells.

CD55 Also called decay accelerating factor, this glycoprotein blocks the assembly of C3 convertase and accelerates its disassembly. It thus protects normal cells against attack by complement. It is broadly distributed on many cell types.

CD56 An adhesion molecule expressed on NK cells and nerve cells.

CD58 Also called LFA-3, this is a glycoprotein found on most cells where it is a ligand for CD2.

CD59 A glycoprotein also called protectin, it is the major inhibitor of the terminal complement pathway by binding to C8 and C9 and blocking the assembly of the terminal complement complex. It is expressed on leukocytes, vascular endothelium, and epithelial cells.

CD61 A $β_3$-integrin that associates with CD41 to bind to extracellular matrix proteins. It is expressed on platelets and macrophages.

CD62 The selectins (S-lectins) bind to carbohydrate structures such as CD15s (sialyl Lewis^x) on neutrophils. CD62E is E-selectin, CD62L is L-selectin, and CD62P is P-selectin. They are expressed on platelets, lymphocytes, and endothelial cells.

CD64 Also called FcγRI, this high-affinity IgG receptor plays a key role in antibody-dependent cellular cytotoxicity. It is expressed on monocytes and interferon-γ-stimulated granulocytes.

CD66e Also called carcinoembryonic antigen, this glycoprotein is expressed in large quantities by malignant intestinal cells. Its detection is therefore diagnostic of intestinal malignancy in humans.

CD71 A transferrin receptor expressed on activated leukocytes. It is required by dividing cells to import iron. It may also act as a selective IgA receptor.

CD72 Found on B cells (but not plasma cells), CD72 is a ligand for CD5. It may participate in an alternative pathway of B cell and T cell activation.

CD74 Also called the γ or invariant chain, this protein associates with intracellular MHC class II molecules. Found in all MHC class II–positive cells. It is believed to prevent the premature binding of endogenous peptides.

CD79 CD79a is an alternative name for the BCR signal-transducing peptide, Ig-α, and CD79b is another name for Ig-β.

CD80 Also called B7-1, this is high-affinity receptor for CD28 and CD152 (CTLA-4). The interaction of CD80 with its ligands is crucial to T cell communication with antigen-presenting cells.

CD81 Also called TAPA-1, CD81 is a widely expressed cell surface protein that regulates both B cell and T cell responses. On B cells it forms a complex with CD19 and CD21 and is involved with co-stimulation of T cells.

CD83 A member of the immunoglobulin superfamily used as a marker for mature dendritic cells. Its function is unknown.

CD85 A family of leukocyte Ig-like receptors (LIRs) that act as receptors for MHC class I molecules. They are expressed on macrophages, dendritic cells, and B cells.

CD86 Related to CD80 and also called B7-2, this co-stimulatory receptor is expressed on antigen-presenting macrophages, activated B cells, and dendritic cells. Its ligands are CD28 and CD152 (CTLA-4).

CD88 The C5a receptor found on granulocytes, macrophages, and mast cells.

CD89 This IgA receptor (FcαRI) is expressed on granulocytes, monocytes, and some subpopulations of T and B cells.

CD90 Otherwise known as Thy-1, this glycoprotein is expressed on thymocytes and T cells in some species. It is also expressed on some brain cells.

CD91 The heat-shock protein receptor. This protein, expressed on macrophages and dendritic cells, is important in the intracellular processing of these molecules.

CD93 The C1q receptor. Found on monocytes and neutrophils, but not lymphocytes. It modulates phagocytosis of apoptotic cells.

CD94 An NK cell receptor that associates with NKG2D and binds target cell MHC class I molecules.

CD95 Otherwise known as Fas, this is a receptor for Fas-ligand (CD95L or CD178) and a signaling component of an important cell death pathway. It is found on myeloid and T cells and plays a key role in the negative selection of self-reactive T cells.

CD102 Also called ICAM-2, a glycoprotein expressed on vascular endothelial cells, resting lymphocytes, and monocytes, but not neutrophils. It is the ligand for the integrin CD11a/CD18.

CD105 The TGF-β receptor expressed on endothelial cells.

CD106 Also called VCAM-1, a glycoprotein expressed on endothelial cells. It is the ligand for CD49d/CD29 (VLA-4).

CD115 The M-CSF receptor expressed on macrophages and their precursors.

CD116 The α chain of the GM-CSF receptor is found on granulocytes, monocytes, and eosinophils. It shares a common β chain with IL-3R and IL-5R.

CD117 Also called c-kit, this is the receptor for stem cell factor. It is an immunoglobulin superfamily tyrosine kinase found on hematopoietic stem cells.

CD119 The IFN-γ receptor is found on B cells, macrophages and monocytes, fibroblasts, and endothelial cells.

CD120 There are two TNF receptors (TNFR-I [CD120a], and TNFR-II [CD120b]. TNFR-I is found at higher levels on epithelial cells, whereas TNFR-II is more highly expressed on myeloid cells.

CD121 These are the two IL-1 receptors, IL-1RI and IL-1RII, expressed on thymocytes, fibroblasts, keratinocytes, endothelial cells (type I), and macrophages and B cells (type II).

CD122 The IL-2 receptor β chain expressed on T cells, activated B cells, NK cells, and monocytes.

CD123 The IL-3 receptor α chain.

CD124 The IL-4 receptor expressed on T and B cells, fibroblasts, endothelial cells, and stem cells.

CD125 The IL-5 receptor α chain

CD126 The α chain of the IL-6 receptor expressed on B cells, plasma cells, epithelial cells, and hepatocytes.

CD127 The IL-7 receptor expressed on stem cells, T cells, and monocytes.

CD128 The IL-8 receptors expressed on leukocytes and keratinocytes. Also called CXCR1 and 2.

CD130 The β chain of the IL-6 (with CD126) and IL-11 receptors is found mainly on B cells but expressed at lower levels on most leukocytes, epithelial cells, hepatocytes, and fibroblasts.

CD131 The common β chain of the IL-3 (with CD123), IL-5 (with CD125), and GM-CSF (with CD123) receptors.

CD132 The common γ chain of IL-2 (with CD25 and CD122), IL-4 (with CD124), IL-7 (with CD127), IL-9 (with CD129), and IL-15 receptors.

CD134 A member of the TNF receptor family that serves as the cell-binding receptor of feline immunodeficiency virus.

CD140 Platelet-derived growth factor (PDGF) receptor.

CD150 Also called SLAM (signaling lymphocyte activation molecule.) The receptor for canine distemper virus.

CD152 Also known as CTLA-4, this is the ligand for CD80 and CD86 and a suppressor of T cell activation. It is expressed on antigen-presenting cells.

CD154 A member of the TNF family. Since it serves as the ligand for CD40, it is also called CD40L. Found on activated Th cells, it plays a key role in T cell activation by cross-linking with CD40 on antigen presenting cells.

CD158 The KIR family of MHC class I receptors expressed on NK cells. They play a key role in NK cell activation in primates and cattle.

CD159 Members of the NKG2 family that serve as inhibitory receptors on NK cells.

CD166 A leukocyte adhesion molecule that acts as a receptor for IL-6.

CD169 Siglec 1 or sialoadhesin, a macrophage lectin-like adhesion molecule.

CD172a A signal regulatory protein expressed on monocytes and a subset of dendritic cells.

CD178 Also called Fas-ligand (CD95-L). A member of the tumor necrosis factor superfamily, this is a key molecule in the induction of cell death by apoptosis.

CD181-CD185 CXCR1-CXCR5 chemokine receptors. CD184 is a coreceptor for feline immunodeficiency virus.

CD191-CD199 CCR1-CCR9 chemokine receptors.

CD206 The mannose-binding receptor found on mature macrophages and immature dendritic cells.

CD209 DC-SIGN found on a subset of dendritic cells. This molecule permits transient binding between T cells and dendritic cells. It is a C-type lectin whose ligand is ICAM-3 (CD50).

CD210 The IL-10 receptor α chain.

CD212 The IL-12 receptor β chain.

CD213 The IL-13 receptor α chain (and a member of the IL-4 receptor complex).

CD215 The IL-15 receptor α chain.

CD217 The IL-17 receptor.

CD218a and b The α and β chains of the IL-18 receptor.

CD230 The prion protein (PrP). A large membrane protein found on neurons. The abnormal form of this protein PrPsc is a transmissible agent causing spongiform encephalopathies.

CD233 An erythrocyte membrane protein that functions as an anion (chloride and bicarbonate) exchanger. Also called band 3 protein. It plays a major role in the removal of aged cells.

CD240 The Rhesus blood group molecules found in humans and some primates.

CD247 The T cell antigen receptor zeta (ζ) chain.

CD256 APRIL, a B cell stimulating cytokine from macrophages and dendritic cells.

CD257 BAFF, another B cell stimulating cytokine expressed on B cells, macrophages, and dendritic cells. It is active in a cell-bound form or as a soluble fragment.

CD281-CD290 The CD designations of the toll-like receptors, TLR1 through TLR10.

CD295 The leptin receptor.

CD314 NKG2D, the NK cell receptor for the cellular stress proteins MICA and MICB.

CD327-CD329 Siglec-6, siglec-7, and siglec-9.

CD335 Also called NKp46. A member of the KIR family and an important molecule expressed on NK cells.

CD360 The IL-21 receptor.

Appendix 2

Some Selected Cytokines

Adiponectin A glycoprotein secreted exclusively by adipocytes. It suppresses inflammatory responses by inhibiting macrophage development and functions. It regulates both glucose and lipid metabolism. (See Chapter 38.)

Granulocyte colony-stimulating factor (G-CSF) A glycoprotein of 20 kDa produced by macrophages, endothelial cells, and fibroblasts that regulates the maturation of granulocyte progenitors into mature neutrophils. The term *colony-stimulating factor* refers to its ability to promote the growth of bone marrow stem cell "colonies" in tissue culture.

Granulocyte-monocyte colony stimulating factor (GM-CSF) A protein of 14 kDa produced by T cells, macrophages, fibroblasts, and endothelial cells. It is the major regulator of granulocyte and macrophage stem cells. It induces phagocytosis, superoxide production, and ADCC by neutrophils.

High-mobility group box protein-1 (HMGB1) A chromatin-binding protein of 28 kDa that is either actively secreted by inflammatory cells such as macrophages or passively released from necrotic cells. HMGB1 acts through TLRs to promote macrophage cytokine release, enhancing inflammation. It is an attractant for vascular smooth muscle cells. It has bactericidal activity and is a potent inducer of fevers. (See Chapter 6.)

Interferon-α Produced in at least 23 different variants, with molecular masses ranging from 19 to 26 kDa. It has a common conserved sequence region but a highly variable amino terminus. It is produced in large quantities by plasmacytic dendritic cells and in much smaller amounts by lymphocytes, monocytes, and macrophages. It activates NK cell–mediated cytotoxic activity and stimulates the differentiation of monocytes into dendritic cells as well as the maturation and activity of dendritic cells. IFN-α also drives certain γ/δ T cell responses. It has, of course, potent antiviral activities. (See Chapter 26.)

Interferon-β A 20-kDa protein produced by fibroblasts and coded for by a single gene in most mammals. Produced in response to viral infections, it has similar properties to IFN-α. (See Chapter 26.)

Interferon-γ The only type II interferon. It is a 17-kDa glycoprotein mainly produced by CD4+ Th1 cells, by some CD8+ T cells, and by NK cells. IFN-γ acts on B cells, T cells, NK cells, and macrophages and is the key mediator of cell-mediated immune responses. (See Chapter 14.)

Interferon-ω A protein of 20 kDa produced by lymphocytes, monocytes, and human, horse, pig, rabbit, and dog trophoblast cells. It has significant antiviral activity.

Interferon-τ A protein of 20 kDa produced by ruminant trophoblast cells during early pregnancy. It regulates immune responses in the placenta.

Interferon-δ A protein of 19 kDa produced by pig trophoblast cells. It probably controls the maternal immune response to the fetus.

Interferon-λ A collective name for IL-28A, IL-28B, and IL-29. All are 20-kDa proteins distantly related to the IL-10 family. All three use a distinct receptor system to trigger antiviral defense.

Interleukin-1 A family of cytokines produced by macrophages, dendritic cells, T cells, B cells, NK cells, vascular endothelium, fibroblasts, and keratinocytes. They originate as 31-kDa procytokines but are cleaved by caspase-1 to 17-kDa active peptides. The two most important forms of IL-1 act on Th2 cells, B cells, NK cells, neutrophils, eosinophils, dendritic cells, fibroblasts, endothelial cells, and hepatocytes. IL-1 is a proinflammatory mediator and a Th2 cell stimulator. (See Chapter 14.)

Interleukin-2 A 15-kDa glycoprotein produced by Th1 and NK cells. Its targets include other T cells, B cells, and NK cells. IL-2 activates helper and cytotoxic T cells and NK cells. IL-2 stimulates T cell proliferation and cytotoxicity. (See Chapter 14.)

Interleukin-3 A 15-kDa protein produced by activated T cells, NK cells, eosinophils, and mast cells. It is a hematopoietic growth factor that stimulates the growth and maturation of bone marrow stem cells for eosinophils, neutrophils, and monocytes.

Interleukin-4 A 15-kDa protein produced by activated Th2 cells, mast cells, and activated basophils. It acts on B cells, T cells, macrophages, endothelial cells, fibroblasts, and mast cells. IL-4 stimulates the growth and differentiation of B cells. (See Chapter 14.)

Interleukin-5 A 26-kDa glycoprotein produced by activated Th2 cells, mast cells, and eosinophils. In humans its main activity is the control of eosinophil production.

Interleukin-6 A 20- to 30-kDa glycoprotein that occurs in at least five isoforms. It is produced by activated macrophages, T and B cells, mast cells, vascular endothelial cells, fibroblasts, keratinocytes, and mesangial cells. It is also produced by muscle cells during exercise. It acts on T cells, B cells, hepatocytes, and bone marrow stromal cells as well as the brain. (See Chapter 6.)

Interleukin-7 A 17-kDa glycoprotein produced by bone marrow and thymic stromal cells. It regulates the activity of lymphoid stem cells. Its major role, however, is to control lymphocyte function by regulating V(D)J recombination in both B and T cells.

Interleukin-8 The prototypical chemokine (CXCL8). Like other chemokines, it is a relatively small (8.4 kDa) protein produced by macrophages and endothelial cells. IL-8 attracts and activates neutrophils.

Interleukin-9 A 14-kDa stem cell growth factor produced by Th2 cells. It promotes the growth of helper T cells and mast cells. It also potentiates the effects of IL-4 on IgE production.

Interleukin-10 An 19-kDa nonglycosylated homodimeric protein that acts as an immunosuppressive and antiinflammatory cytokine and suppresses inflammation as well as T cell, NK cell, and macrophage function. It is mainly produced by Th2 cells but also from M2 cells, NK cells, and some dendritic cells. Its targets are Th1 cells, B cells, macrophages, NK cells, and mast cells. (See Chapter 20.)

Interleukin-11 A 19-kDa nonglycosylated protein produced by bone marrow stromal cells, epithelial cells, and fibroblasts. It stimulates B cell growth in association with IL-6. IL-11 also stimulates megakaryocyte formation in association with IL-3 and promotes the production of acute-phase proteins.

Interleukin-12 A 75-kDa heterodimer consisting of disulfide-linked 35- and 40-kDa subunits (p35 and p40). It is produced by monocytes and macrophages, dendritic cells, B cells, and keratinocytes. It is the major activator of Th1 cells and NK cells. (See Chapter 14.)

Interleukin-13 A 12-kDa glycoprotein produced by Th2 cells, cytotoxic T cells, mast cells, and dendritic cells. It has biological activities similar to those of IL-4 because it acts through a receptor (CD213) that shares a common α chain with the IL-4R.

Interleukin-14 A 53-kDa glycoprotein produced by T cells and some malignant B cells. It is a B cell growth factor that inhibits immunoglobulin secretion and selectively expands some B cell subpopulations.

Interleukin-15 A 14-kDa glycoprotein produced by activated macrophages, dendritic cells, endothelial cells, and fibroblasts. It shares many biological activities with IL-2. IL-15 acts as a T cell, B cell, and NK cell growth factor. IL-15 is essential for the prolonged survival of memory T cells.

Interleukin-16 A 13-kDa protein produced by CD8+ T cells, eosinophils, dendritic cells, and mast cells. Its receptor is CD4, through which IL-16 regulates CD4+ T cell recruitment and activation. It also acts on eosinophils and macrophages.

Interleukin-17 A family of at least six proteins (IL17A to F) produced by Th17 cells and other innate immunity cells. They are 35-kDa disulfide-linked homodimers. IL-17 molecules stimulate macrophages and endothelial cells to secrete proinflammatory cytokines and chemokines, leading to the recruitment and activation of neutrophils. Members of the IL-17 family play a key role in the development of acute inflammation, in autoimmune diseases, and in cancer. (See Chapter 20.)

Interleukin-18 An IL-1 family member that is produced, like IL-1, by antigen-presenting cells. It originates as a 24-kDa pro-protein that is cleaved by caspase-1 to an 18-kDa active molecule. It activates Th1 cells to promote the production of IFN-γ, TNF-α, IL-1, CD95L, and several chemokines. This can lead to positive feedback whereby the IL-18 and IFN-γ reinforce each other's activities. IL-18 is a potent appetite suppressant.

Interleukin-19 An 18-kDa protein and a member of the IL-10 family produced by B cells and activated monocytes. It is a proinflammatory cytokine that acts on monocytes to stimulate production of IL-1, IL-6, and TNF-α.

Interleukin-20 A 35-kDa homodimeric protein and a member of the IL-10 family. It is produced by monocytes and keratinocytes and acts as a hematopoietic growth factor.

Interleukin-21 A protein of 15 kDa produced by activated Th2 cells and structurally related to IL-2 and IL-15. It regulates NK, B, and T cell function. It upregulates production of IL-18R and IFN-γ,

Interleukin-22 A 34-kDa member of the IL-10 family produced by activated Th17 cells and mast cells. It induces acute-phase protein production in the liver. IL-22 acts on cells of the skin and digestive and respiratory systems to increase production of several β-defensins and presumably promotes innate immunity in these tissues. (See Chapter 20.)

Interleukin-23 A heterodimer consisting of a 19-kDa peptide chain (IL-23p19) paired with the IL-12p40 chain. IL-23 is produced by macrophages, dendritic cells, and activated γ/δ T cells. It is a major cytokine produced by activated M1 cells. It stimulates Th17 cells to secrete IL-17 and IL-22, and these T cells in turn promote acute neutrophil-mediated inflammation. (See Chapter 20.)

Interleukin-24 A 37-kDa dimeric protein. It is a member of the IL-10 family produced by activated monocytes and Th2 cells. It is involved in antitumor activity since it stimulates apoptosis in many tumor cell lines and stimulates acute-phase responses in hepatocytes. It may play a role in wound healing.

Interleukin-25 A member of the IL-17 family produced by Th2 cells and mast cells; also called IL-17E. It appears to play an important role in intestinal immunity, in which it promotes Th2 cytokine responses and resistance to helminths.

Interleukin-26 A 37-kDa member of the IL-10 family. It is produced by activated T cells, activated memory cells, and activated NK cells. It induces the proliferation of keratinocytes and T cells. It signals through a novel receptor composed of IL-20R1 and IL-10R2.

Interleukin-27 A heterodimer, with one chain called p28 or IL-30, and the other called EB-13; it is related to IL-12p40. IL-27 is expressed by activated monocytes and dendritic cells. IL-27 suppresses the activation of all three helper T cell subsets and prevents neutrophil activation. It thus serves a major regulatory role. (See Chapter 20.)

Interleukin-28 Two protein isoforms of 22 kDa produced by virus-infected cells. They are also called IFN-λ2 (IL-28A) and IFN-λ3 (IL-28B). They share a common three-dimensional structure with IL-10 but have limited sequence similarity. They have antiviral activity.

Interleukin-29 (IFN-λ1) A 20-kDa member of the IL-10 family produced by virus-infected cells. It is closely related to IL-28A and IL-28B. It has antiviral activity.

Interleukin-30 A 28-kDa protein secreted by antigen-presenting cells. It forms one subunit of heterodimeric IL-27. IL-30 acts on naïve CD4 T cells and synergizes strongly with IL-12 to promote IFN-γ production by Th1 cells.

Interleukin-31 A 15-kDa protein produced by activated Th2 cells. Its receptor is expressed on keratinocytes and induced on monocytes by IFN-γ. It is related to IL-6 and may be involved in the pathogenesis of allergic skin diseases.

Interleukin-32 A protein of 15-kDa produced by activated human lymphocytes, NK cells, and endothelial cells. It induces monocytes to develop into macrophages and acts on macrophages to enhance the production of the proinflammatory cytokines, TNF-α, IL-1β, IL-6, and IL-8. It has significant antiviral activity.

Interleukin-33 An 18-kDa member of the IL-1 family that serves as a matched counterpart to IL-18. IL-33 is produced by many different cells, including macrophages and dendritic cells. It acts through its own receptor to drive production of IL-4, IL-5, and IL-13 by Th2 cells and mast cells. IL-33 is thus a proallergic cytokine and can trigger anaphylaxis. It induces antinematode immunity. (See Chapter 28.)

Interleukin-34 A 39-kDa homodimer expressed in many different tissues and in spleen, liver, heart, brain, and lung. It acts through the macrophage colony-stimulating factor receptor. It promotes monocyte viability and macrophage colony formation in the bone marrow. It is produced in large amounts in the splenic red pulp.

Interleukin-35 A heterodimer consisting of IL-12p35 and a peptide called EBI3 related to IL-12p40. It stimulates the growth of Treg cells while suppressing Th17 cells. It thus has an antiinflammatory effect.

Interleukin-36 A mixture of three IL-1-family members (IL-36α, -36β, and -36γ) that employ the same receptor complex (IL-1Rrp2 and AcP). They have proinflammatory effects. There is also an IL-36RA.

Interleukin-37 An antiinflammatory member of the IL-1 family. It acts by suppressing the production of proinflammatory cytokines induced by TLR agonists.

Leptin A 16-kDa protein produced by adipocytes. This cytokine suppresses appetite by signaling through a receptor in the hypothalamus. It exerts a strong proinflammatory effect and promoting dendritic cell activation and Th1 responses. (See Chapter 38.)

Macrophage colony-stimulating factor (M-CSF) A 80- to 100-kDa glycoprotein. Its active form is a disulfide-linked dimer. It is a hematopoietic factor produced by lymphocytes, macrophages, fibroblasts, epithelial cells, and endothelial cells. These act on monocyte stem cells to induce their proliferation and differentiation and promote macrophage cytotoxicity.

Macrophage migration inhibitory factor (MIF) A 12-kDa protein that associates to form homotrimers. It is produced by macrophages and T cells. It acts on macrophages to prevent their random migration, hence its name. It also activates lymphocytes and lymphocytes. MIF promotes the production of the proinflammatory mediators TNF-α, and IFN-γ.

Transforming growth factor-β (TGF-β) Belongs to a family of at least 45 signaling proteins. It is a 25-kDa protein consisting of disulfide-linked homodimers. There are three isoforms of this protein that act through the same receptor and have identical biological properties. They are produced by platelets, activated macrophages, neutrophils, B cells, and T cells and act on most cell types, including T and B cells, dendritic cells, macrophages, neutrophils, and fibroblasts. The TGF-βs regulate cell division, enhance the deposition of extracellular matrix proteins, and are immunosuppressive. (See Chapter 20.)

Tumor necrosis factor-α (TNF-α) A 17-kDa protein produced by macrophages, mast cells, T cells, endothelial cells, B cells, adipocytes, and fibroblasts. It forms a noncovalently linked trimer in solution. TNF-α is the central inducer of inflammation. (See Chapter 3.)

Tumor necrosis factor-β (TNF-β) A 19-kDa protein produced by Th1 cells and activated CD8+ T cells. It is either secreted in a soluble form or forms a complex with lymphotoxin-β in the T cell membrane. TNF-β kills tumor cells and activates neutrophils, macrophages, endothelial cells, and B cells.

Glossary

Activated macrophage A macrophage in a state of enhanced metabolic and functional activity.

Active immunity Immunity produced as a result of administration of an antigen, thus triggering an immune response.

Acute inflammation Rapidly developing inflammation of recent onset. It is characterized by tissue infiltration by neutrophils.

Acute-phase proteins Proteins, synthesized by the liver and other tissues, whose level in serum rises rapidly in response to acute inflammation and tissue damage.

Adjuvant Any substance that, when given with an antigen, enhances the immune response to that antigen.

Adoptive immunity Immunity that results from the transfer of cells from an immunized animal to an unimmunized recipient.

Affinity The strength of binding between two molecules such as an antigen and antibody. Usually expressed as an association constant (Ka).

Affinity maturation The progressive increase in antibody affinity for antigen that occurs during the course of an immune response as a result of somatic mutation in *V* genes.

Agammaglobulinemia The absence of γ globulins in blood.

Agglutination The clumping of particulate antigens by antibody.

Agnatha A class of jawless fish. It includes the cyclostomes, an order containing the hagfish and lamprey.

Alarmins Molecules released by dead or damaged tissues that trigger innate immune responses, especially inflammation. See also: Damage-associated molecular patterns.

Albumin The major serum protein of 60 kDa.

Alleles Different forms of a gene that occupy the same polymorphic locus.

Allelic exclusion The expression of only one allelic protein by a cell from a heterozygous individual that has the genes to express both allelic proteins.

Allergens Antigens that provoke allergic reactions. Usually type I hypersensitivity.

Allergic contact dermatitis An inflammatory skin reaction mediated by Th1 cells responding to low-molecular-weight chemicals bound to skin cells.

Allergy A hypersensitivity reaction initiated by specific immunologic mechanisms.

Allogeneic Genetically dissimilar animals of the same species.

Allograft An organ graft between two genetically dissimilar animals of the same species.

Allotype Phenotypic (antigenic and structural) differences between the proteins of different individuals of the same species as a result of transcription of different alleles.

Alternative complement pathway The complement pathway triggered by the activation of C3 by the presence of an activating surface.

Amyloid An extracellular, amorphous, waxy protein deposited in the tissues of individuals with a chronic inflammation or a myeloma. It consists of misfolded insoluble fibrillar proteins.

Analog An organ or tissue that has the same function as another but is of different evolutionary origin.

Anamnestic response A secondary immune response.

Anaphylatoxins Complement fragments that stimulate mast cell degranulation and smooth muscle contraction.

Anaphylaxis A severe, life-threatening generalized or systemic hypersensitivity reaction.

Anergy The failure of a sensitized animal to respond to an antigen—a form of immunological tolerance.

Antibiotic A chemical compound, usually obtained from microorganisms, that can prevent growth or kill bacteria. Do not confuse this with antibody.

Antibody An immunoglobulin molecule synthesized on exposure to antigen, which can combine specifically with that antigen.

Antibody-dependent cellular cytotoxicity (ADCC) The killing of antibody-coated target cells by cytotoxic cells with surface Fc receptors.

Antigen Any foreign substance that can bind to specific lymphocyte receptors and so induce an immune response.

Antigen-presenting cells Cells that can ingest, process, and present antigen to antigen-sensitive cells in association with MHC class I and class II molecules.

Antigen processing The series of events that modify antigens so that they bind to MHC molecules and can be recognized by antigen-sensitive cells.

Antigen-sensitive cells Cells that can bind and respond to specific antigen.

Antigenic determinant See Epitope.

Antigenic variation The progressive changes in surface antigens exhibited by viruses, parasites, and some bacteria in order to evade destruction.

Antigenicity The ability of a molecule to be recognized by an antibody or lymphocyte.

Antiglobulin Antibody made against an immunoglobulin, usually by injecting immunoglobulin into an animal of another species.

Antiglobulin test A technique for detecting the presence of nonagglutinating antibody on the surface of a particle.

Antiserum Serum that contains specific antibodies. Synonymous with immune globulin.

Antitoxin Antiserum directed against a toxin and used for passive immunization.

Anurans An order of advanced amphibians that includes the frogs and toads.

Apoptosis The controlled self-destruction of a cell; one form of programmed cell death. (*Apoptosis* is a Greek word describing the falling away of petals from flowers or the leaves from trees.)

Arthus reaction Local inflammation due to a type III hypersensitivity reaction; it is induced by the injection of antigen into the skin of an immunized animal.

Asthma A type I hypersensitivity disease characterized by a reduction in airway diameter, leading to difficulty in breathing (dyspnea).

Atopy A genetic predisposition to become sensitized and produce IgE antibodies in response to allergens commonly occurring in the environment.

Attenuation The reduction of virulence of an infectious agent.

Autoantibodies Antibodies directed against epitopes on normal body tissues.

Autoantigen A normal body component that acts as an antigen.

Autograft A tissue or organ graft made between two sites within the same animal.

Autoimmune disease Disease caused by an immune attack against an individual's own tissues.

Autoimmunity An immune response against normal body components.

Autophagy A process of cellular self-digestion by which cells can ingest and destroy intracellular microbes or damaged organelles.

B lymphocytes (B cells) Lymphocytes that have undergone a period of processing in the bursa or its mammalian equivalent. They are responsible for antibody production.

Bacille Calmette-Guérin (BCG) vaccine An attenuated strain of *Mycobacterium bovis*. This may be used as a specific vaccine or as a nonspecific immune stimulator.

Bacterin A preparation of killed bacteria used for immunization.

Basophil A polymorphonuclear cell that contains granules with a high avidity for basic dyes such as hematoxylin. It participates in type I hypersensitivity reactions.

BCG See Bacille Calmette-Guérin (BCG) vaccine.

Bence Jones protein Immunoglobulin light chains found in the urine of patients with myelomas. They precipitate out of solution when the urine is warmed and redissolve at higher temperatures.

Benign tumor A tumor that does not spread from its site of origin.

Blastogenesis The stimulation of cell division.

Blast cells Actively dividing cells with large amounts of cytoplasm.

Blocking antibody A noncytotoxic, non-complement-activating antibody that, by coating cells, can protect them against immune destruction.

Blood groups Antigens found on the surface of red blood cells. Their expression is inherited.

Bursectomy Surgical removal of the bursa of Fabricius.

C-terminus The end of a peptide chain with a free carboxy (COO-) group.

C3 convertases Enzymes that can cleave native C3 into C3a and C3b fragments.

Capping The clumping of surface structures such as antigens or receptors in a small area on the surface of a cell.

Capsid The protein coat around a virus.

Carcinoma A tumor originating from cells of epithelial origin.

Carrier An immunogenic macromolecule to which a hapten may be bound, making the hapten immunogenic.

Cascade reactions A linked series of enzyme reactions in which the products of one reaction catalyze a second reaction, and so forth.

Cell-mediated cytotoxicity The killing of target cells induced by contact with cytotoxic T cells, NK cells, or macrophages.

Cell-mediated immunity A form of immune response mediated by T lymphocytes and macrophages; it can be conferred on an animal by adoptive transfer.

Cestodes Parasitic tapeworms.

Chemokine A family of proinflammatory and chemotactic cytokines with a characteristic sequence of four cysteine residues. They regulate the emigration of leukocytes from blood into tissues.

Chemotaxis The directed movement of cells under the influence of a chemical concentration gradient.

Chimera An animal that contains cells from two or more genetically different individuals.

Chondrichthyes The class that contains the cartilaginous fishes, including sharks, skates, and rays.

Chromosome translocation A form of mutation in which portions of two chromosomes switch position.

Chronic inflammation Slowly developing or persistent inflammation characterized by tissue infiltration with macrophages and fibroblasts.

Class The five major forms of immunoglobulin molecules common to all members of a species (see Isotype). Each has its own set of heavy chain genes.

Class switch The change in immunoglobulin class that occurs during the course of an immune response as a result of heavy chain gene rearrangement.

Classical complement pathway The complement pathway triggered by activation of C1 by antigen-antibody complexes.

Clonal deletion The elimination of self-reactive T cells in the thymus.

Clonal selection A key concept in immunology. The proliferation of specific lymphocyte clones in response to a specific epitope. The response is triggered through specific antigen-binding receptors.

Clone The progeny of a single cell.

Clonotype A clone of B cells with the ability to bind a single epitope.

Cluster of differentiation (CD) The set of monoclonal antibodies that recognize a single protein on a cell surface. A CD antigen is by extension, therefore, a defined protein on the surface of a cell.

Coelomocyte A phagocytic cell found in the coelomic cavity of invertebrates.

Collectins A family of carbohydrate-binding lectins that depend on calcium for their adhesion.

Colostrum The secretion that accumulates in the mammary gland in the last weeks of pregnancy. It is very rich in immunoglobulins.

Combined immunodeficiency A deficiency in both the T cell– and B cell–mediated components of the immune system.

Complement A group of serum and cell surface proteins activated by factors such as the combination of antigen and antibody and results in the generation of enzyme cascades that have a variety of biological consequences including cell lysis and opsonization.

Complementarity determining region Those areas within the variable regions of antibodies and T cell antigen receptors that bind to antigen and determine the molecule's antigen binding specificity. Synonymous with hypervariable region.

Concanavalin A (Con A) A lectin extracted from the Jack bean that makes T cells divide.

Conglutinin A bovine mannose-binding protein that also combines with C3b.

Constant domains Structural domains with little sequence variability found in antibodies and TCRs.

Constant region The portion of immunoglobulin and TCR peptide chains that consists of a relatively constant sequence of amino acids.

Convertase A protease that acts on a protein to cause its activation.

Cortex The outer region of an organ such as the thymus or lymph node.

Corticosteroids Steroid hormones released from the adrenal cortex that have profound effects on the immune system. Some corticosteroids may be synthetic in origin.

Co-stimulators Molecules required to stimulate an antigen-sensitive cell simultaneously with antigen in order to initiate an effective immune response.

Cross-reaction The reaction of an antibody or an antigen receptor directed against a specific antigen, with a second antigen. This occurs because the two antigens possess an epitope in common.

Cutaneous basophil hypersensitivity A form of delayed hypersensitivity reaction in skin associated with an extensive basophil infiltration.

Cytokine storm The pathological effects induced by the massive activation of T cells, and as a result, the unregulated production of many different cytokines.

Cytokines Secreted proteins that mediate cellular interactions and regulate cell growth and secretion. As a result, they regulate many aspects of the immune system.

Cytolysis Destruction of cells by immune processes.

Cytotoxic cell A cell that can injure or kill other cells.

Damage-associated molecular patterns (DAMPs) Conserved molecular structures derived from damaged cells and tissues that trigger inflammation.

Delayed hypersensitivity A cell-mediated inflammatory reaction in the skin, so called because it takes 24 to 48 hours to reach maximum intensity.

Dendritic cells Specialized antigen-processing cells. They possess long cytoplasmic processes (dendrites), and their primary role is to function as highly effective antigen-trapping and antigen-presenting cells.

Desensitization The prevention of allergic reactions through the use of multiple injections of allergen.

Diapedesis The emigration of cells from intact blood vessels during inflammation.

Disseminated intravascular coagulation Activation of the clotting cascade within the circulation.

Disulfide bonds Bonds that form between two cysteine residues in a protein. They may be either interchain (between two peptide chains) or intrachain (joining two parts of one chain).

Domain Discrete structural units from which protein molecules are constructed. Their sizes, structure, and sequences are very diverse.

Dysgammaglobulinemia The abnormal production of γ-globulins in blood.

Effector cell A cell that is able to "effect" an immune response. These cells include cytotoxic T cells and natural killer cells.

Eicosanoids A family of lipid signaling molecules mainly synthesized from arachidonic acid. They include the prostaglandins and leukotrienes and are involved in inflammation, autoimmunity, and allergic diseases.

Electrophoresis The separation of the proteins in a complex mixture by subjecting them to an electrical potential. They thus migrate in a substrate such as a gel or paper at a rate determined by their charge.

ELISA Enzyme-linked immunosorbent assay. A serologic test that uses enzyme-linked antiglobulins and substrate bound to an inert surface.

Endocytosis The uptake of extracellular substances by cells.

Endogenous antigen Foreign antigen synthesized within body cells. Examples include newly formed virus proteins.

Endosomes Cytoplasmic vesicles formed by invagination of the outer cell membrane. They contain endocytosed substances.

Endothelium The cells that line blood vessels and lymphatics.

Endotoxins Lipopolysaccharide components of Gram-negative bacterial cell walls.

Enhancement Improved survival of grafts or cancer cells mediated by some antibodies.

Eosinophil A polymorphonuclear leukocyte containing characteristic granules that stain intensely with the dye eosin.

Eosinophilia Increased numbers of eosinophils in the blood.

Epithelioid cells Macrophages that accumulate around a tubercle and resemble epithelial cells in histological sections.

Epitope A site on the surface of an antigen that is recognized by an antigen receptor. As a result, immune responses are directed against specific epitopes. Synonymous with antigenic determinant.

Erythema Redness due to inflammation.

Eukaryotic organism An organism characterized by cells possessing a distinct nucleus and containing both DNA and RNA.

Eutherians The placental mammals; the order to which humans and domestic mammals belong.

Exocytosis The export of material from a cell by the fusion of cytoplasmic vesicles with the outer cell membrane.

Exogenous antigen A foreign antigen that originates at a source outside the body; for example, bacterial antigens.

Exon A region within a gene that is expressed.

Exotoxins Soluble protein toxins, usually produced by Gram-positive bacteria, that have a specific toxic effect.

Fab fragment The antigen-binding fragment of a partially digested antibody. It consists of light chains and the N-terminal halves of heavy chains.

Facultative intracellular organism An organism that can, if necessary, grow within cells.

Fc receptor A cell surface receptor that specifically binds antibody molecules through their Fc region.

Fc region That part of an immunoglobulin molecule consisting of the C-terminal halves of heavy chains. It is responsible for the biological activities of the molecule.

Fluorescent antibody An antibody chemically attached to a fluorescent dye.

Framework regions The parts of a variable region of immunoglobulins and TCRs that have a relatively constant amino acid sequence and so form a structure on which the hypervariable, complementarity determining regions may be constructed.

G-proteins Guanosine triphosphate (GTP)-binding proteins that act as signal transducers for many cell surface receptors.

Gamma-globulins (γ-globulins) Serum proteins that migrate toward the cathode on electrophoresis. They contain most of the immunoglobulins.

Gammopathies Abnormal increases in γ-globulin levels.

Gel diffusion An immunoprecipitation technique that involves letting antigen and antibody meet and precipitate in a clear gel such as agar.

Gene complex A cluster of related genes occupying a restricted area of a chromosome.

Gene conversion The exchange of blocks of DNA between different genes.

Gene segment Another term for exon. It tends to be used exclusively to denote the exons that code for immunoglobulin and TCR V, D, and J regions.

Genes Units of DNA that code for the amino acid sequence of a protein.

Germinal center A structure characteristic of many lymphoid organs, in which rapidly dividing B cells form a pale-staining spherical mass surrounded by a zone of dark-staining cells. This is the site where somatic mutation occurs and memory cells are generated.

Globulins Serum proteins precipitated by the presence of a half-saturated solution of ammonium sulfate.

Glomerulonephritis Pathological lesions in the glomeruli of the kidney.

Glycoform Differing molecular forms of a protein resulting from differences in glycosylation.

Glycoprotein A protein that contains carbohydrate.

Graft-versus-host disease Disease caused by an attack of transplanted lymphocytes (usually in the form of a bone marrow allograft) on the cells of a histoincompatible and immunodeficient recipient.

Granulocyte A myeloid cell containing prominent cytoplasmic granules. They include neutrophils, eosinophils, and basophils.

Granuloma An inflammatory lesion characterized by chronic inflammation with mononuclear cell infiltration and extensive fibrosis.

Granzyme A family of proteases found in the granules of cytotoxic T cells.

Growth factors Molecules that promote cell growth.

Haplotype The complete set of linked alleles within a gene complex. They are inherited as a group and determine a specific phenotype.

Hapten A small molecule that cannot initiate an immune response unless first bound to an immunogenic carrier molecule.

Heat-shock proteins Proteins synthesized by cells in response to many different physiological stresses. Their function is to act as chaperones and carry proteins within different sub-compartments of a cell.

Helminths Worms, many of which are parasites and stimulate immune responses.

Helper T cells The subpopulation of T cells that promote immune responses by providing co-stimulation from cytokines and co-stimulatory receptors.

Hemagglutination The agglutination of red blood cells.

Hematopoietic organ An organ in which blood cells are produced.

Hemocytes Phagocytic cells found in invertebrate hemolymph.

Hemolymph The fluid that fills the body cavities of invertebrates. It has functions analogous to those of blood.

Hemolysin An antibody that can lyse red blood cells in the presence of complement.

Hemolytic disease Disease occurring as a result of the destruction of red blood cells by antibodies transferred to the young animal from its mother.

Herd immunity Immunity conferred on a population as a result of the presence of immune individuals within that population.

Heterodimer A molecule consisting of two different subunits.

Heterophile antibodies Antibodies that react with epitopes found on a wide variety of unrelated molecules.

High endothelial venule A specialized blood vessel lined with high epithelium, found in the paracortex of lymph nodes and other lymphoid organs.

Hinge region The region between the first and second constant domains in some immunoglobulin molecules that permits them to bend freely.

Histiocytes Tissue macrophages.

Histocompatibility molecules Cell membrane proteins that are required to present antigen to antigen-sensitive cells.

Homodimer A molecule consisting of two identical subunits.

Homolog A part similar in structure, position, and origin to another organ.

Homology The degree of sequence similarity between two genes (nucleotide sequences) or two proteins (amino acid sequences).

Humoral immunity An immune response mediated by antibodies.

Hybridoma A cell line formed by the fusion of a myeloma cell with a normal antibody-producing cell.

Hypersensitivity Reproducible clinical signs initiated by exposure to an antigen at a dose tolerated by normal individuals.

Hypersensitivity pneumonitis Inflammation in the lung caused by a type III hypersensitivity reaction to inhaled antigen within the alveoli.

Hypervariable regions Areas within immunoglobulin or TCR variable regions where the greatest variations in amino acid sequence occur and which therefore bind antigens.

Hypogammaglobulinemia Low levels of γ-globulins in blood.

Idiotype The collection of idiotopes on an immunoglobulin molecule.

Idiotype networks The series of reactions among idiotypes, antiidiotypes, and anti-antiidiotypes that play a role in controlling immune responses.

Immediate hypersensitivity The hypersensitivity reaction mediated by IgE and mast cells. Otherwise known as type I hypersensitivity.

Immune complex Another term for antigen-antibody complexes.

Immune elimination The removal of an antigen from the body by circulating antibodies and phagocytic cells.

Immune exclusion The prevention of absorption of antigens from body surfaces by immunoglobulin A.

Immune globulin An antibody preparation containing specific antibodies against a pathogen and used for passive immunization.

Immune paralysis Tolerance induced by very high doses of antigen.

Immune response genes MHC class II genes, so called because they regulate the ability of an animal to respond to specific antigens.

Immune stimulants Compounds, commonly bacterial in origin, that stimulate the immune system by promoting cytokine release from macrophages.

Immune surveillance The concept that lymphocytes survey the body for cancerous or abnormal cells and then eliminate them.

Immunity The state of resistance to an infection.

Immunization The administration of an antigen to an individual in order to confer immunity.

Immunoconglutinins Autoantibodies directed against activated complement components.

Immunodeficiency Diseases in which immune function is partially or totally deficient.

Immunodiffusion Another name for the gel diffusion technique.

Immunodominant The epitope on a molecule that provokes the most intense immune response.

Immunoelectrophoresis A procedure involving electrophoresis in gel followed by immunoprecipitation; it is used to identify the proteins in a complex solution such as serum.

Immunofluorescence Immunological tests that make use of antibodies conjugated to a fluorescent dye.

Immunogenetics That portion of immunology that deals with the direct effects of genes on the immune system.

Immunogenicity The ability of a molecule to elicit an immune response.

Immunoglobulin A glycoprotein with antibody activity.

Immunoglobulin superfamily A family of proteins that contain characteristic immunoglobulin domains.

Immunological paralysis A form of immunological tolerance in which an ongoing immune response is inhibited by the presence of large amounts of antigen.

Immunoperoxidase Immunological test that makes use of antibodies chemically conjugated to the enzyme peroxidase.

Immunosuppression Inhibition of the immune system by drugs or other processes.

Inactivated vaccine A vaccine containing an agent that has been treated in such a way that it can no longer replicate in the host.

Incomplete antibody An antibody that can bind to a particulate antigen but cannot make it agglutinate.

Indurated Hardened.

Inflammasome A multiprotein complex that forms in response to triggering of certain pattern-recognition receptors and triggers synthesis of inflammatory cytokines.

Inflammation The responses of tissues to injury. These responses enhance tissue defenses and initiate repair.

Inflammatory macrophage A partially activated macrophage associated with microbial invasion, tissue damage, or inflammation.

Innate immunity Immunity present in all animals that need not be induced by prior exposure to an infectious agent. It is mediated by proteins encoded in the germline.

Inoculation The administration of a vaccine by injection or scratching.

Integral membrane protein Cell surface proteins that are integral components of the cell membrane as opposed to proteins that are passively adsorbed to cell surfaces.

Integrins A family of adhesion proteins found on cell membranes that bind either to ligands on the surface of other cells or to connective tissue proteins such as fibronectin or collagen.

Interchain bond A bond between two different peptide chains. Usually formed by a disulfide linkage between two cysteine residues.

Interdigitating cell A form of dendritic cell found within lymphoid organs.

Interferons Cytokines that can interfere with viral replication. Some interferons play an important role in the regulation of immunity.

Interleukins Cytokines that act as growth and differentiation factors for the cells of the immune system.

Intrachain bond A bond between two cysteine residues on a single peptide chain. Because disulfide bonds are short, its effect is to produce a fold in the peptide chain.

Intraepithelial lymphocytes Lymphocytes, mainly T cells, located among the epithelial cells in the intestinal wall.

Intron A region within a gene that separates exons and is not expressed.

Isoform Different molecular forms of a protein that are generated by differential processing of RNA transcripts of a single gene.

Isogeneic (syngeneic) Genetically identical.

Isograft A graft between two genetically identical animals.

Isotype These are closely related proteins that arise as a result of gene duplication. They are found in all animals of a species. Thus the classes and subclasses of immunoglobulins are actually isotypes.

Isotype switching The change in immunoglobulin class that occurs during the course of the immune response as a result of heavy chain gene switching.

J chain A short peptide that joins units in the polymeric immunoglobulins IgM and IgA.

Joining (J) gene segment A short gene segment that is located 3′ to the *V* gene segments in immunoglobulin and TCR *V* genes and codes for part of the variable region.

K antigens Capsular antigens of Gram-negative bacteria.

Killer cell See Cytotoxic T cell and Natural killer cell.

Kinins Vasoactive peptides produced in injured or inflamed tissue.

Kupffer cells Macrophages lining the sinusoids of the liver.

Lag period The interval between administration of antigen and the first detection of antibody.

Langerhans cells A population of specialized dendritic cells found in the skin. They are effective antigen-presenting cells.

Lectin A protein that can bind specifically to a carbohydrate. Some lectins of plant origin can induce lymphocytes to divide.

Leukemia A cancer consisting of white cells that proliferate within the blood.

Leukocytes White blood cells. This general term covers all the nucleated cells of blood.

Leukopenia The absence of leukocytes.

Leukotrienes Lipid mediators derived from arachidonic acid and responsible for potent proinflammatory responses. Released by degranulating mast cells.

Ligand A generic term for the molecules that bind specifically to a receptor.

Linkage disequilibrium A situation in which a pair of genes is found in a population at an unexpectedly high frequency when compared with the frequency of the individual genes. It occurs when two genes are located close to each other so that recombinations rarely occur.

Linked recognition The necessity for lymphocytes to receive two simultaneous signals to be activated.

Locus The location of a gene in a chromosome.

Looping out A method of excising a segment of intervening DNA (intron) in order to join two gene segments (exons).

Lymph The clear tissue fluid that flows through lymphatic vessels.

Lymphadenopathy Literally, "disease of lymph nodes." In practice it is used to describe enlarged lymph nodes.

Lymphoblast A dividing lymphocyte.

Lymphocyte A small mononuclear cell with a round nucleus containing densely packed chromatin found in blood and lymphoid tissues. Most have only a thin rim of cytoplasm. They recognize foreign antigens through specialized receptors.

Lymphocyte trapping The trapping of lymphocytes within a lymph node during the node's response to antigen.

Lymphokine-activated killer (LAK) cells Lymphocytes activated by exposure to cytokines such as IL-2 in vitro.

Lymphokines Cytokines secreted by lymphocytes.

Lymphopenia Abnormally low numbers of lymphocytes in blood.

Lymphotoxins Cytotoxic cytokines secreted by lymphocytes.

Lysosomal enzymes The complex mixture of enzymes, many of which are proteases, found within lysosomes.

Lysosomes Cytoplasmic organelles found within phagocytic cells that contain a complex mixture of potent proteases.

Lysozyme An enzyme present in tears, saliva, and neutrophils. It attacks carbohydrates in the cell walls of Gram-positive bacteria.

Macrophages Large phagocytic cells containing a single rounded nucleus.

Major histocompatibility complex The gene region that contains the genes for the major histocompatibility molecules, as well as for some complement components and related proteins.

Malignant tumors Tumors whose cells have a tendency to invade normal tissues, break away, and spread by lymphatics or blood to distant tissue sites.

Marsupials The order containing the pouched mammals. These include not only the Australian forms, such as kangaroos and koalas, but also the opossums.

Maternal antibodies Antibodies that originate in the mother but enter the bloodstream of her offspring either by transport across the placenta as in primates, or by adsorption of ingested colostrum in other mammals.

Medulla The region in the center of lymphoid organs such as the thymus or lymph nodes.

Memory cells Lymphocytes formed as a result of exposure to antigen. They have the ability to mount an enhanced response to antigen compared with lymphocytes that have not previously encountered antigen.

Memory response The enhanced immune response that is triggered as a result of exposing a primed animal to antigen.

Mesangial cells Modified muscle cells found within a glomerulus.

MHC molecules Proteins coded for by genes located in the major histocompatibility complex. (See Chapter 11.)

MHC restriction The necessity for a T cell to recognize an antigen in association with an MHC molecule. It is required for helper and cytotoxic T cells to recognize antigen and for helper T cells to cooperate with B cells.

Microglia Macrophages resident within the brain.

Mitogen Any substance that makes cells divide.

Mixed lymphocyte reaction Lymphocyte proliferation induced by contact with foreign lymphocytes in vitro.

Modified live virus A virus whose virulence has been reduced so that it can replicate in the host but cannot cause disease in normal animals.

Molecular mimicry The development by parasites or other infectious agents of molecules whose structure closely resembles molecules found in their host. In this way the invaders may be able to evade destruction by the immune system or perhaps trigger autoimmunity.

Monoclonal Originating from a single clone of cells.

Monoclonal antibody Antibody derived from a single clone of cells and hence chemically homogeneous.

Monoclonal gammopathy The appearance in serum of a high level of a monoclonal immunoglobulin. This is commonly, but not always, associated with the presence of a myeloma.

Monocytes Immature macrophages found in the blood.

Monokines Cytokines secreted by macrophages and monocytes.

Monomer The basic unit of a molecule that can be assembled using repeating subunits.

Mononuclear cells Those leukocytes with a single round nucleus; for example, lymphocytes and macrophages.

Mononuclear-phagocytic system The cells that belong to the macrophage family and their precursors.

Monotremes The order containing the least complex egg-laying mammals. These include the platypus and the spiny anteaters (Echidna).

Myeloid system All the granulocytes and their precursors. These precursor cells are found in the bone marrow.

Myeloma A tumor of plasma cells.

Myeloma protein The immunoglobulin product secreted by a myeloma cell.

N-terminus The end of a peptide chain with a free amino (NH_2) group.

Natural antibodies Antibodies against foreign antigens found in serum in the absence of known antigenic stimulation from immunization or an infection. Most probably arise as a result of exposure to cross-reacting bacterial antigens.

Natural killer cells Large granular lymphocytes that are found in normal, unsensitized individuals and that can recognize and kill abnormal cells such as tumor- and virus-infected cells.

Natural suppressor cells A population of cells found in unimmunized individuals that have the ability to suppress some immune responses.

Necrosis Cell death due to pathological causes.

Negative feedback A control mechanism whereby the products of a reaction act to suppress their own production.

Negative selection The killing of T cells that have the potential to react to self-antigens. A key mechanism in the prevention of autoimmunity.

Nematode A roundworm.

Neutralization Blockage of the activity of an organism or a toxin by antibody.

Neutropenia Low numbers of neutrophils in blood.

Neutrophilia High numbers of neutrophils in blood.

Neutrophils Polymorphonuclear neutrophil granulocytes.

NK cells Natural killer cells.

Noncovalent bonds Chemical bonds, such as hydrogen or hydrophobic bonds, that reversibly link peptide chains. They play a key role in the binding of antigen with antibodies or with T cell antigen receptors.

Normal flora The microbial population consisting mainly of bacteria that colonize normal body surfaces. They play a key role in preventing invasion by pathogenic organisms and regulate development of the immune system.

Nucleocapsid The key structural component of a virus consisting of the viral nucleic acid and its protective capsid coat.

Nude mice A mutant strain of mice that have no thymus and are hairless.

O antigens Somatic antigens of Gram-negative bacteria.

Obligate intracellular parasite An organism that is absolutely required to grow inside cells. Viruses are excellent examples.

Oncofetal antigens Antigens found on fetal and tumor cells.

Oncogene A gene whose protein product plays a key role in cell division. As a result, its uncontrolled production leads to excessive cell growth and tumor formation. Oncogenes may be found in normal cells, as well as in cancer-causing viruses.

Oncogenic virus A virus that causes cancer.

Ontogeny The embryonic development of an organ or animal.

Opportunistic pathogen An organism that, although unable to cause disease in a healthy individual, may invade and cause disease in an individual whose immunological defenses are impaired.

Opsonin A molecule that facilitates phagocytosis by coating foreign particles.

Optimal proportions When antigen and antibody combine, this is the ratio of reactants that generates the largest immune complexes.

Orthologous Genes that are clearly descended from a common ancestral gene.

Osteichthyes The class containing the bony fish. It includes several orders of fish, the most highly evolved of which are the teleosts. The teleosts include such typical fish as the goldfish, catfish, and trout.

Paracortex The region located between the cortex and medulla of lymph nodes in which T cells predominate.

Paralogous Two genes or gene clusters that although likely descended from a single ancestor are located on different chromosomes and have diverged significantly.

Passive agglutination The agglutination of inert particles by antibody directed against antigen bound to their surface.

Passive immunization Protection of one individual conferred by administration of antibody produced in another individual.

Pathogen-associated molecular patterns (PAMPs) Conserved molecular structures widely distributed among pathogenic microbes that trigger inflammation.

Pathogenesis The mechanism of a disease.

Pathogenic organism An organism that causes disease.

Pattern-recognition receptors (PRRs) Cellular receptors that can recognize pathogens or their soluble components. PRRs include toll-like receptors, among others.

Perforin A family of proteins made by T cells and NK cells (and the complement component C9) that, when polymerized, can insert themselves into target cell membranes and provoke cell lysis.

Phagocytes Cells whose prime function is to eat foreign particles, especially bacteria. They include macrophages and related cells, neutrophils, and eosinophils.

Phagocytosis The ability of some cells to ingest foreign particles. Literally, "eating by cells."

Phagolysosome A structure produced by the fusion of a phagosome and a lysosome following phagocytosis.

Phagosome The cytoplasmic vesicle that encloses an ingested organism.

Phenogroup A set of blood group alleles that are consistently inherited as a group.

Phylogeny The evolutionary history of a plant or animal species.

Phytohemagglutinin (PHA) A lectin derived from the red kidney bean. It acts as a T-cell mitogen.

Pinocytosis The endocytosis of small fluid droplets—drinking by cells.

Plasma The clear fluid that forms the liquid phase of blood.

Plasma cell A fully differentiated B cell capable of synthesizing and secreting large amounts of antibody.

Point mutation A mutation resulting from an alteration in a single base in a gene.

Pokeweed mitogen (PWM) A lectin derived from the pokeweed plant that stimulates T and B cells to divide.

Polyclonal gammopathies The appearance in serum of a high level of immunoglobulins of many different specificities originating from many different clones.

Polymorphism Inherited structural differences among proteins from allogeneic individuals as a result of multiple alternative alleles at a single locus.

Polymorphonuclear neutrophil granulocytes Blood leukocytes possessing neutrophilic cytoplasmic granules and an irregular lobed nucleus.

Positive selection The enhanced proliferation of cells within the thymus that can respond optimally to foreign antigen.

Precipitation The clumping of soluble antigen molecules by antibody to reproduce a visible precipitate.

Premunition A form of immunity seen in some parasitic conditions that depends on the continued presence of the parasite in the host.

Prevalence The number of cases of a disease.

Primary binding tests Serological assays that directly detect the binding of antigen and antibody.

Primary immune response The immune response resulting from an individual's first encounter with an antigen.

Primary immunodeficiencies Inherited immunodeficiency diseases.

Primary lymphoid organ An organ that serves as a source of lymphocytes or in which lymphocytes mature.

Primary pathogen An organism that can cause disease without first suppressing an individual's immune defenses.

Primary structure The amino acid sequence of a protein.

Privileged sites Locations within the body where foreign grafts are not rejected. A good example is the cornea of the eye.

Prokaryotic organism An organism composed of cells whose genetic material is free in the cytoplasm and as a result do not contain a recognizable nucleus.

Prostanoids A class of lipid mediators derived from arachidonic acid produced by the actions of the enzyme cyclooxygenase. They include prostaglandins, thromboxanes, and prostacyclin.

Protein kinase An enzyme that phosphorylates proteins.

Proteasome A large complex multienzyme structure found in the cytosol. It acts on ubiquinated cellular proteins to cleave them into small fragments.

Prozone The inhibition of agglutination by the presence of high concentrations of antibody.

Pseudogenes DNA sequences that resemble functional genes but that cannot be transcribed.

Pyrogen A fever-causing substance.

Pyroninophilic Stained by the dye pyronin. This stain preferentially binds to RNA, so a cell whose cytoplasm stains intensely with pyronin is rich in ribosomes and is therefore probably a protein-synthesizing cell.

Radioimmunoassay An immunological test that requires the use of an isotope-labeled reagent.

Reaginic antibody An antibody of the IgE class that mediates type I hypersensitivity.

Recombinant vaccine A vaccine that contains antigen prepared by recombinant DNA techniques.

Respiratory burst The rapid increase in metabolic activity that occurs in phagocytic cells while particles are being ingested. It generates potent oxidants that can kill invading microorganisms.

Reticuloendothelial system All the cells in the body that take up circulating colloidal dyes. Many are macrophages. This term is best avoided because it is not a true body system

Retrovirus An RNA virus that employs the enzyme reverse transcriptase to convert its RNA into DNA.

Reverse transcriptase An enzyme that reversely transcribes RNA to DNA. It is found in retroviruses such as FIV.

Rheumatoid factor An autoantibody directed against epitopes on the immunoglobulin Fc region. Classically found in the blood of patients with rheumatoid arthritis.

Sarcoma A tumor arising from cells of mesodermal origin.

Secondary binding tests Serological tests that detect the consequences of antigen-antibody binding such as agglutination and precipitation.

Secondary immune response An enhanced immune response that results from second or subsequent exposure to an antigen.

Secondary immunodeficiencies Immunodeficiency diseases resulting from a known, nongenetic cause.

Secondary infections Infections by organisms that can invade only a host whose defenses are first weakened or destroyed by other infectious agents or toxins.

Secondary lymphoid organ A lymphoid organ whose function is to trap and respond to foreign antigens.

Secondary response The response of a sensitized animal to foreign antigen.

Secondary structure The way in which a peptide chain is made up of structural components such as α-helices and β-pleated sheets.

Secretory component A protein produced by mucosal epithelial cells; it functions as an IgA receptor and, on binding to IgA, protects IgA against proteases in the intestine.

Selectin A family of cell surface adhesion proteins that bind cells to glycoproteins on vascular endothelium.

Self-cure The elimination of intestinal worms by a localized type I hypersensitivity reaction in the intestinal tract.

Sensitization The triggering of an immune response by exposure to an antigen.

Sepsis The systemic inflammatory response to an infectious agent

Septic shock A severe disease condition that results from the massive release of cytokines such as TNF as a result of infection.

Seroconversion The appearance of antibodies in blood, indicating the onset of an infection.

Serology The science of antibody detection.

Serum The clear, yellow fluid that is expressed when blood has clotted and the clot contracts.

Serum sickness A type III hypersensitivity response to the administration of foreign serum as a result of the development of immune complexes in the bloodstream.

Signal transduction The transmission of a signal through a receptor to a cell by means of a series of linked reactions.

Skin test A diagnostic procedure that induces a local inflammatory response following intradermal inoculation of an antigen or allergen.

Somatic antigens Antigens associated with bacterial bodies.

Somatic mutation Mutations that occur in somatic rather than germline cells. In immunology, this refers to the extensive mutations that occur in the *V* genes of B cells during the course of an immune response.

Specificity A term that describes the ability of a test to give true-positive reactions.

Splice The joining of two DNA or RNA segments (exons) together.

Stem cell A cell that can maintain itself and serve as a source of many different differentiated cell lines.

Stimulation index A measure of the extent to which a cell population is stimulated to divide. It is the ratio of thymidine uptake in a stimulated cell population to the thymidine uptake in an unstimulated population.

Subclass Different immunoglobulin isotypes closely related within a specific class.

Subisotype See Subclass.

Substrate modulation A method of controlling enzyme activity seen in the complement system, by which a protein cannot be cleaved by a protease until it first binds to another protein.

Superantigen A molecule that, as a result of its ability to bind to certain TCR variable regions, can cause certain T cells to divide.

Superfamily A grouping of protein molecules that share common structures. For example, the members of the immunoglobulin superfamily all contain characteristic immunoglobulin domains.

Synapse The area of contact between cells. Within the synapse, cell surface molecules are arranged in a well-defined pattern designed to optimize signaling between the cells.

Syndrome A group of symptoms that together are characteristic of a specific disease.

Syngeneic (isogeneic) Genetically identical.

T lymphocyte A lymphocyte that has undergone a period of processing in the thymus and is responsible for mediating cell-mediated immune responses.

Terminal complement complex A multimolecular structure that formed by complement activation that generates pores in target cell membranes leading to osmotic lysis and cell death.

Tertiary binding tests Serological tests that measure the protective ability of an antibody in living animals.

Thoracic duct The major lymphatic vessel that collects the lymph, draining the lower portion of the body.

Thymectomy Surgical removal of the thymus.

Thymocytes Developing lymphocytes in the thymus.

Thymus-dependent antigen An antigen that requires the assistance of helper T cells to provoke an immune response.

Thymus-independent antigen An antigen that can activate B cells and trigger an antibody response without help from T cells.

Titer The reciprocal of the highest dilution of a serum that gives a reaction in an immunological test.

Titration The measurement of the level of specific antibodies in a serum, achieved by testing increasing dilutions of the serum for antibody activity.

Tolerance A state of specific unresponsiveness to an antigen induced by prior exposure to that antigen.

Tolerogen A substance that induces tolerance.

Toxic shock A disease resulting from exposure to large amounts of staphylococcal superantigen.

Toxoid Nontoxic derivatives of toxins used as antigens.

Transcription The conversion of a DNA nucleotide sequence into an RNA nucleotide sequence by complementary base-pairing.

Transcription factors Specialized proteins that regulate gene activity by binding to the promoter region of a gene. They thus turn gene transcription on or off.

Transduction The conversion of a signal from one form to another.

Translation The conversion of the RNA nucleotide sequence into an amino acid sequence in a ribosome.

Transporter protein Proteins that bind fragments of endogenous antigen and carry them to newly assembled MHC class I molecules in the endoplasmic reticulum.

Trematode A helminth known as a fluke. Trematodes are important human and animal parasites.

Tubercle A persistent inflammatory response to the presence of mycobacteria in the tissues.

Tuberculin An extract of tubercle bacilli used in a diagnostic skin test for tuberculosis.

Tumor necrosis factors Macrophage and lymphocyte-derived cytokines that can exert a direct toxic effect on neoplastic cells.

Tunicates Complex marine invertebrates possessing characteristic outer cuticular coverings, whose embryonic stages possess features that resemble those found in some vertebrates.

Tyrosine kinase An enzyme that phosphorylates tyrosine residues in proteins. It plays a key role in signal transduction.

Urodeles The most primitive order of amphibians; it includes the newts and salamanders.

Urticaria Inflammatory and edematous skin reactions due to allergic mechanisms and associated with intense itching.

Vaccination The administration of an antigen (vaccine) to stimulate a protective immune response against an infectious agent. The term is synonymous with immunization.

Vaccine A suspension of living or inactivated organisms used as an antigen to confer immunity.

Variable region That part of the immunoglobulin or TCR peptide chains in which the amino acid sequence shows significant variation among molecules.

Variolation An early method of protecting an individual against smallpox by inoculation with live smallpox virus.

Vasculitis Inflammation of blood vessel walls.

Vasoactive molecules Molecules that cause changes in local blood flow such as those observed during inflammation.

Virion A virus particle.

Virulence The ability of an organism to cause disease.

Xenograft A graft between two animals of different species.

Xenohybridoma A hybridoma formed by fusing plasma cells and myeloma cells from two different species (e.g., mouse and bovine).

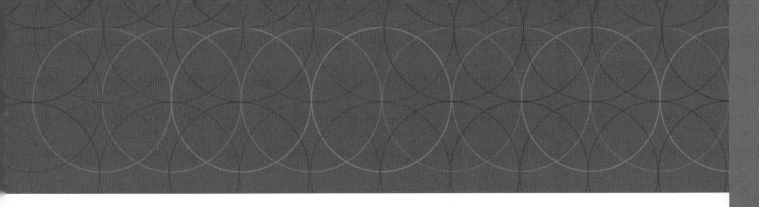

Index

Page numbers follow by "f" indicate figures, "t" indicate tables, and "b" indicate box.

Abbreviations

ADCC	antibody-dependent cell-mediated cytotoxicity
AIDS	acquired immune deficiency syndrome
AIHA	autoimmune hemolytic anemia
AITP	autoimmune thrombocytopenia
ANA	antinuclear antibody
APC	antigen-presenting cell
BALT	bronchus-associated lymphoid tissue
BCG	bacillus Calmette-Guérin *(Mycobacterium bovis)*
BCR	B cell antigen receptor
BLAD	bovine leukocyte adherence deficiency
BLV	bovine leukemia virus
BoLA	bovine leukocyte antigen
C	complement
CAM	cell adhesion molecule
CBH	cutaneous basophil hypersensitivity
CD	cluster of differentiation
CDw	cluster of differentiation (provisional designation)
CDR	complementarity determining region
CFT	complement fixation test
CID	combined immunodeficiency
CLL	chronic lymphoid leukemia
cM	centimorgans, a unit of genetic distance
Con A	concanavalin A
CR	complement receptor
CRP	C-reactive protein
CSF	colony-stimulating factor (or cerebrospinal fluid)
DAF	decay accelerating factor
DAG	diacylglycerol
DAMP	damage-associated molecular pattern
DC	dendritic cell
dsRNA	double-stranded RNA
DTH	delayed-type hypersensitivity
EAE	experimental allergic encephalitis
EAN	experimental allergic neuritis
ELISA	enzyme-linked immunosorbent assay
EPO	eosinophil peroxidase
Fab	antigen-binding fragment
Fc	crystallizable fragment (of immunoglobulin)
FCA	Freund's complete adjuvant
FcR	Fc receptor
FeLV	feline leukemia virus
FOCMA	feline oncornavirus cell membrane antigen
FPT	failure of passive transfer
FITC	fluorescein isothiocyanate
FIV	feline immunodeficiency virus
GALT	gut-associated lymphoid tissue
GM-CSF	granulocyte-macrophage colony-stimulating factor
GPI	glycosyl-phosphatidylinositol
GVH	graft-versus-host (disease)

HAT	hypoxanthine aminopterin thymidine (medium)
HDN	hemolytic disease of the newborn
HEV	high endothelial venule
HI	hemagglutination inhibition
HIV	human immunodeficiency virus
HLA	human leukocyte antigen
HMGB1	high-mobility group box protein-1
HSP	heat shock protein
Ia	mouse MHC class II molecule
ICAM	intercellular adhesion molecule
IDDM	insulin-dependent diabetes mellitus
IEL	intraepithelial lymphocytes
IFA	indirect fluorescence assay
IFN	interferon
Ig	immunoglobulin
IK	immunoconglutinin
IL	interleukin
IMHA	immune-mediated hemolytic anemia
ISCOM	immune-stimulating complex
ISG	immune serum globulin
IU	international unit
IVIG	intravenous (human) immunoglobulins
J	joining
JAK	janus tyrosine kinases
kb	kilobases, a measure of gene size
kDa	kilodalton
LAD	leukocyte adherence deficiency
LAK	lymphokine-activated killer (cells)
LBP	lipopolysaccharide binding protein
LD_{50}	lethal dose 50
LE	lupus erythematosus
LFA	leucocyte function-associated antigen
LGL	large granular lymphocyte
lpr	lymphoproliferation
LPS	lipopolysaccharide
LT	lymphotoxin (or leukotriene)
$\beta_2 M$	β_2-microglobulin
MAC	membrane attack complex
MBL	mannose-binding lectin
M-CSF	macrophage colony-stimulating factor
MHC	major histocompatibility complex
MIP	macrophage inflammatory protein
MLC	mixed lymphocyte culture
MLD	minimal lethal dose
MLR	mixed lymphocyte reaction
MLV	modified live virus
MPGN	mesangioproliferative glomerulonephritis
NF-κB	nuclear factor-κB
NK	natural killer (cell)
NKT	natural killer T cell
NLR	Nucleotide-binding oligomerization domain-like receptor